Psychiatric Care Plans

Psychiatric Care Plans
Guidelines for Individualizing Care
Edition 3

Marilynn E. Doenges, RN, MA, CS, APN

Clinical Specialist, Adult Psychiatric/Mental Health Nursing
Adjunct Faculty
Beth-El College of Nursing
Colorado Springs, Colorado

Mary C. Townsend, RN, MN, CS

Assistant Professor
Kramer School of Nursing
Oklahoma City University
Oklahoma City, Oklahoma

Certified Specialist, Adult Psychiatric/Mental Health Nursing
Private Practice
Oklahoma City, Oklahoma

Mary Frances Moorhouse, RN, CRRN, CLNC

Nurse Consultant
TNT-RN Enterprises
Colorado Springs, Colorado

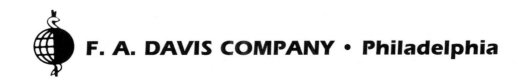

F. A. DAVIS COMPANY • Philadelphia

F. A. Davis Company
1915 Arch Street
Philadelphia, PA 19103

Printed in the United States of America

Last digit indicates print number: 10 9 8 7 6 5 4 3 2

Publisher, Nursing: Robert G. Martone
Production Editors: Stephen D. Johnson/Nancee Morelli
Cover Designer: Louis J. Forgione

As new scientific information becomes available through basic and clinical research, recommended treatments and drug therapies undergo changes. The authors and publisher have done everything possible to make this book accurate, up to date, and in accord with accepted standards at the time of publication. The authors, editors, and publisher are not responsible for errors or omissions or for consequences from application of the book, and make no warranty, expressed or implied, in regard to the contents of the book. Any practice described in this book should be applied by the reader in accordance with professional standards of care used in regard to the unique circumstances that may apply in each situation. The reader is advised always to check product information (package inserts) for changes and new information regarding dose and contraindications before administering any drug. Caution is especially urged when using new or infrequently ordered drugs.

Library of Congress Cataloging-in-Publication Data

Doenges, Marilynn E., 1922–
    Psychiatric care plans : guidelines for individualizing care / Marilynn E. Doenges,
Mary C. Townsend, Mary Frances Moorhouse. — Ed. 3.
      p.   cm.
    Includes bibliographical references and index.
    ISBN 0-8036-0322-3
    1. Psychiatric nursing—Handbooks, manuals, etc.   2. Nursing care plans—Handbooks, manuals, etc. I. Townsend, Mary C., 1941– . II. Moorhouse, Mary
Frances, 1947– . III. Title.
RC 440.D64 1998
610.73′68—DC21

97-24117
CIP

We dedicate this book to ourselves—our own intestinal fortitude, our unfailing optimism, our dogged perseverance, and our own increasing conviction in the value of nursing diagnosis and the future of the profession of nursing.

Special thanks to our husbands, Dean, Jim, and Jan; our families who have continued to support our dreams, fantasies, and obsessions: Nancy, Jim, Jennifer, and Jonathan Daigle; David, Monita, Matthew, and Tyler Doenges; Jim Doenges; Barbara Doenges, and Bob Lanza; John, Holly, Nicole, and Kelsey Doenges; Kerry and Tina Townsend; Paul Moorhouse; and Jason, Ellaina, Alexa, and Mary Moorhouse.

Alice Geissler, for being available when we need help; the staff at Memorial Hospital library, for cheerfully filling in all the blanks and patiently helping us find those elusive references; and our colleagues, who continue to provide a sounding board and feedback for our professional beliefs and expectations.

Kudos to the F. A. Davis staff, Robert Martone and Ruth DeGeorge, who have shown great patience and helped maintain our sanity (or contributed to our insanity); and Robert Butler and Herb Powell, who facilitated the revision process to get this project completed in a timely fashion.

Lastly, to the nurses who have patiently awaited this revision, we hope it will help in applying theory to practice and enhance the delivery and effectiveness of your care.

Contributors

ALICE Y. ANDERSON, CAPTAIN (P), AN, BSN, MSN
Head Nurse, Inpatient Psychiatry
Tripler Army Medical Center, Hawaii

IDA MARLENE BEAM, BSN
Retired, Army Nurse Corps
Private Home Respite Care
Colorado Springs, Colorado

PAULETTE BOTKIN, RN
Institute of Forensic Psychiatry
Colorado State Hospital
Pueblo, Colorado

MARTI DAVIS BUFFUM, RN, MS
Nursing Faculty/Lecturer, San Francisco State
    University
Staff Nurse III, Inpatient Psychiatry, Marin General
    Hospital
Greenbrae, California
Private Practice, Clinical Specialist
San Anselmo, California

WM G. CANTIN, Lt, NC, USN
Consultant/Liaison Nurse
Alcohol Rehabilitation Facility
Tripler Army Medical Center, Hawaii

**VERNA CARSON, RN, MS, DOCTORAL
    CANDIDATE**
Assistant Professor in Psychiatry/Community Health
    Nursing
University of Maryland School of Nursing
Baltimore, Maryland

KATHLEEN K. DUNCANSON, BSN, CRRN, CRC
Senior Rehabilitation Specialist
Intracorp
Woodland Park, Colorado

ROSEMARIE GEISER, RN, MSN, CS
Clinical Nurse Specialist, Adult Psychiatry
Palo Alto Veterans Administration Medical Center
Menlo Park Division
Palto Alto, California

*CHRISTIE A. HINDS, RN, NP
Director
FHL Health Care, Inc.
Colorado Springs, Colorado

MARYANNIE LEWIS HUGHES, MSN, BSN, RN, CS
Captain, US Army Nurse Corps
Clinical Head Nurse
Clinical Specialist at Tri-Services Alcoholism Recovery
    Facility (TRI-SARF)
Tripler Army Medical Center, Hawaii
Nurse Recruiter-Counselor
Ft. Sheridan, Illinois

*NOLA LANGE, RN, MA, CS
Psychiatric Nurse Liaison
Penrose-St. Francis Health Services
Colorado Springs, Colorado

NAOMI K. LEDERACH, RN, BSN, MN
Director of Education
Philhaven Hospital
Mount Gretna, Pennsylvania

MARGARET D. McCOMB, RN, MN, CS
Clinical Specialist for Nursing Process
Nursing Quality Assurance Coordinator
Veterans Administration Medical Center
Portland, Oregon

JILL G. MEIDER, MS, RN, CS
Clinical Specialist Child/Adolescent Psychiatric Nurse
N.E.E.D. Foundation Day Treatment Program and
    Mental Health Clinic
Colorado Springs, Colorado

* Contributor for the Third Edition

JOANNE BARNES MULLANEY, RN, PhD
Associate Professor
Salve Regina College
Newport, Rhode Island

*LESLIE MURTAGH, RN, MS, CS
Certified Child and Adolescent Clinical Nurse
  Specialist
Private Practice
Colorado Springs, Colorado

EARLENE PETERSON, RNC, BSN
Ob/Gyn Nurse Practitioner
Academy Women's Clinic
Colorado Springs, Colorado

LEANN G. RYNIER, RN, BSN Ed, MEd
Patient Care Education Specialist
Philhaven Hospital
Mount Gretna, Pennsylvania

BARBARA THOMAS, RN, BSN, C
CEO, Cheyenne Mesa Residential Treatment Center
Colorado Springs, Colorado

*SANDRA F. YANEY, RN, NM, NPH, CS
Retired, Army Nurse Corps
Family Nurse Practitioner
Collaborative Practice Consultant
Cedar Springs Psychiatric Hospital
Colorado Springs, Colorado

* Contributor for the Third Edition

Contents in Brief

Detailed Contents

xvii

INTRODUCTION

One of the most significant achievements in the healthcare field during the past 20 years has been the emergence of the nurse as an active coordinator and initiator of client care. Although the transition from helpmate to healthcare professional has been painfully slow and is not yet complete, the importance of the nurse within the system can no longer be denied or ignored. Today's nurse designs holistic nursing care interventions that will move the client toward a positive outcome and optimal health. This is especially true in the area of mental health nursing, in which healthcare reform and managed care are attempting to bring more available and affordable care to all clients.

The current state of the theory of Nursing Process, (diagnosis, intervention, and evaluation) has been brought to the clinical setting to be implemented by the nurse. This book defines and gives direction to the development and use of individualized client care for nurses in the psychiatric setting (hospital, clinic, home healthcare, and private practice) who are using critical thinking and the nursing process to identify client needs. A holistic/humanistic focus is presented in which the nurse serves as advocate for the client. Plans of care are formulated using nursing diagnoses with interventions and rationale based on current scientific premises. They encompass psychosocial/psychodynamic concepts and have been organized according to psychiatric diagnoses as listed in the fourth edition of *Diagnostic and Statistical Manual of Mental Disorders (DSM-IV)*. Standards of the American Nurses' Association (ANA) are used as a basis for the nursing process and development of plans of care, which serve as guides to the therapeutic nurse/client relationship. Therefore, this book is not an end in itself but rather a beginning for the future growth and development of the profession.

Advancement of professional care standards and demands of physicians/psychologists, clients, and third-party payors will continue to increase expectations of nurses' performance, as each day brings advances in the struggle to understand the mysteries of normal body/mind function and human response to actual and potential health problems. As knowledge increases, so does the nurse's responsibility. To meet these challenges competently, the nurse must have up-to-date physical and psychiatric assessment skills and a working knowledge of pathophysiological concepts concerning the changes occurring in the healthcare field. This book is a tool—a means of attaining that competency.

In the past, plans of care were viewed principally as learning tools for students and seemed to have little relevance after graduation. However, the need for a written format to communicate and document individualized client care has been recognized in all healthcare settings. In addition, governmental regulations and third-party payor requirements have created the need to validate the appropriateness of the care provided, as well as the need to justify client care charges and staffing patterns. Thus, although the student's "case studies" may have been too cumbersome to be practical in the clinical setting, the client plan of care meets the foregoing identified needs. The practicing nurse, as well as the nursing student, will welcome this text as a ready reference in clinical practice. The primary focus is early intervention to enable the client to maintain quality of life and independent living within individual capabilities. This book is designed for use in the psychiatric setting, serving as a guide for nurses who plan and promote healthcare for the psychiatric client and his or her family. Sample plans of care addressing specific psychiatric illnesses are organized by categories and identified by the *DSM-IV*

1

classification for easy reference. Rationales (which clarify why an intervention is important and provide related pathophysiology when applicable) enhance the reader's understanding of the intervention. This information also serves as a catalyst for thought in planning and evaluating the care being rendered.

Chapter 1 examines current issues/trends and how they apply to the nurse caring for the client and family experiencing emotional difficulties. Trends in healthcare such as cost-containment, shortened hospital stays, outpatient care, and increased use of alternative treatments are examined in light of possible effects on the delivery of care. There has been a dramatic growth of scientific knowledge regarding the biological side of mental illness. Many psychiatric disorders are being reappraised as "diseases of the brain" rather than "disorders of the mind." A growing body of evidence suggests that biochemical dysfunction of the brain and central nervous system causes the development of some disorders—particularly schizophrenia, bipolar disorder, and some anxiety disorders. Research of the genetic factors involved in psychiatric disorders should also provide new insights into mental illness and its treatment.

An overview of cultural, community, sociological, and ethical concepts that have an impact on the psychiatric nurse in a variety of healthcare settings is included. The importance of the nurse's role in cooperation and coordination with other healthcare professionals is integrated throughout the plans of care.

Chapter 2 reviews the historical use of the nursing process in formulating plans of care and the nurse's role in the delivery of that care. Nursing diagnosis is discussed to help the nurse understand its role in the nursing process.

Chapter 3 demonstrates construction of the plan of care and the use and adaptation of the guides for care planning presented in this book. A nursing-based assessment tool is presented with a sample client situation, data base, and corresponding plan of care to help the nurse make the transition from theory to practice. Additionally, a clinical pathway reflecting the sample situation is included to demonstrate another method of evaluating and documenting the client's response to care.

Chapters 4 through 16 provide plans of care that include information from multiple disciplines to help the nurse in providing holistic care for the client/family within the community or acute-care setting. Each plan includes a client assessment data base (presented in a nursing format) and associated diagnostic studies. After the data base is collected, nursing priorities are sifted from the information

to help focus and structure the care provided. Discharge goals are listed to identify which general goals should be accomplished in settings in which care is expected to be terminated and not simply progress to another stage. The nursing diagnoses contain "related to" and "evidenced by" statements that provide an explanation of client problems/needs. Desired client outcomes are stated in behavioral terms that can be measured to evaluate the client's progress and the effectiveness of the care provided. The interventions are designed to promote problem resolution.

A decision-making model is used to organize and prioritize nursing interventions based on the nurse acting independently/collaboratively within the healthcare team. No attempt is made to indicate whether independent or collaborative actions come first, as this must be dictated by the individual situation. Inclusion of rationale for the nursing actions will help the nurse to decide whether the interventions are appropriate for an individual client. A bibliography follows the text to allow for further reference/research as desired. Samples of Critical Pathways have been included to demonstrate alternative plans of care formats and enhance learning experiences. In addition, Therapeutics and Non-Therapeutics Techniques Assessment and Suidical Assessment Tool have been placed in the Appendix.

In summary, each plan of care in this text is an informational guide, designed to provide generalized information on the associated psychiatric/medical condition; therefore, this book is a ready reference for the practicing nurse as well as a catalyst for thought in planning and evaluating care.

Additionally, students will find the plans of care helpful as they learn and develop skills in applying the nursing process, using nursing diagnoses in the psychiatric setting. The plan-of-care guides can be modified either by using portions of the information provided or by adding additional client care information to the existing guides. We appreciate that not all diagnoses presented in these plans may be appropriate for a particular client or locale, in which case alternatives should be chosen to meet individual client needs. We support the belief that practicing nurses and researchers need to study, use, and evaluate the diagnoses as presented. As new nursing diagnoses are developed, the information they encompass must be reflected in the data base. The nurse is encouraged to share insights and ideas with the Diagnosis Review Committee of the North American Nursing Diagnosis Association (NANDA), 1211 Locust St., Philadelphia, PA 19107; 1-800-647-9002.

As a final note, this book is not intended to be a procedure manual, and efforts have been made to avoid detailed descriptions of interventions/protocols that might be viewed as individual or regional in nature. Instead, the reader is referred to a procedure manual/agency standards of care for in-depth direction regarding these concerns.

KEY TO ESSENTIAL TERMINOLOGY

Client Assessment Data Base

This provides an overview of the more commonly occurring etiology and coexisting factors associated with a specific psychiatric diagnosis as well as the signs/symptoms (cues) and corresponding diagnostic findings.

Nursing Priorities

These have established a general ranking of needs/concerns on which the nursing diagnoses are ordered. In constructing an actual plan of care, this ranking would be altered according to the individual client situation.

Discharge Goals

These identify generalized statements that could be developed into short-term and intermediate goals to be achieved by the client before being "discharged" from nursing care. They may also provide guidance for creating long-term goals for the client to work on after discharge.

Nursing Diagnoses

The general problem/concern (diagnosis) is stated without the distinct reasons (etiology) and signs/symptoms, which would be added to create a client diagnostic statement when specific client information is available. For example, when a client develops increased tension, apprehension, quivering voice, and focus on self, the nursing diagnosis *Anxiety* could be stated "Anxiety, severe, related to unconscious conflict, threat to self-concept as evidenced by statements of increased tension, apprehension, observation of quivering voice, focus on self." In addition, diagnoses that have been identified within these guides for planning care as *actual*

or *risk* may be changed or deleted, or diagnoses may be added, depending on specific client information.

May Be Related To/Possibly Evidenced By

Lists the usual/common etiology (related factors) of why a particular problem may occur and the probable signs/symptoms that would be used to create the "related to" and "evidenced by" portions of the client diagnostic statement when the specific client situation is known.

When a risk diagnosis has been identified, signs/symptoms have not yet developed and therefore are not included in the client diagnostic statement. However, interventions are provided to prevent progression to an *actual* problem. The exception to this occurs in the nursing diagnosis *Violence, risk for*, which has possible indicators that reflect the client's risk status.

Client Outcomes/Evaluation Criteria

These give direction to client care as they identify what the client and nurse hope to achieve. They are stated in general terms in this book to let the practitioner modify/individualize them by adding timelines and specific client criteria so that they become "measurable." For example, "Client will appear relaxed and report anxiety is reduced to a manageable level within 24 hours."

Actions/Interventions

Activities are divided into sections designated *independent* and *collaborative,* and are ranked in this book from most to less common. When creating the individual plan of care, these interventions would normally be reordered to reflect the client's specific needs/situation. In addition, the division of independent/collaborative is arbitrary and actually depends on the individual nurse's capabilities and agency/community standards.

Rationale

Although not commonly appearing in client plans of care, rationale has been included here to provide a psychiatric and pathophysiological basis to help the nurse decide about the relevance of a specific intervention for an individual client situation.

CHAPTER 1

ISSUES AND TRENDS IN MENTAL HEALTHCARE

Within the past century, psychiatry began to emerge from behind the veil of mystery and superstition. Primitive societies believed that an individual with mental illness had been dispossessed of his or her soul and that returning the soul would lead to wellness. Some believed that evil spirits or supernatural or magical powers had entered the body. Treatments often involved cruel and torturous methods to exorcize the body of these forces. Still another belief was that the individual may have broken a taboo, or sinned against another individual or God, with various types of retribution being demanded. As understanding of mental illness increased and cultural, religious, and sociopolitical attitudes changed, it gradually came to be regarded as an illness, and special hospitals were established to care for these individuals. In the 19th century, a system of state asylums was developed to provide humanistic therapeutic care. However, the patient population grew faster than the number of facilities, and they became more a place for custodial care than for therapy. In the 1960s, through the initiation of the community health movement, the focus shifted from custodial to more therapeutic care; however, resources today still continue to fall behind the need for them.

Two significant factors in bringing psychiatric care to the arena of scientific study and therapeutic modalities are the work of Sigmund Freud and the advent of psychotropic drugs. Although there now are many theories and techniques of communication therapy, Freud was most responsible for establishing communication as therapy and for studying mental and emotional dysfunction in a scientific manner.

Research of the biological and genetic causes of mental illness has produced a dramatic increase in the scientific knowledge available. Many psychiatric disorders are being reappraised as "diseases of the brain" rather than "disorders of the mind." A growing body of evidence suggests that biochemical dysfunction of the brain and central nervous system is the etiology of some disorders—particularly schizophrenia, bipolar disorder, and some anxiety disorders. Increasing information supports a relationship between stress and immunosuppression, providing insights about the link between stressful life events and the development of physical and emotional illness. Knowledge about substances that can poison the brain and nervous system (neurotoxicology) has enhanced awareness of environmental pollutants and provoked us to look at the kinds of preventive measures that can be taken. Efforts to treat brain diseases by the use of neural transplants and nerve regeneration have led to controversy and ethical discussions about how to accomplish these procedures. In addition, research into what makes the sexes different has exploded. Evidence presents a consistent picture of difference between male and female brains. Although sociological influences are important, it is clear that biological differences, the way in which our brains are organized and perceive data, underlie the way in which the sexes think and act. The genetic code makes us male or female, but hormones are a factor in sex determination and in the distinct male or female organization of the brain as the fetus develops in the womb. None of these differences is better or worse, they are simply differences affecting the way each individual interacts with the world.

Coupled with the ideas of brain disease is a growth in technology that allows sophisticated examination of the structure and function of the brain. Technologies such as computerized tomography (CT) scans, nuclear magnetic resonance imagery (MRI), and positron emission tomography (PET) have provided information about brain functioning that has served to guide diagnosis and intervention with some clients. Computer-assisted enhancements of the information provided by electroencephalograms (EEGs) (e.g., the brain electrical activity map [BEAM]) show distinctive brain patterns associated with dyslexia and other learning problems. Studies of the workplace regarding individual biological rhythms and shift work and the potential for behavioral and neurological harm are ongoing.

Psychotropic drugs, many of which have been available only since the 1950s, have made it possible to control symptoms of psychiatric illnesses. The major psychotropic medications may be used as therapy by themselves, but more often they are used as an adjunct to individual or group psychotherapy. Although these medications do not cure the underlying condition or emotional problem, they do enable the client to benefit from other therapies and live as normal a life as possible. It is widely accepted that combined treatments, using psychopharmacology and other treatments with psychotherapy, are most beneficial.

Within the past 20 to 30 years, a movement has emerged to release chronically ill clients from state hospitals and other mental health institutions. One reason for this was economic: it is expensive to keep people institutionalized and unproductive in large hospital settings. Another reason was the growing awareness of the civil rights of the individual and a belief that the rights of the chronic psychiatric client were being violated. Changes in treatment made it possible to begin to look at what could be done to help this population become more self-sufficient, contributing members of society. Clinics, day treatment programs, and other alternate facilities were proposed, and to some extent established, in an attempt to meet these goals. However, the move in the 1960s to community mental healthcare did not fulfill the promises anticipated at that time. Professional education and payment structures did not fully support the concept of community-based care, and many caregivers did not understand the mission of this movement. Although much has been learned in the past 20 years about how to treat severe mental illnesses effectively in both acute-care and community-based programs, present community facilities are still insufficient to meet the increasing need for mental health treatment and care. Because mental illness can now be defined in the same way as physical illness, effective treatments are usually available. However, access to care remains a problem. Studies indicate that targeting at-risk groups for early intervention, the availability of appropriate treatment, and the use of employee assistance plans have proved cost-effective. Intensive

community services for children, to prevent their separation from the family and the problems that would result from that separation, also provide the opportunity for promoting family interaction and problem-solving. In addition, it has been reliably demonstrated that mental healthcare can reduce costs for physical illnesses (e.g., chronic pain conditions).

Longitudinal studies in this country and those conducted by the World Health Organization are changing the outlook for those individuals with severe and persistent mental illness. For example, long-held myths about schizophrenia have been sufficiently challenged and disproved by two decades of empirical data. Worldwide research shows a 50% rate of recovery and improvement in individuals with symptoms of schizophrenia. Gone is the belief that "once a schizophrenic, always a schizophrenic." Hope promotes the self-healing process in recovery from any illness. Supportive therapy is necessary to move the client and his or her family toward recovery. Clients are benefiting from treatment that is focused on the individual as a *person* who happens to have schizophrenia. Nurses have long embraced the practice model of *care* and *respect for personhood.*

TREATMENT MODALITIES

In spite of these advances, the stigma of mental illness persists, as the mysteries surrounding psychiatry are slow to resolve. True scientific study of the relationship between therapy and change in human behavior is difficult at best, and the etiology of many disorders is still unknown or only partly understood or accepted. Biomedical research has greatly increased recently, providing information about the biological, genetic, and psychological bases for mental illness. However, intervention is still based primarily on theory and on the personality and style of the therapist. Although theoretical approaches are many and varied (e.g., psychoanalytical, family systems, and behavioral), three basic forms of treatment are used today. These are (1) the use of drugs (neuropsychopharmacology), (2) conditioning or behavior modification, and (3) communication therapies. Brief therapy modalities are being widely researched and used. Of particular note are Eye Movement Desensitization and Reprocessing (EMDR) and Thought Energy Synchronization Therapy (TEST). Many economic and social factors also influence the care given to psychiatric clients.

Psychiatric nursing has also been evolving and is currently defined as the diagnosis and treatment of human responses to actual or potential mental health problems. The first school of psychiatric nursing, established in 1882, focused on teaching students to provide custodial care, and psychological concepts were not a part of the curricula. Significant change occurred in 1955 when psychiatric nursing became a requirement for all undergraduate schools of nursing, with an emphasis on the nurse-patient relationship and therapeutic communication techniques. Nurses no longer provide only long-term custodial care but are qualified and expected to provide therapeutic interventions, including facilitating group therapy. The role of the nurse in administering medications has expanded to include prescriptive privileges as well as discussions of side effects and expected therapeutic results to help clients make informed choices about their care. Psychiatric rehabilitation and the use of case management provide the nurse with the opportunity to help those who are disabled by major mental illnesses to relearn skills—how to care for their daily needs, how to become productive (returning to school or the workforce), and how to get along with colleagues and family—thus increasing their ability to live independently.

People who are recovering from a mental illness are excellent sources of knowledge for others who are working on their own mental illness. Self-directed rehabilitation in the form of self-help groups is an important adjunct to professional therapies. The consumer movement is growing across the nation as consumer hotlines direct individuals to seek their own empowerment. Early research on the efficacy of self-help groups shows five reasons why this method works:

1. Creates a social network
2. Changes the perception of *helpless* to the role of *helper*
3. Encourages sharing of effective coping tools based on experience
4. Provides positive role models
5. Gives meaning to people's lives

Family members also benefit from developing their own support network as they learn to set realistic expectations and use more effective coping strategies for themselves. Nurses are often in a position to advocate for the development and use of self-help groups in their practice settings.

FINANCIAL CONSIDERATIONS

The need to provide an economic base for long-term, treatment-oriented psychiatric care remains a challenge for the healthcare system. With healthcare costs escalating, there is a strong push to economize in all areas. A major step in cost-cutting was the passage by Congress of a prospective payment system for all Medicare medical/surgical inpatients. This system uses diagnosis-related groups (DRGs) to determine hospital reimbursement. Although DRGs are not applicable to psychiatry at this time, they do influence reimbursement, as third-party payors use this concept for establishing payment for all healthcare. Additionally, healthcare reform is being debated, with many different options offered to reduce costs while attempting to increase the access to care. It is clear that community settings (e.g., community mental health centers, schools, homes, halfway houses, and even shopping malls) will increasingly be used to deliver care.

This trend indicates to healthcare providers that psychiatric nurses need to develop new methods of providing effective client care. Primary healthcare is an important concept of healthcare reform. The psychiatric/mental health nurse, in addressing the needs of the whole person, promotes optimal mental and physical health by preventing illness, maintaining health, and using referrals and rehabilitation skills. Goal-oriented, time-limited interventions are necessary if we are to provide quality mental healthcare in a timely manner. The nursing process as a model for problem-solving can be used to achieve this goal, providing a framework for systematic nursing care based on scientific knowledge. Additionally, the development of nursing diagnoses has provided the impetus to more effective planning, delivery, and documentation of client care.

CULTURAL FACTORS

The study of mental illness in relation to culture has been limited and often localized. However, available research suggests that both mental illnesses and therapeutic approaches differ among the world's cultures. Thus, there is a growing awareness that cultural factors do affect mental health and that clients from different cultural backgrounds require culturally appropriate diagnosis and care combining different therapeutic modalities. Failure of healthcare providers to be aware of the historical and social similarities and differences between and within cultures or to address the physiological and psychological differences between men and women can result in less than optimal therapeutic results. "Traditional" approaches may encourage changes that are unacceptable to the client, creating conflict or even termination of therapy.

"Normal" behavior is relative to a specific culture, and different psychological characteristics are promoted by each culture. Other variables influencing mental health include family relationships, child-rearing practices, attitudes toward illness, and socioeconomic status. Misdiagnosis may occur because of many factors, including differences in language, mannerisms, personality traits, religious dogma, and acceptability of the presence of and communication with ancestors or supernatural powers. For example, an individual from a gentle, mild, passive culture may create the impression of being guarded or reticent or may even be misdiagnosed as passive-aggressive. Furthermore, when a problem does exist, the culture may dictate that seeking help from outsiders is inappropriate, and the family may choose to tolerate "unusual" behavior or attempt to manage the individual on its own rather than seek treatment, thus delaying therapy. Diagnosis may be further influenced by racial and ethnic differences in the clinical presentation, as variations of biological markers for various psychiatric disorders are identified (e.g., serum creatinine phosphokinase, platelet serotonin, and HLA-A2 determinations).

Once therapy is begun, the practice of self-medication, use of folk remedies, and cultural dietary preferences have an impact on choice and use of drugs, as well as on individual cooperation with the therapeutic regimen. Additionally, racial and ethnic differences in response to psychotropic medications affect dosage requirements and potential side effects. For example, research reveals that as a rule, Asians require low dosages and closer monitoring of several psychotropic drugs (e.g., lithium, antidepressants, and neuroleptics).

Separate from, but in conjunction with, cultural issues, religious beliefs can greatly influence the client's view of the existence and etiology of mental illness and acceptance of therapy needs and options. It is therefore imperative that psychiatric nurses be sensitive to the potential for racial, ethnic, and gender differences or needs and promote awareness by other team members, while remembering that a specific group is not a single entity to be dealt with stereotypically. It is also important for the nurse therapist to understand the client's motivation for seeking psychological help. For example, American men generally seem to seek solutions, whereas American women desire empathy and compassion.

COMMUNITY CONSIDERATIONS

The movement from institutional to community-based care has resulted in a dramatic reduction in the number of long-term clients in institutions. However, new problems have been created, and the system has failed to care adequately for the clients who have been returned to their community. The decrease in cost of care is dubious because many nonfunctional or borderline individuals have been released only to become dependent on other community agencies and/or to wander the streets. Even though studies indicate that lower rates of rehospitalization are related to assertive community treatment and aftercare programs, sufficient funding often has not been allotted to provide an adequate level of care.

Care providers find themselves working with persons who have difficulty adapting to, or who cannot adapt to, society as self-sufficient members because of chronic illness and/or long-term institutionalization. Nurses are challenged to help these clients reach realistic goals with a minimum of dependency on community resources.

Concern for civil rights has also had an impact on involuntary commitment. It must be demonstrated that a person poses a danger to self or others and/or the community before legal commitment to an institution can be accomplished. Although this protects the individual from unjust confinement, there seems to be little recourse for the families of disturbed persons who will not voluntarily seek treatment. Inevitably, some people who would greatly benefit receive no treatment and, without adequate care, join the chronically psychotic or nonfunctional clients in board-and-care facilities or other community agencies. Other individuals fade into the anonymity of "street" or "bag" people, subsisting by whatever means possible. Occasionally much publicity is given to the infrequent case in which a client, after having been discharged from the psychiatric system, commits violent acts creating in the general populace fear, anger, and a demand for tighter controls.

AGE-RELATED FACTORS

Ours is an aging society. More and more people are reaching middle and late years. An increasing awareness of "midlife crisis" and the emotional impact that it has on the individual has encouraged more people to seek help with the problems that may be created at this time. Additionally, more individuals are willing to disrupt their lives (e.g., change relationships or careers) to seek happiness and "find themselves," which also affects those around them. As a person ages, many losses may occur—e.g., jobs, loved ones, health, and ability to function (sexually and otherwise)—and often the individual's self-image suffers. Chronic depression and substance abuse are increasing problems in the older population. The suicide rate also increases in this neglected segment of our society, as depression may go unnoticed simply because no one pays attention. Nurses are in an excellent position to detect these problems and initiate goal-setting and treatment referrals for the elderly. In the past, because of limited life expectancy, goals for the elderly were not given much consideration. Obviously, this view is short-sighted and clearly discriminating. With this awareness comes a need for more programs to meet the needs of this group.

On the other end of the spectrum, children's and adolescents' psychiatric needs are growing also, requiring the expansion of facilities and programs. More recognition is being given to the reality that delinquent youngsters are often troubled and may in fact be mentally ill. Issues of physical and sexual abuse, incest, neglect, changes in family configuration, and gender identity concerns create the additional need for both inpatient and community treatment. Although facilities and programs specifically designed for children and/or adolescents and their families are becoming more available, there is still a reluctance to acknowledge the reality of mental illness, substance abuse, and suicide in young people, resulting in insufficient resources to meet the need.

SUBSTANCE ABUSE

Substance abuse has come full-force to national and worldwide attention. Society's awareness of this problem has brought to the forefront both legal and therapeutic means of solving it. Specific modalities have been developed to work with the addicted client. Increased knowledge of the frequency of issues of dual diagnosis (presence of psychiatric illness in combination with substance abuse) has led to more effective treatment for these individuals. Additionally, recognition of the effect on the family, as well as issues of enabling/codependent behavior, has led to a broader approach to what was once believed to be an individual problem. With the substance abuser, psychiatric nurses need to be aware of such specific concerns as chemical imbalances, as well as the unique problems and needs of the individual or family unit, as many of the therapy needs for addicted individuals remain unfulfilled.

SUICIDE

As mentioned previously, suicide is on the increase. The statistical rise may be attributed in part to the identification today of some deaths as suicide that formerly may have been labeled accidental. To-

day we also live in a world in which television brings the reality of global concerns into the home daily, fears about debilitating and/or terminal illnesses prevail, stress about developmental stages of life (including adolescent, midlife concerns, issues of independence, and gender identity) overwhelm us, and financial/employment insecurities are a constant concern. The pressures of life in such a world present individuals with problems of coping that may lead to suicide. With an alarming rise in the incidence of suicide among children, adolescents (suicide is currently the second cause of death in this group), and the elderly, specific interventions are necessary in determining what kinds of preventive actions can be helpful. The nurse is often in a position to recognize the potential for suicide in a client and to take effective action.

STRESS

An increased awareness of the effects of stress on our lives is emerging. Of special interest is the influence of stress in the development of many psychological problems. Manifestations of stress (e.g., ulcers, asthma, and perhaps any or all of the physical illnesses humans experience) have also been acknowledged. Although many psychiatric treatment modalities (e.g., biofeedback, relaxation skills, and guided imagery) are directed at stress reduction/management, stress is often a neglected area for the client with physical illness.

As life stessors have increased, the numbers of people who are victims of physical, sexual, and emotional abuse continue to rise in epidemic proportions. In psychiatry, the phenomenon of delayed stress reactions (the belated response of victims to violence or chronic deprivation) is being given more attention. This is now recognized as a significant cause of many disorders, which may appear years after the occurrence of the stressor. Identification of victims of, or those at risk for, abuse, and intervention to prevent further victimization, are also within the scope of nursing practice. Family intervention, crisis intervention, and group support can help interrupt the pattern of violence, as well as provide assistance for the victim's recovery.

Societal changes, such as the increase in the number of divorces and remarriages, which result in single-parent homes and stepfamilies, create problems that demand new and creative approaches to treatment. Role changes include fathers taking on more child-rearing responsibilities and mothers combining careers with homemaking. Increased mobility of individuals often results in the lack of extended family available for role-modeling and assistance, leaving nuclear families vulnerable to added stress. Watching unrealistic television models of the "perfect" family and the "quick" solution of the 30-minute situation comedy lead people to believe that there is something wrong with them when problems persist. In addition, with the wide use of television, rapid travel, and the opening of Third World countries to the West, our world is shrinking, and things that happen in one area affect and influence all other areas. Changes in manufacturing, including the decline in the number of jobs available and downsizing of major companies, which also affect the healthcare industry, have the workforce in a constant state of turmoil. As a result, workers fear layoffs, look for other positions, and/or decide to return to school to train for new jobs, often at lower salary levels. Finally, advances in science and technology fuel changes in all areas of life.

TRENDS AFFECTING DELIVERY OF CARE

The Role of the Nurse

New developments and changes in the nursing profession are having an impact on the psychiatric nursing field. One of these changes is the development and implementation of nursing diagnoses, which is making written plans of care more useful for the provision and documentation of care. Identification of specific problems and determination of individual interventions necessary for reaching timely goals have enhanced the care-planning process. Additionally, more recognition is being given to the need for the client to be an active participant in the therapeutic process. Nurses develop therapeutic relationships with clients, which become the cornerstone of quality care. Assessments are made, nursing diagnoses are identified, and nursing care is planned, implemented, and evaluated with the active involvement of the client.

Psychiatric nursing is a specialized area of nursing that uses theories of human behavior as its science and the purposeful use of self as its art. The development of Standards of Psychiatric and Mental Health Nursing Practice (ANA, 1994) and identification of Psychiatric–Mental Health Nursing's Phenomena of Concern (Table 1–1) provide a beginning framework for the nurse to use to guide professional practice. In conjunction with the growth of specialty professional groups and the expansion of the psychiatric nursing practice arena, nursing involvement in the interdisciplinary team approach to psychiatric care is now more frequently acknowledged and valued. Nursing organizations such as the ANA have established programs to credential nurses (e.g., Clinical Specialist in Psychiatric/Mental Health Nursing). These specialty certification programs share common goals: to provide consumer protection, to enhance nursing knowledge and competency, to increase nursing autonomy, and to strengthen collaboration. Specialty certification will take on more importance in this cost-conscious era as managers seek to hire competent professionals.

TABLE 1–1. Psychiatric–Mental Health Nursing's Phenomena of Concern

Actual or potential mental health problems of clients pertaining to:

The maintenance of optimal health and well-being and the prevention of psychobiological illness

Self-care limitations or impaired functioning related to mental and emotional distress

Deficits in the functioning of significant biological, emotional, and cognitive systems

Emotional stress or crisis components of illness, pain, and disability

Self-concept changes, developmental issues, and life-process changes

Problems related to emotions such as anxiety, anger, sadness, loneliness, and grief

Physical symptoms that occur along with altered psychological functioning

Alterations in thinking, perceiving, symbolizing, communicating, and decision-making

Difficulties in relating to others

Behaviors and mental states that indicate the client is a danger to self or others or has a severe disability

Interpersonal, systemic, sociocultural, spiritual, or environmental circumstances or events that affect the mental and emotional well-being of the individual, family, or community

Symptom management, side effects/toxicities associated with psychopharmacological intervention, and other aspects of the treatment regimen

Adapted from *A Statement on Psychiatric–Mental Health Clinical Nursing Practice and Standards of Psychiatric–Mental Health Clinical Nursing Practice*, ANA, 1994.

Furthermore, independent roles for the nurse, such as private practice and liaison/consultant positions in institutions or community settings, and prescriptive authority for advanced practice nurses, are beginning to affect how psychiatric care is delivered. These nursing roles require greater clinical expertise, maturity, critical thinking ability, assertiveness, and client-management skills to meet the challenges of functioning as a first-line provider. The ANA (1996) has listed the following competencies as important to success:

1. A strong clinical, specialty preparation in multiple modalities—individual, family, group
2. Effective written and oral communication abilities
3. Treatment planning, goal-setting, and evaluation skills
4. Community orientation
5. Family-centered and diverse population experience
6. Psychopharmacology and crisis intervention competencies

The ability to be a partner in the multidisciplinary team and to maintain a holistic perspective with an emphasis on wellness promotion will be a nursing strength.

Managed Mental Healthcare

The next generation of managed mental healthcare is here with more than 40 million lives covered by managed-care companies nationwide. Virtually all corporations have entered into health maintenance organizations (HMOs), preferred provider organizations (PPOs), and carve-out plans to provide employees and their dependents with psychiatric and substance abuse treatment benefits. Privatization of Medicaid behavioral health and substance abuse services are in operation in growing proportions as state and federal government entities contract with private-sector managed-care companies. Federal legislation has been in effect to reduce discrimination in health plans whereby insurance companies are now mandated to provide mental health services with the same amount of benefits as was previously allowed for medical healthcare.

Managed care is purposely designed to control the balance between cost and quality of care. However, many view it as a two-edged sword. The emphasis is on ease of access and accountability for delivery of effective treatment in a timely fashion. Fifty-four percent of all HMOs undergo accreditation. This is one way to ensure that health plans are providing appropriate levels of care while monitoring the performance of the providers in the delivery

of quality services. Managed-care "report cards" are the latest yardstick that rate access to care, consumer satisfaction, and quality of care. On the one hand, it is a way to provide attention to goal-oriented brief therapy, strengthen accountability, and focus on treatment and outcomes. On the other hand, healthcare provider autonomy and client choices are restricted in managed care. Additionally, many in the multidisciplinary settings have high and perhaps unrealistic expectations and may become discouraged or sabotage the efforts when problems arise. Problems of disagreements between disciplines may also become more apparent, creating further conflict and interfering with establishment of the system. Each discipline must satisfy multiple masters—consumers, insurance plan managers, and private payors.

With the advent of managed care, opportunities for nurses to practice in different settings have been abundant. Nurses have the administrative and clinical skills to function as practice managers for various provider groups. Many nurses have assumed the role of case manager, whereas others have established private case management practices. In these endeavors, they consider the client's health status and diagnosis, treatment plans, payment resources, and healthcare options. Nurses are often the stop-gap measure to control costly delivery of services as more and more responsibility for direct care is shifted to them. Referrals are being made to these nurses to run preventive healthcare clinics and to provide home-based treatment to manage the client's recovery/rehabilitation. Expansion of the continuum of care in this managed-care era has been especially beneficial to clients with chronic physical or mental disorders. The ANA has developed Managed Care Curriculum Guidelines for Psychiatric–Mental Health and Addictions Nurses, which can be a helpful tool for the nurse in dealing with these issues.

Case Management

Case management is the actual coordination of services required to meet the needs of the client. Social service–based case management began in the social welfare system in the 1970s. Although these case managers were often social workers, many were also nurses who coordinated the long-term care needs in the community for the elderly or deinstitutionalized clients. Today, strategies to bring expenditures under control by managing the care include preauthorization, concurrent review, and ongoing case management. The ANA describes 12 different models of care management, with the goals being:

1. To determine what the expected clinical outcomes would be in an individual with a specific illness at a specific time
2. To ensure that use of resources is appropriate to contain healthcare costs
3. To promote collaborative practice among multidisciplinary team members and provide continuity of care for the patient
4. To discharge the client within a designated length of time (often determined by insurance company designations)

In the acute-care setting, case management is viewed as "a methodology for organizing client care through an episode of illness so that specific clinical and financial outcomes are achieved within an allotted timeframe" (Zander, 1988). Hospitals use care management to establish early identification of high-risk clients who may require extensive use of services. By initiating case-finding, the case manager becomes responsible not only for the client's clinical outcome but also for the institution's financial outcome. This disparity in goals can lead to conflict. Limiting the length of care is a departure from traditional psychiatric practice. However, with the managed-care mandate for the clinical goals of returning the client to a "reasonable level" of functioning as soon as possible and preventing recurrence, *how many* visits/days of hospitalization becomes the debate.

With nurse case managers often acting as gatekeepers for managed care, dealing with the reduction in the length of stay and episodic nature of the care provided, they are required to focus on how clients will benefit from a particular type or level of intervention. During this process, the nurse must identify elements of the client's care that are critical. For example, if the client is "authorized" to be in a facility for only 5 days, what are the critical components of care that must be addressed at this level of care delivery? These critical components of care become the established guidelines for the provision of care by the healthcare team. Such guidelines become the clinical (critical) pathway or "blueprint" for the care. Clinical pathways are most effective in guiding acute-care needs, for those problems that have predictable outcomes within a specific time frame, and in improving the quality of client care and significantly containing costs during the shorter stays. However, the application of these methods to the client who needs long-term treatment is still evolving and needs to be resolved.

Thus, case management has emerged as one method to ensure coordination and integration of both the clinical and fiscal needs of the client. Nurses have the knowledge and are well positioned to meet the ever-changing demands to improve the quality of care while controlling the costs and use of finite resources.

Computer Applications

Many nurses believe that their limited time can be better spent with the client, giving care, rather than generating written plans of care. Computerization can decrease time spent in generating and maintaining these plans and improve the quality of record-keeping. Computerized plans of care provide psychiatric nurses with a more efficient means to develop comprehensive, continuous, individualized, and legible plans for each client. Nurses may quickly enter, display, evaluate, update, and print a revised plan.

Standardized plans of care establish priorities of care and define minimum standards of safe practice. They provide an outline for documentation of the care that has been given and the way the client responded to that care. They also serve to jog the nurse's memory when caring for clients not usually seen in that nurse's area of clinical practice. However, standardized plans are not intended to be all-inclusive, and nursing judgment is required to individualize the plan of care for each specific client.

Easy access to computerized plans of care provides information and promotes safe, effective care. Many computerized systems providing standardized client plans of care use the nursing diagnoses accepted for testing by NANDA. These basic plans of care reflect standards of care for particular client problems and are designed to meet specific needs. Because the plans reflect a wealth of varied nursing experience, they allow even novice practitioners to formulate effective care strategies and individualize care.

CONCLUSION

Up to this time, the major focus of psychiatric care has been largely on inpatient treatment. As we travel into the 21st century, psychiatric services are moving out of the inpatient arena and into the ambulatory care setting. Today the community mental healthcare system is the fastest-growing subgroup of healthcare. As previously noted, the factors affecting mental health and the healthcare system are many and varied. In this era of rapid change with the public expectation of instant cures and the demand to contain healthcare costs, increasing pressure is placed on healthcare providers. New and inventive approaches are being developed in an attempt to find effective solutions and improve the delivery of mental healthcare.

There is no doubt that psychiatric/mental health nursing will change as a result of these developments in the healthcare arena. Nursing is in a position to assist with care planning and to contribute to the provision of cost-effective care. Psychiatric nurses can work in the community to provide preventive therapy, as well as to provide supportive, transitional, or continued therapy for clients discharged from inpatient settings. To meet these challenges, nurses must continue their professional growth and accept accountability for their practice. To this end, psychiatric nurses need to incorporate new knowledge from the fields of neuroanatomy, physiology, psychoneuroendocrinology, immunology, and psychopharmacology to develop the most effective treatment interventions. Nurses need to assist consumers of mental health services in their efforts to become self-reliant and to empower those with severe and persistent mental illness to overcome the stigma of having a mental disorder. The nursing profession shares in the role of client advocate by participating in legislative action and education of the public concerning the needs of children and their families regardless of socioeconomic and cultural background. Nurses are responsible for ensuring access to community services and availability of resources for ongoing psychiatric treatment. They also need to increase their participation in research to determine the efficacy of nursing therapy strategies and the cost-effectiveness of treatment by clinical nurse specialists/advanced practitioners.

CHAPTER 2

THE NURSING PROCESS: PLANNING CARE WITH NURSING DIAGNOSIS

Nursing care is a key factor in client recovery and in the maintenance, rehabilitation, and prevention aspects of mental healthcare. To this end, the nursing profession has identified a problem-solving process that "combines the most desirable elements of the art of nursing with the most relevant elements of systems theory, using the scientific method" (Shore, 1988). Publication of the ANA Social Policy Statement (ANA, 1980), which defined nursing as the diagnosis and treatment of human responses to actual and potential health problems, in combination with the ANA Standards of Clinical Nursing Practice (1991) and the ANA Psychiatric/Mental Health Standards (1994) have provided the impetus and support for the use of nursing diagnosis in the practice setting. Prospective payment plans, movement from acute care (inpatient) to community settings (outpatient services in mental health centers, group homes/foster care), and other changes in the healthcare system are highlighting the need for a common framework of communication and documentation. This framework promotes continuity of care of the client who moves from one area of the healthcare system to another, while it maintains the confidentiality of the client.

The delivery of quality care involves planning and coordination. Medicine, psychiatry, and nursing, as well as other health disciplines (the multidisciplinary team), are interrelated with implications for each other. This interrelationship optimally includes exchanging data, sharing ideas or thoughts, and developing plans of care that include all data pertinent to the individual client/family. The plan of care helps coordinate care given by all disciplines, as the different activities are combined into a functional plan providing holistic care for the client. Properly written and used, plans of care provide tools for client care assessment, guidelines for evaluation and documentation, and direction for continuity of care among

nurses and other caregivers. This is particularly true in the routinely multidisciplinary approach of psychiatric care. The written plan of care communicates the past and present status and needs of the client to all members of the healthcare team. It identifies problems that have been solved and those yet to be solved, approaches that have been successful, and patterns of client responses. The written plan provides a mechanism to help ensure continuity of care and can document client care in the areas of accountability, quality improvement, and liability.

NURSING PROCESS

The concept of nursing process was introduced in the 1950s, but it has taken many years to develop national acceptance of the process as an integral part of nursing care. It is adapted from the scientific approach to problem-solving and requires the skills of (1) assessment (systematic collection of data relating to clients and their problems), (2) problem identification (analysis/interpretation of data), (3) planning (setting goals and choice of solutions), (4) implementation (putting the plan into action), and (5) evaluation (assessing the effectiveness of the plan and changing the plan as indicated by the client's current needs). Although nurses use these terms separately, in reality they are interrelated and form a continuous circle of thought and action, providing an efficient method of organizing thought processes for clinical decision-making. Nursing process is now included in the conceptual framework of nursing curricula and accepted in the legal definition of nursing in most nurse practice acts. It is also the basis of the Standards of Psychiatric and Mental Health Clinical Nursing Practice (ANA, 1994) (Table 2–1).

TABLE 2–1. Standards of Psychiatric–Mental Health Clinical Nursing Practice

STANDARD I. Assessment
THE PSYCHIATRIC–MENTAL HEALTH NURSE COLLECTS CLIENT HEALTH DATA
Rationale
The assessment interview—which requires linguistically and culturally effective communication skills, interviewing, behavioral observation, data base record review, and comprehensive assessment of the client and relevant systems—enables the psychiatric–mental health nurse to make sound clinical judgments and plan appropriate interventions with the client.
STANDARD II. Diagnosis
THE PSYCHIATRIC–MENTAL HEALTH NURSE ANALYZES THE ASSESSMENT DATA
   IN DETERMINING DIAGNOSES
Rationale
The basis for providing psychiatric–mental health nursing care is the recognition and identification of patterns of response to actual or potential psychiatric illnesses and mental health problems.
STANDARD III. Outcome Identification
THE PSYCHIATRIC–MENTAL HEALTH NURSE IDENTIFIES EXPECTED OUTCOMES
   INDIVIDUALIZED TO THE CLIENT
Rationale
Within the context of providing nursing care, the ultimate goal is to influence health outcomes and improve the client's health status.
STANDARD IV. Planning
THE PSYCHIATRIC–MENTAL HEALTH NURSE DEVELOPS A PLAN OF CARE THAT PRESCRIBES
   INTERVENTIONS TO ATTAIN EXPECTED OUTCOMES
Rationale
A plan of care is used to guide therapeutic intervention systematically and achieve the expected client outcomes.
STANDARD V. Implementation
THE PSYCHIATRIC–MENTAL HEALTH NURSE IMPLEMENTS THE INTERVENTIONS
   IDENTIFIED IN THE PLAN OF CARE
Rationale
In implementing the plan of care, psychiatric–mental health nurses use a wide range of interventions according to their level of practice, designed to prevent mental and physical illness, and promote, maintain, and restore mental and physical health.
   Va. Counseling—Uses counseling interventions to assist clients in improving or regaining their previous coping abilities, fostering mental health, and preventing mental illness and disability
   Vb. Milieu Therapy—Provides, structures, and maintains a therapeutic environment in collaboration with the client and other healthcare providers
   Vc. Self-Care Activities—Structures interventions around the client's activities of daily living to foster self-care and mental and physical well-being
   Vd. Psychobiological Interventions—Uses knowledge of psychobiological interventions and applies clinical skills to restore the client's health and prevent further disability
   Ve. Health Teaching—Through health teaching, assists clients in achieving satisfying, productive, and healthy patterns of living
   Vf. Case Management—Provides case management to coordinate comprehensive health services and ensure continuity of care
   Vg. Health Promotion and Health Maintenance—Employs strategies and interventions to promote and maintain mental health and prevent mental illness
ADVANCED PRACTICE INTERVENTIONS FOR THE CERTIFIED SPECIALIST
   Vh. Psychotherapy—Uses individual, group, and family psychotherapy, child psychotherapy, and other therapeutic treatments to assist clients in fostering mental health, preventing mental illness and disability, and improving or regaining previous health status and functional illness

14

continued

Vi. Prescription of Pharmacological Agents—Uses prescription of pharmacological agents in accordance with the state nursing practice act to treat symptoms of psychiatric illness and improve functional health status

Vj. Consultation—Provides consultation to healthcare providers and others to influence the care plans for clients and to enhance the abilities of others to provide psychiatric and mental healthcare and affect change in systems

STANDARD VI. Evaluation

THE PSYCHIATRIC–MENTAL HEALTH NURSE EVALUATES THE CLIENT'S PROGRESS IN ATTAINING EXPECTED OUTCOMES

Rationale

Nursing care is a dynamic process involving change in the client's health status over time, giving rise to the need for new data, different diagnosis, and modifications in the plan of care. Therefore, evaluation is a continuous process of appraising the effect of nursing interventions and the treatment regimen on the client's health status and expected health outcomes.

Adapted from *A Statement on Psychiatric–Mental Health Clinical Nursing Practice and Standards of Psychiatric–Mental Health Clinical Nursing Practice,* ANA, 1994.

To use this process, the nurse must demonstrate fundamental abilities of knowledge, intelligence, and creativity, as well as expertise in interpersonal and technical skills. Some critical assumptions for the nurse to consider in the decision-making process are that:

- The client is a human being with worth and dignity.
- Individuals have basic human needs that must be met. When they are not, problems arise requiring intervention by another person until the individual can resume responsibility for self.
- The client has a right to quality health and nursing care delivered with concern, compassion, and competence, and focusing on wellness, prevention, and restoration.
- The therapeutic nurse-client relationship is a critical element in this process.

NURSING DIAGNOSIS

Nurses have struggled for years to define nursing by identifying its parameters with a goal of attaining/verifying professional status. To this end, nurses have been meeting and conducting research to develop nursing diagnoses. NANDA has accepted the following working definition:

Nursing diagnosis is a clinical judgment about individual, family, or community responses to actual and potential health problems/life processes. Nursing diagnoses provide the basis for selection of nursing interventions to achieve outcomes for which the nurse is accountable.

Nursing diagnosis, which provides a framework for using the nursing process, is the crux of the plan of care, as it focuses attention on client needs/responses (identifying problems, nursing interventions, and evaluation tools) and serves as the prime determinant of the style of nursing care to be delivered. Historically, nursing actions have often been based on variables such as signs and symptoms, tests, and medical diagnosis. However, at this time, the accurate diagnosis of a client problem, using the critical thinking process, can become a standard for nursing practice, understood by all who are using the plan of care, and thus can lead to improved delivery of care. The nursing diagnosis is as precise as the data will allow. It communicates the client's current situation and reflects changes as they occur. It is necessary to seek, incorporate, and synthesize all the relevant data and make the statement meaningful to provide appropriate direction for nursing care.

The affective tone of the nursing diagnosis can shape expectations of the client's response and influence the nurse's behavior toward the client. For instance, if the nurse sees the client as noncompliant, the nurse's attitudes and behavior may reflect anger and mistrust, and judgmental decisions may be made that do not accurately treat the client's problem. However, accurate identification of a client's problem (e.g., Ineffective Management Therapeutic Regimen: Individual related to medication side effects) can be understood by all who are using the plan of care, leading to improved delivery of care.

The nurse needs to be aware of the biases that may interfere with reaching an accurate diagnosis. Keeping one's mind open to numerous possibilities and not getting stuck on a single symptom/thought will facilitate this process. For example, from cues that are identified (e.g., restlessness), the nurse may infer that the client is anxious. If the nurse as-

15

sumes that this is only psychological, the possibility of its being physiologically based may be overlooked.

As previously noted, nursing diagnosis provides a common language for identifying client problems, nursing interventions, and evaluation and documentation tools. This common language is important, as it facilitates communication among nurses, shifts, units, and alternate care settings, as well as among healthcare professionals. It also provides a base for clinicians, educators, and researchers to document, validate, and/or alter the nursing process.

COMPONENTS OF THE PLAN OF CARE

For each plan of care presented, the *Client Assessment Data Base* is constructed from information obtained from the *History, Physical Examination,* and *Diagnostic Studies. Nursing Priorities* are then determined, serving as a general ranking system for the nursing diagnoses in the plan of care. In any given client situation, nursing priorities differ on the basis of specific client needs and can vary over time. In this book, each psychiatric condition has established *Discharge Goals,* which are broadly stated and reflect the desired general status of the client on discharge from care or on transfer from one setting to another. An example of discharge goals for a client with panic disorder would include:

1. Stays in feared situation even when discomfort is experienced
2. Identifies techniques to lower/maintain fear at manageable level
3. Confronts the phobia and is desensitized to the stimulus
4. Demonstrates greater independence, with an increasingly freer lifestyle
5. Develops plan to meet needs after discharge

Nursing priorities, along with the discharge goals, may be reworded and reorganized with timelines, according to individual client needs or situation, to create short-/long-term goals. The *Client Diagnostic Statement* is validated by the *Related to/Evidenced By* statements, which reflect the etiology and defining characteristics (signs and symptoms, or cues) most consistent with a specific psychiatric situation. *Desired Outcomes/Evaluation Criteria* for each diagnostic statement are followed by appropriate independent and collaborative interventions (with accompanying rationales) in this text.

Assessment

The critical element for providing effective planned nursing care is its relevance as identified in client assessments. Therefore, construction of the plan begins with the collection of data (assessment). According to the Standards of Clinical Nursing Practice (ANA, 1991), client assessment is required in the following areas: physical, psychological, sociocultural, spiritual, cognitive, functional abilities, developmental, economic, and lifestyle. These assessments, combined with the results of medical findings and diagnostic studies, are documented in the client data base.

The *Assessment Data Base* consists of subjective and objective information encompassing the various nursing concerns reflected in the current list of nursing diagnoses developed by NANDA. Subjective data are those reported by the client and/or significant other(s). This information includes any perceptions the individual may want to share. It is important to accept what is reported, because the client/significant other is the "expert" in this regard. However, the nurse needs to note any incongruencies/dissonances that may indicate the presence of other factors, such as lack of knowledge, myths, misconceptions, or fear.

Objective data are those that are observed (quantitatively or qualitatively) and may be verified by others (family, social network, other healthcare providers/medical records, and community agencies), as well as findings from the physical examination and diagnostic testing, including standardized instruments such as the Minnesota Multiphasic Personality Inventory and intelligence tests. Analysis (using the critical thinking process) of the subjective and objective data will lead to the identification of problems and areas of concern or need.

Problem Identification/Analysis

The second step involves examining assessment findings, grouping related findings, and comparing the findings against established normal parameters. The key, then, to accurate nursing diagnosis is problem identification, which focuses attention on a current or high-risk physical, psychological, or behavioral response that interferes with the quality of life the client desires or to which he or she is accustomed. Problem identification addresses the concerns of the client, significant other(s), and/or nurse that require nursing intervention and management. In this text, the choice of individual nursing diagnosis is validated by the "related to/risk factors" and "evidenced by" statements most consistently associated with a specific psychiatric situation/medical condition.

Even though nurses may feel at risk in committing themselves to documenting a nursing diagnosis, many references are currently available to help identify and formulate the diagnostic statement. (Refer to Table 2–2 for a list of NANDA-approved diagnostic labels.) In addition, unlike medical diagnoses, nursing diagnoses change as the client progresses through various stages of illness or maladaptation to problem resolution. From the specific information obtained in the client assessment data base, the related factors, signs, and symptoms can be identified, and an individualized statement of the client's problem/need (diagnosis) can be formulated. For example, a client may report fear of becoming obese and recurrent family focus on eating habits/changes in weight, leading to a choice of the following nursing diagnosis: Body Image, disturbance related to morbid fear of obesity as evidenced by negative feelings about body/view of self as fat in presence of normal body weight.

Planning

Goals are established and outcome statements formulated to aid in choosing interventions to give direction to nursing care. *Desired Outcomes* emerge from the diagnostic statement and are defined as the results of nursing interventions and client responses that are achievable, desired by the client and/or caregiver, and attainable within a defined time, given the present situation and resources. The desired outcomes are the measurable steps toward achieving the previously established discharge goals and are used to evaluate the client's response to nursing interventions. They have been stated in general terms in this book to permit the practitioner to modify/individualize them by adding timelines, dependent on the client's projected length of stay/involvement in therapy, and other client-specific data as appropriate. The terminology needs to be concise, realistic, measurable, and stated in words that the client can understand. Beginning the outcome statement with an action verb provides direction that is measurable (e.g., Client will: *verbalize* an increased sense of self-worth within 4 visits). Psychiatric nurses often work in settings in which they are members of a multidisciplinary team, requiring highly coordinated and frequently interdependent planning based on the separate and distinct roles of each team member. In this setting, it is important that the goals of the disciplines do not conflict. When outcomes are properly written, they provide direction for choosing and validating the selected interventions. Additionally, the nurse should plan care *with* the client/significant other, as

TABLE 2–2. Nursing Diagnoses Accepted for Use and Research (1997)

Activity Intolerance [specify level]
Activity Intolerance, risk for
Adaptive Capacity: Intracranial, decreased
Adjustment, impaired
*Airway Clearance, ineffective
Anxiety [specify level]
Aspiration, risk for

Body Image disturbance
Body Temperature, altered, risk for
Bowel Incontinence
Breastfeeding, effective
Breastfeeding, ineffective
Breastfeeding, interrupted
*Breathing Pattern, ineffective

*Cardiac Output, decreased
Caregiver Role Strain
Caregiver Role Strain, risk for
Communication, impaired, verbal
Community Coping, potential for enhanced
Community Coping, ineffective
Confusion, acute
Confusion, chronic
Constipation
Constipation, colonic
Constipation, perceived
Coping, defensive
*Coping, Individual, ineffective

Decisional Conflict (specify)
Denial, ineffective
Diarrhea
Disuse Syndrome, risk for
Diversional Activity deficit
Dysreflexia

Energy Field disturbance
Environmental Interpretation Syndrome, impaired

*Family Coping, ineffective, compromised
*Family Coping, ineffective, disabling
Family Coping: potential for growth
Family Process, altered: alcoholism
Family Processes, altered
Fatigue
Fear
*Fluid Volume deficit [Hyper/Hypotonic]

continued

*Fluid Volume deficit [Isotonic]
Fluid Volume deficit, risk for
*Fluid Volume excess

*Gas Exchange, impaired
*Grieving, anticipatory
*Grieving, dysfunctional
Growth & Development, altered

Health Maintenance, altered
Health-Seeking Behaviors (specify)
Home Maintenance Management, impaired
Hopelessness
Hyperthermia
Hypothermia

Incontinence, functional
Incontinence, reflex
Incontinence, stress
Incontinence, total
Incontinence, urge
Infant Behavior, disorganized
Infant Behavior, disorganized, risk for
Infant Behavior, organized, potential for
    enhanced
Infant Feeding Pattern, ineffective
Infection, risk for
Injury, risk for

*Knowledge deficit [Learning Need] (specify)

Loneliness, risk for

Memory, impaired

Noncompliance, [Compliance, altered] specify
Nutrition: altered, less than body requirements
Nutrition: altered, more than body requirements
Nutrition: altered, risk for more than body
    requirements

Oral Mucous Membrane, altered

*Pain [acute]
*Pain, chronic
Parental Role conflict
Parent/Infant/Child Attachment, altered, risk for
Parenting, altered
Parenting, altered, risk for
Perioperative Positioning Injury, risk for
Peripheral Neurovascular dysfunction, risk for
Personal Identity disturbance
Physical Mobility, impaired
Poisoning, risk for
Post-Trauma Response
Powerlessness
Protection, altered

Rape-Trauma Syndrome
Rape-Trauma Syndrome: compound reaction
Rape-Trauma Syndrome: silent reaction
Relocation Stress Syndrome
Role Performance, altered

Self Care deficit, feeding, bathing/hygiene,
    dressing/grooming, toileting
*Self Esteem, chronic low
*Self Esteem disturbance
*Self Esteem, situational low
Self-Mutilation, risk for
Sensory/Perceptual alterations (specify): visual,
    auditory, kinesthetic, gustatory, tactile, olfactory
Sexual dysfunction
Sexuality Patterns, altered
Skin Integrity, impaired
Skin Integrity, impaired: risk for
Sleep Pattern disturbance
Social Interaction, impaired
Social Isolation
Spiritual Distress (distress of the human spirit)
Spiritual Well-Being, potential for enhanced
Spontaneous Ventilation, inability to sustain
Suffocation, risk for
Swallowing, impaired

Therapeutic Regimen: Community, ineffective
    management
Therapeutic Regimen: Families, ineffective
    management
Therapeutic Regimen: Individual, effective
    management
Therapeutic Regimen: Individuals, ineffective
    management
Thermoregulation, ineffective
*Thought Processes, altered
Tissue Integrity, impaired
Tissue Perfusion, altered (specify): cerebral,
    cardiopulmonary, renal, gastrointestinal,
    peripheral
Trauma, risk for

Unilateral Neglect
Urinary Elimination, altered
Urinary Retention [acute/chronic]

Ventilatory Weaning Response, dysfunctional
    (DVWR)
*Violence, risk for, directed at self
*Violence, risk for, directed at others

[ ] Author recommendations
*Revised 1996
Permission from North American Nursing Diagnosis
Association (1997). NANDA Nursing Diagnoses:
Definitions and Classifications 1997–1998. Philadelphia:
NANDA. Copyright 1996 by the North American
Nursing Diagnosis Association.

appropriate, because all are accountable for that care and for achieving the desired outcomes.

Interventions communicate actions to be taken to achieve desired client outcomes and discharge goals. The expectation is that the prescribed behavior (interventions/action) will benefit the client and family in a predictable way, related to the identified problem and chosen outcomes. These interventions have the intent of individualizing care by meeting a specific client need and should incorporate identified client strengths when possible. Again, using an action verb (e.g., "instruct" or "demonstrate") provides direction for the nurse. The rationale for each intervention needs to be sound and feasible, focusing on providing individualized care. Actions may be independent or collaborative and may encompass orders from nursing, medicine/psychiatry, and other disciplines. In this book, collaborative actions in conjunction with other disciplines are identified to help the nurse choose appropriate interventions for the individual/ setting. The nurse's educational background/ expertise, standing protocols, and areas of practice (rural/urban, acute-care inpatient, or community-care settings) can influence whether an individual intervention is actually an independent nursing function or requires collaboration. Finally, the written interventions need to be dated and signed to identify the person initiating and coordinating the care.

Implementation

Once the goals, outcomes, and interventions have been identified, the nurse is ready to perform the activities recorded in the client's plan of care. In putting the plan into action and providing cost-effective and timely care, the nurse first identifies the priorities for providing that care. To determine the current priorities, the nurse reviews resources (such as diagnostic studies and progress reports from other healthcare providers), while consulting with and considering the desires of the client.

Next, many activities, ranging from simple tasks to complex procedures, can be involved in carrying out interventions to provide the planned care. The nurse needs to consider which interventions can be combined to facilitate accomplishing the activities within the given time constraints. Then, as care is provided, data on the client's response to each of the interventions is noted. The nurse also monitors the client and related resources for changes in status/development of complications.

Evaluation

Evaluation of the client's response to the care delivered and achievement of the desired outcomes (which were developed in the planning phase and documented in the plan of care) constitute the final step of the nursing process. The evaluation phase, which is an ongoing process, is necessary for the determination of how well the plan of care is working. As implied, this reassessment occurs not just when a desired client outcome is due to be reviewed or when it must be determined whether or not a client is ready for discharge; instead, it is a constant monitoring of the client's status. Based on the findings of each evaluation, the plan of care is revised to meet the changing needs of the client.

Rationale

Although rationales do not appear on agency plans of care, they are included in this book to assist the student and practicing nurse in associating the psychological and/or pathophysiological principles with the selected nursing intervention.

DOCUMENTING THE NURSING PROCESS

In general, the goals of the documentation system are to:

- Facilitate the quality of client care
- Ensure documentation of progress with regard to client-focused outcomes
- Facilitate interdisciplinary consistency and the communication of treatment goals and progress

Two recent publications provide the nurse with guidelines for documenting the nursing process and support the need for a written (or computer-generated) plan of care. The Standards of Clinical Nursing Practice (ANA, 1991) ". . . delineate care that is provided to all clients of nursing services," and each standard includes a measurement criterion addressing documentation. In addition, the Nursing Care Standards (Joint Commission on Accreditation of Healthcare Organizations [JCAHO], 1995) also focus attention on documentation, as presented in Table 2–3. These revised standards delineate the professional responsibilities of all registered nurses and provide criteria to assist in measuring achievement of identified standards.

From a nursing focus, documentation provides a record of the use of the nursing process for the delivery of individualized client care. The initial *assessment* is recorded in the client history or data base. The identification or diagnosis of client problems/needs and the *planning* of client care are recorded in the plan of care. The *implementation* of the plan is recorded in progress notes and/or flow

TABLE 2–3. A Sample Portion of One Nursing Care Standard from the Joint Commission on Accreditation of Healthcare Organizations

NC.1. Patients receive nursing care based on a documented assessment of their needs.

NC.1.3.4. The patient's medical record includes documentation of:

NC.1.3.4.1 The initial assessments and reassessments

NC.1.3.4.2 The nursing diagnosis and/or patient care needs

NC.1.3.4.3 The interventions identified to meet the patient's nursing care needs

NC.1.3.4.4 The nursing care provided

NC.1.3.4.5 The patient's response to, and the outcomes of, the care provided

NC.1.3.4.6 The abilities of the patient and/or, as appropriate, his/her significant other(s) to manage continuing care needs after discharge

Adapted from Accreditation Manual for Hospitals, JCAHO, 1995.

sheets. Finally, the *evaluation* of care is documented in progress notes and/or the plan of care.

The maintenance of a medical record is one of the most essential requirements for accreditation of healthcare facilities by JCAHO and/or other credentialing and licensing agencies. JCAHO standards state that the medical record should be documented accurately and in a timely manner. Therefore, the importance of completing notes on schedule and in manner that facilitates retrieval of data should be emphasized.

Documentation is not only a requirement for accreditation but also a permanent record of what happens with each client. It is a legal requirement in any healthcare setting. In our society, with its many lawsuits and aggressive malpractice emphasis, all aspects of the psychiatric medical record may be important for legal documentation. The plan of care that has been developed for a particular client serves as a framework or outline for charting administered care. Progress notes and flow sheets therefore reflect implementation of the treatment plan by documenting that appropriate actions have been carried out, precautions taken, and so forth. Both the implementation of interventions and progress toward the measurable outcomes need to be documented in the progress notes. These notes should be written clearly and objectively and in a manner that reflects progress toward desired measurable outcomes with the use of planned staff interventions. These notations also need to be date- and time-specific and to be signed by the person making the entry. Any errors in the document must be crossed out with one line so that the original entry is still legible, identified by the author as "error," and then initialed. White-outs or cross-outs that make the original information unreadable are not acceptable because this could be construed to mean that the individual or facility is trying to alter facts.

The psychiatric medical record is also the primary source of providing proof of services, which is necessary for maintaining revenues. Third-party reimbursers insist that the *why, when, where, how, what,* and *who* of services be clearly documented. Absence of such documentation may result in loss of funding for individual clients and possibly in termination of treatment. Therefore, progress notes must document what is happening to the client during all phases of treatment—acute-care/inpatient, outpa-

TABLE 2–4. Contents of a Progress Note

Unsettled or unclear problems or "issues" that need to be dealt with, including attempts to contact other client care providers

Noteworthy incidents or interviews involving the client that would benefit from a more detailed recording

Other pertinent data such as notes on phonecalls, home visits, and family interactions

Additional critical incident data such as seemingly significant or revealing statements made by the client, an insight you have into a client's patterns of behavior, client injuries, the use of any special treatment procedure, or other major events such as episodes of pain, respiratory distress, panic attacks, medication reactions, or suicidal comments

Administered care, activities, or observations if not recorded elsewhere on flow sheets (e.g., physician visits, completion of ordered tests, PRN medications)

tient, and rehabilitation. It is important to record information and observations that will assist both the oncoming nurse and other healthcare providers in maintaining the continuity of planned care. Table 2–4 provides examples of information to be documented in the client's record.

There are several charting formats that are currently used for documentation (e.g., problem-oriented medical record [POMR] and Focus® Charting). Regardless of the form you use, entries should be concise and consistent in style and format, to avoid confusion and to comply with existing agency policies and procedures. Examples of documentation formats are included in Chapter 3.

SUMMARY

The nurse's therapeutic relationship with the client creates a milieu in which the art of nursing can be practiced. As the primary coordinator of overall client care, the nurse strives to ensure that the client receives quality and cost-effective care through the use of the nursing process. Creation of, and effective use of, the client plan of care helps ensure that the psychiatric client receives individualized quality care in the midst of cost-containment. The plan further serves as the vehicle for, and documentation of, ongoing communication among nurses and other providers, as well as the impact of nursing care on the client. Although nursing diagnosis is an essential component of nursing practice in the acute-care setting, the use of nursing diagnosis within the nursing case management delivery system has yet to realize its full potential. Its value will come to be appreciated as the concept of case management evolves and is continually refined. Additionally, other disciplines will come to realize what the nursing profession has discovered: that nursing diagnosis is the key to executing and preserving the independent practice component of nursing.

Given the rapid changes affecting the healthcare system, nurses need resources to help them stay current and provide quality care for their clients. This book is designed to help the psychiatric nurse plan and deliver care to the client in the hospital and/or community setting, with consideration of family/significant other(s). The plan of care guidelines provided are intended to facilitate the use of the nursing process and identify nursing diagnoses for many of the most common psychiatric conditions the nurse/student deals with in daily practice. Chapter 3 will assist you in applying and adapting theory to practice.

CHAPTER 3

APPLYING THEORY TO PRACTICE

The previous chapter discussed the theory of nursing process, incorporating nursing diagnosis. In this chapter, given the evolving nature of nursing diagnosis, the nurse is encouraged to learn to tailor the plan of care to the individual client. The plans presented here are guides for the nurse in the use of this process. They are designed to give the nurse a sampling of information about general client situations and to identify many factors that may or may not need to be given consideration in caring for any particular client.

Client assessment is the foundation on which identification of individual needs, responses, and problems is based. To facilitate the steps of assessment and diagnosis in the nursing process, a psychiatric assessment tool (Fig. 3–1) has been constructed using a nursing focus instead of the familiar medical approach ("review of systems"). This has the advantage of identifying and validating nursing diagnoses as opposed to medical diagnoses.

To achieve this nursing focus, we have grouped the current NANDA nursing diagnoses into related categories titled Diagnostic Divisions (Table 3–1), which reflect a blending of theories, primarily Maslow's hierarchy of needs and self-care philosophy. These divisions serve as the framework or outline for data collection and clustering that focuses attention on the nurse's concerns—the human responses to actual and potential health problems—and directs the nurse to the corresponding nursing diagnosis label. Because these divisions are based on human responses/needs and not on specific "systems," the information gathered may occasionally be recorded in more than one area. For this reason, the nurse is encouraged to keep an open mind, pursue leads, and collect as much data as possible before choosing the nursing diagnosis label. For example, when the nurse identifies the cue of restlessness in a client, the nurse may infer that the client is anxious. The nurse may believe that the restlessness is psychologically based, overlooking the possibility that it is physiologically based. The results (synthesis) of the collected data are written concisely in a client diagnostic statement that best reflects the client's situation.

Recognizing and reflecting on current changes in the delivery and utilization of healthcare, and realizing that many people may not be seen in the healthcare system except when their illness has become exacerbated, this assessment tool is not restricted to *psychiatric data* but includes general health information. Physiological well-being may affect or be affected by the individual's psychological state, and baseline information is necessary to assist in recognizing changes that may occur in relation to subsequent therapies or state of wellness. From the specific data recorded in the data base, the related/risk factors (etiology) and signs/symptoms or cues can be identified. Then an individualized client diagnostic statement can be formulated, using the problem, etiology, signs/symptoms (PES) format to represent the client's situation accurately. The plan of care guidelines in this text were developed using the nursing diagnosis labels recommended by NANDA, except in a few examples in which the authors felt that more clarification and enhancement were required. In the ongoing controversy on the validity of the NANDA-approved nursing diagnosis, "Knowledge Deficit" is one example in which further clarification was added. The term "Learning Need" has been added to the diagnostic label "Knowledge Deficit." For example, the diagnostic statement may read: "Knowledge Deficit [Learning Need] regarding condition, prognosis, and treatment needs, related to learned maladaptive coping skills, lack of exposure to/misunderstanding of information presented evidenced by

This is a suggested tool for development by an individual or institution to create a data base reflecting diagnostic divisions of nursing diagnoses. Although the divisions are alphabetized for ease of presentation, they can be prioritized or rearranged to meet individual needs. **Note:** Although medical evaluation has been abbreviated in this assessment tool, it is important to remember that this may be the client's only contact with the healthcare profession and a more complete physical examination may be needed.

General Information

Name: _____

Age: _____   DOB: _____   Sex: _____   Race: _____

Admission Date: _____   Time: _____   From: _____

Source of Information: _____   Reliability (1–4 with 4 very reliable): _____

Activity/Rest

REPORTS (SUBJECTIVE)

Energy Level/Pattern: _____
  Fatigue: _____
Occupation: _____
Usual Activities/Hobbies: _____
Leisure Time Activities: _____
Exercise Program: _____
Feelings of Boredom/Dissatisfaction: _____
Limitations Imposed by Condition(s): _____
Sleep: Hours: _____   **Naps:** _____   **Aids:** _____
Insomnia: _____   **Related to:** _____
  Dreams: _____   **Nightmares:** _____
  Rested Upon Awakening: _____
  Excessive Grogginess: _____
  Feelings of Boredom/Dissatisfaction: _____

EXHIBITS (OBJECTIVE)

Observed Response to Activity:
  Cardiovascular: _____
  Respiratory: _____
Mental Status (e.g., withdrawn/lethargic):
  _____
Neuro/Muscular Assessment:
  Muscle Mass/Tone: _____
  Posture: _____   **Tremors:** _____
  ROM: _____   **Strength:** _____
  Deformity: _____

Circulation

REPORTS (SUBJECTIVE)

History of: Hypertension: _____
  Heart Trouble: _____
  Rheumatic Fever: _____
  Ankle/Leg Edema: _____
  Phlebitis: _____   **Slow Healing:** _____
  Bleeding Tendencies/Episodes: _____
  Palpitations: _____   **Syncope:** _____
Extremities: Numbness: _____ **Tingling:** _____
Cough/Hemoptysis: _____
Change in Frequency/Amount of Urine: _____

EXHIBITS (OBJECTIVE)

B/P: _____   **R and L:** _____
Peripheral Pulses (palpation): —————
Heart Sounds: _____
Breath Sounds: _____
Jugular Vein Distention: _____
Extremities: _____   **Temperature:** _____
  Color: _____   **Capillary Refill:** _____
  Edema: _____
Color: _____ **Mucous Membranes:** _____
  Nail Beds: _____
  Conjunctiva: _____   **Sclera:** _____
Diaphoresis: _____

Ego Integrity

REPORTS (SUBJECTIVE)

**What kind of person are you (positive/
  negative, etc.)?:** _____
What do you think of your body?: _____

EXHIBITS (OBJECTIVE)

**Emotional Status (check those that
  apply):**
  Calm: _____   **Friendly:** _____

Figure 3–1: Psychiatric Nursing Assessment Tool

How would you rate your self-esteem (1–10)?: _____

What are your moods?:

Depressed: _____   Guilty: _____

Unreal: _____   Ups/Downs: _____

Apathetic: _____   Detached: _____

Separated from the World: _____

Are you a nervous person?: _____

Are your feelings easily hurt?: _____

Report of Stress Factors: _____

Previous Patterns of Handling Stress: ___

Financial Concerns: _____

Relationship Status: _____

Work History/Military Service: _____

Cultural Factors: _____

Religion: _____   Practicing: _____

Lifestyle: _____   Recent Changes: _____

Significant Changes (date): _____

Stages of Grief/Manifestations of Loss: _____

Feelings of: Helplessness: _____

Hopelessness: _____

Powerlessness: _____

Cooperative: _____   Evasive: _____

Anxious: _____   Angry/hostile: _____

Withdrawn: _____   Fearful: _____

Irritable: _____   Restive: _____

Passive: _____   Dependent: _____

Euphoric: _____   Other (specify): ___

Defense Mechanisms: Projection: ___

Denial: _____   Undoing: _____

Rationalization: ___   Repression: ___

Passive-aggressive: ___   Sublimation: ___

Intellectualization:

Somatization: _____   Regression: ___

Identification: _____   Introjection: __

Reaction formation: __   Isolation: __

Displacement: ___   Substitution: ___

Consistency of Behavior: _____

Verbal: _____   Nonverbal: _____

Characteristics of Speech: _____

Motor Behaviors: _____   Posturing: ___

Under/Overactive: _____   Stereotypic: ___

Observed Physiological Response(s): _____

Elimination

REPORTS (SUBJECTIVE)

Usual Bowel Pattern: _____

Laxative Use: _____   Last BM: _____

Character of Stool: _____

History of Bleeding (urine/stool): _____

Hemorrhoids: _____

Usual Voiding Pattern: _____

Character of Urine: _____

Pain/Burning/Difficulty Voiding: _____

History of Kidney/Bladder Disease: _____

Diuretic Use: _____

EXHIBITS (OBJECTIVE)

Abdomen: Tender: _____   Soft/Firm: ___

Palpable Mass: _____

Bowel Sounds: _____

Food/Fluid

REPORTS (SUBJECTIVE)

Usual Diet (type): _____

Number of Meals Daily: _____

Last Meal/Intake: _____

Dietary Pattern/Content: _____

Loss of Appetite: _____

Nausea/Vomiting: _____

Heartburn/Indigestion: _____

Related to: _____   Relieved by: _____

Allergy/Food Intolerance: _____

Mastication/Swallowing Problems: _____

Dentures: _____

Usual Weight: _____

Changes in Weight: _____

Diuretic Use: _____

EXHIBITS (OBJECTIVE)

Current Weight: _____   Height: _____

Body Build: _____

Skin Turgor: _____

Mucous Membranes Moist/Dry: _____

Edema: _____

Jugular Vein Distention: _____

Condition of Teeth/Gums: _____

Appearance of Tongue: _____

Halitosis: _____

Thyroid Enlarged: _____

Bowel Sounds: _____

Breath Sounds: _____

Hygiene

REPORTS (SUBJECTIVE)

Activities of Daily Living:
  Independent/Dependent: _____
  Mobility: _____   Feeding: _____
  Hygiene: _____   Dressing: _____
  Toileting: _____
Equipment/Prosthetic Devices Required:

_____
  Assistance Provided by: _____

EXHIBITS (OBJECTIVE)

General Appearance: _____
Manner of Dress: _____
Personal Habits: _____
Body Odor: _____
Presence of Vermin: _____

Neurosensory

REPORTS (SUBJECTIVE)

Dreamlike States: _____
  Walking in Sleep: _____
  Automatic writing: _____
Believe/Feel You Are Another Person:

_____

Perception Different Than Others:

_____

Fainting Spells/Dizziness: _____
  Blackouts: _____
Ability to Follow Directions: _____
  Perform Calculations: _____
  Accomplish ADLs: _____
Seizures: Type: _____ Aura: _____
  Frequency: _____ Postictal State: _____
  How Controlled: _____
  Changes in Vision/Hearing: _____

EXHIBITS (OBJECTIVE)

Mental Status (note duration of change):
  Oriented/Disoriented: Time: _____
  Place: _____   Person: _____
Check All That Apply:
  Alert: _____   Drowsy: _____
  Lethargic: _____   Stuporous: _____
  Comatose: _____   Cooperative: _____
  Combative: _____   Delusions: _____
  Hallucinations: _____
  Affect (describe): _____
Memory: Immediate: _____
  Recent: _____
  Remote: _____
Comprehension: _____
Thought Processes (assessed through speech):
  Patterns of Speech (e.g., spontaneous/ sudden silences): _____   Content: _____
  Change in Topic: _____
  Delusions: _____ Hallucinations: _____
  Illusions: _____   Rate or Flow: _____
  Clear, Logical Progression: _____
  Expression: _____
  Mood: _____   Affect: _____
  Appropriateness: _____   Intensity: _____
  Range: _____
  Insight: _____   Misperceptions: _____
Attention/ Calculation Skills: _____
  Judgment: _____
  Ability to Follow Directions: _____
  Problem-solving: _____

Pain/Discomfort

REPORTS (SUBJECTIVE)

Location: _____   Intensity (0–10 with 10 most severe): _____
  Frequency: _____   Quality: _____
  Duration: _____   Radiation: _____
Precipitating/Aggravating Factors:

_____

EXHIBITS (OBJECTIVE)

Facial Grimacing: _____
  Guarding Affected Area: _____
Emotional Response: _____
  Narrowed Focus: _____

How Relieved: _____
Associated Symptoms: _____
Effects on Activities: _____
   Relationships: _____

Respiration

REPORTS (SUBJECTIVE)

Dyspnea: _____   Related to: _____
Cough/Sputum: _____
History of Bronchitis: _____
   Asthma: _____   Tuberculosis: _____
   Emphysema: _____
   Recurrent Pneumonia: _____
   Exposure to Noxious Fumes: _____
Smoker: Pack/Day: _____
   Number of Years: _____
Use of Respiratory Aids: _____
Oxygen: _____

EXHIBITS (OBJECTIVE)

Respiratory: Rate: ___   Depth: ___
Use of Accessory Muscles: _____
Breath Sounds: _____
Cyanosis: _____
Clubbing of Fingers: _____
Sputum Characteristics: _____
Mentation/Restlessness: _____

Safety

REPORTS (SUBJECTIVE)

Allergies/Sensitivity: _____
   Reaction: _____
Exposure to Infectious Diseases: _____
History of Sexually Transmitted Disease
   (date/type): _____
Previous Alteration of Immune System:

   _____
   Cause: _____
Blood Transfusion/Number: _____
   When: _____   Reaction: _____
   Describe: _____
High-Risk Behaviors (work/hobby/
   sexual): _____
Seat Belt/Helmet Use: _____
History of Accidental Injuries: _____
   Fractures/dislocations: _____
   Arthritis/Unstable Joints: _____
   Back Problems: _____
Changes in Moles: _____
Enlarged Nodes: _____
Delayed Healing: _____
Impaired Vision: _____   Hearing: _____
Prosthesis: _____ Ambulatory Devices: _____
Expressions of Ideation of Violence
   (self/others): _____
Suicidal Plan: _____
   Means Available: _____

EXHIBITS (OBJECTIVE)

Temperature: _____   Diaphoresis: _____
Skin Integrity: Scars: _____   Rashes: _____
   Lesions (describe): ___   Lacerations: ___
   Ecchymosis: _____
   Drainage: _____
General Strength: _____   Muscle Tone: _____
   Gait: _____   ROM: _____
   Paresthesia/Paralysis: _____
Immune System Testing: _____
TB Testing: _____

Sexuality [Component of Social Interaction]

REPORTS (SUBJECTIVE)

Sexually Active: _____   Age: _____
   Use of Condoms: _____
Birth Control Method: _____
Sexual Concerns/Difficulties: _____
Recent Change in Frequency/ Interest: _____
Sexual Orientation/Variant Preferences:

_____

EXHIBITS (OBJECTIVE)

Comfort Level with Subject Matter: _____

Female

Age at Menarche: _____
   Length of Cycle: _____
   Duration: _____   No. of Pads Used/Day:____

_____
   Last Menstrual Period: _____
Pregnant?: _____   Menopause: _____
Vaginal discharge: _____
Bleeding Between Periods: _____
Practices Breast Self-Exam: _____
Frequency/Last Mammogram: _____
Frequency/Last PAP Smear: _____
Hormone Therapy/Calcium Use: _____

Breast Exam: _____
Genital Warts/Lesions: _____
Discharge: _____

Male

Penile Discharge: ____
Prostate Disorder: ____
Circumcised: _____   Vasectomy: _____
Practice Self-Exam: Breast: ___ Testicles: ___
Last Proctoscopic/Prostate Exam:

_____

Breast: _____   Penis: _____
Testicles: _____
Genital Warts/Lesions: _____
Discharge:_____

Social Interactions

REPORTS (SUBJECTIVE)

Marital Status: ____ Years in Relationship: ____
   Living with: _____
Concerns/Stresses: _____
Extended Family: _____
   Other Support Person(s): _____
Role Within Family Structure: _____
Perception of Relationships with Family: ____
Genogram (separate form): Y/N _____
   Memory of Early Years: _____
Family Dynamics: _____
Performance/Interactions: Work: _____
   School: _____   Social: _____
Problems Related to Illness/Condition:

_____

Change in Speech: _____
   Use of Communication Aids:
Feelings of Mistrust: _____   Rejection: _____
Loneliness/Isolation: _____

EXHIBITS (OBJECTIVE)

Verbal/Nonverbal Communication with
   Family/SO(s): _____
   Family Interaction (Behavioral)
   Pattern: _____
Speech: Clear: _____   Slurred: _____
   Unintelligible: _____   Aphasic: _____
   Unusual Speech Pattern/Impairment:_____
   Use of Speech Aids: _____

Teaching/Learning:

Dominant Language (specify): _____
  Literate: _____   Education Level: _____
  Learning Disabilities (specify): _____
  Cognitive Limitations: _____
Employment/Education Goals: _____
Health Beliefs/Practices: _____
Special Healthcare Concerns
  (e.g., impact of religious, cultural
  practices): _____
Familial Risk Factors (indicate relationship):
  Mental Illness: _____
  Depression: _____   Diabetes: _____
  Thyroid (specify): _____
  Tuberculosis: _____
  Heart disease: _____
  Strokes: _____   High B/P: _____
  Neuromuscular Conditions: _____
  Epilepsy: _____
  Kidney Disease: _____
  Cancer: _____
Prescribed Medications: Drug: _____
  Dose: _____   Times: _____
  Take Regularly: _____
  Purpose: _____
Nonprescription Drugs:
  OTC: _____   Street: _____
  Tobacco: _____   Smokeless Tobacco: _____
  Use of Alcohol (amount/frequency): _____
Initial Diagnosis Per Psychiatrist/
  Primary Therapist: _____
Reason for Seeking Therapy Per Client:
  _____

History of Current Complaint: _____
  Client Expectations of Therapy: _____
Previous Illnesses and/or
  Hospitalizations/Surgeries: _____
Evidence of Failure to Improve: _____
Last Complete Physical Exam: _____

Date Information Obtained: _____
Anticipated Date of Discharge: _____
  Resources Available: _____
  Persons (specify): _____   Financial: _____
Anticipated Changes in Living Situation
After Discharge: _____
Assistance Required:
  Self-Care (specify): _____
  Homemaker/Maintenance Assistance: ___
  Other: _____
Living Facility Other Than Home (specify):
  _____

Vocational Rehabilitation: _____
  Interest/Abilities: ___   Resources: ___
Community Supports: _____   Groups: _____
  Socialization: _____
Referrals: Therapy: _____
  Social Services: _____

TABLE 3–1. Diagnostic Divisions

After data are collected, and areas of concern/need identified, the nurse is directed to the Diagnostic Divisions to review the list of nursing diagnoses that fall within the individual categories. This will help the nurse choose the specific diagnostic label to describe the data accurately. Then, with the addition of etiology or related/risk factors (when known) and signs and symptoms or cues (defining characteristics), the patient diagnostic statement emerges.

ACTIVITY/REST

Ability to engage in necessary/desired activities of life (work and leisure) and to obtain adequate sleep/rest
- Activity intolerance
  - Activity intolerance, risk for
  - Disuse Syndrome, risk for
  - Diversional Activity deficit
  - Fatigue
  - Sleep Pattern disturbance

CIRCULATION

Ability to transport oxygen and nutrients necessary to meet cellular needs
- Adaptive Capacity: Intracranial, decreased
- Cardiac Output, decreased
- Dysreflexia
- Tissue Perfusion, altered, (specify) renal, cerebral, cardiopulmonary, gastrointestinal, peripheral

EGO INTEGRITY

Ability to develop and use skills and behaviors to integrate and manage life experiences
- Adjustment, impaired
- Anxiety [specify level]
- Body Image disturbance
- Coping, defensive
- Coping, Individual, ineffective
- Decisional Conflict (specify)
- Denial, ineffective
- Energy Field disturbance
- Fear
- Grieving, anticipatory
- Grieving, dysfunctional
- Hopelessness
- Personal Identity disturbance
- Post-Trauma Response
- Powerlessness
- Rape-Trauma Syndrome
- Rape-Trauma Syndrome: compound reaction
- Rape-Trauma Syndrome: silent reaction
- Relocation Stress Syndrome
- Self Esteem, chronic low
- Self Esteem disturbance
- Self Esteem, situational low
- Spiritual Distress (distress of the human spirit)
- Spiritual Well-Being, potential for enhanced

ELIMINATION

Ability to excrete waste products
- Bowel Incontinence
- Constipation
- Constipation, colonic
- Constipation, perceived
- Diarrhea
- Incontinence, functional
- Incontinence, reflex
- Incontinence, stress
- Incontinence, total
- Incontinence, urge
- Urinary Elimination, altered
- Urinary Retention [acute/chronic]

FOOD/FLUID

Ability to maintain intake of and use nutrients and liquids to meet physiological needs
- Breastfeeding, effective
- Breastfeeding, ineffective
- Breastfeeding, interrupted
- Fluid Volume deficit [hyper/hypotonic]
- Fluid Volume deficit [isotonic]
- Fluid Volume deficit, risk for
- Fluid Volume excess
- Infant Feeding Pattern, ineffective
- Nutrition: altered, less than body requirements
- Nutrition: altered, more than body requirements
- Nutrition: altered, risk for more than body requirements
- Oral Mucous Membrane, altered
- Swallowing, impaired

HYGIENE

Ability to perform activities of daily living
- Self Care deficit: feeding, bathing/hygiene, dressing/grooming, toileting

NEUROSENSORY

Ability to perceive, integrate, and respond to internal and external cues
- Confusion, acute
- Confusion, chronic
- Infant Behavior: disorganized
- Infant Behavior: disorganized, risk for
- Infant Behavior: organized, potential for enhancement
- Memory, impaired
- Peripheral Neurovascular dysfunction, risk for

Sensory/Perceptual alterations (specify) visual, auditory, kinesthetic, gustatory, tactile, olfactory

Thought Processes, altered

Unilateral Neglect

PAIN/DISCOMFORT

Ability to control internal/external environment to maintain comfort

Pain [acute]

Pain, chronic

RESPIRATION

Ability to provide and use oxygen to meet physiological needs

Airway Clearance, ineffective

Aspiration, risk for

Breathing Pattern, ineffective

Gas Exchange, impaired

Spontaneous Ventilation, inability to sustain

Ventilatory Weaning Response, dysfunctional (DVWR)

SAFETY

Ability to provide safe, growth-promoting environment

Body Temperature, altered, risk for

Environmental Interpretation Syndrome, impaired

Health Maintenance, altered

Home Maintenance Management, impaired

Hyperthermia

Hypothermia

Infection, risk for

Injury, risk for

Perioperative Positioning Injury, risk for

Physical Mobility, impaired

Poisoning, risk for

Protection, altered

Self-Mutilation, risk for

Skin Integrity, impaired

Skin Integrity, impaired, risk for

Suffocation, risk for

Thermoregulation, ineffective

Tissue Integrity, impaired

Trauma, risk for

Violence, risk for, directed at others

Violence, risk for, self-directed

SEXUALITY [Component of Ego Integrity and Social Interaction]

Ability to meet requirements/characteristics of male/female role

Sexual dysfunction

Sexuality Patterns, altered

SOCIAL INTERACTION

Ability to establish and maintain relationships

Caregiver Role Strain

Caregiver Role Strain, risk for

Communication, impaired verbal

Community Coping, ineffective

Community Coping, potential for enhanced

Family Coping, ineffective: compromised

Family Coping, ineffective: disabling

Family Coping: potential for growth

Family Process, altered: alcoholism

Family Processes, altered

Loneliness, risk for

Parent/Infant/Child Attachment, altered, risk for

Parental Role conflict

Parenting, altered

Parenting, altered, risk for

Role Performance, altered

Social Interaction, impaired

Social Isolation

TEACHING/LEARNING

Ability to incorporate and use information to achieve healthy lifestyle/optimal wellness

Growth and Development, altered

Health Seeking Behaviors (specify)

Knowledge deficit [Learning need] (specify)

Noncompliance [Compliance, altered] (specify)

Therapeutic Regimen: Community, ineffective management

Therapeutic Regimen: Families, ineffective management

Therapeutic Regimen: Individual, effective management

Therapeutic Regimen: Individual, ineffective management

questions and expressions of concern." Additionally, some diagnoses have been combined for convenience, indicating that two or more factors may be involved (e.g., Body Image disturbance/Self Esteem, chronic low). We anticipate that the nurse will choose what is applicable in the individual situation, or leave the two diagnoses combined if both diagnoses are appropriate, as the interventions address both problems.

Desired client outcomes are identified to facilitate choosing appropriate interventions and to serve as evaluators of both nursing care and client response. These outcomes also form the framework for documentation.

Interventions are designed to specify the action of the nurse, the client, and/or significant other(s). Sometimes controversial issues or treatments are presented for the sake of information or because alternate therapies may be used in different care settings or geographical locations.

In addition to achieving psychological and physiological stability, interventions need to promote the client's movement toward health and independence. This requires that the client be involved in his or her own care, including participation in decisions about care activities and projected outcomes. This promotes client responsibility, negating the idea that healthcare providers control clients' lives. It is also important to remember that, although the individual is the primary client, significant other(s)/family members will also need consideration and inclusions in care.

To help you visualize the tailoring of a plan of care, a prototype Client Situation (p 32) is provided as an example of data collection and construction of the plan of care. As you review the client assessment data base, you can identify the etiological risk factors and other characteristics that we used to formulate the client diagnostic statements. Timelines were added to specific client outcomes to reflect anticipated length of therapy and individual client/nurse expectations. The choice of interventions is based on the concerns and needs identified by the client and nurse during data collection, in addition to psychiatrist/physician orders and input from the rest of the interdisciplinary team. Although not normally included in a plan of care, rationales are included in this sample for the purpose of explaining or clarifying the choice of interventions and enhancing the nurse's learning. Additionally, because the diagnosis of anorexia is an acute problem with predictable outcomes to be achieved within a predetermined time frame (e.g., 28 days), a sample clinical pathway is also provided. Finally, to complete the learning experience, samples of documentation based on the client situation are presented.

SAMPLE CLIENT SITUATION: Anorexia Nervosa/Bulimia Nervosa

MJB, a 33-year-old female, presented at the doctor's office with reports of lightheadedness, fatigue, and weakness, as well as a history of eating disorders. She was admitted to the eating disorders program on referral by her family physician for psychiatric care, controlled environment, and monitoring of physiological well-being.

ADMITTING PSYCHIATRIST'S ORDERS

CBC, electrolytes, blood sugar on admission
ECG in AM
Endocrine studies, dexamethasone suppression test (DST) in AM
Urinalysis in AM
Regular diet with selective menu; schedule dietary consult
Weight on admission and per protocol
Trilafon 8 mg/tid

CLIENT ASSESSMENT DATA BASE

Name: Mary Jane B.
Age: 33
DOB: 2/13/1964
Sex: F   **Race:** W   **Admission Date:** 6/23/97
Time: 3:30 PM
From: Home
Source of Information: Self-reliability: 2–3 (1–4 scale)
Family Member/Significant Other(s): Family not in area, no contact
Friend: Mrs. CP

Activity/Rest

SUBJECTIVE

Energy Level: Low; works hard, tires easily
Fatigue: Always
Occupation: Receptionist, city government office
Usual Activities/Hobbies: Volunteers for church; has lots of projects, but can't get them completed; would like to learn new vocation
Leisure Time Activities: "Not much. I don't like to get out with people, and I just don't seem to have the energy."
Exercise Program: Aerobics irregularly, sometimes twice a day, 5 days/wk (7 times last 2 wk)
Limitations imposed by condition: "Afraid people will know about my problem."
Sleep: "Not enough, maybe 4–5 hours/night."

OBJECTIVE

Observed Response to Activity:
Respiratory: Tachypnea/28
Cardiovascular: Elevated pulse/120
Mental Status: Withdrawn
Posture: Sits hunched over, not looking up

Insomnia: "I have some problem, usually because I don't get to bed." This is her binge time, finds things to do to avoid going to bed. Not rested on awakening, tired all the time.

Circulation

SUBJECTIVE

History of: Occasional ankle/leg edema
Palpitations: Occasional
Syncope: "Fainting spells" several times a week, feels lightheaded/weak

OBJECTIVE

B/P: 106/68 lying; 90/63 sitting
Pulse: 104 at rest
Heart/Breath Sounds: Deferred
Color: Skin, pale
Conjunctiva/Mucous Membranes/Lips: Pale

Ego Integrity

SUBJECTIVE

What kind of person are you?: "I'm a nothing, a zero."
What do you think of your body?: "I don't like my body, it's too fat." Doesn't do anything in which she has to expose her body. Would like to learn massage but doesn't want to have a man touch her body (a requirement of the class is that students practice on one another).
How would you rate your self-esteem (1–10)?: "Zero"
What are your moods?: "Depressed, lonely, feel tense and anxious, empty."
Are you a nervous person? "Yes"
Are your feelings easily hurt?: "Yes. I'm afraid I'm a bother to other people. They think I'm not doing a good job." (Denies any direct knowledge of criticism.)
Report of Stress Factors: Worries about everything: binge eating, having to deal with people in her job, limited income, no savings/health insurance.
Previous Patterns of Coping with Stress: "I was anorectic, avoided eating," distance running (frequently 10 miles a day), withdrawal (ran away from the hospital last time she was hospitalized).
Financial Concerns: Is in a low-paying job, no resources
Relationship Status: Single; has never been married or had a relationship. "I don't like men, can't trust them."
Cultural Factors: White, middle class
Lifestyle: Has no home of her own, house-sits for people who are gone,

OBJECTIVE

Emotional Status: Calm, cooperative, fearful, anxious, dependent
Behavior: Consistent; verbal responses congruent; speech modulated, congruent; voice low
Defense Mechanisms: Rationalization ("I ate lunch, some lettuce and sunflower seeds."); denial ("I'm not a worthwhile person."); and projection ("I don't like the way people act. They lie, cheat, and steal.")
Body Language: Sitting quietly with head down; looks up occasionally and maintains eye contact when she does; playing with a tissue

stays with church friends between house-sitting jobs ("helps with the money"), is alone a lot in this situation.

Significant Losses/Changes (Date): Left home and moved to another state 10 years ago (7/1986); does not have contact with family. Father died 4 years ago (3/1993); did not see him or return for funeral.

Stage of Grief/Manifestations of Loss: (Stated matter-of-factly) "I don't want to have any contact with my family. I was glad to get away from them and really don't want to have any contact with them now."

Religion: Catholic   **Practicing:** Yes

Elimination

SUBJECTIVE

Usual bowel pattern: Irregular, constipation an ongoing problem; uses herbal laxative once or twice a week

Last BM: 2 days ago

Character: Dry, light-colored

Usual Voiding Pattern: No problem, but voiding less frequently (once/twice a day)

Character of Urine: Dark yellow

OBJECTIVE

Examinations: Deferred

Food/Fluid

SUBJECTIVE

Usual diet: Vegetarian, does not eat eggs or chicken. Eats 1 meal a day; no breakfast; snacks on lettuce, nuts; may have tuna for lunch. Afraid to eat for fear she cannot stop. Binges on whatever is available, usually carbohydrates (candy bars, cookies)

Fluids: Drinks occasional glass of water, diet colas (2–3/day)

Usual Weight: 130 pounds, no recent weight changes. Weighed 85 pounds when she was hospitalized for anorexia the first time, 12 years ago (10/1984)

Vomiting: Usually once a day; sometimes only 2–3 times/wk

Swallowing Problem: Sore mouth and throat frequently

OBJECTIVE

Current Weight: 128 pounds
Height: 5 feet 4 inches
Body Build: Slight
Skin Turgor: Tight
Mucous Membranes/Lips: Dry
Edema: None
Halitosis: Sour breath
Condition of Teeth/Gums: Tooth decay/ erosion evident, gums inflamed, salivary glands slightly swollen
   Bowel/breath sounds: Deferred

Hygiene

SUBJECTIVE

Independent in Self-Care

OBJECTIVE

General Appearance: Neatly dressed in boxy-style blue suit; oxford-type shoes, in good condition; dark, short hair curled around face; eye makeup lightly applied; nails well kept, no nail polish; no jewelry noted

Neurosensory

SUBJECTIVE

Perception Different From Others: Reports sees self as fat, even though others do not

Fainting Spells/Dizziness: Several times a week

Headaches: Occasionally all over head, 2–3 times/wk past 3 months. Says did not have headaches until recently when vomiting became more frequent.

Ability to Follow Directions: Concerned because she is not remembering things, being forgetful. States she has a problem concentrating, difficulty making decisions.

Eyes: No reports of eye strain or change in acuity; no glasses

OBJECTIVE

Mental Status: Alert and oriented to time, place, and person

Memory: Intact

Intellectual Functioning: Testing deferred

Thought Processes: Speech pattern normal. Thinking fairly rational/logical with organized, coherent flow of ideas. Occasional evidence of distorted thinking (e.g., "I'm afraid my electrolytes are out of balance, but I take vitamins every day."). Speaks in a quiet voice. Defensive thinking apparent—occasional ideas of reference ("People will say I'm weird if they find out about me.").

Mood: Depressed, fearful, consistent; verbalizes feelings appropriate to the situation

Affect: Behavior consistent with expression of feelings

Insight: Demonstrates some awareness of extent of condition ("I think my electrolytes are out of balance."). Verbalizes awareness of not being sure she wants to give up behavior ("What will I have if I don't binge/purge anymore?"). States it makes her feel, knows she is alive, in control.

Pain/Discomfort

SUBJECTIVE

No reports of pain at present, has headaches occasionally

OBJECTIVE

None noted

Respiratory

SUBJECTIVE

Dyspnea Related to: Exertion
Does not smoke
Cough: With colds

OBJECTIVE

Respiratory Rate: 28 with activity/22 at rest
Breath Sounds: deferred

Safety

SUBJECTIVE

Accidents/Injuries: None
Allergies: None
　　(Frequent colds every few months)
Delayed Healing: Notes accidental injuries
　　(e.g., cut finger chopping celery)
　　slow to heal.
**Expressions of Ideation of Violence
　　(Self/Others):** Has suicidal thoughts
　　occasionally and recognizes behavior
　　as suicidal; no specific plan.

OBJECTIVE

Temperature: 99.4 tympanic
Exam of Skin: Deferred, though hands
　　dry/flaky
Physical Evidence of Self-Harm: None noted

Sexuality

SUBJECTIVE

Is not sexually involved with anyone,
　　states she is a virgin and does not
　　need birth control.
Age at Menarche: 12 years
Length of Cycle: Irregular
Duration: 2 days
Last Menstrual Period: 2 months ago
Breast Self-Exam: No
Routine Pap Smear: No, refuses
　　gynecological exams

OBJECTIVE

Deferred

Social Interactions

SUBJECTIVE

Memory of Early Years: Father alcoholic,
　　mother rejecting person who often
　　told the children she wished she had
　　not gotten married or had children.
　　Physical abuse common in family.
　　Reports father occasionally "belted"
　　mother (struck her with open hand);
　　children were frequently beaten
　　when they had displeased parents
　　or done something wrong.
Marital Status: Single. Living with church
　　friends, house-sitting.
Genogram: Deferred to 6/25/97
Family Dynamics: Mother was angry with
　　father most of the time. Sister and
　　brother are 2 and 5 years younger, says
　　she felt responsible for them when they
　　were little, grew apart as she became
　　older. Has not had contact with them
　　in past 10 years.
Extended Family: None
Other Support Persons: Employer, church
　　friends, including Mrs. CP and Mr. and
　　Mrs. S, an older couple described as
　　surrogate parents.

OBJECTIVE

Not observed with family/significant
　　other(s)

Role Within Family Structure. Oldest child with younger sister and brother

Performance/Interaction–Work: Excellent job ratings, states she is a perfectionist. Talks with coworkers, but not about self/personal issues; rarely socializes with coworkers.

Report of Problems: Feels lonely, does not have friends, knows she has to stop the binging/vomiting cycle. Does not trust people. Does have limited relationship with church friends; does not want them to know about her problem.

Coping Behaviors: Preoccupation with food and compulsive need to binge/purge, withdrawal from interaction with others

Frequency of Social Contacts (Other Than Work): None other than church, attends mass once or twice a week

Teaching/Learning

SUBJECTIVE

Dominant Language: English

Education Level: HS, graduated from business program, secretarial

Learning Disabilities/Cognitive Limitations: Not aware of any

Employment/Education Goals: Wants a job with less public contact; no specific plan

Health Beliefs/Practices: Vegetarian. Believes if she eats something, cannot stop. Believes if she eats sugar, her body craves it and she will just keep on eating.

Familial Risk Factors: Father died of stroke, age 67; maternal grandmother had a bad heart. Not aware of any other significant family history, although mother was not well.

Prescribed Medications: None

Nonprescription Drugs: Does not take any OTC or illicit drugs. Takes an herbal laxative once or twice a week. Takes vitamins because "I know I don't eat right."

Use of Alcohol: None

Admitting Diagnosis (Psychiatrist): Anorexia/bulimia

Reason for Seeking Therapy (Client): "To get my electrolytes under control."

History of Current Complaint: Long-standing eating problems (20 years), anorectic as an adolescent, binging and purging for past 10 years

Discharge Considerations

Date Data Obtained: 6/23

Anticipated Date of Discharge: 7/21 (28 days)

Resources Available:

Persons: Employer and church friends

Financial: Has job (not doing what she was trained to do), which employer will hold for her

Anticipated Changes in Living After Discharge: None, at the moment. Would like to get her own place as soon as feasible but would continue to house-sit (helps financially).

Community Supports: Church

Socialization: No social activities

Client Expectations of Therapy: "I want to begin to feel good about myself and my work, spiritually, mentally, and physically."

Previous Hospitalization: Twice, 10 and 12 years ago. Ran away from the hospital the last time and moved to another state.

Evidence of Failure to Improve:

Physical: Having blackouts, fainting spells, says electrolytes are out of balance

Mental: States has difficulty thinking, relaxing; complains of feelings of inferiority

Date of Last Physical Exam: 1987

Sample Plan of Care: Ms MJB

NURSING PRIORITIES

1. Reestablish adequate/appropriate nutritional intake.
2. Correct fluid and electrolyte imbalance.
3. Assist MJB to develop realistic body image/improve self-esteem.
4. Encourage identification and expression of feelings, especially anger.
5. Coordinate total treatment program with other disciplines.
6. Provide information about disease, prognosis, and treatment to MJB/significant others (Mr. and Mrs. S and her employer).

DISCHARGE GOALS (ANTICIPATED LENGTH OF STAY: 28 DAYS)

1. Adequate nutrition and fluid intake maintained.
2. Maladaptive coping behaviors and stressors that precipitate anxiety recognized.
3. Adaptive coping strategies and techniques for anxiety reduction and self-control implemented.
4. Self-esteem increased.
5. Plan in place to meet needs after discharge.

CLIENT DIAGNOSTIC STATEMENT: Altered nutrition, less than body requirements

Related To: Inadequate food intake and self-induced vomiting
Evidenced By: Verbal reports of intake less than RDA, pale conjunctiva and mucous membranes, poor skin turgor, inflamed gums, tooth decay/erosion, slightly swollen salivary glands, reports of sore mouth/throat

DESIRED OUTCOME/EVALUATION CRITERIA—MJB WILL:

1. Establish a dietary pattern with caloric intake adequate to maintain appropriate weight within 72 hours (6/26, 4 PM).
2. Verbalize/demonstrate understanding of nutritional needs within 2 weeks (7/7).
3. Select and consume appropriate foods for healthy diet 80% of the time within 3 weeks (7/14).
4. Maintain weight between 125 and 135 pounds throughout program (ongoing).

ACTIONS/INTERVENTIONS	RATIONALE
Establish a minimum weight goal to be maintained. (6/24 Client conference: minimum goal 125 pounds.)	When this is agreed on, psychological work can begin. Malnutrition is a mood-altering condition leading to depression and agitation so that adequate nutrition is important for psychological well-being.
Maintain a regular weighing schedule (Mon/Fri immediately on arising and following first voiding in same attire; graph results).	Provides accurate ongoing record of weight loss and/or gain. Also diminishes obsession about changes/fluctuations.
Provide selective menu and review MJB's choices with her.	Client needs to gain confidence in self and feel in control of environment. More likely to eat preferred foods but may require guidance to make healthy choices.
Be alert to choices of low-calorie foods; hoarding food; disposing of food in various places such as pockets or wastebaskets.	Client may try to avoid taking in what she views as excessive calories.

ACTIONS/INTERVENTIONS	RATIONALE
Provide dietary information per teaching plan.	Understanding nutritional needs, clarifying misconceptions may enhance client's willingness to choose a more balanced diet.
Use a consistent approach. Present and remove food without persuasion and/or comment. Sit with MJB while eating (30 minutes maximum), also without comment.	Client detects urgency and reacts to pressure. When staff responds consistently, client can begin to trust her responses. Client avoids manipulative games. Any comment that might be seen as coercion provides focus on food. Client may experience guilt if forced to eat. The one area in which she has exercised power and control is food/eating. Structuring meals and decreasing discussions about food will decrease power struggles with client.
Provide 1:1 supervision. Have MJB remain in the dayroom with no bathroom privileges for 1 hour following eating, or involve in group program as scheduled.	Prevents vomiting during/after eating. **Note:** Sometimes clients desire food and use a binge-purge syndrome to maintain weight. Purging may occur for the first time in a client as a response to establishment of weight pro-gram.
Avoid room checks and control devices.	Reinforces feelings of powerlessness and are usually not helpful.
Establish controlled exercise program with MJB (e.g., walking, aerobics, swimming); discuss likes and dislikes.	A gradually increasing exercise program can help client begin to improve muscle tone and control weight in a more satisfactory manner. MJB's excessive exercising has been counterproductive to her overall well-being.
Monitor exercise program and set limits on physical activities. Chart activity/level of work (pacing, etc.).	Client may exercise excessively to burn calories.
Provide regular diet and snacks with substitutes and preferred foods available.	Having a variety of foods available will enable client to have a choice of potentially enjoyable foods/may enhance intake.
Carry out program of behavior modification. Involve MJB in setting up program. Provide reward for maintaining weight, ignore gains/losses.	Provides structured eating situation while allowing client some control in choices. **Note:** Behavior modification may be effective only in mild cases or for short-term weight maintenance.
Avoid giving laxatives. Encourage use of bran or provide Metamucil as indicated.	Use of laxatives is counterproductive, as they may be used by client to try to rid body of food/calories. May require short-term use of Metamucil initially to assist with the management of constipation.
Schedule dietary consultation (6/24 AM).	Helpful in establishing individual dietary needs/program and provides educational opportunity.
Administer Trilafon 8 mg tid (8 AM, 2 and 10 PM).	Antipsychotic drug that blocks postsynaptic dopamine receptors in the brain. Given to manage underlying pathology (e.g., depression/anxiety.).
Review laboratory studies, blood sugar, CBC, endocrine studies.	Provides information about dietary status/needs and effectiveness of therapy.

40

CLIENT DIAGNOSTIC STATEMENT: Fluid Volume deficit, isotonic

Related To: Inadequate intake of food and liquids, consistent self-induced vomiting
Evidenced By: Dry skin/mucous membranes, decreased skin turgor, increased pulse rate (104), body temperature (99.4°F), orthostatic hypotension (90/63), concentrated urine/decreased urine output, change in mental state (states she is "flaky," forgets things she ought to remember)

DESIRED OUTCOMES/EVALUATION CRITERIA—MJB WILL:

1. Report fluid intake of 2000 ml/day with increased urine output within 40 hours (6/25, 8 AM).
2. Demonstrate improvement in vital signs, skin turgor, and moisture of mucous membranes within 72 hours (6/26, 4 PM).
3. Verbalize understanding of causative factors and behaviors necessary to correct fluid deficit within 1 week (6/30).

ACTIONS/INTERVENTIONS	RATIONALE
Discuss strategies to stop vomiting (e.g., verbalizing positive affirmation of "I can stop vomiting," talking to friend/therapist, use of imagery/ relaxation).	Helping the client to deal with anxiety feelings that lead to vomiting and supporting decision to stop will prevent continued fluid loss.
Have MJB measure urine output accurately each day.	Reduced urinary output may be a direct result of reduced food/fluid intake and continued vomiting.
Monitor amount and types of fluid intake. Be aware of use of caffeinated beverages and diet soft drink intake.	Increased intake of diet soft drinks results in adequate output even though there is no protein/ calorie intake. Caffeine can promote output, negatively affecting fluid balance.
Monitor vital signs per protocol, check capillary refill, and note episodes of dizziness. Recommend rising slowly, sitting, then standing.	Orthostatic hypotension can occur with fluid deficit.
Note reports of muscle pain/cramps, generalized weakness, paresthesia, nausea.	These are signs of potassium deficit and may reflect inadequate intake, starvation state, deficit from self-induced vomiting.
Discuss actions necessary to regain optimal fluid balance (e.g., drinking a glass of fluid every 2 hours). Encourage use of calorie-containing beverages as well as water.	Involving client in plan to correct fluid imbalances may enhance success and provide sense of control over what is happening to her.
Review diagnostic studies, electrolytes, CBC, urinalysis, ECG.	Syndrome may result in electrolyte imbalances, hemoconcentration.

CLIENT DIAGNOSTIC STATEMENT: Altered Thought Processes

Related To: Malnutrition/electrolyte imbalance, psychological conflicts (e.g., sense of low self-worth, perceived lack of control)
Evidenced By: Impaired ability to make decisions and to problem-solve; non–reality-based verbalizations ("I need to lose 30 pounds"; "I ate a lot of food today—sesame seeds and lettuce"); ideas of reference (says people think she is not doing a good job); altered attention span, distractibility, delay in seeking healthcare, does not perceive personal relevance of symptoms/danger of behavior

DESIRED OUTCOMES/EVALUATION CRITERIA—MJB WILL:

1. Verbalize awareness and understanding of relationship of lack of food intake to problems of concentration and decision-making within 48 hours (6/25, 4 PM).
2. Demonstrate improved ability to make decisions, problem-solve, and remember daily/recent events, within 3 weeks (7/14).
3. Acknowledge reality of situation that eating behaviors are maladaptive within 3 weeks (7/14).
4. Verbalize ways to gain control in life situation within 4 weeks (7/21).
5. Decrease use of manipulative behaviors in interactions with others within 2 weeks (7/7).

ACTIONS/INTERVENTIONS	RATIONALE
Establish a therapeutic nurse/client relationship.	Within a helping relationship, the client can begin to trust and try out new thinking and behaviors.
Be aware of MJB's distorted thinking ability.	Allows the caregiver to lower expectations (when indicated) and provide information and support appropriate to MJB's current needs/abilities.
Listen to but do not challenge irrational, illogical thinking. Present reality concisely and briefly.	It is not possible to respond logically when thinking ability is physiologically impaired. The client needs to hear reality, but challenging leads to distrust and frustration.
Encourage strict adherence to nutrition regimen.	Improved nutrition is essential to improved brain functioning.
State limits matter-of-factly. Avoid arguing/bargaining.	Client who denies reality of the situation often uses manipulation to achieve control. Consistency and firmness of staff help decrease use of these behaviors.

CLIENT DIAGNOSTIC STATEMENT: Body Image disturbance/Self-Esteem, chronic low

Related To: Morbid fear of obesity; perceived loss of control in some aspect of life (e.g., ability to interact satisfactorily with others, eating); unmet dependency needs; dysfunctional family system

Evidenced By: Distorted body image, view of self as fat, even in the presence of normal body weight (states needs to lose 30 pounds); expresses concern, uses denial as a defense mechanism, and feels powerless to prevent binge/purging and make changes in her life; perceptual disturbances with failure to recognize hunger; reports of fatigue, anxiety, and depression

DESIRED OUTCOMES/EVALUATION CRITERIA—MJB WILL:

Identify/be involved in other life interests within 1 week (6/30).
Identify individual assets/strengths, accept compliments within 2 weeks (7/7).
Verbalize a more realistic body image within 3 weeks (7/14).
Acknowledge self as an individual who has responsibility for own actions and voluntarily stops binging and purging by the end of the 4-week program (7/21).
Recognize reality of areas of life in which she has control, within 4 weeks (7/21).

ACTIONS/INTERVENTIONS	RATIONALE
Identify individual strengths and reflect positives noted without moral judgment. Encourage MJB to recognize positive characteristics related to self.	Promotes self-worth. Individual often sees self as weak-willed, even though a part of the person may feel a sense of power and control. Discussion of

42

ACTIONS/INTERVENTIONS	RATIONALE
	positive aspects of the self-system, such as social skills, work abilities, education, talents, and appearance, can reinforce client's feelings of being a worthwhile/competent person.
Explore MJB's expectation of self regarding need to "be perfect."	Recognizing unrealistic expectations may enhance ability to accept self as fallible.
State rules regarding weighing schedule, remaining in sight during medication and eating times, and make known the consequences of not following the rules. Be consistent in carrying out rules, without undue comment.	Client is obsessed with fear of weight gain. Regular monitoring of client's weight is important to nutritional status. Consistency is important in establishing trust. As part of the behavior modification program, client knows the risks involved in not following established rules (e.g., decrease in privileges). Failure to do so is viewed as client's choice and accepted by staff in matter-of-fact manner so as not to provide reinforcement for the undesirable behavior.
Respond (confront) with reality when MJB makes unrealistic statements, such as, "I've stopped vomiting so there's nothing really wrong with me."	Client needs to be confronted because she denies the psychological aspects of her situation and often expresses a sense of inadequacy and depression. Confrontation provides opportunity for constructive feedback about how improving nutrition will give her energy to look at other aspects of her life so that the issue of food will not be so all-consuming.
Be aware of own reaction to MJB's behavior. Avoid arguing.	Feelings of disgust, hostility, and fury are not uncommon when caring for these clients. Prognosis remains poor even with stabilization of weight, as other problems may remain. Many continue to see themselves as fat, and there is also a high incidence of affective disorders, social phobias, obsessive-compulsive symptoms, substance abuse, and psychosexual dysfunction. The nurse needs to deal with own response/feelings so they do not interfere with care of the client.
Help MJB assume control in areas other than dieting/weight loss, (e.g., management of own daily activities, work/leisure choices).	Feelings of personal ineffectiveness, low self-esteem, and perfectionism are often part of the problem. Client feels helpless to change and requires assistance to problem-solve methods of control in life situations.
Assist MJB to formulate goals for self not related to eating (e.g., choice of a satisfying vocation/ avocation), and formulate a manageable plan to reach those goals, one at a time, on a short-/ long-term basis.	Client needs to recognize ability to control other areas in life and may need to learn problem-solving skills to achieve this control. Client may not know how to set realistic goals, and choices may be influenced by altered thought processes.
Encourage MJB to consider disclosing illness to someone of her choosing. Role-play anticipated situation.	Fear of having others know about this illness and being judgmental is a major concern and affects her involvement with others. Practicing with trusted therapist can help MJB to take this important step.
Help MJB confront sexual fears. Provide sex education as necessary.	Major physical/psychological changes in adolescence can contribute to development of this

problem. Feelings of powerlessness and loss of control of feelings (particularly sexual feelings, sensations, and physical development) lead to an unconscious desire to desexualize self. Client often believes that sexual fears can be overcome by taking control of bodily appearance/development/function.

Encourage MJB to take charge of her own life in a more healthful way by making her own decisions and accepting herself "as is." Encourage acceptance of inadequacies as well as strengths. Let MJB know that it is acceptable to be different from family, particularly mother.

Client often does not know what she may want for herself. Parents (i.e., mother) made decisions for her. Client also believes she has to be the best in everything and holds herself responsible for being perfect. She needs to develop a sense of control in other ways, besides dieting and weight loss.

Involve in personal development program.

Learning about proper application of makeup and methods of enhancing personal appearance may be helpful to achieving long-range sense of self-esteem.

Use interpersonal psychotherapy rather than interpretive therapy.

More helpful for the client to discover feelings/impulses/needs from within own self. Client has not learned this internal control as a child.

Encourage MJB to express anger and acknowledge when it is verbalized.

Important to know that anger is part of self and as such is acceptable. Expressing anger may need to be taught to client, as anger is generally considered unacceptable in the family and therefore client does not express it appropriately.

Assist MJB to learn strategies other than eating for dealing with feelings. Have MJB keep a diary of feelings, particularly when thinking about food.

Feelings are the underlying issue, and clients often use food instead of dealing with feelings appropriately. May need to learn to recognize feelings and how to express them.

Assess feelings of helplessness/hopelessness.

54% of clients with anorexia have a history of major affective disorder, 33% have a history of minor affective disorder.

Be alert to suicidal ideation/behavior.

Intensity of anxiety/panic about weight gain, depression, hopeless feelings may lead to suicidal attempts, particularly if client is impulsive.

Collaborative

Involve a group therapy daily to include Goals Group and Creative, Occupational, and Recreational sessions, per protocol.

Provides an opportunity to talk about feelings and try out new behaviors.

CLIENT DIAGNOSTIC STATEMENT: Knowledge Deficit [Learning Need] regarding condition, prognosis, therapy, self-care, and discharge needs

Related To: Learned maladaptive coping skills, lack of exposure to/unfamiliarity with new information

Evidenced By: Verbalization of misconception of relationship of behaviors (preoccupation with extreme fear of obesity and distortion of own body image, refusal to eat, binging and purging; and current hospitalization), request for new information, and expressions of desire to learn more adaptive ways of coping with stressors

DESIRED OUTCOMES/EVALUATION CRITERIA—MJB WILL:

1. Identify relationship of signs/symptoms (e.g., weight loss, tooth decay, skin problems) to behaviors of not eating or binge-purging within 3 days (6/26 4 PM).
2. Verabalize awareness of and plans for lifestyle changes to maintain normal weight without aberrant eating pattern within 2 weeks (7/7).
3. Assume responsibility for own learning within 2 weeks (7/7).
4. Verbalize intention to attend community support group within 4 weeks (7/21).

ACTIONS/INTERVENTIONS	RATIONALE
Orient to unit. Discuss rules/behavior modification program, involving MJB in establishing parameters.	Helps allay anxiety. Client involvement in establishing treatment program increases likelihood of success.
Determine level of knowledge and readiness to learn.	Learning is easier when it begins where the learner is.
Note blocks to learning (e.g., physical/intellectual/emotional).	Malnutrition, family problems, affective disorders, and obsessive-compulsive symptoms can interfere with learning.
Review dietary needs, answering questions as indicated.	May need assistance with planning for new way of eating.
Encourage MJB to keep a diary of feelings, especially when thinking about food.	Provides avenue for client to identify feelings associated with maladaptive behaviors. Promotes discussion of more appropriate coping methods.
Provide information about and encourage the use of relaxation and other stress-management techniques.	New ways of coping with feelings of anxiety and fear will help client to manage these feelings more effectively, assisting in giving up maladaptive behaviors of not eating/binging-purging.
Help establish a sensible exercise program. Caution client regarding overexercise.	Exercise can assist with developing a positive body image and combat depression. Client may overexercise in attempt to "control" weight, depress appetite.
Review appropriate skin care needs. Encourage bathing every other day. Use skin cream twice a day and after bathing; gently massage skin, especially over bony prominences. Observe for reddened/blanched areas.	Frequent baths contribute to dryness of the skin. Supplemental lubrication of the skin decreases itching/flaking and reduces risk for breakdown. Massage improves circulation to the skin and skin tone. Involves client in monitoring and intervening in own therapy.
Discuss importance of adequate nutrition/fluid intake.	Improved nutrition will improve skin and oral condition, maintain electrolyte balance, and help clear thought processes.
Provide written information for MJB.	Helpful as reminder of and reinforcement for learning.
Encourage MJB to ask friends and coworkers to provide support for necessary changes.	Can serve as a support system to help client make necessary lifestyle changes.
Refer for dental consult/care.	Emesis of stomach acids (purging) can damage gum tissues and tooth enamel.
Refer to local affiliate of the National Association of Anorexia Nervosa and Associated Disorders.	May be helpful source of support and information for client and significant others (Mr. and Mrs. S and employer).

45

EVALUATION

As nursing care is provided, ongoing assessments determine the client's response to therapy and progress toward accomplishing the desired outcomes. This activity serves as the feedback and control part of the nursing process, through which the status of the individual client diagnostic statement is judged to be resolved, continuing, or requiring revision.

This process is visualized in Figure 3–2. Discussion with MJB reveals she has reviewed dietary materials and completed the posttest (9 of 10 correct). She displays increased understanding of general dietary needs and is ready to progress to focusing on her

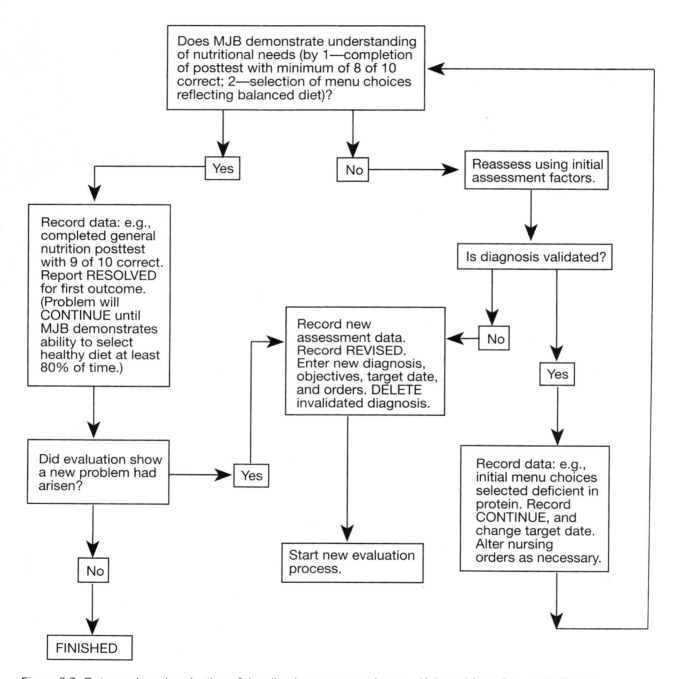

Figure 3-2. Outcome-based evaluation of the client's response to therapy. (Adapted from Cox, et al: Clinical Applications of Nursing Diagnosis: Adult, Child, Women's, Mental Health, Gerontic, and Home Health Considerations, ed 3. FA Davis, Philadelphia, 1997, p 445)

Sample Clinical Pathway of Care for MJB

Estimated Length of Stay: 28 days—Variations from Designated Pathway Should Be Documented in Progress Notes

Nursing Diagnoses and Categories of Care	Time Dimension	Goals and/or Actions	Time Dimension	Goals and/or Actions	Time Dimension	Discharge Outcome
Altered nutrition: Less than body requires Fluid volume deficit	Ongoing	Client will establish adequate dietary pattern and maintain adequate state of hydration			Day 28	Patient will exhibit no signs/symptoms of malnutrition or dehydration
Referrals	Day 1 and ongoing	Consult dietitian	Days 2–28	Fulfill nutritional needs. Client will consume 80% of food provided and at least 2000 ml fluid/day		
Diagnostic studies	Day 1	Electrolytes Electrocardiogram Blood urea nitrogen/creatine Urinalysis Complete blood count Thyroid function	Day 14	Repeat of selected diagnostic studies	Day 28	All laboratory values are within normal limits
Additional assessments	Day 1–5 (and PRN)	Vital signs	Day 3	Vital signs within normal limits	Days 22–28	Client will refrain from self-induced vomiting and binging
	Day 1–5	Input and output	Day 3	Appropriate balance is achieved		
	Day 1	Weight	Days 2–28	Client will maintain weight between 125 and 135 pounds		

47

Nursing Diagnoses and Categories of Care	Time Dimension	Goals and/or Actions	Time Dimension	Goals and/or Actions	Time Dimension	Discharge Outcome
	Day 1 and ongoing	Monitor for purging following meals	Days 1–21	Client bathroom is locked for 1 hour following meals		
Patient education	Day 1	Unit orientation; behavior modification plan	Days 7–14	Principles of nutrition; foods for maintenance of wellness	Days 15–18	Client will demonstrate ability to select appropriate foods for healthy diet 80% of time
Altered Thought Processes	Day 1	Client will cooperate with orientation to unit and explanation of behavior modification plan	Days 2–28	Client will cooperate with therapy to restore nutritional status; verbalizes understanding of relationship between nutritional status and thought processes	Days 18–28	Client will acknowledge that eating behaviors are maladaptive and demonstrate improved ability to make decisions, problem-solve
Referrals	Day 7 (or when physical condition is stable)	Psychologist, social worker, psychodramatist	Days 8–28	Client will attend group psycho-therapies daily	Day 28	Client will verbalize ways to gain control in life situation
Additional assessments	Days 1–17	Assess client's ability to trust; set limits on manipulative behavior	Day 14	Client will develop trusting relationship with at least one staff member each shift	Day 28	Client will demonstrate decreased use of manipulation in interactions with others

Patient education	Day 1 and ongoing as required	Describe privileges and responsibilities of behavior modification program; explain consequences of altered compliance	Day 21	Discuss role of support groups for individuals with eating disorders	Day 28	Client and family will verbalize intention to attend community support group
Body Image/Self Esteem chronic low	Day 7	Client will acknowledge that attention will not be given to the discussion of body image and food, shift focus to other life interests	Days 14–21	Client will acknowledge misperception of body image as fat and verbalize positive self-attributes	Day 28	Client will verbalize more realistic body image and recognize areas of control within own life
Referrals	Day 1 (or when physical condition is stable)	Occupational therapy, recreational therapy, music	Days 2–28	Client attends therapy sessions on a daily basis	Day 28	Through self-expression, client has gained self-awareness, verbalizes positive attributes of self
Additional assessments	Day 7	Compare specific measurements of client's body with client's perceived calculations; clarify discrepancies	Days 8–28	Discuss strengths and weaknesses; client will strive to achieve self-acceptance	Day 28	Client will verbalize acceptance of self, including "imperfections"
Patient education	Days 7–14	Client will verbalize plans for lifestyle changes and assume responsibility for own learning	Days 14–28	Discuss alternative coping strategies for dealing with feelings; have client keep diary of feelings, particularly when thinking about food	Day 28	Client will demonstrate adaptive coping strategies unrelated to eating behaviors dealing with feelings

TABLE 3-2. Comparison of SOAP and Focus Charting (DAR) Formats

Documenting Specific Client Situation
Example 1. Sample of SOAP/SOAPIER Charting:**S(Subjective) O(Objective) A(Analysis) P(Plan)**
I (Implementation) E(Evaluation) R(Revision)

Date	Time	Number (Problem)*	Note
6/24/97	0900	#4 (Self Esteem)	**S:** "I see myself as a 'zero.' I'm not able to control my eating." **O:** Sits in group (3 members), shoulders hunched, looking down, fidgeting with hands **A:** Believes she is unable to control maladaptive eating behavior **P:** To identify individual strengths and encourage her to recognize positive characteristics related to self **I:** Was instructed to start a list, noting individual strengths, talents, and abilities that will be reviewed daily with therapist. Was encouraged to attend and participate in recreational/occupational therapy activities. Signed: *M Davis,* RNC
7/6/97	1800	#1 (Nutrition)	**S:** "I've seen the dietitian 3 times now and reviewed the material she gave me. I've finished this quiz and think I did well." **O:** Appears tentative, displays slight smile, fidgets with pencil. Postquiz result: 9 out of 10 correct. **A:** Following through with assignments. Displaying improved knowledge regarding dietary needs and achievement of Outcome #2. **P:** Continue teaching plan as outlined. **I:** MJB's select menu choices for next day were reviewed. **E:** Choices met dietary guidelines formulated with dietitian regarding fruits, vegetables, and grains. Protein deficiency noted. MJB added 1/2 cup 1% milk for breakfast and peanut butter with graham crackers for HS snack. Signed: *B Briner,* RNC

Example 2. Sample of Focus Charting: **D (Data) A (Action) R (Response)**

Date	Time	Focus	Note
7/6/97	1800	Nutrition	**D:** Completed 3 sessions with dietitian, and post-test. Tentatively stated "think I did well" while fidgeting with pencil. **A:** Test reviewed, 9 of 10 correct. Applied learning to select individual menu choices for next day. **R:** Choices met dietary guidelines formulated with dietitian except for protein. MJB added 1/2 cup 1% milk to breakfast and peanut butter to HS snack of graham crackers. Demonstrated achievement of Outcome #2. Signed: *B Briner,* RNC

50

The following is an example of documentation of a client need/concern that currently does not require identification as a client problem (nursing diagnosis) or inclusion in the plan of care and therefore is not easily documented in the SOAP format:

Date	Time	Focus	Note
6/27/96	1920	Gastric distress	**D:** Reports "indigestion/burning sensation" with hand over epigastric area. Skin warm, dry, and pink, pulse 88 and regular. Noted she ate broccoli for dinner.
			A: Given Mylanta 30 ml PO. Head of bed elevated approximately 15 degrees.
	1945		**R:** Reports pain relieved. Appears relaxed, resting quietly.
			Signed: *B Briner,* RNC

*As noted on plan of care.

individual needs as outlined in the plan of care. No revision in the treatment plan is required at this time.

DOCUMENTATION

There are several charting formats currently used for documentation. These include block notes, with a single entry covering an entire shift (e.g., 7 AM to 3 PM) or visit; narrative timed notes (e.g., 9:30 AM, Participated in group activity); and the problem-oriented record (POMR or POR) using the SOAP/SOAPIER approach, to name a few. The latter can provide thorough documentation. However, it was designed by physicians for episodic care and requires that the entries be tied to a client problem identified from a problem list.

A different format created by nurses for documentation of frequent/repetitive care is Focus Charting. This was designed to encourage viewing the client from a positive rather than a negative (or problem-oriented) perspective by using precise documentation to record the nursing process. Recording of assessment, interventions, and evaluation information in data, action, and response (DAR) categories facilitates tracking and following what is happening to the client at any given moment. Charting focuses on client and nursing concerns with the focal point being client status and the associated nursing care. The focus is always stated in a way that reflects the *client's* concern/need rather than reflecting a *nursing* task or *psychiatric/medical* diagnosis. Thus, the focus can be a client problem/concern or nursing diagnosis, signs/symptoms of potential importance (e.g., increasing agitation, fever), a significant event or change in status (e.g., use of "time-out," seclusion, or application of restraints), or a specific standard of care/hospital policy. Based on the client situation of MJB, Table 3–2 provides examples of documentation and the problem-oriented medical record system (POMR or POR) using the SOAP/SOAPIER approach.

CHAPTER 4

CHILDHOOD AND ADOLESCENT DISORDERS

PERVASIVE DEVELOPMENTAL DISORDERS

DSM-IV
299.00 Autistic disorder
299.80 Rett's disorder
299.80 Asperger's disorder
299.10 Childhood disintegrative disorder
299.80 Pervasive developmental disorder NOS (including atypical autism)

The category of pervasive developmental disorders is organized in terms of the qualitative degree of impairment in social and communicative functioning. Autism comprises extremely varied manifestations that encompass deficits in cognition, social awareness, communication, affective expression, and motor control. Because of the continuity of the symptomatology, the term *autistic spectrum disorder (ASD)* is recognized in the current literature. ASD may occur with or without a neurological substrate, as in the case of *idiopathic autism*. Age of onset and whether the child developed normally from birth through the first 5 years of life are factors that help differentiate between Rett's disorder or childhood disintegrative disorder. The intractable anxiety, mood liability, perseveration of thought and behavior, and odd social presentation of these children may mimic other psychiatric disorders, including anxiety disorders, schizophrenia, obsessive-compulsive disorder, and the manic phase of bipolar affective disorder. When neurological impairment coexists with the diagnosis, the individual is often low functioning.

ETIOLOGICAL THEORIES

Psychodynamics

Autistic children are fixed in the presymbiotic stage of development. These children do not achieve a symbiotic attachment, nor do they differentiate self from mother. Psychotic-like behaviors are based on abnormal primary development rather than on a regression from a higher level of functioning. Children with autism lack the intuitive skills to engage in and sustain meaningful social contact, particularly in new situations, and they have a marked inability to generalize.

Biological

Neurological evaluation, including family history, electroencephalogram (EEG), magnetic resonance imaging (MRI), karyotyping, and positron emission tomography (PET), reveals strong evidence of a familial pattern of organic neurological impairment and psychiatric illness. Several research studies estimate the coexistence of neuropsychiatric illness in extended family members to be as high as 50% in individuals with ASD.

Research to confirm brain anatomical abnormalities suggests that neurons in the amygdala (the area responsible for processing emotions and behavior) and the hippocampus (involved in learning and memory) are smaller, more densely packed in some areas, and have shorter, less-developed branches than normal. Low blood circulation in some parts of the cerebral cortex during certain intellectual functions and a reduced number of cells relaying inhibitory messages have been demonstrated. It has been hypothesized that these severe developmental disorders of childhood are the result of a disturbance in the central nervous system integration and in the biological process of maturation. Predisposing organic factors include maternal rubella, phenylketonuria, encephalitis, meningitis, hydrocephalus, hypothyroidism, and tuberous sclerosis.

Family Dynamics

This disorder has been viewed in the past as a result of a severe disturbance in parent-child interaction. Lack of bonding and stimulation as well as maternal deprivation have been listed as causative factors. More recently, dysfunctional parenting has been seen less as contributing to the disorder (not accepted) and more as a response to the disturbed behavior.

CLIENT ASSESSMENT DATA BASE

Activity/Rest

Problems in sleeping

Ego Integrity

Detached, separated from work, withdrawn, restive, may be passive
Verbal/nonverbal communication may be incongruent
Demonstrates repetitive stereotypical motor behaviors (hand flicking, head banging, complex whole-body movements)

Elimination

Disturbances in bowel and bladder functioning

Food/Fluid

Disturbed eating patterns

Hygiene

Generally dependent
Eccentric preoccupation with one area of hygiene and neglect of another (e.g., showering repeatedly but never brushing teeth)

Neurosensory

Abnormalities noted in almost every sphere of development
Delayed motor, perceptual, cognitive, and language development
Soft neurological signs are often seen (e.g., slight tremors, slowed responses)
Varied/bizarre responses to the environment, with resistance or extreme behavioral reactions to minor occurrences; ritualistic behaviors; extreme fascination with moving objects; special interests in music (although heightened hearing/inability to filter or dampen sounds may result in intolerance)
Bizarre facial expressions
Alterations in mood—lacking the gradations in range of fear, sadness, joy

Unreasonable insistence on following routines in precise detail; marked distress over changes in trivial aspects of environment

Difficulty communicating verbally, with delays in/no development of speech; may mimic sounds made by others, incorrect use of words, echolalia, inability to understand abstract terms; consistent reversal of pronouns "I" and "you"

May show periods of extreme agitation in which behavior becomes disruptive and unmanageable

Does not initiate social imitative play appropriate for stage of development

Safety

Self-mutilative behaviors (e.g., head banging, hair pulling)

Lack of appropriate fear/ignoring signs of danger (e.g., running into street with heavy traffic); fearing harmless objects such as shrinking from touch, going limp or stiffening when held (autism), putting people off by abrupt/awkward approaches (Asperger's)

Social Interactions

Poor eye contact, impaired responsiveness/communication when interacting with others

Severely disturbed/impaired development in social relationships; may be barely able to distinguish parents from strangers (autism)

Marked impairment in use of nonverbal gestures associated with social interactions

Lack of social or emotional reciprocity, does not express pleasure toward or in response to other people's happiness; indifference or aversion to physical contact

Teaching/Learning

High association with mental retardation; normal or high verbal intelligence (Asperger's)

Onset during infancy or early childhood before age 3 (autism) with telltale symptoms possibly noted during first months; marked regression following at least 2 years of apparently normal development, and before age 10 (disintegrative disorder), predominantly males; diagnosis of Rett's made at about 5 months of age, occurring only in females

DIAGNOSTIC STUDIES

Neurological examination to determine presence and/or extent of organic impairment.

BEAM/PET Scans: May reveal abnormalities in cerebellum (regulates motion and some aspects of memory) and the limbic region (controls much of emotional life).

EEG: May be abnormal, reflecting presence/extent of organic impairment.

Psychological Testing/Intelligence Quotient (IQ): Provides information about cognitive and personality functioning; IQ below 70 may be noted.

Biochemical Studies: Abnormalities not consistently noted.

Laboratory Tests: As indicated by antipsychotic drug therapy.

Auditory Testing: To rule out deafness as a cause of speech problems.

Vision Testing: To differentiate responses to auditory and visual stimuli as abnormal reactions versus distorted perceptions.

Developmental Testing (e.g., Denver Developmental): May reveal delays.

Determine physical causes for disturbances in age-appropriate functions and behaviors (e.g., toileting problems).

NURSING PRIORITIES

1. Facilitate control/decrease of behavioral symptoms.
2. Enhance communication skills and social interaction.
3. Promote family involvement in treatment process and acceptance of child's disability.

DISCHARGE GOALS

1. Current behavior problems or troublesome symptoms for which treatment is being sought are effectively managed.
2. Treatment within the community is maintained; institutional placement is avoided, when possible.
3. Family verbalizes knowledge about resources to meet the need for a long-term structured therapeutic program.
4. Plan is in place to meet needs after discharge.

NURSING DIAGNOSIS	SOCIAL INTERACTION, impaired
May Be Related to:	Disturbance in self-concept
	Delayed development of secure attachment and altered behavioral expression indicating the degree of attachment
	Inadequate sensory stimulation or abnormal response to sensory input, organic brain dysfunction
	Lack of intuitive skills to comprehend and accurately respond to social cues
Possibly Evidenced by:	Lack of responsiveness to others, lack of eye contact or facial responsiveness
	Treating persons as objects, lack of awareness of feelings in others or empathy for them
	Indifference or aversion to comfort, affection, or physical contact
	Failure to develop cooperative social play and peer friendships in childhood
Desired Outcomes/Evaluation Criteria—Client Will:	Increase periods of eye contact.
	Tolerate short periods of physical contact with another person.
	Initiate interactions between self and others.

ACTIONS/INTERVENTIONS	RATIONALE
Independent	
Assign limited number of caregivers to child and monitor interactions.	Consistent approach by familiar persons, and evaluating the appropriate match of providers increases chances for establishing trust.
Convey warmth, acceptance, and availability.	These characteristics encourage nonthreatening interaction.
Have personal items (favorite toy, blanket) available and use in interactions as appropriate.	These items can provide sense of security when child feels distressed.
Reinforce eye contact with something acceptable to the child (e.g., food, object). Eventually replace with social reinforcement.	Establishing eye contact is essential before interventions for other symptoms can succeed.

Gradually increase proximity and planned intrusion into child's isolation (e.g., touch, smiling, hugging, and verbal positive reinforcement).

Client will likely feel threatened by onslaught of unaccustomed stimuli. Caregivers need to initiate interaction as avenue toward social response.

Be available as support during child's attempts to interact with others.

Presence of a trusted person provides a feeling of security.

Give careful directions, maintain reliable, consistent rules of behavior and constant checks on reality of child's thoughts and perceptions

Provides structure to help child maintain control/follow the program. Feedback helps child differentiate between fantasy and reality.

Organize and plan time carefully. Manage tasks so child makes as few mistakes and suffers as few disappointments as possible.

Promotes successful experiences and encourages repetition of desired behaviors.

Provide social coaching of the rules of social behavior, including pictures of facial expressions and videos of social situations.

Didactic instruction supplements the lack of intuitive skills necessary to analyze social situations.

Collaborative

Work with others who are involved (e.g., teachers) to maintain a structured environment with the emphasis on continual interpretation of social needs and interactions.

Coordinated, consistent efforts help the child learn new behaviors.

Maintain contact with social services caseworker and involve in team conferences.

Provides continuity of care when child/family is involved with social services system.

NURSING DIAGNOSIS	COMMUNICATION, impaired, verbal
May Be Related to:	Inability to trust others
	Withdrawal into self
	Organic brain dysfunction
	Inadequate sensory stimulation; maternal deprivation
Possibly Evidenced by:	Lack of interactive communication mode; does not use gestures or spoken language
	Absent or abnormal nonverbal communication; lack of eye contact or facial expression
	Peculiar patterns in form, content, or speech production (if speech is present)
	Impaired ability to initiate or sustain conversation despite adequate speech
Desired Outcomes/Evaluation Criteria— Client Will:	Use sounds, words, or gestures in an interactive way with others.
	Communicate needs/desires to significant others/caregivers.
	Initiate verbal or nonverbal interaction with others.

ACTIONS/INTERVENTIONS	RATIONALE

Independent

Maintain consistency in caregivers assigned to child.

Familiarity helps child to develop trust and helps caregivers to learn ways child attempts to communicate.

Anticipate and fulfill needs until communication can be established.	Reduces frustration while child is learning communication skills. Some therapists believe this process should be limited to force verbal requests for wants beyond basic needs.
Assess previously used words or sounds. Seek validation and clarification to decode communication attempts.	Facilitates recognition of speech efforts. These techniques are useful in determining accuracy of messages received.
Use face-to-face (eye-to-eye) approach to convey correct nonverbal expressions by example.	Expresses genuine interest in, and respect for, client.
Reinforce eye contact with something acceptable to the child (e.g., food, object).	Eye contact is essential to capture child's attention, to successfully initiate conversation.
Repeat and reinforce approximations of sounds or words whenever used by child.	"Shaping" gives child information about the caregiver's expectations and may encourage attempts to communicate.
Engage in alternative forms of communication such as picture exchange, sign language, or use of computers for children with minimal language development.	Three-fourths of children trained in the picture exchange communication system eventually communicate by speech or by speech with pictures. Signing may produce less anxiety than verbal expression for some children, and the use of computers can be helpful to engaging the child in interaction.

Collaborative

Refer for assessment and testing in cooperation with special education teachers and speech pathologists.	Provides for treatment planning with appropriate specialized interventions/techniques.

NURSING DIAGNOSIS	**SELF-MUTILATION, risk for**
Risk Factors May Include:	Organic brain dysfunction
	Inability to trust others
	Disturbance in self-concept
	Inadequate sensory stimulation or abnormal response to sensory input (sensory overload)
	History of physical, emotional, or sexual abuse
	Response to demands of therapy, realization of severity of condition
	History of self-injury/destructive behavior
	Indifference to environment or marked distress over changes in environment
Possibly Evidenced by:	[Not applicable; presence of signs and symptoms establishes an *actual* diagnosis]
Desired Outcomes/Evaluation Criteria— Client Will:	Recognize angry feelings and underlying anxiety.
	Decrease incidence of self-mutilating behaviors by "x" times per day.

Demonstrate alternative behavior (e.g., initiate interaction between self and caregiver) in response to anxiety.

ACTIONS/INTERVENTIONS	RATIONALE

Independent

Note prior history of violent behaviors and relationship to anxiety or stressful events. Identify events or stimuli that precipitate self-mutilating behavior, and intervene before these occur.	Useful in determining patterns and predicting and controlling violent behavior. Self-harm may be prevented if causes can be determined and averted. **Note:** May be first priority if this behavior is a prominent symptom.
Reinforce acceptable behavior; provide other satisfying activities (e.g., rocking, swinging, clapping hands to music).	Diversion or replacement activities may become substitutes for self-harm/destructive behaviors.
Involve in sensory integration therapy.	Flooding the child with sensations (e.g., swinging, rolling around in a foam rubber container) helps to train the child to recognize where each stimulus originates and how to mentally organize the stimulus.
Apply protective devices (e.g., helmet, padded arm covers, bandages over sores or scabs).	Provides protection when potential for self-harm is present. **Note:** The inability to tune out unimportant sounds results in sensory overload. The child may engage in repetitive activities or harmful behaviors to vent the frustration and associated anxiety.
Stay with child during times of increasing anxiety.	Helps maintain feelings of trust and security, reducing frequency/severity of destructive behaviors.
Avoid physical restraint if possible, but hold child as necessary until agitation subsides.	Restriction of movement may increase anxiety. Protection from self-harm is essential for safety. **Note:** Some therapists advocate use of aversive conditioning to eliminate life-threatening behaviors.
Establish individualized exercise program.	Exercise therapy as an adjunct to psychotherapy provides outlets for anxious feelings/frustrations to decrease symptoms and thought disturbances.

Collaborative

Administer antipsychotic medications or lithium, as indicated.	May control symptoms of agitated behaviors. **Note:** Current research suggests that medication may neither extinguish behaviors nor be helpful.

NURSING DIAGNOSIS	PERSONAL IDENTITY disturbance
May Be Related to:	Organic brain dysfunction
	Lack of development of trust

May Be Related to (cont.):	Maternal deprivation
	Fixation at presymbiotic phase of development
Possibly Evidenced by:	Lack of awareness of the feelings or existence of others
	Increased anxiety resulting from physical contact with others
	Absent or impaired imitation of others; repeats what others say
	Persistent preoccupation with parts of objects; obsessive attachment to objects
	Marked distress over changes in environment
	Severe panic reactions to everyday events
	Autoerotic, ritualistic behaviors; self-touching, rocking, swaying
Desired Outcomes/Evaluation Criteria— Client Will:	Show signs of developing awareness of self as separate from others and environment (e.g., discontinuing echolalia, knows body boundaries).
	Tolerate separations and environmental changes without signs/reports of undue anxiety.
	Modify eccentric behaviors into strengths.

ACTIONS/INTERVENTIONS	RATIONALE
Independent	
Use positive reinforcement to encourage eye contact.	Eye contact focuses child on the recognition of another person.
Assist child in learning to name own body parts. Provide mirrors and pictures for self-identification.	This activity may increase awareness of self as separate from others.
Encourage appropriate exploratory touching of others and touching by caregivers.	If done gradually, child can feel the differences between self and others without excessive anxiety.
Encourage self-care activities that differentiate child from environment (self-feeding, washing, dressing, etc.). Divide activity into individual actions or steps, and reinforce completion of each step.	Activities may help child to identify body boundaries. Reinforcement encourages learning. Behavior-modification techniques provide framework for learning.
Engage in imaginative play behavior. Provide modeling and reinforcement both in the home and therapeutic setting.	Pretend play is a cognitively complex form of play that relates to social understanding and the ability to assume roles later in care.

NURSING DIAGNOSIS	**FAMILY COPING, ineffective: compromised/disabling**
May Be Related to:	Family members unable to express feelings related to having a severely disturbed child
	Excessive guilt, anger, or blaming among family members regarding child's condition

Possibly Evidenced by:

Ambivalent or dissonant family relationships; disagreements regarding treatment, coping strategies

Prolonged coping with problem exhausts supportive ability of family members

Denial of existence or severity of disturbed behaviors

Preoccupation with personal emotional reaction to situation (anger, guilt)

Persistent lack of acceptance of chronic nature of child's disorder; rationalization that problem is developmental and will eventually be outgrown

Attempts to intervene with child achieving increasingly ineffective results

Withdraws from or becomes overly protective of child

Desired Outcomes/Evaluation Criteria— Family Will:

Verbalize knowledge and appropriate understanding of child's disorder.

Express feelings appropriately with decreased defensive behavior (denial, projection, rationalization).

Demonstrate more consistent, effective methods of coping with child's behavior.

Seek outside therapeutic support as needed.

ACTIONS/INTERVENTIONS	RATIONALE
Independent	
Meet regularly with family members to discuss feelings and attitudes.	Supportive counseling can help family members express feelings, explore own reactions to child's disorder.
Assess underlying circumstances that may be contributing to ineffective family coping (e.g., financial problems, health of other members, needs of other children).	Identification of stressors may help parents sort out feelings related to child and other issues.
Assist family to develop new methods for dealing with the child's behaviors. Reinforce effective parenting methods. (Refer to CP: Parenting.)	Effective intervention skills can assist family to regain self-esteem and control of their environment.
Collaborative	
Refer to other resources as necessary (e.g., psychotherapy, financial aid, respite care, clergy, support groups [e.g., National Society for Autistic Children]).	Developing a support system can sustain family coping skills and integrity; provide role models and hope for the future.
Encourage parental involvement in training program to serve as cotherapists as appropriate.	Promotes greater involvement and continuation of therapeutic milieu on a full-time basis. Allows for ongoing monitoring of therapy and child's development.

ATTENTION-DEFICIT/HYPERACTIVITY DISORDER (ADHD)

DSM-IV
314.00 ADHD predominantly inattentive type
314.01 ADHD predominantly hyperactive-impulsive type
314.01 ADHD combined type
314.9 ADHD NOS

This disorder is associated with inattentive, impulsive, and hyperactive behavior that is maladaptive and inconsistent with developmental level. This behavior creates clinically significant impairment in social/academic functioning. Accurate diagnosis is difficult, as symptoms resemble depression, learning disabilities, or emotional problems. The diagnosis is made through extensive observation of the child's behavior; however, contact with health professionals is limited and the child's activity may be misleading during short office visits. Reports from parents and teachers are often used to make the diagnosis, and their observations may be distorted, as they assume a problem exists and often predetermine the diagnosis themselves.

ETIOLOGICAL THEORIES

Psychodynamics

The child with this disorder has impaired ego development. Ego development is retarded and manifested impulsive behavior represents unchecked id impulses, as in severe temper tantrums. Repeated performance failure, failure to attend to social cues, and limited impulse control reinforce low self-esteem. Some theories suggest that the child is fixed in the symbiotic phase of development and has not differentiated self from mother.

Genetic/Biological

The disorder may be gender-linked as the incidence is higher in boys than in girls (3:1). ADHD is also more prevalent among children whose siblings have been diagnosed with the same disorder. Recent studies have established that the fathers of hyperactive children are more likely to be alcoholic or to have antisocial personality disorders. Affected children have shown the presence of subtle chromosomal changes and mild neurological deficits with irregular brain function including too little activity in the area that inhibits impulsiveness. Hyperactivity may result from fetal alcohol syndrome, congenital infections, and brain damage resulting from birth trauma or hypoxia. Cognitive distractibility and impulsivity are associated with other disorders involving brain damage or dysfunction, such as mental retardation, seizure disorder, and brain lesions.

Physiological conditions that can mimic the symptoms include constipation, hypoglycemia, lead toxicity, and thyroid and other metabolic diseases.

Family Dynamics

This theory suggests that disruptive behavior is learned as a means for a child to gain adult attention. It is likely that whether or not the impulsive irritability seen in individuals with ADHD was present from birth, some parental reactions tend to reinforce and thus maintain or increase its intensity. Anxiety generated by a dysfunctional family system, marital problems, and so forth, could also contribute to symptoms of this disorder. Parents become frustrated with the child's poor response to limit-setting. Parents may become overly sensitive or may give up and provide no external structure.

CLIENT ASSESSMENT DATA BASE

Activity/Rest

Very active, "always on the move," does not slow down when should/must
Difficulty playing or engaging in leisure activities quietly

Ego Integrity

Emotional liability, hot temper, mood changes

Hygiene

Forgetful in daily activities

Neurosensory

Reports from parents and teachers of:
  Being easily distracted, unable to sustain attention to remain on task or complete projects
  Having difficulty sitting still, sometimes physically overactive, fidgets with hands/feet, may engage in disruptive behavior or dangerous activities without considering the consequences
  Difficulty following instructions, organizing tasks/activities

Social Interactions

Does not seem to listen/attend to what is being said
Significant distress or impairment in social, academic, or occupational functioning

Teaching/Learning

Onset before age 7
Family history of alcohol abuse

DIAGNOSTIC STUDIES

(ADHD is a diagnosis by exclusion, and studies are done to rule out other conditions having similar symptoms.)
Thyroid Studies: May reveal hyperthyroid/hypothyroid conditions contributing to problems.
Neurological Testing (e.g., EEG, CT Scan): Determines presence of organic brain disorders.
Psychological Testing as Indicated: Rules out anxiety disorders; identifies gifted, borderline-retarded, or learning-disabled child; and assesses social responsiveness and language development.
Individual Diagnostic Studies dependent on presence of physical symptoms (e.g., rashes, upper respiratory illness, or other allergic symptoms, CNS infection [cerebritis]).

NURSING PRIORITIES

1. Facilitate child's achievement of more consistent behavioral self-control and improvement in self-esteem.
2. Promote parents' development of effective means of coping with and interventions for their child's behavioral symptoms.
3. Participate in the development of a comprehensive, ongoing treatment approach using family and community resources.

DISCHARGE GOALS

1. Disruptive and/or dangerous behavior minimized or eliminated.
2. Able to function in a structured learning environment.

3. Parents have gained or regained the ability to cope with internal feelings and to intervene effectively in their child's behavioral problems.
4. Plan in place to meet needs after discharge.

NURSING DIAGNOSIS	COPING, INDIVIDUAL, ineffective/ COPING, defensive
May Be Related to:	Situational or maturational crisis; denial of obvious problems
	Mild neurological deficits/retardation
	Retarded ego development; low self-esteem
	Projection of blame/responsibility; rationalization of failure
	Dysfunctional family system, negative role models; abuse/neglect
Possibly Evidenced by:	Easy distraction by extraneous stimuli; shifting from one uncompleted activity to another; difficulty reality-testing perceptions
	Inability to meet age-appropriate role expectations
	Excessive motor activity; cannot sit still
	Inability to delay gratification; manipulation of others in environment to fulfill own desires
Desired Outcomes/Evaluation Criteria—Client Will:	Demonstrate a decrease in disruptive behaviors, expressing anger in socially acceptable manner.
	Show improvements in attention span, concentration, and appropriate activity level.
	Delay gratification without resorting to manipulation of others.

ACTIONS/INTERVENTIONS	RATIONALE
Independent	
Provide quiet atmosphere; decrease amount of external stimuli. Maintain atmosphere of calm.	Reduction in environmental stimulation may decrease distractibility. Calm approach helps prevent transmission of anxiety between individuals.
Provide area and activities for gross motor movement (e.g., gym and/or outdoor area for running, large balls, climbing equipment).	Appropriate outlets are necessary to discharge motor activity.
Reinforce attending, concentrating, and completing tasks.	Desired behaviors will increase with positive reinforcement.
Set limits on disruptive behaviors (e.g., talking incessantly); suggest alternative competing behaviors such as playing quietly.	Child needs to know expectations and to learn competing acceptable behaviors (e.g., raising hand vs. shouting out, keeping hands to self vs. pushing others).

Encourage discussion of angry feelings and identity of true object of the hostility.

Dealing with the feelings honestly and directly helps discourage displacement of the anger onto others.

Explore alternative ways for handling frustration with client.

Promotes learning how to interact in society with others in more productive ways.

Provide positive feedback for trying new coping strategies.

Supports efforts and encourages use of acceptable behaviors.

Evaluate with client the effectiveness of new behaviors. Discuss modifications for improvement.

As client has limited problem-solving skills, assistance may be required to reassess and develop strategies.

Assist client to recognize signs of escalating anxiety. Explore ways client can intervene before behavior becomes disabling.

Helps client recognize ineffective behaviors and develop new coping skills to effect positive change.

Provide information and assist parents in learning positive ways of handling problem behaviors.

Behaviors can often be minimized and/or averted by consistent, positive approaches.

Involve in individual counseling.

Medication alone or in combination with a behavior modification program is insufficient. Children with ADHD do not outgrow their problems and many continue to have difficulties into adulthood. Research suggests about 25% of children with ADHD have or will soon develop bipolar disorder with a volatile mix of symptoms (e.g., distractibility, anxiety, depression, irritability, and violent outbursts), often requiring hospitalization. Counseling helps the individual modify their behavior, works to improve social skills and self-esteem, and addresses depression or other emotional issues.

Collaborative

Administer medication as indicated, e.g.: methylphenidate [Ritalin], imipramine [Tofranil],

Psychostimulants and antidepressants may improve attention and reduce impulsiveness in hyperactive children.

pemoline [Cylert], dextroamphetamine [Dexedrine]; diazepam [Valium], chlordiazepoxide [Librium], alprazolam [Xanax].

Antianxiety medications provide relief from immobilizing effects of anxiety, facilitating cooperation with therapy.

Investigate alternative treatments (e.g., diet, allergy).

Some children seem to respond favorably to control of refined sugar, food dyes, and allergens. **Note:** Current research has failed to show a correlation between sugar use and hyperactive behavior/cognitive problems.

NURSING DIAGNOSIS	SOCIAL INTERACTION, impaired
May Be Related to:	Retarded ego development; low self-esteem
	Dysfunctional family system, negative role models; abuse/neglect

May Be Related to (cont.):	Neurological impairment; mental retardation
Possibly Evidenced by:	Discomfort in social situations
	Difficulty waiting turn in games or group situations; interrupts or intrudes on others
	Does not seem to listen to what is being said
	Difficulty playing quietly, maintaining attention to task or play activity; often shifts from one activity to another
Desired Outcomes/Evaluation Criteria— Client Will:	Identify feelings that lead to poor social interactions.
	Participate appropriately in interactive play with another child or group of children.
	Develop a mutual relationship with another child or adult.

ACTIONS/INTERVENTIONS	RATIONALE
Independent	
Develop trust relationship with child, show acceptance of child separate from unacceptable behavior.	Acceptance and trust encourage feelings of self-worth.
Encourage client to verbalize feelings of inadequacy and need for acceptance from others. Discuss how these feelings affect relationships by provoking defensive behaviors such as blaming and manipulating others.	Recognition of problem is first step toward resolution.
Offer positive reinforcement for appropriate social interaction. Ignore ineffective methods of relating to others; teach competing behaviors.	Behavior modification can be an effective method of reducing disruptive behaviors in children by encouraging repetition of desirable behaviors. Attention to unacceptable behavior may actually reinforce it.
Identify situations that provoke defensiveness and role-play more appropriate responses.	Provides confidence to deal with difficult situations when they occur.
Provide opportunities for group interaction and encourage a positive and negative peer feedback system.	Appropriate social behavior is often learned from age-mates.
Collaborative	
Arrange staffings with other professionals (e.g., social workers, teachers). Include parents and child when possible.	Cooperation and coordination among those working with these children enhance treatment program. Including child and parents provides them with understanding of the total problem and proposed treatment program.

NURSING DIAGNOSIS	SELF ESTEEM disturbance
May Be Related to:	Retarded ego development
	Lack of positive feedback with repeated negative feedback
	Dysfunctional family system; abuse/neglect; negative role models
	Mild neurological deficits
Possibly Evidenced by:	Lack of eye contact
	Derogatory remarks about self
	Lack of self-confidence; hesitance to try new tasks
	Engagement in physically dangerous activity
	Distraction of others to cover up own deficits or failures (e.g., acting the clown)
	Projection of blame/responsibility for problems; rationalization of personal failure, grandiosity
Desired Outcomes/Evaluation Criteria—Client Will:	Verbalize increasingly positive self-regard.
	Demonstrate beginning awareness and control of own behavior.
	Participate in new activities without extreme fear of failure.

ACTIONS/INTERVENTIONS	RATIONALE
Independent	
Convey acceptance and unconditional positive regard.	This may help child to increase own sense of self-worth.
Assist child to identify basic ego strengths/positive aspects of self; give immediate feedback for acceptable behavior.	Focusing on positive aspects of personality may help improve self-concept. Positive reinforcement enhances self-esteem and increases likelihood of repetition of desired behavior.
Spend time with client in 1:1 and group activities.	Conveys to client that you believe he or she is worthy of time and attention.
Provide opportunities for success; plan activities with short time span and appropriate ability level.	Repeated successes can help improve self-esteem.
Discuss fears, encourage involvement of new activities/tasks.	Confronting concerns and engaging in new tasks promote personal growth and new skills.
Help client set realistic, concrete goals and determine appropriate actions to meet these goals.	Provides a structure to develop sense of hope for the future and framework for reaching desired goals.
Collaborative	
Provide learning opportunities, structured learning environment (e.g., self-contained classroom, individually planned educational program).	Successful school performance is essential to preserve a child's positive self-image.

67

NURSING DIAGNOSIS	FAMILY COPING, ineffective: compromised/disabling
May Be Related to:	Excessive guilt, anger, or blaming among family members regarding child's behavior
	Parental inconsistencies; disagreements regarding discipline, limit-setting, and approaches
	Exhaustion of parental resources due to prolonged coping with disruptive child
Possibly Evidenced by:	Unrealistic parental expectations
	Rejection or overprotection of child
	Exaggerated expressions of anger, disappointment, or despair regarding child's behavior or ability to improve or change
Desired Outcomes/Evaluation Criteria— Parent(s)/Family Will:	Demonstrate more consistent, effective intervention methods in response to child's behavior.
	Express and resolve negative attitudes toward child.
	Identify and use support systems as needed.

ACTIONS/INTERVENTIONS	RATIONALE
Independent	
Provide information and materials related to child's disorder and effective parenting techniques. (Refer to CP: Parenting.)	Appropriate knowledge and skills may increase parental effectiveness.
Encourage individuals to verbalize feelings and explore alternative methods of dealing with child.	Supportive counseling can assist family in developing coping strategies.
Provide feedback and reinforce effective parenting methods.	Positive reinforcement can increase self-esteem and encourage continued efforts.
Involve siblings in family discussions and planning for more effective family interactions.	Family problems affect all members and treatment is more effective when everyone is involved in therapy.
Collaborative	
Involve in family counseling.	Family therapy may help resolve global issues affecting the whole family structure. Disruption in one family member inevitably affects the rest of the family.
Refer to community resources as indicated including parent support groups, parenting classes (e.g., Parent Effectiveness).	Developing a support system can increase parental confidence and effectiveness. Provides role models/hope for the future.

NURSING DIAGNOSIS	KNOWLEDGE deficit [LEARNING NEED] regarding condition, prognosis, self care and treatment needs
May Be Related to:	Lack of knowledge; misinformation/misinterpretation
	Mild neurological deficits; associated developmental learning disabilities; inability to concentrate; cognitive deficits
Possibly Evidence by:	Verbalization of problem/misconceptions
	Poor school performance; purposefully losing necessary articles to complete schoolwork (e.g., homework assignments, pencils, books)
	Shifting from one uncompleted activity to another
	Unrealistic expectation of medication management
Desired Outcomes/Evaluation Criteria— Client/Parent(s) Will:	Verbalize understanding of reasons for behavioral problems, treatment needs within developmental ability.
	Participate in learning and begin to ask questions and seek information independently.
Client Will:	Achieve cognitive goals consistent with level of temperament.

ACTIONS/INTERVENTIONS	RATIONALE

Independent

Provide quiet environment, self-contained classrooms, small-group activities. Avoid overstimulating places, such as school bus, busy cafeteria, crowded hallways.	Reduction in environmental stimulation may decrease distractibility. Small groups may enhance ability to stay on task and help client learn appropriate interaction with others, avoid sense of isolation.
Give instructional material in written and verbal form with step-by-step explanations.	Sequential learning skills will be enhanced. Instruct child in problem-solving skills, practice situational examples. Effective skills may increase performance levels.
Educate child and family on the use of psychostimulants and behavioral response anticipated.	Use of psychostimulants may not result in improved school grades without accompanying changes in child's study skills.
Coordinate overall treatment plan with schools, collateral personnel, the child, and the family.	Cognitive effectiveness will most likely be advanced when treatment is not fragmented, nor significant interventions missed because of lack of interdisciplinary communication.

CONDUCT DISORDER

DSM-IV

312.XX Conduct disorder
312.81 Childhood-onset type
312.82 Adolescent-onset type

Conduct disorder is most distinguishable by the degree of repetitive and persistent violation of the basic rights of others. Common antisocial behaviors acted out in the home and school setting include physical aggression toward people and animals, destruction of property, lying, and theft. There is a total disregard for age-appropriate social norms as the child purposely engages in criminals acts, truancy from school, and breaking curfew. The *DSM-IV* criteria rates the level of severity as *mild, moderate, to severe.* The greater the level of delinquency and frequency in early childhood, the greater the risk for chronic offending into adulthood. Other prognostic factors leading to the continuation of the disorder include age of onset and the variation in problem behaviors displayed in multiple settings. Co-morbid diagnoses often associated with this condition are hyperactivity, depression, and chemical abuse and dependence.

ETIOLOGICAL THEORIES

Psychodynamics

According to psychoanalytical theory, these children are fixated in the separation-individuation phase of development. The mother figure projects her view of the child's needs as an unrealistic demand on her. The child cannot solidify attachment with the maternal object and compensates for the mother's narcissistic need for gratification by *overidealizing* the image of the mother. The child fails to build up identification and differentiation between self and others to support sufficient superego development. The id behavior is prominent.

Biological

Temperamental abnormalities have been observed in infants at birth in terms of excitability, attention span, and adaptability. Heredity influences such traits as the tendency to seek risks and obey authority. One possibility is the biological influence of heightened arousal in the CNS and abnormally high levels of testosterone, leading to aggression. Differences in the lack of sufficient serotonin transmission is evidenced.

Current research suggests that negative experiences in infancy cause biological and neurological damage to the brain tissue. When persistent stress results in an internal perception of a constant state of danger, the *"fight-or-flight"* hormones (adrenaline and cortisol) are released, reaching dangerously high levels that can cause neurological impairment. These damaged brain cells react in unusual ways to the stimuli, possibly resulting in epileptic seizures or depression.

Family Dynamics

Certain family patterns contribute to the disruptive behavior. A high correlation exists between chronic conflict and neglect in the parent–child relationship. Poor parental management skills, inconsistent or rigid and harsh discipline practices increase the risk for acting out by the child. Changes in caretakers, unstable spousal relationships, and parental rejection are all contributing/causal factors. These children lack strong emotional bonds or reliable role models to promote prosocial behavior. Socioeconomic conditions may also play a part, with poverty being a risk factor.

CLIENT ASSESSMENT DATA BASE

Ego Integrity

Feelings of rejection, powerlessness
Blames others for what happens to self

Displays maladaptive coping behaviors; uses manipulation to get needs met
Engages in unacceptable behaviors in response to stressors (e.g., staying out at night, running away)
May have had frequent/recurrent life changes, (e.g., multiple moves, change of schools, lifestyle changes, placement in foster homes)

Food/Fluid

Skips meals, eats excessive amounts of junk foods
Eats in response to external cues/stressors
Reports of nausea
May have excessive weight for height; recent weight gain may be noted

Hygiene

Poor hygiene/personal habits
Style of dress may reflect fashion trends or be atypical (antisocial/gang attire)

Neurosensory

Nervousness, worry, and jitteriness/excessive psychomotor activity
May be depressed, angry, or react with ambivalence or hostility; poor impulse control
Affect may be labile
Physical characteristics/development may not be normal for age range

Safety

Engages in risk-taking behavior (e.g., gang involvement, exposure to STDs, drug use)
Overt aggressive acts
Suicidal ideation; may have plan/means, previous suicide attempts

Sexuality

Early onset of sexual behavior, may have forced others into sexual activity

Social Interactions

Symptoms most often appear during prepubertal to pubertal period and may predispose the child to conduct or adjustment disorders in adolescence
Family disharmony/disruption, little contact with absent parent/separation from extended family may be reported
Individual may have history of poor school/work performance
Parents may report client isolates self, plays stereo loudly, does not participate in family activities; shows little empathy or concern for others
Displays hostility toward authority figures; intimidates others
Participation in social activities may be nonexistent or sporadic, or gang-related
Client may be involved with legal system/juvenile court, have record of antisocial behavior (e.g., fire-setting, cruelty to people/animals, stealing, use of a weapon)

Teaching/Learning

Onset usually between age 5 to early adolescence; rare after age 16
May be involved in drug use/abuse (e.g., alcohol, inhalants, cigarettes/chewing tobacco)
May have had previous psychiatric hospitalization for same or other problems

DIAGNOSTIC STUDIES

Drug Screen: To identify substance use/abuse.

NURSING PRIORITIES

1. Provide a safe environment and protect client from self-harm.
2. Promote development of strategies that regulate impulse control, regain sense of self-worth and security.
3. Facilitate learning of appropriate and satisfying methods of dealing with stressors/feelings.
4. Promote client's ability to engage in satisfying relationships with family members and peer group.
5. Increase the client's behavioral response repertoire.

DISCHARGE GOALS

1. Exhibits effective coping skills in dealing with problems.
2. Understands need and strategies for controlling negative impulses/acting-out behaviors.
3. Expresses anger in appropriate/nonviolent ways.
4. Family involved in group therapy; participating in treatment program.
5. Plan in place to meet needs after discharge.

NURSING DIAGNOSIS	VIOLENCE, risk for, directed at self/others
Risk Factors May Include:	Retarded ego development; loss of self-esteem; antisocial character
	Dysfunctional family system and loss of significant relationships; feelings of rejection, sense of powerlessness
	Poor impulse control
	History of suicidal/acting-out behavior
[Possible Indicators:]	Behavior changes (e.g., absenteeism, poor grades, hostility toward authority figures, stealing)
	Increased motor activity, increasing anxiety level, anger
	Overt aggressive acts directed at the environment
	Self-destructive behavior, active suicidal threat/gestures
Desired Outcomes/Evaluation Criteria—Client Will:	Verbalize understanding of behavior and factors that precipitate violent actions.
	Express anger in appropriate ways, avoiding hostile or suicidal gestures/statements or harm to self or others.
	Demonstrate self-initiated intervention strategies that facilitate more effective coping skills.
	Identify and use resources and support systems in an effective manner.

ACTIONS/INTERVENTIONS	RATIONALE

Independent

Establish trusting relationship with client. Encourage exploration and verbalization of feelings.	Client's expression of internal conflicts, in words rather than action, will more likely be made to knowledgeable and accepting staff.

Strike a balance in the intimacy of the therapeutic relationship.

Children who are more disturbed respond best to a less-intrusive relationship in the beginning.

Monitor stressors and warning signals such as behavior changes, anger, anxiety, and recently disrupted family.

Impulsive reactions to stressful situations, directed toward harm to self or others, may be a cry for help.

Observe/assist client to recognize mood (e.g., anger, sadness, anxiety).

Identifying own feelings is the first step in the change process. Signs and symptoms of anxiety need to be identified before client can begin to make constructive changes.

Identify antecedents to violent behavior.

Correct assessment and interpretation of premonitory conditions provide for timely intervention to reduce risk of violent/acting-out behavior.

Support client's exploration to identify behaviors or interventions that offer relief.

Connecting feelings with behaviors that afford relief will encourage the development of more productive behaviors.

Determine seriousness of suicidal tendency, gestures, threats, or previous attempts. (Use scale of 1–10 and prioritize according to severity of threat, availability of means.)

Knowledge of past and present behavior in reference to suicidal ideation will assist in assessing client's tolerance for stress, degree of concern. **Note:** This may be first-priority nursing diagnosis if suicide risk is rated in the 8–10 range.

Provide information regarding suicidal ideation/ warnings. Include significant other(s) in discussions.

Client may be unaware or/ignorant of meaning of warning signals when suicidal ideation exists.

Maintain a therapeutic milieu that includes a safe environment (e.g., suicide precautions, behavioral contract).

Internal controls may be inadequate, requiring some external controls and interventions until internal control is learned.

Observe client unobtrusively for signs of potential violence toward others.

Intervention before the onset of violence can prevent injury to the client and others. Overt monitoring may be interpreted negatively and potentiate acting-out behavior.

Explore and offer more satisfying alternatives to aggressive behavior (e.g., physical outlets for redirection of angry feelings; use of quiet room, or "Soft Spot" with soft balls/pillows to pound).

Increased ability to discover satisfying alternatives in coping with stressors will decrease need for aggressive behavior. Physical outlets help relieve pent-up tension and anxiety.

Engage in action-oriented recreational therapy (e.g., exercise activities [jogging in the gym, etc.], outdoor program, wall climbing, noncompetitive games/supervised sports).

Recreational therapy helps discharge nervous, pent-up energy, releasing tension and reducing anxiety. Sustained activity stimulates release of endorphins, enhancing sense of well-being. Formal exercise therapy programs are an adjunct to psychotherapy, decreasing symptoms related to anxiety, depression, and thought disturbances. Exercise does not need to be aerobic or intensive to achieve desired effect. **Note:** Competitive games may increase anxiety.

Establish hierarchy of responses to aggressive behaviors (e.g., Time out). Have sufficient staff available to indicate a show of strength to client if it becomes necessary.

This conveys to client evidence of control over the situation and provides some sense of security for the client and staff.

Encourage client to ask for time with staff, give permission to express angry feelings. Be alert to "acting out" to please peers or nursing staff.

Early interventions can interrupt the pattern prior to seriously escalating behavior. Recognizing feelings and taking responsibility by asking for

Assess how unit functioning affects adolescent behaviors.

Milieu stressors like vacations, personnel changes, and staff conflict can affect client's own issues (e.g., abandonment). It is important to look at the psychodynamics as well as the unique meaning of individual behavior.

time to discuss them helps the adolescent learn more effective ways of dealing with problems that can lead to anger and acting-out behaviors.

Have staff member stay with client when necessary. Encourage client to choose own "Time out," going to room for alone time, taking medications; or choosing room schedules, use of seclusion and/or restraints.

Staff member can help client to express feelings and begin to recognize value of appropriate handling of anger. Adolescent may see "Time out" as punishment if staff imposes, but begins to take responsibility for self by recognizing and choosing own quiet/alone time.

Include whole community/classroom in reinforcing positive behaviors. Use daily goal-setting group or problem-solving group.

Peer interaction is effective in this age group to help client control own behavior.

Collaborative

Place in seclusion or apply restraints as necessary.

External restraints may be needed until client regains control of own behavior.

Administer/supervise medications and monitor effects of therapy.

Helps client to maintain impulse control. Neuroleptic medications decrease aggressive outbursts and improve impulse control.

NURSING DIAGNOSIS	THOUGHT PROCESSES, altered
May Be Related to:	Physiological changes—damage to brain tissues
	Lack of psychological conflicts
	Biochemical changes—substance use/abuse
Possibly Evidenced by:	Inaccurate interpretation of stimuli; tendency to interpret the intentions and actions of others as blaming and hostile
	Deficits in problem-solving skills, perceptions, and self-statements; demonstrating fewer solutions to interpersonal problems—physical aggression is the solution most often chosen
Desired Outcomes/Evaluation Criteria— Client Will:	Describe how thoughts and emotions relate to own behavior.
	List characteristics of the antisocial personality that client sees in self.
	Explain the concept of thinking error, how it leads to antisocial behavior, and name those that personally apply.
	Practice new cognitive problem-solving skills that will lead to social competence and adjustment.

ACTIONS/INTERVENTIONS	RATIONALE
Independent	
Assign primary nurse to develop a therapeutic relationship.	Continuity of care for client builds trust and clarifies expectation.
Discuss characteristics of the antisocial personality with the client.	Some common beliefs of the person with an antisocial personality are as follows: does not have to conform to society's rules or norms, believes the world revolves around self, and believes that others should meet client's needs rather than client meeting society's expectations.
Provide written handout and allow time for client to review information, ask questions, and clarify understanding	Allows client to internalize information and prepares for restructuring activities to change behavior.
Discuss the concept of thinking errors.	A thinking error occurs when a person has a thought that is extremely different from the way most people under the same circumstances would think. If the person acts on the thought, the behavior will be outside of societal norms.
Relate concept to client's own thinking errors and behavior.	Common thinking errors are as follows: victim stance ("He started it/I couldn't help it"); doesn't stop to think how actions will hurt others; lack of effort; unwillingness to do anything perceived as boring or disagreeable; refusal to accept obligation, ("I forgot/I don't have to"); gaining power through anger; refusal to acknowledge fear; blaming others when criticized; "I can't" attitude—statement of refusal, not inability.
Have client keep a "thinking log," emphasizing the importance of writing actual thoughts and not trying to "con" the staff with what the client thinks they want to hear. Explain responsibility for daily entry and attendant consequence.	Provides opportunity for client to "see" thoughts and compare with reality, connect outcomes/consequences with specific behaviors, and begin to take responsibility for change process.
Promote client responsibility for the review process. Help client identify the thinking errors and relate them to the client's pattern of thinking in everyday life. Reinforce that the thinking errors are only the "tip of the iceberg."	Helps client begin to assume inner-directed self-control. Promotes attention to content and conformity to process, allowing client to begin to identify ineffective methods of getting needs met.
Observe for shame reactions. Explain that the process is not judgmental and discuss behavioral responses.	Thinking log is a tool for client to identify thinking errors and choose not to act on them.
Require attendance at Thinking Error Group. Facilitate honest noncritical feedback from group members. Continuously evaluate the group process and identify thinking errors as they occur in the group.	Sharing information from the log promotes awareness and opportunities to change behavior in safe environment of the group.
Review entire log with client before discharge. Provide feedback regarding improved behavioral responses and areas in which continued work is needed. Encourage client to continue thinking log after discharge.	This provides opportunity for client to identify predominant pattern of thinking errors and recognize new ways to respond that have been learned in treatment.

ACTIONS/INTERVENTIONS	RATIONALE

Independent

Assess individual causes and contributing factors (e.g., disruption of the family, frequent moves during child's/adolescent's life, individual's poor coping and adjustment to developmental stage).	Although learning social skills is one of the maturational tasks, many factors can interfere with the client's ability to interact satisfactorily with others in social situations.
Review medical history.	Long-term illness/accident may have interfered with development of social skills at earlier stages.
Observe family patterns of relating and social behaviors. Explore possible family scripting of expectations of the child/adolescent. Note prevalent patterns.	Family may not have effective patterns of relating to others, and the child learns these skills in this setting. Often child reflects family expectations rather than own desires. Identification of patterns will help with plan for change.
Encourage client to verbalize feelings about discomfort in social settings, noting recurring factors or precipitating patterns.	Client identifies areas of concern and suggests ways to learn new skills.
Active-listen verbalizations indicating hopelessness, powerlessness, fear, anxiety, grief, anger, feeling unloved or unlovable, problems with sexual identity, and/or hate (directed or not).	Client may believe that nothing can be done to change the way things are and that own actions do not make a difference. Active-listening client's words and feelings conveys a message of confidence in the individual's own abilities.
Assess client's coping skills and defense mechanisms.	Although skills may have helped client to "survive" in the past, their use was often based on thinking errors/misinterpretation of the situation. These skills may be effective for dealing with restructured reality and/or provide a base for learning new skills.

Have client identify behaviors that cause discomfort and review negative behaviors others have identified.

Listing specific behaviors will help the client know where change is possible. Knowing what others see can help the client accept and effect change.

Explore with client and role-play new ways of handling identified behaviors/situations.

Active involvement is the most effective way to create change.

Provide reinforcement for positive social behaviors and interactions.

Promotes feelings of self-worth and helps reinforce desired behaviors.

Work with client to correct basic negative self-concept (Refer to ND: Self Esteem, chronic low).

Negative self-concepts may be a major factor impeding positive social interactions.

Help client identify responsibility for own behavior. Encourage keeping a daily journal of social interactions and feelings.

Enhances self-esteem and provides feedback to improve skills. Journaling can provide an ongoing record to note improvement and/or areas of need for change.

Collaborative

Involve in group therapy as indicated.

Helpful arena to practice new social skills and to receive feedback with support for efforts to improve.

Encourage reading, attendance at classes (e.g., positive image, self-help, assertiveness), and community support groups.

Assists in alleviating negative self-concepts that lead to impaired social interactions.

NURSING DIAGNOSIS	COPING, defensive
May Be Related to:	Inadequate coping strategies; maturational crisis; multiple life changes/losses
	Lack of control of impulsive actions; personal vulnerability
Possibly Evidenced by:	Denial of obvious problems/weaknesses; projection of blame/responsibility; rationalizing failures
	Difficulty in reality-testing perceptions; grandiosity
	Inappropriate use of defense mechanisms (e.g., stealing and other acting-out behaviors, excessive smoking/drinking)
	Inability to meet role expectations
	Difficulty establishing/maintaining relationships; hostile laughter at, or ridicule of, others; superior attitude toward others; hypersensitivity to slight or criticism
Desired Outcomes/Evaluation Criteria— Client Will:	Verbalize and recognize significance of losses in life.
	Verbalize understanding of the relationship between emotional needs and acting-out impulsive behaviors and the consequences thereof.

Desired Outcomes/Evaluation Criteria—Client Will (cont.):	Develop ego strength sufficient to cope with inner impulses.
	Identify and demonstrate ways to meet own needs.
	Participate in treatment program/therapy.

ACTIONS/INTERVENTIONS	RATIONALE

Independent

Establish level of authority of primary nurse; monitor the need for nurturance and limit-setting.	Consistent "parent figure" can uniformly reinforce consequences of behaviors of the client.
Provide explanation of the rules of the treatment setting and develop consequences with the client for his or her lack of cooperation.	Clear explanation of the rules allows the client to make choices about participating. Involvement in setting of the consequences promotes an investment in which the client is more apt to comply.
Encourage client to express fears and concerns.	Self-understanding and further exploration are enhanced when verbalizations of concern and anxiety are received in a nonjudgmental manner.
Listen to client's perception of inability to adapt to situations occurring at present.	Provides clues to reality of these perceptions and avenues to assist in dealing with them.
Help client to recognize significance of losses and express feelings regarding these.	Grief work cannot begin until losses are acknowledged (e.g., divorce, relocation, loss of friends/extended family/support systems).
Encourage exploration of the relationship of behavior, anxiety, and somatic symptoms to the grief process.	Knowledge regarding possible psychological and physiological manifestations of the grief process helps identify etiology of existing symptoms and to alleviate denial.
Discuss appropriateness and desirability of the grief process as it relates to the loss(es). Discuss stages of the grief process and behaviors associated with each stage.	Grief work is necessary and a natural reaction to loss. Time is required (at least 6–12 months) to work through grief. The process gives the client permission to grieve and offers hope for eventual acclimation to the loss.
Determine coping mechanisms used (e.g., projection, rationalization) and how these affect current situation.	Provides a beginning point for client to see how use of ineffective coping methods causes problems in life/relationships.
Assist client to recognize the reality and nonproductivity of maladaptive behaviors (e.g., failing grades, trouble with the law, running away). Offer support and confront client when appropriate.	Old patterns of behavior tend to recur under stress. Continuous monitoring of behavior is necessary to avoid old, nonproductive methods of coping and problem-solving. Therapeutic confrontation can help client to look at incongruencies of behavior and own responsibility for actions.
Describe all aspects of the problems using therapeutic communication skills (e.g., Active-listening).	This clarifies problems and promotes understanding by the client and nurse.
Focus on specific behaviors (e.g., poor academic performance, antisocial behavior) that are amenable to change.	Energy is best used when focus is on those areas that can be altered.

Set limits on manipulative behavior by telling client what will be tolerated; be consistent in enforcing consequences when rules are broken and limits tested.

Reinforce client positively when change in behaviors indicates effective coping through behavior-modification system. Anticipate and accept occasional regressive behavior.

Identify past and present support systems.

Explore religious beliefs/affiliations. Encourage client to draw again on spiritual resources that had been useful in the past.

Explore possible ways to rekindle relationships with positive peer/role models, influential adults, organizations/church youth group, as appropriate.

Encourage the development of a positive relationship with an adult.

Being clear and confronting these behaviors in a consistent manner will help client begin to change ways of getting needs met.

Adolescence is a time of stress and vulnerability because of a lack of well-developed coping skills. Positive reinforcement encourages continuing personal growth. Hospitalization may precipitate periodic regression.

Reinforces availability of resources to aid the client to develop new coping skills.

When these ties have been previously established, they may be helpful in providing resources for the adolescent to enhance inner controls.

Attaining peer acceptance is of primary importance during adolescence. Peer groups that share common values promote the formation of belonging and identity.

A quality relationship with an adult (preferably a parent) reinforces the strength and supportive function of the relationship (family) and is a positive factor when setting limits with the adolescent.

NURSING DIAGNOSIS	**FAMILY COPING, ineffective: compromised/disabling**
May Be Related to:	Loss of significant relationship (parent/child); lack of effective parent management skills
	Highly ambivalent family relationships; family disorganization/role changes
	Presence of other situational/developmental crises affecting family members
Possibly Evidenced by:	Client states feelings of abandonment, rejection, and guilt about parent's response to adolescent's problems
	Client expresses sense of powerlessness and lack of control
	Parents describe preoccupation with own reactions (e.g., fear, guilt, anxiety)
	Parents withdraw or have limited communication with adolescent or display protective behavior disproportionate (too little or too much) to client's abilities or need for autonomy
Desired Outcomes/Evaluation Criteria—Family Will:	Express feelings openly and honestly.
	Evaluate individual role in family problems.
	Initiate positive/amicable relationship with one another.

ACTIONS/INTERVENTIONS	RATIONALE

Independent

Foster trust through 1:1 family/nurse relationship.	Basic trust and stability can be established through continuity and consistency of care.
Identify underlying family dynamics and determine how they are operating in the present.	Established family patterns affect how current situation has arisen, as well as how problems need to be resolved and changed now.
Encourage open communication between client and family.	Communication patterns affect the functional level of each family member.
Encourage client to identify and appropriately verbalize feelings of rejection, abandonment, and ambivalence related to individual situation.	Verbalizing feelings tends to alleviate tensions that may be internalized or somatized (e.g., reports of nausea). Client lacks emotional attachment to others and may be charming and engaging, which is a pretense to deceive others/facilitate exploitation.
Discuss reasons for client behaviors, including the relationship between differences in the client's thoughts/beliefs and how others in the family think and behave.	Understanding of childhood/adolescent tasks, ambivalent feelings, etc., can help individual(s) accept and deal more appropriately with difficult behaviors. As a rule, client is easily bored and has a low frustration tolerance when desires are not immediately gratified. Emotional reactions can be erratic and demonstrate a lack of concern for others. When the client acts on his or her thoughts, behavior will be outside of societal norms.
Explore feelings of self-blame and guilt related to problems/changes in the family system. Assist individuals in realistic appraisal and verbalization of own role in situation.	Change or disruption in the family system affects all other parts of the system. Children may incorrectly assume that they were instrumental in family problems/marital disruption.
Guide client/family in correlating anger and feelings that are centered around lack of influence in family behavior.	Understanding internal dynamics of anger leads to acceptance of locus of control within self.
Encourage client/family to make as many decisions as are possible within the milieu. **Example:** Client decision to participate in choice of evening activity.	An increase in autonomy and decision-making enhances feeling of self-worth and competency.
Focus on specific behaviors that are amenable to change.	Changing some behaviors can enhance feelings of self-esteem and encourage willingness to make other changes.
Help family recognize and set limits on manipulative behavior.	Stating rules clearly and being consistent in maintaining them helps establish family boundaries and allows the client to recognize when they are violated.
Explore ways client and family can be mutually supportive without fostering overdependence on each other.	Security and trust provide a climate for growth and risk-taking.

ACTIONS/INTERVENTIONS	RATIONALE
Give immediate, consistent, and positive reinforcement when desired behaviors are observed. Conversely, withhold reinforcement/ignore negative behaviors.	Consistent reinforcement of appropriate behaviors fosters continuation of those behaviors. Consequences for inappropriate behaviors and no reinforcement (ignoring) tend to extinguish undesired behaviors.

Collaborative

Explore potential sources of assistance available to meet needs. Refer to social services and other agencies as indicated.	Knowledge of resources available if they are needed tends to decrease fears regarding postdischarge functioning.
Encourage family to participate in family therapy.	Enables family to work on issues that affect all of the family system. **Note:** Family rift may be so severe that the most that can be expected is a neutral relationship in which parties agree to disagree. (Refer to CP: Parenting.)

NURSING DIAGNOSIS	**SELF ESTEEM, chronic low**
May Be Related to:	Life choices perpetuating failure (e.g., runaway behavior)
	Personal vulnerability (loss of family member/ friends; poor school performance, relocation)
	Fixation in earlier level of development (lack of movement toward independence)
Possibly Evidenced by:	Self-negating verbalizations, self-blame, anger
	Rationalizing away/rejecting of positive feedback and exaggeration of negative feedback about self, feelings of rejection
	Frequent lack of success in school/other life events
Desired Outcomes/Evaluation Criteria— Client Will:	Verbalize beginning understanding of negative evaluation of self and reasons for problems.
	Participate in treatment program to promote change in self-evaluation.
	Demonstrate behaviors/lifestyle changes to promote positive self-esteem.
	Verbalize increased sense of self-esteem in relation to current situation.

ACTIONS/INTERVENTIONS	RATIONALE

Independent

Continue the trust relationship that is reliable, supportive, and reassuring.	Communication, growth, and insight flourish in an atmosphere of acceptance and trust.
Schedule time for 1:1 client/nurse interaction and communication.	Individual attention conveys the importance of the individual. Communication skills are refined with frequent interaction.

Explore and discuss feelings of rejection and anger related to individual situation.	Recognition and expression of feelings eliminate need for displacement and denial. This directs focus of energy to problems and alternative solutions.
Point out past academic/personal successes.	Assists in preserving self-esteem. Past performance is a more accurate portrayal of ability than that indicated by recent evaluations/grades.
Assist client in understanding transient nature of poor academic performance related to current stressors.	High-anxiety levels affect motivation, attention to task, and performance.
Work with client to develop a plan of action to meet immediate needs (e.g., physical safety, hygiene, emotional support).	Provides opportunity for client to learn sense of control and fosters self-esteem.
Maintain positive attitude toward the client, providing opportunities for client to exercise control as much as possible.	Cooperation can be enhanced when client feels accepted and included in problem-solving and decision-making.
Encourage activities in areas of client's interest, tasks that can be completed successfully, and reinforce when these are accomplished.	Success in accomplishing goals builds sense of self and diminishes need for disruptive acting-out behaviors.
Provide opportunities for client to make short-term attainable goals (e.g., crafts, activities).	Promotes feelings of self-worth, which can lead to increased appropriate risk-taking and the development of more elaborate future-oriented goals.
Encourage participation in activities with peer group (e.g., outings, hikes, swimming).	Social interaction and peer acceptance are among the tasks of this developmental stage. Participation helps to develop social skills.
Involve in activities to improve personal appearance (e.g., makeup, hairstyling, clothing choices).	How an individual looks affects feelings about inner self and can improve sense of self.
Use the technique of role rehearsal to help the client develop new skills to cope with changes.	Active participation in activity enhances learning.

Collaborative

Consult with resident educational therapist (teacher) regarding academic pursuits while client is hospitalized (residential treatment program).	Keeping up with class work can help to lessen further loss of self-esteem. Can be an opportunity to form a positive relationship with teacher and experience learning successes fostering personal growth and improved self-worth.
Schedule staffings with "home" school counselors, social worker, teachers, and client/parents as possible.	This maintains contact with own public/private school setting; fosters continuity for return and sense of importance for the student.

NURSING DIAGNOSIS	**NUTRITION, altered: less than/more than body requirements**
May Be Related to:	Inadequate intake of balanced, nutritional meals because of lifestyle
Possibly Evidenced by:	Reported/observed inadequate food intake and lack of weight gain, or excessive intake in relation to metabolic need with subsequent weight gain

Desired Outcomes/Evaluation Criteria—Client Will:	Satisfaction of hunger through consumption of excessive amounts of junk food
	Verbalize understanding of the relationship of food intake, exercise, and metabolism.
	Demonstrate positive eating habits with appropriate nutritional intake.
	Achieve desired weight level.

ACTIONS/INTERVENTIONS	RATIONALE

Independent

Encourage client to eat well-balanced meals on a regular basis.	Hunger can be satisfied with nutritous food intake, eliminating empty calories.
Provide information regarding nutritional intake and selection of appropriate foods that will encourage weight loss/gain as indicated.	The correlation of food intake and weight gain/loss, if understood, can lead to food choices that result in achieving appropriate weight. Foods that are self-selected are more likely to be eaten and enjoyed.
Assist client in developing insight into eating habits as they relate to feelings of anxiety. Encourage keeping a diary of food intake and related feeling(s).	Increased anxiety may lead to anorexia or frequent snacking as a response to feelings of tension.
Review daily intake diary, activity level.	This identifies reality of adequate intake in relation to energy output and helps child/family to make decision for change.
Identify blocks to adequate nutritional intake.	Factors such as substance abuse, smoking, limited/inappropriate use of financial resources, and poor family patterns may interfere with child developing healthy eating habits.

Collaborative

Refer to dietitian as needed.	Helps determine individual caloric needs while considering child/adolescent dietary preferences.

OPPOSITIONAL DEFIANT DISORDER

DSM-IV
313.81 Oppositional defiant disorder
312.9   Disruptive behavior disorder NOS

A pattern of negativistic, hostile, and defiant behavior lasting at least 6 months, in which the child loses temper, argues with adults, often actively defies or refuses adult requests or rules, blames others, deliberately does annoying things, and swears or uses obscene language. This behavior creates significant impairment in academic/social functioning but does not meet the criteria for conduct disorder. (Disruptive behavior disorder NOS reflects clinical features that constitute the subthreshold for both oppositional defiant and conduct disorders.)

ETIOLOGICAL THEORIES

Psychodynamics

The oppositional youth is fixed in the separation-individuation stage of development. The youth insists on autonomy by negative adaptive maneuvers in which he or she continually provokes adults or peers. As the youth develops internal controls, he or she will eventually grow out of these behaviors.

Genetic/Biological

Similar to the predisposition for conduct disorder, heredity contributes to individual temperament, frustration, tolerance, and the tendency to seek risks or disobey authority. The disorder may be gender-linked, as the incidence is higher in boys than in girls.

Family Dynamics

Familial and cultural norms may prohibit the degree of individual differentiation among the family members. Attempts to maintain conformity are met by negativism, disobedience, and quarrelsome defiance. Parenting skills are ineffective and/or inconsistent with reactive and emotionally charged interchanges between parent and child. Some parents interpret average or increased levels of developmental oppositionalism as hostility and as the child's deliberate effort to be in control. If power and control are issues for parents, or if they exercise authority for their own needs, a power struggle can be established between the parents and the child that sets the stage for the development of oppositional defiant disorder.

A relationship between life events and the development of anxiety disorders has been identified. This theory suggests that disruptive behavior is learned as a means for a child to gain adult attention. Anxiety generated by a dysfunctional family system, marital problems, etc., could also contribute to symptoms of this disorder. Parents become frustrated with the child's poor response to limit-setting. Parenting intervention become oversensitive or the reverse, with no external structure provided.

CLIENT ASSESSMENT DATA BASE

Activity/Rest

Difficulty playing or engaging in leisure activities quietly

Ego Integrity

Feelings of rejection, powerlessness, fear of abandonment
Blames others for what happens to self; easily annoyed by others
Passive-dependent or demanding attitude of entitlement
Family may report emotional lability

Food/Fluids

Dawdling at mealtime
Oppositional battles over food choices and at mealtimes

Hygiene

Rebellious display of defiance in personal appearance, adherence to hygiene, and personal
    habits

Neurosensory

May be depressed, angry, or react with ambivalence or hostility
Dawdling, passive resistance to time schedules, missing school bus, etc.

Social Interactions

Displays impaired social and academic functioning
Shows provocative display of defiance of adult authority figures
Deliberately engages in annoying behaviors; ignores verbal instructions/requests
Often bullies or bosses others (peers, siblings)
Aggressively interrupts play activity of others; breaking toys, making up own rules for
    games, etc.
May/may not participate in social activities
Interpersonal relationships impaired (e.g., loses temper, argues, refuses to comply with
    requests or rules, is spiteful or vindictive, projects blame for own mistakes or
    misbehavior, interrupts or intrudes on others)

Teaching/Learning

Onset usually before age 8, and not later than early adolescence
Family history of alcohol abuse

DIAGNOSTIC STUDIES

(Studies are done to rule out other conditions that may contribute to presenting problems.)
Thyroid Studies: May reveal hyperthyroid/hypothyroid conditions contributing to problems
Neurological Testing (e.g., EEG, CT Scan): Determines presence of organic brain disorders
Psychological Testing (as indicated): Rules out anxiety disorders; identifies gifted,
    borderline-retarded, or learning-disabled child; and assesses social responsiveness and
    language development.
    Note presence of physical symptoms that might indicate the existence of physical illness
(e.g., rashes, upper respiratory illness, or other allergic symptoms, CNS infection [cerebritis]
requiring appropriate diagnostic studies).

NURSING PRIORITIES

1. Promote client's ability to engage in satisfying relationships with family members, peer
    group.
2. Facilitate parents' development of effective means of coping with and interventions for
    their child's behavioral symptoms.
3. Participate in the development of a comprehensive, ongoing treatment approach using
    family and community resources.

DISCHARGE GOALS

1. Demonstrates appropriate response to limits, rules, and consequences.
2. Parents have gained (or regained) the ability to cope with internal feelings and to
    intervene effectively in their child's behavioral problems.

3. Therapeutic plan developed, with family and client participating in treatment program.
4. Plan is in place to meet needs after discharge.

NURSING DIAGNOSIS	COPING, INDIVIDUAL, ineffective
May Be Related to:	Situational or maturational crisis
	Mild neurological deficits/retardation
	Retarded ego development; low self-esteem
	Family system with dysfunctional coping methods, negative role models; abuse/neglect
Possibly Evidenced by:	Inability to meet age-appropriate role expectations
	Hostility toward others; defiant response to requests/rules
	Inability to delay gratification; manipulation of others in environment to fulfill own desires
Desired Outcomes/Evaluation Criteria— Client Will:	Demonstrate appropriate ways to assert self and establish self-worth.
	Identify adaptive coping skills that will achieve a healthy balance between independence and dependence.
	Delay gratification without manipulating others.

ACTIONS/INTERVENTIONS

Independent

Allow flexibility in shifting from one activity to another, particularly transitioning at bedtime for younger children.

Reinforce all efforts of the child when displaying appropriate efforts to establish autonomy.

Provide opportunities for imaginary play, including use of puppets, clay, sand.

Set limits on disruptive behaviors (e.g., talking incessantly); suggest alternative competing behaviors such as playing quietly.

Encourage discussion of angry feelings and identity of true object of hostility.

Explore with client alternative ways for handling frustration.

Provide positive feedback for trying new coping strategies.

Evaluate with client the effectiveness of new behaviors. Discuss modifications for improvement.

RATIONALE

Recognizing the onset of anxiety and providing flexibility will decrease likelihood of child taking an oppositional stance.

This decreases pattern of negative attention-seeking behavior.

The medium of play materials provides physical displacement of feelings and visualization of dynamics.

Child needs to know expectations and to learn competing acceptable behaviors (e.g., raising hand vs. shouting out, keeping hands to self vs. pushing others).

Dealing with feelings honestly and directly helps discourage displacement of anger onto others.

Promotes learning how to interact in society with others in more productive ways.

Supports efforts and encourages use of acceptable behaviors.

Because client has limited problem-solving skills, assistance may be required to reassess and develop strategies.

Assist client to recognize signs of escalating anxiety. Explore ways client can intervene before behavior becomes disabling.

Helps client to recognize ineffective behaviors and develop new coping skills to effect positive change.

Collaborative

Administer medication as indicated, e.g.:
imipramine (Tofranil), paroxetine (Paxil), sertraline (Zoloft);

diazepam (Valium), chloridiazepoxide (Librium), alprazolam (Xanax).

Antidepressants may be used when depression is a factor in the disorder.

Antianxiety medications provide relief from effects of anxiety, facilitating cooperation with therapy and enhancing sense of self-control.

NURSING DIAGNOSIS	SOCIAL INTERACTION, impaired
May Be Related to:	Retarded ego development; low self-esteem
	Family system with dysfunctional coping methods, negative role models; abuse/neglect
	Neurological impairment; mental retardation
Possibly Evidenced by:	Discomfort in social situations
	Difficulty playing/interacting with others; aggressive, loses temper, argues, bullies/bosses others
	Interrupts or intrudes on others; refuses to comply with requests or rules
Desired Outcomes/Evaluation Criteria—Client Will:	Identify feelings that lead to poor social interactions.
	Participate appropriately in interactive play with another child or group of children.
	Develop a mutual relationship with another child or adult.

ACTIONS/INTERVENTIONS	RATIONALE

Independent

Develop trust relationship with child, show acceptance of child separate from unacceptable behavior.

Acceptance and trust encourage feelings of self-worth.

Encourage client to verbalize feelings of inadequacy and need for acceptance from others. Discuss how these feelings affect relationships by provoking defensive behaviors such as blaming and manipulating others.

Recognition of problem is first step toward resolution.

Engage in play activities, board games, sports, team-building exercises.

Learning appropriate cooperative play activities provides outlet for healthy interactions, leadership skills.

Offer positive reinforcement for appropriate social interaction. Ignore ineffective methods of relating to others; teach competing behaviors.

Behavior modification can be an effective method of reducing disruptive behaviors in children by encouraging repetition of desirable behaviors.

87

Identify situations that provoke defensiveness and role-play more appropriate responses.

Provide opportunities for group interaction and encourage a positive and negative peer feedback system.

Collaborative

Encourage participation in psychoeducation groups on assertiveness training, problem-solving, social skills.

Arrange staffings with other professionals (e.g., social workers, teachers). Include parents and child when possible.

Attention to unacceptable behavior may actually reinforce it.

Provides confidence to deal with difficult situations when they occur.

Appropriate social behavior is often learned from age-mates.

This is a helpful arena in which to practice new social skills, receive feedback with the support for efforts to improve.

Cooperation and coordination among those working with these children will enhance the treatment program. Including the child and parents provides them an opportunity to understand the total problem and proposed treatment program.

NURSING DIAGNOSIS	**SELF ESTEEM disturbance**
May Be Related to:	Retarded ego development
	Lack of positive feedback with repeated negative feedback
	Family system with dysfunctional coping methods; abuse/neglect; negative role models
	Mild neurological deficits
Possibly Evidenced by:	Lack of eye contact
	Lack of self-confidence
	Engagement in physically dangerous activity; refusal to engage in activities or involvement without consideration of consequences
	Derogatory remarks about self and/or bragging about self
	Distraction of others to cover up own deficits or failures (e.g., acting the clown)
	Projection of blame/responsibility for problems; rationalization of personal failures, grandiosity
Desired Outcomes/Evaluation Criteria— Client Will:	Verbalize increasingly positive self-regard.
	Demonstrate beginning awareness and control of own behavior.
	Participate in new activities without extreme fear of failure.

ACTIONS/INTERVENTIONS	RATIONALE

Independent

Convey acceptance and unconditional positive regard.	May help child increase own sense of self-worth.
Assist child to identify basic ego strengths/positive aspects of self; give immediate feedback for acceptable behavior.	Focusing on positive aspects of personality may help improve self-concept. Positive reinforcement enhances self-esteem and increases desired behavior.
Spend time with client in 1:1 and group activities.	Conveys to client that you believe he or she is worthy of time and attention.
Provide opportunities for success; plan activities based on ability level (including noncompetitive and team building), set agreed-upon time limits for task completion.	Repeated successes can help to improve self-worth.
Discuss fears, encourage involvement in new activities/tasks.	Confronting concerns and engaging in new tasks promotes personal growth and new skills.
Identify possible consequences of actions (e.g., refusal to follow rules, engaging in activities for high-risk behaviors without forethought).	Helps client begin to recognize own responsibility for consequences of behavior and provides opportunity to consider alternatives.
Help client set realistic, concrete goals and determine appropriate actions to meet these goals.	Provides a structure to develop sense of hope for the future and framework for reaching desired goals.

Collaborative

Provide learning opportunities, structured learning environment (e.g., self-contained classroom, individually planned educational program).	Successful school performance is essential to preserve a child's positive self-image.

NURSING DIAGNOSIS	FAMILY COPING, ineffective: compromised/disabling
May Be Related to:	Excessive guilt, anger, or blaming among family members regarding child's behavior
	Parental inconsistencies; disagreements regarding discipline, limit-setting, and approaches
	Exhaustion of parental resources due to prolonged coping with disruptive child
Possibly Evidenced by:	Unrealistic parental expectations
	Rejection or overprotection of child
	Exaggerated expressions of anger, disappointment, or despair regarding child's behavior or ability to improve or change
Desired Outcomes/Evaluation Criteria—Family/Parent(s) Will:	Demonstrate more consistent, effective intervention methods in response to child's behavior.

Desired Outcomes/Evaluation Criteria—Family/Parent(s) Will (cont.):	Express and resolve negative attitudes toward child.
	Identify and use support systems appropriately.

ACTIONS/INTERVENTIONS	RATIONALE
Independent	
Provide information and materials related to child's disorder and effective parenting techniques. (Refer to CP: Parenting.)	Appropriate knowledge and skills may increase parental effectiveness.
Encourage parents to verbalize feelings and explore alternative methods of dealing with child.	Supportive counseling can assist parents in developing coping strategies.
Provide feedback and reinforce effective parenting methods.	Positive reinforcement can increase self-esteem and encourage continued efforts.
Involve siblings in family discussions and planning for more effective family interactions.	Family problems affect all members, and treatment is more effective when everyone is involved in therapy.
Collaborative	
Refer to community resources as indicated including psychotherapy, parent support groups, parenting classes (Parent Effectiveness).	Developing a support system can increase parental confidence and effectiveness.

NURSING DIAGNOSIS	**KNOWLEDGE deficit [LEARNING NEED] regarding condition, prognosis, and treatment needs**
May Be Related to:	Lack of knowledge; misinformation/misinterpretation
	Mild neurological deficits; associated developmental learning disabilities; inability to concentrate; cognitive deficits
Possibly Evidenced by:	Verbalization of problem/misconceptions
	Poor school performance; repeated school suspensions
	Inappropriate or exaggerated behaviors
	Development of untoward consequences of behavior
Desired Outcomes/Evaluation Criteria—Client/Parent(s) Will:	Verbalize understanding of reasons for behavioral problems, treatment needs within developmental ability.
	Participate in learning and begin to ask questions and seek information independently.
Client Will:	Achieve cognitive goals consistent with level of temperament.

90

ACTIONS/INTERVENTIONS	RATIONALE

Independent

Provide quiet environment, self-contained classrooms, small-group activities. Avoid overstimulating places, such as school bus, busy cafeteria, crowded hallways.

Reduction in environmental stimulation may decrease distractibility and diminish onset of temper tantrums. Small groups may prevent opportunity for power struggles/control, enhancing ability to stay on task and helping client learn appropriate interaction with others, avoiding sense of isolation.

Give instructional material in written and verbal form with step-by-step explanations.

Sequential learning skills will be enhanced.

Instruct child in problem-solving skills; practice situational examples.

Effective skills may increase performance levels.

Educate child and family about the use of medications and response anticipated.

Lessening of depression and/or anxiety may promote cooperation in therapy, resulting in more acceptable behavior.

Coordinate overall treatment plan with schools, collateral personnel, child, and family.

Cognitive effectiveness will most likely be advanced when treatment is not fragmented and significant interventions are not missed because of lack of interdisciplinary communication.

ELIMINATION DISORDERS:
Enuresis/Encopresis

DSM-IV
307.6 Enuresis (not due to a general medical condition)
307.7 Encopresis without constipation and overflow incontinence
787.6 Encopresis with constipation and overflow incontinence

The *DSM-IV* defines enuresis/encopresis as repeated involuntary (or, much more rarely, intentional) voiding/passage of feces into places not appropriate for that purpose, after attaining the developmental level at which continence is expected. If continence has not been achieved, the condition can be termed "functional" or "primary." The period of continence necessary to differentiate between primary and secondary enuresis/encopresis is now considered to be 1 year. There does seem to be a significant relationship between enuresis and encopresis, although neither condition can be the direct effect of a general medical condition (e.g., diabetes, spina bifida, seizure activity) to be included in this category.

ETIOLOGICAL FACTORS
Psychodynamics

Numerous psychological interpretations exist speculating on the dynamics of toilet training and the significance of flushing bodily fluids down the toilet. Freudian theory places the fixation at the anal stage of development whereby the child fails to neutralize libidinal urges, and the aggressive impulses are fused with the pleasure of controlling bodily functions. Expulsion of feces or urination and untimed feces or urination or intentionally placing the feces in inappropriate places elicits hostility from parents. Loss of bodily functions leads to loss of self-respect, loss of friends, and feelings of shame and isolation.

Biological

Learning to control urination/defecation is a developmental task most likely achieved by age 4 or 5 and requires a mechanically effective anatomy. In some enuretic children, abnormalities in regulation of vasopressor/antidiuretic hormone (ADH) have been evidenced, with ADH regulation being linked to both the dopaminergic and serotonergic systems. A theory of developmental delay suggests there is a common underlying maturational factor that predisposes children to manifest both enuresis and behavioral disturbances. Enuresis and encopresis are normal responses to environmental stresses that occur in certain situations (e.g., when a child is separated from his or her family or is abused). In either case, as the child matures and the environmental stressors are alleviated, normal bodily control is resumed. Children who are hyperactive may have occasional accidents, as they do not attend to the sensory stimuli until it is too late.

Enuresis and its relationship to bladder capacity and urinary tract infections has been explored, as has nocturnal enuresis occurring during deep sleep with no response to arousal signals. In addition, research has been conducted to investigate the physiological basis for encopresis. These studies indicate that the act of bearing down led to decreased anal sphincter control in almost all cases.

Soiling may result from excessive fluid buildup caused by diarrhea, anxiety, or the retention overflow process, whereby leakage occurs around a retentive fecal mass. This mechanism is responsible for 75% of encopretic children.

Genetically, a child is at risk for enuresis if the parent has a history of enuresis after the age of 4. Recent research suggests a genetic mutation on chromosome 13.

Family Dynamics

As mentioned previously, the parental attitude toward cleanliness and the rigidity with which this behavior is controlled may perpetuate the fear associated with loss of bodily control. Parents often get caught up in the volitional aspects, blaming the child for "acting like a baby." Further social embarrassment ensues when school personnel target the problem in terms of "the dirty child from a dirty family." Attempts to deny the problem lead to covert behaviors such as hiding soiled clothing in lockers, under the bed, or in the trash. The child may in fact be using the only weapon available, as in the case of severe neglect and/or sexual assault.

CLIENT ASSESSMENT DATABASE

Activity/Rest

May/may not be awakened when bed-wetting occurs
Unusual sleep habits, increased incidence of sleepwalking or sleep terror disorders

Ego Integrity

Expressions of poor self-esteem (e.g., "I am bad")
Shy, withdrawn, feelings of isolation, shame
Overly anxious around adult figures
Stressors may include family conflicts/change in structure (e.g., divorce, birth of a sibling)

Elimination

History of delayed or difficult toilet training
Inattention to cues of need for elimination
Episodes of urinary incontinence twice a week for at least 3 consecutive months in child of at least 5 years of age (or equivalent developmental level)
Pattern of diurnal and/or nocturnal enuresis
One episode of soiling per month over a 3-month period in child at least 4 years of age (or equivalent developmental level)
Fecal incontinence; seepage secondary to fecal retention/colorectal loading
Anal self-stimulation may be noted in nocturnal pattern of soiling

Hygiene

Deliberate attempts to hide evidence of soiled clothing

Neurosensory

May have developmental (neuromuscular or gross motor) delays
Less than 1/3 of enuretic children have documented emotional disorders (regression is rarely reason for problem)
Acting-out behaviors (e.g., placing feces or defecating in inappropriate places for retaliation)

Safety

History/evidence of abuse may be present (condition may be related to abuse and/or the cause of abuse)

Sexuality

Avoidance of sexual activity in older adolescents

Social Interactions

Impaired social, academic functioning
Power struggles with family/school to maintain personal hygiene, change bed linens
Reluctance to engage in peer activities; social rejection (body odor)
Uncomfortable spending the night with friends either in own home or away

93

Teaching/Learning

Usual age of onset 5–7 years, developmental age of at least 4 (encopresis) or 5 (enuresis) years
Prevalence as high as 22% of 5-year-olds, 10% of 10-year-olds
Boys more often affected than girls (3:1)
History of parental enuresis
Bed-wetting suppressed only as long as medication is taken; relapse usually occurring within 3 months

DIAGNOSTIC STUDIES

Urinalysis: Rule out UTI.
Electrolytes: Identify imbalance in presence of chronic diarrhea.
Abdominal, Lower GI X-Rays: Evaluate anatomical abnormalities such as anal fissure, obstruction.
Cystometrogram (CMG): Test for bladder capacity when in question.
Detailed Toilet Training History: Baseline continence data clarifying problem and evaluating for secondary vs. primary enuresis/encopresis.
ECG: To provide baseline when starting antidepressant medication.

NURSING PRIORITIES

1. Promote understanding of condition.
2. Identify and support change in parent/child patterns of interaction.
3. Enhance self-esteem.
4. Assist client in achieving continence.

DISCHARGE GOALS

1. Condition/therapy needs are understood.
2. All parties are participating in therapeutic regimen.
3. Achieves as near a normal pattern of bowel/bladder functioning as individually possible.
4. Plan in place to meet needs after discharge.

NURSING DIAGNOSIS	URINARY ELIMINATION, altered/ BOWEL incontinence
May Be Related to:	Situational/maturational crisis
	Psychogenic factors: predisposing vulnerability; threat to physical integrity (child/sexual abuse)
	Constipation
Possibly Evidenced by:	Nocturnal and/or diurnal enuresis
	Involuntary passage of stool at least once monthly
	Strong odor of urine/feces on client
	Hiding fecal material/soiled clothing in inappropriate places
Desired Outcomes/Evaluation Criteria— Client/Family Will:	Verbalize understanding of contributing factors and appropriate interventions.
	Participate in appropriate toileting program.
Client Will:	Achieve continence.

ACTIONS/INTERVENTIONS	RATIONALE

Independent

Identify times of occurrence, preceding/precipitating events, amounts of oral fluids, and family/client response to incontinence.

Baseline data will help identify patterns and document improvement after treatment begins

Check for fecal impaction.

This may be a contributing factor.

Discuss measures client/family have tried and successes/failures to date.

Typically, parents/caregivers have tried various methods, usually getting child up periodically at night, limiting fluids before bedtime, and having older children change soiled bed linens. These methods are not very effective and usually lead to frustration, power struggles/battles.

Suggest use of bladder-stretching exercises (e.g., ask child to drink favorite beverage and wait to urinate until the urge becomes very strong, then measure the amount of urine voided). Gradually increase amount of liquid and waiting period.

Although this method can have good results, the length of time needed may be discouraging and result in the family discontinuing the program.

Discuss use of conditioning programs and ask parents/caregivers to maintain a record of occurrences for a specified period before either program begins.

The use of conditioning therapy and/or behavior modification usually does not begin until the child is age 7 or older. The child needs to make a commitment to be involved for the program to succeed. Information regarding the current individual pattern provides a baseline for future evaluation.

Instruct client/family in use of electronic nighttime monitoring device (bell and pad).

Urine alarms (e.g., Wet-Stop) have an effective cure rate of 75% to 90%. Once treatment is started, the alarm should be used every night.

Instruct parents/caregiver initially to get child up each time the urine alarm buzzer sounds, shifting the responsibility gradually to child by stating, "I want you to know you can do this all by yourself." Keep a record of how often the alarm sounds and how sound the child's sleep is.

Client may be fearful at first because of previous family interactions. In the beginning, the parents will probably awaken before the child and take the child to the bathroom. However, as the program progresses, the child will awaken more quickly and assume control. Empowerment promotes feelings of being in control.

Active-listen and involve client in developing the plan for remaining dry/clean. Institute a system of positive reinforcement. Use rewards that the child would like or agrees to. Use the previously determined baseline data to determine parameters of the reward system and when to increase schedule.

Establishing a plan to which the client agrees has more chance of success than using aversive operant behavioral interventions (e.g., bell alarm) alone. Behavioral therapy may be useful when client is included in the planning, with rewards, such as tokens having value, if client agrees to their use. **Note:** If client is not involved in planning/vested in behavioral program, then therapy becomes an external control manipulating the client rather than promoting internal control and growth.

Establish toileting routine with positive reinforcement for "sitting time" and depositing urine/feces in lavatory appropriately.

Client may begin to establish bowel/bladder habits often missing prior to treatment.

Treat occasional relapses with matter-of-fact attitude and follow through with procedures for self-hygiene.

Relapse (whether intentional or not) is to be expected but may be minimized when the client does not feel pressured/blamed for lack of cooperation.

Discuss length of treatment with parents/client and make plans for maintaining dry/clean status.

Knowing that treatment is ongoing prevents becoming discouraged and giving up treatment.

Collaborative

Administer medications as appropriate, e.g:
Imipramine (Tofranil);

May be used after age 7 for enuresis. However, drug therapy is only a temporary treatment, not a cure, as condition recurs within 3 months after medication is discontinued. Pharmacological studies indicate improvement in encopresis with relatively low doses over 2-week period. **Note:** Factors such as child's age, duration of problem, and child's motivation to change are factors that affect decision to include pharmacological agents in combination with behavioral interventions.

Desmopressin acetate (DDAVP);

Used for enuresis that has been intractable to other approaches.

Amphetamines;

These drugs lighten sleep; therefore, client is more likely to awaken to arousal signals.

Laxatives and/or mineral oil.

Given daily for a specific period of time, these agents may promote bowel motility, ease evacuation of stool.

Refer for evaluation of other therapies (e.g., hypnotherapy).

Used alone or in conjunction with conditioning, the use of hypnosis can help the child access the subconscious mind allowing the child to work through emotional conflicts and develop positive suggestions that he or she has good muscle control and will be dry in the morning. **Note:** This technique is contraindicated in the presence of child abuse.

NURSING DIAGNOSIS	BODY IMAGE disturbance/SELF ESTEEM, chronic low
May Be Related to:	Negative view of the self, maturational expectations
	Social factors; stigma attached to loss of bodily functions in public
	Family's belief that soiling/ enuresis is volitional
	Shame related to body odor
Possibly Evidenced by:	Angry outbursts/oppositional behavior
	Verbalization of powerlessness to change/control bodily functions
	Reluctance to take social risks with friends (e.g., overnights, dancing)
Desired Outcomes/Evaluation Criteria— Client Will:	Verbalize acceptance of self in situation.
	Acknowledge own responsibility and control over situation.
	Participate in treatment program to effect change.
	Engage in social activities.

ACTIONS/INTERVENTIONS	RATIONALE
Independent	
Establish a therapeutic nurse/client relationship.	Within a helping relationship, the individual will begin to trust and try out new thinking and behaviors.
Promote self-concept without moral judgment by use of therapeutic communication skills. Discuss how elimination habits are formed and fact that new habits can be learned.	Individual may see self as weak, even though he or she acts as if in control. Age-appropriate information can help the child/family understand there is nothing wrong with the child and the problem can be solved.
Explain to child/family that many children have this problem. Suggest stories child can read (e.g., *Clouds and Clock*, by M. Galvin [1989]).	There is an increased risk for poor self-esteem/isolation when client views self as being "the only one." Use of bibliotherapy can help child to identify with others.
Promote active problem-solving and self-hygiene behaviors around some of the disagreeable aspects of enuresis/encopresis (e.g., control of odor, management of laundry, and successful overnight visits with friends).	Gives sense of control, supports ability to overcome stigma, enhancing self-esteem.
Be aware of own reaction to client's behavior. Avoid controlling attitude or arguing with child about hygiene or toileting routine.	Feelings of disgust, hostility, and wanting distance from these clients are not uncommon. The child may in fact be projecting his or her own negative feelings onto the caretaker. The nurse needs to deal with own responses/feelings to avoid having them interfere with care of the child.
Give positive reinforcement and encouragement for all attempts to join in peer activities or take additional risks in social situations.	Promotes repetition of desired behaviors, strengthens client's willingness to change, and enhances self-esteem.

NURSING DIAGNOSIS	**FAMILY COPING: ineffective (specify)**
May Be Related to:	Inadequate/incorrect information or understanding by primary person; belief that behavior is volitional
	Disagreement regarding treatment, coping strategies
Possibly Evidenced by:	Attempts to intervene with child are increasingly ineffective
	Significant person describes preoccupation with personal reaction (excessive guilt, anger, blame regarding child's condition/behavior)
	Significant person displays protective behavior disproportionate (too little or too much) to client's abilities or need for autonomy
Desired Outcomes/Evaluation Criteria— Family Will:	Express feelings openly and honestly.
	Identify resources within self to deal with situation.

Desired Outcomes/Evaluation Criteria—Family Will (cont.):	Verbalize realistic understanding and expectations of client.
	Provide opportunity for client to deal with situation in own way, as appropriate.

ACTIONS/INTERVENTIONS	RATIONALE

Independent

Identify behaviors of/interactions between family members.	Withdrawal, anger/hostility toward client/others, ways of touching among family members, and expressions of guilt provide clues to problems within family related to or contributing to problem.
Assess for signs of child/sexual abuse.	These issues may be contributing factors to this problem. (Refer to CP: Problems Related to Abuse or Neglect.)
Note verbal/nonverbal expressions of frustration, guilt/blame.	Problems of enuresis/encopresis are difficult for family members to deal with because of the long-term aspect of the problem. More support may be needed to deal with high level of frustration.
Determine willingness of family members to be involved in treatment program.	Success of any program depends on all members being positively committed to therapy. Uncommitted members may sabotage the program.
Encourage expression of feelings openly and honestly.	Feelings of frustration and fear are common and, unless discussed, can interfere with progress of therapy.
Discuss with the parents/caregivers the importance of being neither too strict nor too permissive in dealing with this problem.	Effective use of "win-win" methods (e.g., Active-listening, I-messages, and problem-solving) can enhance the parent/child relationship and promote good feelings about selves and others. (Refer to CP: Parenting.)
Recommend avoidance of spanking or other harsh punishment.	The use of harsh discipline usually results in power struggles where no one wins, making the problem worse and damaging the relationship between adult and child.
Help parents recognize they are not responsible for, and need to separate themselves from, the child's behavior.	Parents often believe they have been "bad" parents and are responsible for the child's failure to achieve what they view as a "natural" behavior. When they see the child as a separate individual who has responsibility for own self, they can let go and be more comfortable in resolving the problem.

ANXIETY DISORDERS

DSM-IV

309.21 Separation anxiety disorder
313.23 Selective mutism
313.89 Reactive attachment disorder of infancy or early childhood
309.24 Adjustment disorder with anxiety
307.3 Stereotypic movement disorder (stereotypy/habit disorder)

Anxiety is distinguished from fear when the emotional response to danger is not within conscious awareness, even though the anxiety may be focused on specific situations. Anxiety disorders are diagnosed when their symptoms cause significant distress or impairment. The more chronic and generalized anxiety states are called *Generalized Anxiety Disorder* (see CP). Nonphobic anxiety reactions to specific stressors are included under the diagnosis of Adjustment Disorder With Anxiety for children and adolescents. In the very young, the diagnosis would include Reactive Attachment Disorder of Infancy or Early Childhood. Separation Anxiety Disorder is the most common diagnosis.

Untreated anxiety can contribute to physical disease and stress-related disorders. Chronic anxiety potentiates the development of depression and substance abuse and increases the risk of suicide.

ETIOLOGICAL THEORIES

Psychodynamics

Anxiety arises unconsciously as internalized conflicts are brought into awareness. By age 8 months, the infant displays separation distress, an indication of the capacity for a healthy infant to differentiate self from significant others and strangers. Clinging behavior and mild separation distress are seen as appropriate and adaptive responses to stressful situations throughout childhood. When the child experiences intense and diffuse symptoms in anticipation of separation, the immature ego is not strong enough to resolve the conflict.

Biological

Anticipatory anxiety is generated physiologically within the limbic system of the brain. Several neurotransmitters including serotonin and norepinephrine are associated with the anxiety response within the CNS. Evidence suggests that children who meet behavioral criteria for anxiety disorders may not manifest panic symptoms because of the immaturity of the norepinephrine system. Should this be proved, panic disorders may emerge in later stages of childhood or in adolescence. The biological response can be elicited and maintained by modifying external events. Current research indicates an increased risk for children in families with a history of anxiety disorders (e.g., panic disorder, agoraphobia) to develop these disorders themselves. The genetic mode of transmission has not been determined. Temperamental characteristics may be related to the acquisition of fear and anxiety disorders in childhood, referred to as anxiety "proneness" or "vulnerability," and may indicate an inherited disposition to these disorders. Anxiety disorders are often associated with physical complaints of stomach aches and chest pains or palpitations. On average, the child will exhibit up to eight somatic complaints associated with the anxiety disorder. Potential medical causes for the pain should not be overlooked. However, a pattern of physical symptoms often coincides with attendance at school or other anticipated events. Stereotypic behaviors may also develop in an attempt to deal with overwhelming feelings of anxiety.

Family Dynamics

The child with separation anxiety is seen as the contagion or compensation for anxiety within the family system. The child experiences distress/anxiety in response to family events, such as life-threatening illness or change in family situation (divorce, moving). The parents, in turn, may become distressed by the child's clinging behavior, and a vicious cycle begins. Often the child refuses to go to school or to sleep alone. Mutism may be a conscious or unconscious response to these stressors.

Parents may instill anxiety in their children by overprotecting them from expectable dangers or by exaggerating the dangers of the present and future. Role-modeling may also transfer fears and anxiety to children. Eldest children, children in small families or upper-socioeconomic groups, and children in families in which there is a concern about achievement, as well as children who come from single-parent homes and a slightly lower socioeconomic class, may be at increased risk.

CLIENT ASSESSMENT DATABASE

Activity/Rest

Reluctance to sleep alone or to go to sleep away from home
Frequent reports of nightmares involving theme of separation
Insomnia
Reluctance to engage in activities with any possible danger; alternatively, engaging in excessive risk-taking (counterphobic)

Ego Integrity

Acute behavioral expression of distress (i.e., crying loudly, shaking, having tantrums, displaying anxious mood, being fretful)
Feeling "different" or left out when social inhibition is present
Being described as nervous or "high-strung" by others
Fearing loss (e.g., getting lost, being kidnapped, dying) or that harm will befall major attachment figure

Elimination

Frequent urination
Diarrhea

Food/Fluid

Nausea, vomiting
Stomach aches
Possible malnourishment (reactive attachment)

Neurosensory

Dizziness, fainting with panic attacks
Headaches
Startles easily
Repetitive, driven, nonfunctional motor behavior, such as body-rocking, head-banging, mouthing of objects (stereotypic movement)
Inhibition of responses, hypervigilance or high level of ambivalence and contradictory behavior (reactive attachment)
Depressed mood

Safety

Self-destructive behaviors (e.g., head-banging, self-biting, picking at skin, hitting own body [stereotypic movement])
Evidence of bodily injury (e.g., bruising [stereotypic movement], physical abuse [reactive attachment])

Social Interactions

Difficulty being alone or participating in activities without significant adult
Appearing clingy, needy, dependent (leading to parental frustration/family conflict); displaying indiscriminate sociability, having excessive familiarity with relative strangers (reactive attachment)
May be shy, withdrawn, avoid social contact; fails to speak in specific situations
Impairment in social, academic/occupational, or other important areas of functioning
Family displaying gross negligence in caretaking with disregard of emotional/physical needs; repeated changes of primary caregiver (reactive attachment)

Teaching/Learning

Early-age onset before 18 years (separation anxiety), with early onset before age 6, or age 5 for reactive attachment disorder, with equal gender distribution
Behaviors persist for 4 weeks or more (separation anxiety, selective mutism)
Reluctance/refusal to go to school out of fear of separation
Frequent visits to school nurse for somatic complaints
Persistent failure to initiate or respond in a developmentally appropriate fashion; growth delayed (reactive attachment)

DIAGNOSTIC STUDIES

Dexamethasone Suppression Test: Children with severe separation anxiety are nearly as likely as severely depressed children to have an abnormal test result.
Laboratory Tests: As indicated by antidepressant drug therapy, nutritional state.
Neurological Testing (EEG, CT/other scans): Rules out presence of organic brain disorders.

NURSING PRIORITIES

1. Facilitate reduction in symptoms and relieve distress.
2. Prevent injury associated with the disorder, particularly with the presence of panic attacks.

DISCHARGE GOALS

1. Somatic complaints/physical symptoms decreased or alleviated as a response to distressful activities or thoughts.
2. Age-appropriate activities engaged in without fear or distress in the absence of the parent.
3. Understanding of the contagion effect of anxiety is verbalized and effective coping skills used.
4. Parent(s) enforce regular school attendance/sleeping alone, while providing positive feedback and encouragement.
5. Plan is in place to meet needs after discharge.

NURSING DIAGNOSIS	ANXIETY [severe/panic]
May Be Related to:	Situational/maturational crisis; internal transmission/contagion
	Threat to physical integrity or self-concept; unmet needs

May Be Related to (cont.):	Dysfunctional family system; independence conflicts
Possibly Evidenced by:	Somatic complaints; nightmares; excessive psychomotor activity
	Refusal to attend school; reluctance to engage in activities without presence of specific adult figure
	Persistent worry/fear of catastrophic doom to family or self
Desired Outcomes/Evaluation Criteria— Client Will:	Appear relaxed and report/demonstrate relief from somatic manifestations of anxiety.
	Engage in age-appropriate activities in absence of parent/primary caregiver without fear or distress noted.
	Demonstrate a decrease in somatic complaints and physical symptoms when faced with impending separation from significant other.

ACTIONS/INTERVENTIONS	RATIONALE
Independent	
Establish an atmosphere of calmness, trust, and genuine positive regard.	Trust and unconditional acceptance are necessary for satisfactory nurse/client relationship. Calmness is important because anxiety is easily transmitted from one person to another.
Identify a primary nurse for client/family.	Often the caregiver will experience separation anxiety at the same level as the child, and trust is necessary to begin to deal with these issues. **Note:** Disorder may be related to loss of family of origin/frequent moves and/or foster care.
Ensure client of his or her safety and security (e.g., listen to client, identify needs, be available for support).	Symptoms of panic anxiety are very frightening, and providing information regarding safety can be reassuring.
Discuss with family members contagious nature of anxious feelings.	Understanding of this contagion allows the participants to begin to recognize and deal with anxiety other is exhibiting.
Explore the child/adolescent's fears of separating from the parent(s)/caregiver. Explore with the adults possible fears they may have of separation from the child.	Some parents may have an underlying fear of separation from the child, of which they are unaware and which they are unconsciously transferring to the child.
Observe/assist client to recognize manifestations of anxiety (e.g., stomachaches, dizziness, frequent urination).	Identifies relationship of symptoms so client can make constructive changes.
Explain to child that feelings are normal bodily reactions to stress—not harmful or dangerous, just unpleasant.	Prevents adding to panic with overexaggeration or misconception about the consequences of acknowledging feeling state.
Identify factors that precede symptoms of anxiety.	Allows client to plan coping strategy and determine level of self-control.

Encourage child to bring transitional object from home (e.g., familiar toys, special pillow or blanket, pictures, posters, or music).

Use of age-appropriate object when child or adolescent is hospitalized or in treatment setting; enhances sense of security.

Use play materials (e.g., puppets, doll house, doctor/nurse kits, fairy tale stories, clay, sand tray).

Play therapy enables child to explore conflicts, express fears, and release tension.

Encourage family visitation while structuring length and frequency of contact when child is hospitalized.

Repeated reunions and separations without disastrous consequences will help to desensitize the child to separation.

Emphasize the importance of staff/family giving verbal prompts in anticipation of absences. Maintain honest information about when the caregiver will leave and when he or she will return.

Avoidance of discussion around impending separation only increases likelihood of anxiety response.

Provide information for family/siblings regarding the typical responses of childhood anxiety during critical stages of development.

Knowledge of "anticipatory anxiety state" will decrease guilt experienced by other family members while they are entering school/separating from home/family.

Help adults and child initiate realistic goals (e.g., child to stay with sitter for 2 hours with minimal anxiety, or child to stay at friend's house without own parents until 6 PM without experiencing panic anxiety).

Parents may be so frustrated with child's clinging and demanding behaviors that a different perspective and assistance with problem-solving may be helpful.

Give, and encourage parent(s)/caregiver to give, positive reinforcement for desired behaviors.

Positive reinforcement encourages repetition of desirable behaviors.

Collaboration

Administer medications as appropriate, e.g.:
Tricyclic antidepressants (e.g., imipramine [Tofranil]); Antihistamines: diphenhydramine (Benadryl); Antianxiety agents: benzodiazepines such as alprazolam (Xanax), clonazepam (Klonopin).

Use of medication can be effective in ameliorating symptoms of anxiety and enhancing child's receptiveness to therapeutic approaches.

Engage in exercise therapy program and monitor activity closely.

Useful adjunct to psychotherapy, as it decreases symptoms relating to anxiety, thought disturbances. Exercise does not need to be aerobic or intensive to achieve desired effect. **Note:** May induce panic attack for patients with panic disorder.

NURSING DIAGNOSIS	**COPING, INDIVIDUAL, ineffective**
May Be Related to:	Maturational crisis; multiple life changes and/or losses
	Personal vulnerability; inadequate coping strategies
Possibly Evidenced by:	Inability to cope/problem-solve
	Persistent, overwhelming fears and anxieties
	Inability to meet role expectations; refusal to attend school

Possibly Evidenced by (cont.):	Social inhibition; shy, withdrawn demeanor
	Panic attacks
Desired Outcomes/Evaluation Criteria— Client Will:	Demonstrate use of more effective coping techniques in response to stressful situations.
	Verbalize understanding of the need for strategies to control frightening thoughts.
	Demonstrate level of autonomy to maximize developmental potential.

ACTIONS/INTERVENTIONS

RATIONALE

Independent

Encourage child/adolescent to discuss specific situations in life that produce the most distress and describe his or her response to these situations. Include parent(s)/caregiver(s) in the discussion.

Client and family may be unaware of the correlation between stressful situations and the exacerbation of physical symptoms.

Encourage client to express fears and concerns. Avoid arguing about client's perception of situation.

Self-understanding and further explanation are enhanced when verbalizations of anxiety and distress are received in a nonjudgmental manner.

Have client envision situation in which fear commonly occurs. Assist client to accept fear, listening to bodily reactions, giving the fear time to pass.

Allows client to recognize that fears are not catastrophic or harmful. Practicing in nonstressful situation will enhance ability to deal with separation/other stressors.

Help the child/adolescent who is perfectionistic to recognize that self-expectations may be unrealistic. Connect times of unmet self-expectations to the exacerbation of physical symptoms.

Recognition of maladaptive patterns is the first step in the change process.

Assist client to learn relaxation techniques (e.g., breathing exercise, visualization, and guided imagery skills).

Enables client to manage uncomfortable manifestations of fears/anxiety, increasing self-reliance.

Encourage parent(s)/caregiver(s) and child to identify more adaptive coping strategies that the child could use in the face of anxiety that feels overwhelming. Practice behaviors through role-playing.

Practice facilitates use of the desired behavior when the individual is actually faced with the stressful situation.

Reinforce client positively when change in behavior indicates effective coping. Anticipate and accept occasional setbacks.

Positive reinforcement encourages personal growth. Consistency in effective coping is a maturational process requiring time and patience.

NURSING DIAGNOSIS	**SOCIAL INTERACTION, impaired**
May Be Related to:	Excessive self-consciousness
	Inability to interact with unfamiliar people
	Self-concept disturbance; altered thought processes

Possibly Evidenced by:	Verbalized/observed discomfort in social situations
	Verbalized/observed inability to receive or communicate a satisfying sense of belonging, caring, interest, or shared history
	Observed use of unsuccessful social interaction behaviors
Desired Outcomes/Evaluation Criteria— Client Will:	Identify feelings that lead to poor social interactions.
	Interact within therapy peer group.
	Verbalize intention of attending school and follow through with action.
	Give self positive reinforcement for changes that are achieved.

ACTIONS/INTERVENTIONS	RATIONALE
Independent	
Develop trusting relationship with client.	This is the first step in helping the client learn to interact with others.
Attend group with the child and support efforts to interact with others. Give positive feedback.	Presence of a trusted individual provides security during times of distress. Positive feedback encourages repetition.
Convey to the child that although attendance in group is expected it is acceptable not to actively participate or contribute until he or she is ready.	Small successes will gradually increase self-confidence and decrease self-consciousness, so that client will feel less anxious in the group situation.
Help client set small personal goals (e.g., "Today I will speak to one person I don't know.").	Simple, realistic goals provide opportunities for success that increase self-confidence and may encourage the client to attempt more difficult objectives in the future.

NURSING DIAGNOSIS	**VIOLENCE, self-directed/ SELF-MUTILATION, risk for**
Risk Factors May Include:	Panic states
	Emotionally disturbed child; presence of separation anxiety
	Dysfunctional family
	History of self-destructive behaviors (e.g., head-banging, self-biting, picking at skin, hitting own body)
[Possible Indicators:]	Increasing anxiety level; increased motor activity (e.g., excitement, agitation)
Desired Outcomes/Evaluation Criteria— Client Will:	Identify precipitating factors/awareness of arousal state that occurs prior to incident.

ACTIONS/INTERVENTIONS	RATIONALE
Independent	
Determine underlying dynamics of individual situation. Review previous episodes of acting-out/self-destructive behavior.	Information is necessary to promote individual-ized planning of care.
Identify situations that interfere with ability to control own behavior (e.g., panic state).	Additional restraints may be needed to control behavior until self-control is regained.
Observe for early signs of distress/increasing anxiety. (Refer to ND: Anxiety [severe/panic]/Fear.)	Allows for early interventions to prevent exacerbation of situation.
Provide external controls/limit-setting. Hold client, speak in low commanding voice, tell client to STOP behavior.	Helps client to regain self-control in a safe setting, maintains dignity, promotes self-esteem.
Assist client to identify feelings that precede negative behaviors.	Provides opportunity for client to institute controls/ask for help before losing control.
Assist client to learn assertive/healthy behavior rather than use of aggression. Role-play situations and responses.	Promotes positive ways of responding to stress, lessening need for anxious/nonproductive behaviors.
Provide protective headgear as indicated. Use restraints with caution.	Client may need this additional protection when behavior is severe/persists. Restraints may result in injury when client fights against them.

NURSING DIAGNOSIS	**FAMILY COPING, ineffective: compromised/disabling**
May Be Related to:	Presence of other situational/developmental crises affecting family members (e.g., divorce, addition/loss of family member, midlife crisis)
	Frequent disruptions in living arrangements
	Unrealistic parental expectations for child's achievement in areas of sports, academics, etc.
	High-risk family situations (e.g., history of neglect/abuse, substance abuse, panic disorder, depression)
Possibly Evidenced by:	SO reports frustration with clinging behaviors; colludes with truancy
	SO displays emotional lability; harsh or punitive response to tyrannical behaviors
	Neglectful care of child with regard to basic human needs

Desired Outcomes/Evaluation Criteria—Family/Caregiver Will:	SO displays protective behavior disproportionate (too little or too much) to child's abilities or need for autonomy
	Verbalize knowledge and understanding of child's condition.
	Verbalize more realistic understanding and expectations of client.
	Develop strategies to help child begin to deal with stressful situations (e.g., attending school, sleeping alone, etc).
	Provide opportunity for child to deal with situation in own way.

ACTIONS/INTERVENTIONS

RATIONALE

Independent

Establish rapport with family members/caregivers. Acknowledge difficulty of the situation for the family by Active-listening.	Promotes trust, opens lines of communication, and provides feeling of being understood.
Identify current and past behaviors of family members(s) (e.g., overprotectiveness, withdrawal, anger toward child, neglect of emotional/physical needs).	Provides beginning point to create plan of care for individual client and family/caregiver.
Provide information and materials related to child's disorder including discussion of developmental stages and growth.	Promotes knowledge and skills that help parents understand and may increase parental effectiveness.
Encourage parents/caregivers to verbalize feelings and explore alternative methods of dealing with child.	Supportive counseling can assist adults in developing coping strategies.
Provide feedback and reinforce effective parenting methods. (Refer to CP: Parenting.)	Positive reinforcement can increase self-esteem and encourages continued efforts.
Formulate plan for regular school attendance/ sleeping alone.	Provides specific interventions to help family resolve problem and goals to measure effectiveness of actions/additional needs.
Involve siblings in family discussions and planning for more effective family interactions.	Family problems affect all members and treatment is more effective when everyone is involved in therapy.

Collaborative

Refer to community resources as indicated including psychotherapy, parent support groups, parenting classes (Parent Effectiveness).	Developing a support system and learning new skills can increase parental confidence and effectiveness.

PARENTING: Growth-Promoting Relationship

DSM-IV
V61.20 Parent-child relational problem

Many parents are concerned about how to raise responsible children who have high self-esteem, demonstrate self-control, and display skills of cooperation and consideration of others. Most people believe that we somehow know how to "parent" instinctively. Usually, this attitude results in parenting the same way we were parented. However, it is clear that the traditional authoritarian or permissive methods of parenting create inner conflict for most parents, and praise, punishment, and rewards do not have the desired effects of positive relationships with children. Conflicts in the parent/child relationship can lead to dysfunctional/abusive relationship patterns. In addition, when children are experiencing mental health crises requiring therapeutic intervention, learning different ways of parenting becomes essential to developing positive relationships between parent and child. It is generally accepted that primary prevention activities (e.g., parenting classes, support for new parents) produce more functional families and are cost-effective for society over the long run.

ETIOLOGICAL THEORIES

Psychodynamics

Effective parenting is a learned skill and is not a set of instinctive behaviors. Parental roles are derived from many factors (e.g., the family of origin, family myths and scripts, parental skills, knowledge and level of differentiation, socioeconomic and cultural factors, and the marital relationship). Family interactional patterns develop in a predictable pattern over time. The family rules that develop out of these patterns can be functional or dysfunctional. Functional rules are workable and constructive, promoting the needs of all family members. Dysfunctional rules are contradictory, self-defeating, and destructive.

Biological

There is a genetic plan for the growth and development of the physical body. In the same way, there is a biological plan for intelligence that is genetically encoded within the individual and drives the child from within. At the same time, parents provide an anxiety-conditioned view of the world that conflicts with the child's nature. Many of the problems of parenting are caused by people ignoring this plan of nature. When parental expectations of child behavior are inconsistent with the reality of a developmental stage (i.e., bladder/bowel training) conflicts arise that may result in dysfunctional parenting.

Family Dynamics

A family is seen as a natural social system, with its own set of rules, definition of roles, power structure, and methods of communicating, negotiating, and problem-solving that provides a means of dealing with the process of daily living. These family patterns are largely unconscious and set the emotional tone. These systems are multigenerational, with underlying family dynamics affecting all members in some way. These patterns may be functional or dysfunctional.

PARENT ASSESSMENT DATA BASE

Activity/Rest

Difficulty sleeping
Exhaustion

Ego Integrity

Broad range of feelings (e.g., calm to hysterical) may be noted

May display increasing tension and disorganization (e.g., anger, frustration, crying, depression); may repeat the same question over and over

Defense mechanisms (e.g., denial, rationalization, defensiveness, intellectualization, projection)

Multiple stress factors, changes in relationships

Feelings of helplessness, hopelessness, powerlessness

Food/Fluid

Difficulty eating, loss of appetite

Hygiene

General appearance of family members (neat or disheveled; clean or odious) may be indicators of coping ability, state of denial, presence of crisis

Neurosensory

Behavior: Upset, anxious, rapid speech or quiet and withdrawn; appropriate or inappropriate

Social Interactions

Family Genogram: Determine patterns between family members and generations and identify potential positive and negative dynamics

Family structure: May be traditional 2-parent, or single-parent (mother or father as head), blended (stepfamily), or other nontraditional structure

Lack of/limited support (presence of/geographic distance and degree of involvement of extended family)

Some family member(s) may not seem to be experiencing symptoms of stress or may possibly have changed their usual patterns of interacting

Varied socioeconomic/cultural factors (e.g., financial status, inclusion of extended family, family myths and beliefs, sense of community)

Multiple losses/crises (e.g., death, divorce, other separations, frequent relocation)

History of period of family disorganization often present

Child-rearing practices may be ineffective; dysfunctional/ineffective communication patterns present

History of child abuse/sexual abuse

NURSING PRIORITIES

1. Promote positive feelings about parenting abilities.
2. Involve parents in problem-solving solutions for current situation.
3. Provide assistance to enable family to develop skills to deal with present situation.
4. Facilitate learning of new parenting skills.

DISCHARGE GOALS

1. Parenting role, expectations, and responsibilities understood.
2. Aware of own strengths, individual needs, and methods/resources to meet them.
3. Demonstrates appropriate attachment/parenting behaviors.
4. Involved in activities directed at family growth.
5. Plan in place to meet needs after discharge.

NURSING DIAGNOSIS	PARENTING, altered, actual (or risk for)
May Be Related to:	Lack of/ineffective role model; lack of support between or from significant other(s)
	Interruption in bonding process
	Lack of knowledge; unrealistic expectations for self, child, partner
	Presence of stressors: recent crisis, financial, legal, household move, change in family structure
	Physical/psychosocial/sexual abuse by nurturing figure
	Lack of appropriate response of child to parent/parent to child
Possibly Evidenced by:	Frequent verbalization of disappointment in child; resentment toward child; inability to care for/discipline child
	Lack of parental attachment behaviors (e.g., negative characterizations of child; lack of touching; inattention to child's needs)
	Inappropriate or inconsistent discipline practices and/or caretaking behaviors
	Growth and/or developmental lag in child
	Presence of child abuse or abandonment
Desired Outcomes/Evaluation Criteria— Parent(s) Will:	Verbalize realistic information and expectations of parenting role and acceptance of situation.
	Identify own needs, strengths, and methods/resources to meet them.
	Demonstrate appropriate attachment and effective parenting behaviors.

ACTIONS/INTERVENTIONS	RATIONALE

Independent

Determine existing situation and parental perception of the problems, noting presence of specific factors such as psychiatric/physical illness, disabilities of child or parent.	Identification of the individual factors will aid in focusing interventions and establishing a realistic plan of care.
Identify developmental stage of the family (e.g., first child/new infant, school-age/adolescent children, stepfamily).	These factors affect how family members view current problems and how they will solve them.
Determine cultural/religious influences on parenting expectations of self/child, sense of success/failure.	This information is crucial to helping the family to identify and develop a treatment plan that meets its needs.
Assess parenting skill level, considering intellectual, emotional, and physical strengths and limitations.	Identifies areas of need for further education, skill training, and factors that might interfere with ability to assimilate new information.

Note attachment behaviors between parent and child(ren), recognizing cultural background. Encourage the parent(s) to hold and spend time with the child, particularly the newborn/infant.	Lack of eye contact and touching may indicate bonding problems. (Behaviors such as eye-to-eye contact, use of en face position, talking to the infant in a high-pitched voice are indicative of attachment behaviors in American culture but may not be appropriate in another culture.) Failure to bond effectively is thought to affect subsequent parent-child interaction.
Observe interactions between parent(s) and child(ren).	Identifies relationships, communication skills, feelings about one another.
Note presence/effectiveness of extended family/support systems.	Provides role models for parent(s) to help them develop own style of parenting. **Note:** Role models may be negative and/or controlling.
Stress the positive aspects of the situation, maintaining a positive attitude toward the parents' capabilities and potential for improving.	Helping the parent(s) to feel accepting about self and individual capabilities will promote growth.
Involve all members of the family in learning activities.	Learning new skills is enhanced when everyone is involved and interacting.
Provide specific information about limit-setting, time management, and conflict resolution.	New information and skills can help manage parenting responsibilities more effectively.
Encourage parent(s) to identify positive outlets for meeting own needs (e.g., going to a movie or out to dinner). (Refer to ND: Self Esteem disturbance/Role Performance, altered.)	Parent often believes it is "selfish" to do things for own self, that children are primary. However, parents are important, children are important, and the family is important. As a rule, when parents take care of themselves, they are better parents.
Discuss issues of stepparenting and ways to achieve positive relationships in a blended family. Refer to resources such as books, classes for stepfamilies.	Blending two families can be a very demanding task and preconceived ideas can be counterproductive. Providing information can help people learn to negotiate and develop skills for living together in a new configuration.

NURSING DIAGNOSIS	SELF ESTEEM, disturbance [specify]/ROLE PERFORMANCE, altered
May Be Related to:	View of self as "poor," ineffective parent(s)
	Problems of child(ren), including psychiatric/physical illness of the child
	Belief that seeking help is an admission of defeat/failure
Possibly Evidenced by:	Change in usual patterns/responsibility
	Expressions of lack of information about parenting skills
	Lack of follow-through of therapy; not keeping appointments; nonparticipation in therapy
Desired Outcomes/Evaluation Criteria— Parent(s) Will:	Verbalize acceptance of selves as parents who are not perfect.
	Verbalize understanding of role expectations/obligations.

111

ACTIONS/INTERVENTIONS	RATIONALE

Independent

Assess level of parent's anxiety, and determine the parent's perception and reality of the situation.	Identification of how family members view the situation and their role in what is happening is essential to the development of the plan of care. The difference between what is actually happening and individual perception can provide helpful clues to family problems and defense mechanisms.
Discuss parental perceptions of their skills and roles as parents. Give information as needs are identified.	Parent may see self as a "bad parent" when children have problems and do not live up to expectations of either the parents or society. **Note:** Information can be given and may be more readily accepted in casual learning environment.
Listen to expressions of concern about others' reactions to child's behavior/problems, sense of their control over self/situations.	Parent(s) may allow themselves to be influenced by "what others think" rather than establishing own actions, beliefs, and control.
Note previous and current level of adaptive behaviors/defense mechanisms.	Identifies positive/negative skills and establishes baseline for assisting parents to identify things they already do well and to learn new ways of parenting.
Encourage open discussion of situation/expression of feelings.	Helps individuals identify areas of concern, hear own ideas, and share with other members of the family.
Acknowledge and accept feelings of anger and hostility.	Parents may believe that expression of negative feelings is not acceptable. However, feelings are OK and are signals of something that needs to be acknowledged and dealt with.
Set limits on maladaptive behaviors and suggest alternative actions, such as hitting pillows, pounding a mattress, taking a walk.	Anger may be expressed by unacceptable actions such as hitting/breaking objects in the environment or in violence toward themselves or others.
Have parents identify positive behaviors they already use (e.g., positive I-messages, hugging one another, use of listening skills).	Improves feelings of self-worth and increases sense of self-esteem when parents recognize that they do have strengths on which to build/establish more positive family interactions.
Encourage individuals to become aware of own responsibility for dealing with what is happening.	Each person has control only over own self and cannot control or make another do anything.
Assist parent(s) to look at own role(s) as actor/reactor to what has been happening in the family.	May limit own options by reacting to situations rather than taking action to make things better.
Help parent(s) avoid comparisons with others.	Each family and the individuals involved have unique ways of dealing with own problems, and comparisons are usually used in a negative way to prove own lack of self-worth.

Assist parents to learn therapeutic communication skills (e.g., I-messages, Active-listening.) Discuss the use of positive I-messages instead of praise.	Improving skills for talking to others offers the opportunity to enhance relationships. Positive I-messages help the individual to develop own internal sense of self-worth, self-esteem.
Provide empathy, not sympathy.	Empathy is objective and communicates an understanding of the other's problems as viewed by that individual, promoting the "I-Thou" relationship. Sympathy is subjective and expresses concern for the nurse's own feelings.
Use positive words of encouragement for improvements noted.	Can help to reinforce development of positive coping behaviors.
Discuss inaccuracies in perception as they become apparent.	Encourages parents to identify areas of needed action.

Collaborative

| Encourage attendance at group therapy (family and multifamily), assertiveness training, and positive self-esteem classes. | Learning new skills helps individuals develop an improved sense of self-worth. |

NURSING DIAGNOSIS	FAMILY PROCESSES, altered
May Be Related to:	Situational crisis of child/adolescent (e.g., illness/hospitalization, delinquency)
	Maturational crisis (e.g., adolescence, midlife)
Possibly Evidenced by:	Expressions of confusion and difficulty coping with situation
	Family system not meeting physical, emotional, and/or security needs of members
	Difficulty accepting help, not dealing with traumatic experiences constructively
	Parents not respecting each other's parenting practices
Desired Outcomes/Evaluation Criteria— Parent(s) Will:	Express feelings appropriately.
	Demonstrate individual involvement in problem-solving.
	Verbalize understanding of child/family problems.
	Take responsibility for own words/actions.

ACTIONS/INTERVENTIONS	RATIONALE

Independent

| Assess family components, roles, dynamics, developmental stage (e.g., young/adolescent children, divorced with stepparents, children leaving home), and cultural influences. | Information is essential to development of plan of care. |

Identify patterns of communication within family.	Helps establish areas of positive and negative patterns.
Determine boundaries within the family system.	Boundaries need to be clear so individual family members are free to be responsible for themselves.
Assess use of addictive substances by members of the family.	Alcoholism and other drug use may be a critical issue in the interacting of the family as well as in developing a treatment plan. **Note:** Individuals may be reluctant to share this information until they feel safe within the therapeutic relationship.
Identify patterns of communication between individual members and the family as a whole.	May be ineffective in accomplishing family tasks and may be maintaining the maladaptive behaviors/relationships.
Identify and encourage previously successful coping mechanisms.	Using these behaviors will be comfortable for the individual, and a sense of competence and assurance will be gained.
Acknowledge differences among family members with open dialogue about how these differences have been derived.	Conveys an acceptance of these differences among individuals and helps to look at how the differences can be used to facilitate the family process.
Identify effective parenting skills already being used and suggest new ways of handling difficult behaviors.	Allows the individual to realize that some of what has been done already has been helpful and assists in learning new skills to manage the situation in a more effective manner.
Encourage participation in role-reversal activities.	Helps to gain insight and understanding of the other person's feelings and point of view.

NURSING DIAGNOSIS	**FAMILY COPING, ineffective: compromised/disabling**
May Be Related to:	Individual preoccupation with own emotional conflicts and personal suffering/anxiety about the crisis
	Temporary family disorganization; situational crisis
	Exhausted supportive capacities of family members
	Chronically unexpressed feelings of guilt, anger, etc.
	Highly ambivalent family relationships
	Arbitrary handling of a family's resistance, which solidifies defensiveness
Possibly Evidenced by:	Expressions of concern
	Complaints about SO(s)' response to problem; expressions of despair about family reactions
	Withdrawal and/or display of protective behavior; distortion of reality about problems; denial
	Intolerance, agitation, depression, hostility, aggression
	Neglecting relationships
	Detrimental decisions/actions

Desired Outcomes/Evaluation Criteria—Family Will:	Express more realistic expectations of themselves and situation.
	Identify internal and external resources.
	Interact with each other realistically and with understanding.
	Participate in activities to promote improved coping.

ACTIONS/INTERVENTIONS	RATIONALE

Independent

Establish rapport with family members.	Helps family members to feel comfortable and talk freely about the problems they are experiencing.
Identify premorbid behaviors and interactions. Compare with current behaviors.	Necessary baseline to help establish treatment goals and measure progress. Family members may be withdrawn, angry, hostile, and ignoring each other (or one specific member).
Note readiness of family to be involved in treatment.	Readiness and willingness are important for the success of therapy.
Encourage communication, free expression of feelings without judgment.	Promotes understanding of how others are feeling, perceiving what is happening.
Note other stressors having an impact on the family (e.g., financial, legal, physical illness).	May need assistance with these factors before the family can begin to deal with the issues at hand.
Encourage questions, provide accurate information, involve family in treatment planning. (Refer to ND: Knowledge deficit.)	Personal involvement by client and family enhances learning and promotes cooperation with/success of therapy.
Reframe individual's negative statements when possible.	Provides a different way of looking at the problem/situation.
Encourage dealing with the problems in small increments.	One moment at a time can seem more manageable than looking at the whole picture.

Collaborative

Refer to social services, support group, marriage counselor, community/spiritual resources as indicated.	Family may need additional help and support to resolve issues, incorporating new techniques and problem-solving.

NURSING DIAGNOSIS	FAMILY COPING: potential for growth
May Be Related to:	Surfacing of self-actualization goals
Possibly Evidenced by:	Expressing interest in making contact with another person experiencing a similar situation
	Moving in direction of health promoting/enriching lifestyle, auditing, negotiating therapy program, generally choosing experiences that optimize growth

Desired Outcomes/Evaluation Criteria—Family Will:	Express willingness to look at own role in the situation.
	Verbalize desire to change, and feelings of self-confidence, satisfaction with progress.
	Identify/use resources appropriately.

ACTIONS/INTERVENTIONS	RATIONALE

Independent

Determine situation and stage of growth family is experiencing. Note verbalizations of awareness of the growth, impact of the situation/crisis, and expressed interest in learning opportunity.	Baseline data required to establish plan of assistance and measure progress/growth.
Listen to expressions of hope, planning, and so forth.	Acknowledgment by the nurse provides reinforcement of hopes and desires for positive change for the future.
Discuss values/beliefs, note expression of change or "rethinking" of values.	Willingness to look at own values, discuss meanings, and make decisions about own beliefs is helpful to growth of family members.
Role-model/identify individual(s) for parent(s) to observe and be involved with.	Provides opportunity to learn new behaviors.
Role-play new ways of interacting.	Allows client and family to "practice" how they will respond in stressful situations, in an effort to prevent future crises.
Encourage open communication within the family (no "family secrets") and use of effective communication skills (e.g., I-messages, Active-listening).	Open acceptance of a variety of feelings and attitudes is necessary for growth within the family system.
Assist individuals to learn new effective ways of dealing with feelings.	Learning to identify and express feelings provides opportunity to act in different ways.

Collaborative

Identify with others who have had similar experiences (e.g., multifamily group therapy, support groups, stepfamily group).	Sharing of experiences provides opportunities to develop empathy and understanding of parenting roles; helps family members realize others have same dilemmas.
Refer to educational resources (e.g., parenting classes, assertiveness training, headstart program).	Helps individuals to see how they and others solve problems, effectively or ineffectively, and provides role models and opportunities to learn new skills.

NURSING DIAGNOSIS	KNOWLEDGE deficit [LEARNING NEED] regarding parenting skills, developmental stages
May Be Related to:	Lack of information/unfamiliarity with resources about child growth and development; information misinterpretation

Possibly Evidenced by:	Ineffective parenting skills
	Angry expressions about parenting role
	Verbalization of problems in dealing with child(ren)
	Statements of misconceptions about how to parent
	Inappropriate or exaggerated behaviors (e.g., hostile, agitated, apathetic)
Desired Outcomes/Evaluation Criteria— Parents Will:	Participate in learning process/activities.
	Assume responsibility for learning new parenting skills.
	Identify stressors and actions to deal effectively with them.
	Initiate necessary lifestyle changes.

ACTIONS/INTERVENTIONS

RATIONALE

Independent

ACTIONS/INTERVENTIONS	RATIONALE
Determine level of knowledge of parenting skills and beliefs.	Individual needs are based on current information and/or beliefs and misconceptions.
Note level of anxiety and signs of avoidance; cultural beliefs about parents and children; feelings about self as a parent.	Moderate to severe anxiety, level of self-esteem, cultural beliefs can interfere with desire/ability to learn new information.
Review information about developmental level of child(ren), expected maturational progression, and individual nature of process. Discuss parental expectations.	This knowledge helps parents to recognize and accept behavior related to growth process and promotes realistic individual expectations.
Provide information and help parent(s) learn new communication skills of Active-listening and declarative, responsive, preventive, and positive I-messages. Discuss conflict-resolution concepts of "who owns the problem," problem-solving and resolving of value collisions.	Learning new methods of interaction promotes improved relationships among family members and helps to resolve current situation/conflicts. Conflict is inevitable in relationships with others, and learning to understand the other person's point of view and effective ways to deal with differences can strengthen and enhance the relationship between family members.
Be aware of "teachable moments" that occur during interaction with the family and/or individual members.	Taking advantage of opportunities as they present themselves can enhance the learning situation.
Promote active participation in learning by the use of role-play, participant discussion, and other activities.	Learning is enhanced when the individual is actively engaged in the process.
Provide positive reinforcement for attempts to learn new behaviors/communication skills.	Parent frequently feels guilty and critical of self when a child has difficulties, and positive feedback can help individual to be more realistic about own self, the child, and the situation.
Provide information about additional resources (e.g., books on related topics, tapes).	Bibliotherapy can be a helpful adjunct to information given by other means as well as providing a continuation of learning in informal/home setting.
Refer to social workers, clergy, psychotherapy, and/or classes such as parent effectiveness and assertiveness training.	Additional resources may help with resolution of other, deeper problems/concerns (e.g., divorce, stepfamily issues).

117

CHAPTER 5

DEMENTIA AND AMNESTIC AND OTHER COGNITIVE DISORDERS

DEMENTIA OF THE ALZHEIMER'S TYPE/VASCULAR DEMENTIA

DSM-IV
DEMENTIA OF THE ALZHEIMER'S TYPE (DAT)
Early Onset (At or Below Age 65)
290.10 Uncomplicated
290.11 With delirium
290.12 With delusions
290.13 With depressed mood
Late Onset (After Age 65)
290.0 Uncomplicated
290.3 With delirium
290.20 With delusions
290.21 With depressed mood
(Note: DAT should also be coded on Axis III, 331.0.)
VASCULAR DEMENTIA
290.40 Uncomplicated
290.41 With delirium
290.42 With delusions
290.43 With depressed mood
Note: In the presence of vascular dementia, the specific underlying medical cause, such as stroke, should be coded on Axis III.
(For dementias due to other general medical conditions, refer to DSM-IV for specific code listing.)

Dementia of the Alzheimer's type is a specific degenerative process occurring primarily in the cells located at the base of the forebrain that send information to the cerebral cortex and hippocampus. It is the most common form of dementia and is characterized by a steady and global decline. In comparison, vascular dementia reflects a pattern of intermittent deterioration related to multiple infarcts to various areas of the brain. Although the etiologies differ, these two forms of dementia share a common symptom presentation and therapeutic intervention.

118

ETIOLOGICAL THEORIES

Psychodynamics

These forms of dementia reflect a chronic organic mental disorder with progressive cognitive losses caused by damage to various areas of the brain, depending on underlying pathology. Personality change is common and may be manifested by either an alteration or accentuation of premorbid characteristics with primary deficits in memory and planning and a predisposition to confusion.

Biological Theories

Vascular dementia reflects a pattern of intermittent deterioration in the brain. Symptoms fluctuate and are determined by the area of the brain that is affected. Deterioration is thought to occur in response to repeated infarcts of the brain. Predisposing factors include cerebral and systemic vascular disease, hypertension, cerebral hypoxia, hypoglycemia, cerebral embolism, and severe head injury.

Several studies have shown that antibodies are produced in the brains of individuals with Alzheimer's disease. Although the triggering mechanism is not known, the reactions are actually autoantibody production, suggesting a possible alteration in the body's immune system. Although the exact cause of Alzheimer's disease is unknown, several hypotheses have been supported by varying amounts and quality of research data. The exception is research on environmental causes, such as the ingestion of aluminum, which to date have not been supported by research findings. Research has revealed that, in DAT, the enzyme required to produce acetylcholine is dramatically reduced, especially in the areas of the brain where the senile plaques and neurofibrillary tangles occur in the greatest numbers. This decrease in acetylcholine production reduces the amount of neurotransmitter that is released to cells in the cortex, hippocampus, and nucleus basalis, resulting in a disruption of memory processes. Additionally, the neuritic plaques that accumulate are composed of beta-amyloid, an insoluble protein that is an abnormal breakdown product of the cell membrane constituent amyloid precursor protein (APP). Furthermore, the formation of the customary plaques and tangles appears to be related to the cholesterol-transporting protein, apolipoprotein-E (ApoE), which has been associated with an earlier-than-average age of onset for the common form of Alzheimer's disease for individuals who carry the $ApoE_4$ genetic variant.

Thus, genetics appears to play a role. Studies suggest a familial pattern of transmission that is four times greater than in the general population. Familial, or early-onset Alzheimer's, has been linked to defects of genes on chromosomes 1, 14, or 21, with some families exhibiting a pattern of inheritance that suggests possible autosomal-dominant gene transmission. Furthermore, Down syndrome (extra chromosome 21) may have some relationship to Alzheimer's disease. At autopsy, both have many of the same pathophysiological changes, and a high percentage of individuals with Down syndrome who survive to adulthood develop Alzheimer's lesions by age 50. (Incidentally, these individuals carry two copies of the gene for APP.)

Current research suggests that Alzheimer's disease may actually be a lifelong process, with changes in the brain developing decades before the onset of dementia. Other researchers theorize that a rich education may increase a person's reserve of brain cells or connections between nerve cells, either of which could reduce the risk of dementia.

CLIENT ASSESSMENT DATA BASE

Activity/Rest

Feeling tired; fatigue may increase severity of symptoms, especially as evening approaches

Day/night reversal; wakefulness/aimless wandering, disturbance of sleep rhythms

Lethargy; decreased interest in usual activities, hobbies; inability to recall what is read/follow plot of television program; possibly forced to retire

Impaired motor skills; inability to carry out familiar, purposeful movements

Content sitting and watching others

Main activity may be hoarding inanimate objects; repetitive motions (e.g., fold-unfold-refold linen), hiding articles, or wandering

Circulation

Possible history of systemic/cerebral vascular disease, hypertension, embolic episodes (predisposing factors)

Ego Integrity

Behavior often inconsistent; verbal/nonverbal behavior may be incongruent

Suspicious or fearful of imaginary people/situations; clinging to significant other(s)

Misperception of environment, misidentification of objects/people, hoarding objects; belief that misplaced objects are stolen

Multiple losses; changes in body image and self-esteem

Emotional lability (cries easily, laughs inappropriately); variable mood changes (apathy, lethargy, restlessness, short attention span, irritability); sudden angry outbursts (catastrophic reactions)

May deny significance of early changes/symptoms, especially cognitive changes, and/or describe vague, hypochondriacal reports (e.g., fatigue, diarrhea, dizziness, occasional headaches)

May conceal limitations (e.g., make excuses for not being able to perform tasks; thumbing through a book without reading it)

Feelings of helplessness; strong, depressive overlay; delusions; paranoia

Elimination

Urgency (may indicate loss of muscle tone)

Incontinence of urine/feces

Prone to constipation/impaction, with diarrhea

Food/Fluid

Hypoglycemic episodes (predisposing factor)

Lack of interest in/forgetting of mealtimes; dependence on others for food cooking and preparation at table, feeding, using utensils

Changes in taste, appetite; denial of hunger/refusal to eat (may be trying to conceal lost skills)

Loss of ability to chew (silent aspiration)

Weight loss; decreased muscle mass; emaciation (advanced stage)

Hygiene

May be dependent on SO to meet basic hygiene needs

Appearance disheveled, unkempt; body odor present; poor personal habits

Clothing may be inappropriate for situation/weather conditions

Misinterpretation of, or ignoring, internal cues, forgetting steps involved in toileting self, or inability to find the bathroom

Neurosensory

Concealing inabilities (may make excuses not to perform task, may thumb through a book without reading it)

Family members may report a gradual decrease in cognitive abilities, impaired judgment/

inappropriate decisions, impaired recent memory but good remote memory, behavioral changes/individual personality traits altered or exaggerated
Loss of proprioception sense (location of body/body parts in space)
Primitive reflexes (e.g., positive snout, suck, palmar) may be present
Facial signs/symptoms dependent on degree of vascular insults
Seizure activity (secondary to the associated brain damage) may be reported/noted
Mental status (may laugh at or feel threatened by exams)

    Disoriented to time initially, then place; usually oriented to person until late in disease process

    Impaired recent memory, progressive loss of remote memory

    May change answers during the interview

    Difficulty in comprehension, abstract thinking

    Unable to do simple calculations or repeat the names of three objects, short attention span

    Hallucinations, delusions, severe depression, mania (advanced stage)

    May have impaired communication: difficulty with finding correct words (especially nouns); conversation repetitive or scattered with substituted meaningless words; speech may become inaudible; gradually loses ability to write (fine motor skills) or read

Safety

History of recent viral illness or serious head trauma, drug toxicity, stress, nutritional deficits (may be predisposing/accelerating factors)
Incidental trauma (falls, burns, etc.); presence of ecchymosis, lacerations
Disturbance of gait
Striking out/violence toward others

Social Interactions

Possibly fragmented speech, aphasia, and dysphasia
May ignore rules of social conduct/inappropriate behavior
Prior psychosocial factors (individuality and personality influence present altered behavioral patterns)
Family roles possibly altered/reversed as individual becomes more dependent

Teaching/Learning

Family history of DAT (4 times greater than general population); incidence of primary degenerative dementia is more common in women (who live longer) than in men; vascular dementia occurs more often in men than in women
May present a total healthy picture except for memory/behavioral changes
Use/misuse of medications, OTC drugs, alcohol

DIAGNOSTIC STUDIES

Note: Although no diagnostic studies are specific for Alzheimer's disease, these studies are used to rule out reversible problems that may be confused with these types of dementia.

Antibodies: Abnormally high levels may be found (leading to a theory of an immunological defect).

ApoE$_4$: Screens for the presence of a genetic defect associated with the common form of DAT.

CBC, RPR, Electrolytes, Thyroid Studies: May determine or eliminate treatable/reversible dysfunctions (e.g., metabolic disease processes, fluid/electrolyte imbalance, neurosyphilis).

Vitamin B$_{12}$: May disclose a nutritional deficit, if low.

Folate Levels: Low level can affect memory function.

Dexamethasone Suppression Test (DST): Rules out treatable depression.

ECG: Rules out cardiac insufficiency.

EEG: May be normal or show some slowing (aids in establishing treatable brain dysfunctions), they may also reveal focal lesions (vascular).

Skull X Rays: Usually normal but may reveal signs of head trauma.

Vision/Hearing Tests: Rule out deficits that may be the cause of or contribute to disorientation, mood swings, altered sensory perceptions (rather than cognitive impairment).

Positron-Emission Tomography (PET) Scan, Brain Electrical Activity Mapping (BEAM), Magnetic Resonance Imaging (MRI): May show areas of decreased brain metabolism characteristic of DAT. (In the future, scans may become a screening tool to reveal early changes, such as plaque formation or development of neurofibrillary tangles, for those at risk of developing dementia.)

CT Scan: May show widening of ventricles, or cortical atrophy.

CSF: Presence of abnormal protein from the brain cells is 90% indicative of DAT.

Tropicamide (Mydriacyl) Pupil Response Test: Hypersensitive to drugs that block the action of acetylcholine. Pupil dilation response to the eyedrops seems equal in clients with mild or early-stage DAT as in severe stage; therefore, this test may provide an early screening tool but is still being researched.

Alzheimer's Disease–Associated Protein (ADAP): Postmortem studies have yielded positive results in more than 80% of DAT patients. Adaptation of ADAP for live testing is being investigated.

NURSING PRIORITIES

1. Provide safe environment; prevent injury.
2. Promote socially acceptable responses; limit inappropriate behavior.
3. Maintain reality orientation/prevent sensory deprivation/overload.
4. Encourage participation in self-care within individual abilities.
5. Promote coping mechanisms of client/significant other(s).
6. Support client/family in grieving process.
7. Provide information about disease process, prognosis, and resources available for assistance.

DISCHARGE GOALS

1. Adequate supervision/support systems available.
2. Maximal level of independent functioning achieved.
3. Coping skills developed/strengthened and SOs using available resources.
4. Disease process/prognosis and client expectations/needs understood by SO.
5. Plan in place to meet needs after discharge.

NURSING DIAGNOSIS	INJURY/TRAUMA, risk for
Risk Factors May Include:	Inability to recognize/identify danger in environment, impaired judgment
	Disorientation, confusion, agitation, irritability, excitability
	Weakness, muscular incoordination, balancing difficulties, altered perception (missing chairs, steps, etc.)
	Seizure activity

Possibly Evidenced by:	[Not applicable; presence of signs and symptoms establishes an *actual* diagnosis.]
Desired Outcomes/Evaluation Criteria— Family/Caregiver(s) Will:	Recognize potential risks in the environment Identify and implement steps to correct/compensate for individual factors.
Client Will:	Be free of injury.

ACTIONS/INTERVENTIONS	RATIONALE
Independent	
Assess degree of impairment in ability/competence, presence of impulsive behavior. Assist SO to identify any risks/potential hazards and visual-perceptual deficits that may be present.	Identifies potential risks in the environment and heightens awareness of risks so caregivers are more alert to dangers. Clients demonstrating impulsive behavior are at increased risk of injury because they are less able to control their own behavior/actions. Visual-perceptual deficits increase the risk of falls.
Eliminate/minimize identified hazards in the environment.	A person with cognitive impairment and perceptual disturbances is prone to accidental injury because of the inability to take responsibility for basic safety needs or to evaluate the unforeseen consequences (e.g., may light a stove/cigarette and forget about it, mistake plastic fruit for the real thing and eat it, misjudge distance involving chairs and stairs).
Monitor behavior routinely, note timing of behavioral changes, increasing confusion, hyperactivity. Initiate least restrictive interventions before behavior escalates.	Early identification of negative behaviors with appropriate action can prevent need for more stringent measures. **Note:** "Sundown syndrome" (increased restlessness, wandering, aggression) may develop in late afternoon/early evening, requiring programmed interventions and closer monitoring at this time to redirect and protect client.
Distract/redirect client's attention when behavior is agitated or dangerous (e.g., climbing out of bed).	Maintains safety while avoiding a confrontation that could escalate behavior/increase risk of injury.
Obtain identification jewelry (bracelet/necklace) showing name, phone number, and diagnosis.	Facilitates safe return of client if lost. Because of poor verbal ability and confusion, these persons may be unable to state address, phone number, etc. Client may wander, exhibit poor judgment, and be detained by police, appearing confused, irritable, or having violent outbursts.
Dress according to physical environment/ individual need.	The general slowing of metabolic processes results in lowered body heat. The hypothalamic gland is affected by the disease process, causing person to feel cold. Client may have seasonal disorientation and may wander out in the cold. **Note:** Leading causes of death in these clients are pneumonia and accidents.

123

Lock outside doors as appropriate, especially in evening/night. Do not allow access to stairwell or exit. Provide supervision and activities for client who is regularly awake during night.

Preventive measures can contain client without constant supervision. Activities promote involvement and keep client occupied.

Be attentive to nonverbal physiological symptoms.

Because of sensory loss and language dysfunction, may express needs nonverbally (e.g., thirst by panting; pain by sweating, doubling over). **Note:** Wandering may be a coping mechanism as client seeks a change in environment (too hot/cold, bored/overstimulated), searches for food/bathroom, or relief from discomfort (pain/adverse drug reaction).

Be alert to underlying meaning of verbal statements.

May direct a question to another, such as, "Are you cold/tired?" meaning client is cold/tired.

Monitor for medication side effects, signs of over-medication (e.g., extrapyramidal signs, orthostatic hypotension, visual disturbances, GI upsets).

Client may not be able to report signs/symptoms, and drugs can easily build up to toxic levels in the elderly. Dosages/drug choice may need to be altered.

Recommend use of "child-proof locks", secure medications, cleaning products, poisonous substances, tools, sharp objects, etc. Remove stove knobs, burners.

As the disease worsens, the client may fidget with objects/locks (hypermetamorphosis) or put small items in mouth (hyperorality), which potentiates possibility of accidental injury/death.

Provide quiet room/activity.

Overstimulation increases irritability/agitation, which can escalate to violent outbursts.

Avoid continuous use of restraints. Have SO/others stay with client during periods of acute agitation.

Endangers the individual who succeeds in partial removal of restraints. May increase agitation and potentiate fractures in the elderly (owing to reduced calcium in the bones).

Collaborative

Administer medications as appropriate, e.g., thioridazine hydrochloride (Mellaril).

Short-term use of low-dose neuroleptics may moderate "sundowning" behaviors. **Note:** Condition may be related to deterioration of the suprachiasmatic nucleus of the hypothalamus (controls the sleep-wake cycle) with disturbance of circadian rhythms.

NURSING DIAGNOSIS	**CONFUSION, chronic**
May Be Related to:	Irreversible neuronal degeneration
Possibly Evidenced by:	Altered interpretation/response to stimuli
	Progressive/long-standing cognitive impairment; impaired short-term memory
	Altered personality; impaired socialization
	Clinical evidence of organic impairment
Desired Outcomes/Evaluation Criteria—Client Will:	Experience a decrease in level of frustration, especially when participating in ADLs.

Family/Caregiver Will:	Verbalize understanding of disease process and client's needs.
	Identify/participate in interventions to deal effectively with situation.
	Provide for maximal independence while meeting safety need of clients.
	Initiate behaviors/lifestyle changes to maximize client's cognitive functioning.

ACTIONS/INTERVENTIONS	RATIONALE

Independent

Assess degree of cognitive impairment (e.g., changes in orientation to person, place, time; attention span; thinking ability). Talk with SO about changes from usual behavior/length of time problem has existed.	Provides baseline for future evaluation/comparison, and influences choice of interventions. **Note:** Repeated evaluation of orientation may actually heighten negative responses/client's level of frustration.
Maintain a pleasant, quiet environment.	Reduces distorted input, whereas crowds, clutter, and noise generate sensory overload that stresses the impaired neurons.
Approach in a slow, calm manner.	This nonverbal gesture lessens the chance of misinterpretation and potential agitation. Hurried approaches can startle and threaten the confused client who misinterprets or feels threatened by imaginary people and/or situations.
Face the individual when conversing.	Maintains reality, expresses interest, and arouses attention, particularly in persons with perceptual disturbances.
Address client by name.	Names form our self-identity and establish reality and individual recognition. Client may respond to own name long after failing to recognize SO.
Use lower voice register and speak slowly to client.	Increases the chance for comprehension. High-pitched, loud tones convey stress and anger, which may trigger memory of previous confrontations and provoke an angry response.
Give simple directions, one at a time, or step-by-step instructions, using short words and simple sentences.	As the disease progresses, the communication centers in the brain become impaired, hindering the individual's ability to process and comprehend complex messages. Simplicity is the key to communicating (both verbally and nonverbally) with the cognitively impaired person.
Pause between phrases or questions. Give hints and use open-ended phrases when possible.	Invites a verbal response and may increase comprehension. Hints stimulate communication and give the person a chance for a positive experience.
Listen with regard despite content of client's speech.	Conveys interest and worth to the individual.
Interpret statements, meanings, and words. If possible, supply the correct word.	Assisting the client with word processing aids in decreasing frustration.

125

Reduce provocative stimuli: negative criticism, arguments, confrontations.	Any provocation decreases self-esteem and may be interpreted as a threat, which may trigger agitation or increase inappropriate behavior.
Use distraction. Talk about real people and real events when client begins ruminating about false ideas, unless talking realistically increases anxiety/agitation.	Rumination promotes disorientation. Reality orientation increases client's sense of reality, self-worth, and personal dignity.
Refrain from forcing activities and communications. Change activity if client loses interest in present activity.	Force decreases cooperation and may increase suspiciousness, delusions. Changing activity maintains interest and reduces restlessness and possibility of confrontation.
Use humor with interactions.	Laughter can assist in communication and help reverse emotional lability.
Focus on appropriate behavior. Give verbal feedback, positive reinforcement (e.g., a pat on the back, applause). Use touch judiciously and respect individual's personal space/response.	Reinforces correctness, appropriate behavior. A focus on inappropriate behavior can encourage repetition. Although touch frequently transcends verbal interchange (conveying warmth, acceptance, and reality), the individual may misinterpret the meaning of touch, and intrusion into personal space may be interpreted as threatening because of the client's distorted perceptions.
Respect individuality and evaluate individual needs.	Persons experiencing a cognitive decline deserve respect, dignity, and recognition of worth as an individual. Client's past and background are important in maintaining self-concept, planning activities, communicating, etc.
Allow personal belongings.	Familiarity enhances security, sense of self, and decreases feelings of loss/deprivation.
Permit hoarding of safe objects.	This activity may preserve security and counter-balances irrevocable losses.
Create simple, noncompetitive activities paced to the individual's abilities. Provide entertaining, memory-stimulating music, videos, TV programs. Engage in old hobbies, preferred activities (e.g., arts/crafts, music, supervised cooking, gardening, spiritual programs).	Motivates client in ways that will reinforce usefulness and self-worth and stimulate reality.
Make useful activities (jobs) out of hoarding and repetitive motions, (e.g., collecting junk mail, creating scrapbook, folding/unfolding linen, bouncing balls, dusting, sweeping floors).	May decrease restlessness and provide option for pleasurable activity. Having a "job" helps client feel useful.
Provide several drawers/baskets that are acceptable to rummage through. Fill with safe items that would be of interest to client, e.g., yarn balls, quilt blocks, fabrics with different texture and colors; baby clothes, pictures, costume jewelry (without pins), small tools, sports magazines.	Availability of this kind of assortment provides stimulation that enhances the sense and promotes memories of past life experiences.
Help client find misplaced items, label drawers/belongings. Do not challenge client.	May decrease defensiveness when client believes he or she is being accused of stealing a misplaced, hoarded, or hidden item. To refute the accusation will not change the belief and may invite anger.

126

Monitor phone use closely. Post significant phone numbers in prominent place, secure long-distance numbers.

Can be used as reality orientation. However, client may forget time of day when making calls, try to call dead relative, etc. Impaired judgment does not allow for distinguishing long-distance numbers and makes client easy prey for phone sales pitches.

Evaluate sleep/rest pattern and adequacy. Note lethargy, increasing irritability/confusion, frequent yawning, dark circles under eyes.

Lack of sleep can impair cognitive function and coping abilities. (Refer to ND: Sleep Pattern disturbance.)

Monitor for medication side effects, signs of overmedication.

Drugs can easily build up to toxic levels in the elderly, aggravating confusion. Dosages/drug choice may need to be altered.

Collaborative

Administer medications as individually indicated:
  Antipsychotic: e.g., haloperidol (Haldol), thioridazine (Mellaril);

Small dosages may be used to control agitation, delusions, hallucinations. Mellaril is often preferred because there are fewer extrapyramidal side effects (e.g., dystonia, akathisia), visual problems, and especially gait disturbances.
Note: Phenothiazines may cause oversedation, excitation, or bizarre reactions. Presence of postural hypotension increases the risk of falls and development of constipation, requiring inclusion of a bowel program.

  Vasodilators: e.g., cyclandelate (Cyclospasmol);

May improve mental function but requires further research.

  Ergoloid meyslates (Hydergine LC);

A metabolic enhancer (increases brain's ability to metabolize glucose and use oxygen) that has few side effects. Although it does not increase cognition and memory, it may make client more alert and less anxious/depressed. However, it may be of little value in dementia therapy because there is usually only a limited degree of improvement.
Note: This drug is expensive, and families need accurate information to make informed therapy decisions and avoid false hopes and disappointment resulting from a lack of dramatic improvement.

  Tacrine (Cognex);

Elevates acetylcholine levels in the cerebral cortex to improve cognition and functional autonomy in mild to moderate dementia. Cognex does not appear to alter the course of the disease, and its effects may lessen as the disease advances.
Note: Drug may be toxic to liver, but effect is reversible.

  Donepezil hydrochloride (Aricept);

Clinical trials have demonstrated improvement in clients with mild to moderately severe Alzheimer's disease by blocking the breakdown of acetylcholine; this drug, however, has fewer side effects than cognex.

  Anxiolytic agents: diazepam (Valium), lorazepam (Ativan), chlordiazepoxide (Librium), oxazepam (Serax);

More useful in early/mild stages, for relief of anxiety. It can increase confusion/paranoia in the elderly. **Note:** Serax may be preferred because it is shorter-acting.

127

Thiamine;

Studies are currently underway to verify the usefulness of high doses of thiamine during the early phase of the disease to slow progression of impairment/slightly improve cognition.

Investigational use of drugs approved for other uses, e.g.: NSAIDs, such as ibuprofen (Motrin); estrogen; vitamin E, selegiline (Eldepryl); and prednisone.

These drugs are being studied for possible benefit of treatment or for delaying the onset/progression of DAT.

NURSING DIAGNOSIS	SENSORY-PERCEPTUAL alterations (specify)
May be Related To:	Altered sensory reception, transmission, and/or integration (neurological disease/deficit)
	Socially restricted environment (homebound/institutionalized)
	Sleep deprivation
Possibly Evidenced by:	Changes in usual response to stimuli (e.g., spatial disorientation, confusion, rapid mood swings)
	Change in problem-solving abilities; altered abstraction/conceptualization
	Exaggerated emotional responses (e.g., anxiety, paranoia, and hallucinations)
	Inability to tell position of body parts
	Diminished/altered sense of taste
Desired Outcomes/Evaluation Criteria—Client Will:	Demonstrate improved/appropriate response to stimuli.
Caregiver(s) Will:	Identify/control external factors that contribute to alterations in sensory/perceptual abilities.

ACTIONS/INTERVENTIONS

RATIONALE

Independent

Assess degree of impairment and how it affects the individual, including hearing/visual deficits.

Although brain involvement is usually global, a small percentage of clients may exhibit asymmetrical involvement, which may cause the client to neglect one side of the body (unilateral neglect). Client may not be able to locate internal cues, recognize hunger/thirst, perceive external pain, or locate body within the environment.

Encourage use of corrective lenses and hearing aids, as appropriate.

May enhance sensory input, limit/reduce misinterpretation of stimuli.

Maintain a reality-oriented relationship and environment.

Reduces confusion and promotes coping with the frustrating struggles of misperception and being disoriented/confused.

Provide clues for 24-hour reality orientation with calendars, clocks, notes, cards, signs, music, seasonal hues, scenic pictures; color-code rooms.

Dysfunction in visual-spatial perception interferes with the ability to recognize directions and patterns, and the client may become lost, even in

Provide quiet, nondistracting environment when indicated (e.g., soft music, plain but colorful wallpaper/paint).

Helps to avoid visual/auditory overload, by emphasizing qualities of calmness, consistency. (**Note:** Patterned wallpaper may be disturbing to the client.)

Provide touch in a caring way.

May enhance perception to self/body boundaries.

Engage client in individually meaningful activities, supporting remaining abilities and minimizing failures (e.g., daily living skills including meal preparation, setup/cleaning activities, making bed, gardening/watering plants).

Supports client's dignity, familiarizes individual with home/community events and enables him or her to experience satisfaction and pleasure.

Use sensory games to stimulate reality (e.g., smell mentholated ointment and tell of the time mother used it on client; use of spring/fall nature boxes).

Communicates reality through multiple channels.

Indulge in periodic reminiscence (old music, historical events, photos/mementoes, videos).

Stimulates recollections, awakens memories, aids in the preservation of self/individuality via past accomplishments; increases feelings of security, while easing adaptation to a changed environment.

Provide intellectual activities (e.g., word games, review of current events, storytime, travel discussions).

Stimulates remaining cognitive abilities and provides a sense of normalcy.

Include in Bible study group, church activities, TV services for shut-ins; or arrange for visitation by clergy/spiritual advisor as appropriate.

Provides opportunity to meet spiritual needs and to maintain connection with religious beliefs; may help reduce sense of isolation from humanity.

Encourage simple outings, short walks. Monitor activity.

Outings refresh reality and provide pleasurable sensory stimuli, which may reduce suspiciousness/ hallucinations caused by feelings of imprisonment. Motor functioning may be decreased, because nerve degeneration results in weakness, decreasing stamina.

Promote balanced physiological functions using colorful Nerfballs/beachballs or beanbags for tossing; target games; marching, dancing, or arm dancing with music.

Preserves mobility (reducing the potential for bone loss and muscle atrophy); provides diversional activity and opportunity for interaction with others.

Involve in activities with others as dictated by individual situation (e.g., one-to-one visitors; animal visitation; socialization groups at an Alzhemier center; occupational therapy to include crafts, paintings/finger paints, modeling clay, etc).

Provides opportunity for the stimulation of participation with others and may maintain some level of social interaction.

familiar surroundings. Clues are tangible reminders that aid recognition and may permeate memory gaps, increasing independence.

NURSING DIAGNOSIS	FEAR
May Be Related to:	Decreases in functional abilities
	Public disclosure of disabilities
	Further mental/physical deterioration

Possibly Evidenced by:	Social isolation
	Apprehension, irritability; defensiveness; suspiciousness
	Aggressive behavior
Desired Outcomes/Evaluation Criteria—Client Will:	Demonstrate more appropriate range of feelings and lessened fear.

ACTIONS/INTERVENTIONS	RATIONALE

Independent

Note change of behavior, suspiciousness, irritability, defensiveness.	Change in moods may be one of the first signs of cognitive decline, and the client, fearing helplessness, tries to hide the increasing inability to remember and engage in normal activities.
Identify strengths the individual had previously.	Facilitates assistance with communication and management of current deficits.
Deal with aggressive behavior by imposing calm, firm limits.	Acceptance can reduce fear and lessen progression of aggressive behavior.
Provide clear, honest information about actions/events.	Assists in maintaining trust and orientation as long as possible. When the client knows the truth about what is happening, coping is often enhanced, and guilt over what is imagined is decreased.
Discuss feelings of SO/caregivers. Acknowledge normalcy of feelings/concerns and provide information as needed.	Client senses but may not understand reaction of others. This may heighten client's sense of anxiety/fear.

NURSING DIAGNOSIS	GRIEVING, anticipatory
May Be Related to:	Client awareness of something "being wrong" with changes in memory/family reaction, physiopsychosocial well-being
	Family perception of potential loss of loved one
Possibly evidenced by:	Expressions of distress/anger at potential loss
	Choked feelings, crying
	Alteration in activity level, communication patterns, eating habits, and sleep patterns
Desired Outcomes/Evaluation Criteria—Client/Family Will:	Express concerns openly.
	Discuss loss and participate in planning for the future.

ACTIONS/INTERVENTIONS	RATIONALE

Independent

| Assess degree of deterioration/level of coping. | Information is helpful to understand how much the client is capable of doing to maintain highest |

Provide open environment for discussion. Use therapeutic communication skills of Active-listening, acknowledgment, etc.

level of independence and to provide encouragement to help individuals deal with losses.

Encourages client/SOs to discuss feelings and concerns realistically.

Note statements of despair, hopelessness, "nothing to live for," expressions of anger.

May be indicative of suicidal ideation. Angry behavior may be client's way of dealing with feelings of despair.

Respect desire not to talk.

May not be ready to deal with or share grief.

Be honest; do not give false reassurances or dire predictions about the future.

Honesty promotes a trusting relationship. Expressions of gloom, such as, "You'll spend the rest of your life in a nursing home," are not helpful. (No one knows what the future holds.)

Discuss with client/SOs ways they can plan together for the future.

Having a part in problem-solving/planning can provide a sense of control over anticipated events.

Assist client/SO to identify positive aspects of the situation.

Ongoing research, possibility of slow progression may offer some hope for the future.

Identify strengths client and SO see in self/situation and support systems available.

Recognizing these resources provides opportunity to work through feelings of grief.

Collaborative

Refer to other resources (e.g., support groups, counseling, spiritual advisor).

May need additional support/assistance to resolve feelings.

NURSING DIAGNOSIS	SLEEP PATTERN disturbance
May Be Related to:	Sensory impairments
	Pyschological stress (neurological impairment)
	Changes in activity pattern
Possibly Evidenced By:	Changes in behavior and performance, irritability
	Disorientation (day/night reversal)
	Wakefulness/interrupted sleep, increased aimless wandering; inability to identify need/time for sleeping
	Lethargy, dark circles under eyes, frequent yawning
Desired Outcomes/Evaluation Criteria— Client Will:	Establish adequate sleep pattern, with wandering reduced.
	Report/appear rested.

ACTIONS/INTERVENTIONS	RATIONALE

Independent

Provide for adequate rest. Restrict daytime sleep as appropriate; increase interaction time between client

Although prolonged physical and mental activity results in fatigue, which can increase confusion,

131

and family/staff during day, then reduce mental activity late in the day.

Avoid use of continuous restraints.

Evaluate level of stress/orientation as day progresses.

Adhere to regular bedtime schedule and rituals. Tell client that it is time to sleep.

Provide evening snack, warm milk, bath, back rub/ general massage with lotion.

Reduce fluid intake in the evening. Toilet before retiring.

Provide soft music or "white noise."

Allow to sleep in shoes/clothing if client demands.

Collaborative

Administer medications as indicated for sleep:
  Antidepressants: e.g., amitriptyline (Elavil), doxepin (Sinequan), and trazodone (Desyrel);

  Sedative-hypnotics, e.g., chloral hydrate (Noctec), oxazepam (Serax), triazolam (Halcion).

Avoid use of diphenhydramine (Benadryl).

---

programmed activity without overstimulation promotes sleep.

Potentiates sensory deprivation, increases agitation, and restricts rest.

Increasing confusion, disorientation, and uncooperative behaviors ("sundowner's syndrome") may interfere with attaining restful sleep pattern.

Reinforces that it is bedtime and maintains stability of environment. **Note:** Later-than-normal bedtime may be indicated to allow client to dissipate excess energy and facilitate falling asleep.

Promotes relaxation and drowsiness and helps to address skin-care needs.

Decreases need to get up to go to the bathroom/incontinence during the night.

Reduces sensory stimulation by blocking out other environmental sounds that could interfere with restful sleep.

Providing no harm is done, altering the "normal" lessens the rebellion and allows rest.

May be effective in treating pseudodementia or depression, improving ability to sleep. However, the anticholinergic properties can induce confusion or worsen cognition and side effects (e.g., orthostatic hypotension, constipation) may limit usefulness.

Used sparingly, low-dose hypnotics may be effective in treating insomnia or "sundowner's syndrome."

Once used for sleep, this drug is now contraindicated because it interferes with the production of acetylcholine, which is already inhibited in the brains of clients with DAT.

NURSING DIAGNOSIS	SELF CARE DEFICIT (specify level)
May Be Related to:	Cognitive decline, physical limitations
	Frustration over loss of independence, depression
Possibly Evidenced by:	Impaired ability to perform ADLs (e.g., frustration; forgetfulness, misuse/misidentification of objects; inability to bring food from receptacle to mouth; inability to wash body part(s), regulate water temperature; impaired ability to put on/take off clothing; difficulty completing toileting tasks)

Desired Outcomes/Evaluation Criteria—Client Will:	Perform self-care activities within level of own ability.
Caregiver Will:	Identify and use personal/community resources that can provide assistance; support client's independence.

ACTIONS/INTERVENTIONS	RATIONALE

Independent

Identify reason for difficulty in self-care, e.g., physical limitations in motion, apathy/depression, cognitive decline (such as apraxia), or room temperature ("too cold to get dressed").	Underlying cause affects choice of interventions/strategies. Problem may be minimized by changes in environment or adaptation of clothing, etc.; or may be more complex, requiring consultation from other specialists. Important to distinguish between partial and total dependence to avoid creating excess disability. **Note:** Clients reported to be unable to perform specific ADLs are often able to do so given the right circumstances (e.g., adequate/knowledgeable caregiver support).
Determine hygienic needs and provide assistance as needed with activities, including care of hair/nails/skin, brushing teeth, cleaning glasses.	As the disease progresses, basic hygienic needs may be forgotten. Infection, gum disease, disheveled appearance, or harm may occur when client/caregivers become frustrated, irritated, or intimidated by degree of care required.
Inspect skin regularly.	Presence of ecchymoses, lacerations, rashes, etc. may require treatment, as well as signal the need for closer monitoring/protective interventions.
Incorporate usual routine into activity schedule as possible. Wait or change the time to initiate dressing/hygiene if a problem arises.	Maintaining routine may prevent worsening of confusion and enhance cooperation. Because anger is quickly forgotten, another time or approach may be successful.
Be attentive to nonverbal physiological symptoms.	Sensory loss and language dysfunction may cause client to express self-care needs in nonverbal manner (e.g., thirst by panting; need to void by holding self/fidgeting).
Be alert to underlying meaning of verbal statements.	May direct a question to another, such as "Are you cold?" meaning, "I am cold and need additional clothing."
Supervise, but allow as much autonomy as possible.	Eases the frustration over lost independence.
Allot plenty of time to perform tasks.	Tasks that were once easy (e.g., dressing, bathing) are now complicated by decreased motor skills or cognitive and physical changes. Time and patience can reduce chaos resulting from trying to hasten this process.
Assist with neat dressing/provide colorful clothes.	Enhances esteem; may diminish sense of sensory loss and convey aliveness.
Offer one item of clothing at a time, in sequential order. Talk through each step of the task one at a time. Allow the wearing of extra clothing if client demands.	Simplicity reduces frustration and the potential for rage and despair. Guidance reduces confusion and allows autonomy. Altering the "normal" may lessen rebellion.

Provide reminders for elimination needs. Involve in bowel/bladder program as appropriate.

Assist with and provide reminders for pericare after toileting/incontinence.

Loss of control/independence in this self-care activity can have a great impact on self-esteem and may limit socialization. (Refer to ND: Constipation.)

Good hygiene promotes cleanliness and reduces risks of skin irritation and infection.

NURSING DIAGNOSIS	NUTRITION: altered, risk for less/more than body requirements
Risk Factors May Include:	Sensory changes
	Impaired judgment and coordination
	Agitation; forgetfulness, regressed habits, and concealment
Possibly Evidenced by:	[Not applicable; presence of signs and symptoms establishes an *actual* diagnosis.]
Desired Outcomes/Evaluation Criteria— Client Will:	Ingest nutritionally balanced diet.
	Maintain/regain appropriate weight.

ACTIONS/INTERVENTIONS	RATIONALE

Independent

Assess SO/client's knowledge of nutritional needs.

Identifies needs to assist in formulating individual teaching plan. A role-reversal situation can occur (e.g., child now cooking for parent, husband taking over "duties" of wife), increasing the need for information.

Determine amount of exercise/pacing client does.

Nutritional intake may need to be adjusted to meet needs related to individual energy expenditure.

Offer/provide assistance in menu selection.

Poor judgment may lead to poor choices; client may be indecisive/overwhelmed by choices and/or unaware of the need to maintain elemental nutrition. **Note:** In general, metabolic rate decreases with age, requiring caloric adjustment that must be balanced with activity.

Provide privacy when eating habits become an insoluble problem. Accept eating with hands, spills, and whimsical mixtures (e.g., salad dressing in milk, salt and pepper on ice cream). Avoid solo dining or separating client from other people too early in the disease process.

Socially unacceptable and embarrassing eating habits develop as the disease progresses. Acceptance preserves esteem; decreases irritability or refusal to eat as a result of anger, frustration. Early separation can result in client feeling upset and rejected and can actually result in decreased food intake.

Offer small feelings and/or snacks of 1 or 2 foods around the clock as indicated.

Large feedings may overwhelm the client, resulting either in complete abstinence or gorging. Small feedings may enhance appropriate intake. Limiting number of foods offered at a single time reduces confusion regarding which food to choose.

Simplify steps of eating (e.g., serve food in courses). Anticipate needs, cut foods, provide soft/finger foods.

Promotes autonomy and independence; decreases potential frustration/anger over lost abilities. Coordination decreases as the disease progresses,

134

Provide ample time for eating.

Place food items in pita bread/paper sack for the client who paces.

Avoid baby food and excessively hot foods.

Observe swallowing ability; monitor oral cavity.

Stimulate oral-suck reflex by gentle stroking of the cheeks or stimulating the mouth with a spoon.

Collaborative

Refer to dietitian.

which impairs the client's ability to chew and handle utensils.

A leisurely approach aids digestion and decreases the chance of anger precipitated by rushing.

Carrying food may encourage client to eat.

Baby foods lack adequate nutritional content, fiber, and taste for adults, and can add to client's humiliation. Hot foods may result in mouth burns and/or refusal to eat.

Diminished abilities may result in client/caregiver repeatedly placing food in client's mouth, which is not swallowed, increasing risk of aspiration.

As the disease progresses, the client may clench teeth and refuse to eat. Stimulating the reflex may increase cooperation/intake.

Assistance may be needed to develop nutritionally balanced diet individualized to meet client needs/food preferences.

NURSING DIAGNOSIS	CONSTIPATION (specify)/BOWEL INCONTINENCE/URINARY ELIMINATION, altered
May Be Related to:	Disorientation; inability to locate the bathroom/recognize need
	Lost neurological functioning/muscle tone
	Changes in dietary/fluid intake
Possibly Evidenced by:	Urgency/inappropriate toileting behaviors
	Incontinence/constipation
Desired Outcomes/Evaluation Criteria—Client Will:	Establish adequate/appropriate pattern of elimination.

ACTIONS/INTERVENTIONS	RATIONALE

Independent

Assess prior pattern and compare with current situation.

Locate bed near a bathroom when possible; make signs for/color-code door. Provide adequate lighting, particularly at night.

Take client to the toilet at regular intervals. Dictate each step one at a time and use positive reinforcement.

Provides information about changes that may require further assessment/intervention.

Promotes orientation/finding bathroom. Incontinence may be attributed to inability to find a toilet.

Adherence to a daily and regular schedule may prevent accidents. Frequently the problem is forgetting how to toilet (e.g., pushing pants down, positioning).

135

Establish bowel/bladder training program. Promote client participation to level of ability.	Stimulates awareness, enhances regulation of body function, and helps to avoid accidents.
Encourage adequate fluid intake during the day (at least 2 liters, as appropriate), diet high in fiber and fruit juices. Limit intake during the late evening and at bedtime.	Essential for bodily functions and prevents potential dehydration/constipation. Restricting intake in evening may reduce frequency/incontinence during the night.
Avoid a sense of hurrying/being rushed.	Hurrying may be perceived as intrusion, which leads to anger and lack of cooperation with activity.
Be alert to nonverbal cues (e.g., restlessness, holding self, or picking at clothes).	May signal urgency/inattention to cues and/or inability to locate bathroom.
Be discreet and respect person's privacy.	Although the client is confused, a sense of modesty is often retained.
Convey acceptance when incontinence occurs. Change promptly; provide good skin care.	Acceptance is important to decrease the embarrassment and feelings of helplessness that may occur during the changing process. Prompt changing reduces risk of skin irritation/breakdown.
Record frequency of voidings/bowel movements.	Provides visual reminder of elimination and may indicate need for intervention.
Monitor appearance/color of urine; note consistency of stool.	Detection of changes provides opportunity to alter interventions to prevent complications or acquire treatment as indicated (e.g., constipation/urinary infection).

Collaborative

Administer stool softeners, bulk expanders (e.g., Metamucil), or glycerin suppository, as indicated.	May be necessary to facilitate/stimulate regular bowel movement.

NURSING DIAGNOSIS	SEXUAL dysfunction, risk for
Risk Factors May Include:	Altered body function/progression of disease: decrease in habit/control of behavior, confusion; forgetfulness and disorientation to place or person
	Lack of intimacy/sexual rejection by SO
	Lack of privacy
Possibly Evidenced by:	[Not applicable; presence of signs and symptoms establishes an *actual* diagnosis.]
Desired Outcomes/Evaluation Criteria—Client Will:	Meet sexuality needs in an acceptable manner.
	Experience fewer/no episodes of inappropriate behavior.

ACTIONS/INTERVENTIONS

RATIONALE

Independent

Assess individual needs/desires/abilities of client and partner.	Alternative methods need to be designed for the individual situation to fulfill the need for intimacy and closeness.

Encourage partner to show affection/acceptance.	The cognitively impaired person retains the basic needs for affection, love, acceptance, and sexual expression.
Ensure privacy, or encourage home visitation as appropriate.	Sexual expression or behaviors may differ. The individual may masturbate, expose self. Privacy allows sexual expression without embarrassment and the objections of others.
Use distraction, as indicated. Remind client that, when in a public area, current behavior is unacceptable.	This tool is useful when there is inappropriate/objectionable behavior (e.g., self-exposure).
Provide time to listen/discuss concerns of SO.	SO may need information and/or counseling about alternatives for sexual activity/aggression.

NURSING DIAGNOSIS	FAMILY COPING, ineffective: compromised/disabling
May Be Related to:	Disruptive behavior of client
	Family grief about their helplessness watching loved one deteriorate
	Prolonged disease/disability progression that exhausts the supportive capacity of SO
	Highly ambivalent family relationships
Possibly Evidenced by:	Family becoming embarrassed and socially immobilized
	Home maintenance becoming extremely difficult, leading to difficult decisions with legal/financial considerations
Desired Outcomes/Evaluation Criteria— Family Will:	Identify/verbalize resources within themselves to deal with the situation.
	Acknowledge client's condition and demonstrate positive coping behaviors in dealing with situation.
	Use outside support systems effectively.

ACTIONS/INTERVENTIONS	RATIONALE
Independent	
Include SOs in teaching and planning for home care.	Can ease the burden of home management and increase adaptation. A comfortable and familiar lifestyle at home helps preserve the client's need for belonging.
Review past life experiences, role changes, and coping skills.	Identifies skills that may help individuals cope with grief of current situation more effectively.
Focus on specific problems as they occur, the "here and now."	Disease progression follows no set pattern. A premature focus on the possibility of long-term care or possible incontinence, for example, impairs the ability to cope with present issues.

137

Establish priorities.	Helps to create a sense of order and facilitates problem-solving.
Be realistic and honest in all matters.	Decreases stress that surrounds false hopes (e.g., that client may regain past level of functioning from advertised or unproven medication).
Reassess family's ability to care for client at home on an ongoing basis.	Behaviors like hoarding, clinging, unjust accusations, angry outbursts, etc. can precipitate family burnout and interfere with ability to provide effective care.
Help caregiver/family understand the importance of maintaining psychosocial functioning.	Embarrassing behavior, the demands of care, etc. may cause withdrawal from social contact.
Provide time to listen with regard to concerns/anxieties.	SOs require constant support with the multifaceted problems that arise during the course of this illness to ease the process of adaptation and grieving.
Discuss possibility of isolation. Reinforce need for support systems.	The belief that a single individual can meet all the needs of the client increases the potential for physical/mental illness (caregiver role strain). **Note:** Mortality rate for primary caregivers is actually higher than for the client with DAT.
Provide positive feedback for efforts.	Reassures individuals that they are doing their best.
Acknowledge concerns generated by consideration/decision to place client in LTC facility. Answer questions honestly, explore options as appropriate.	Constant care requirements may be more than can be managed by the SO and support systems. Support is needed for this difficult guilt-producing decision, which may create a financial burden as well as family disruption/dissension.
Encourage unlimited visitation by family/friends as tolerated by client.	Contact with/and familiarity forms a base of reality and can provide a reassuring freedom from loneliness. Recurrent contact helps family members realize and accept situation. **Note:** Family members may require ongoing support in dealing with visitation and issues of client's deterioration and their own personal needs.

Collaborative

Involve SO/family members in planning care/problem-solving. Verify presence of Advance Directives/Durable Medical Power of Attorney.	Consensus may be more readily achieved when family participates in decision-making. It is important, however, to keep client's wishes in mind when making choices and to be aware of who actually has the power to make decisions for the cognitively impaired client.
Refer to local resources, e.g., adult day care, respite care, homemaker services, or a local chapter of Alzheimer's Disease and Related Disorders Association (ADRDA), National Family Caregivers Association (NFCA).	Coping with these clients is a full-time, frustrating task. Respite/day care may lighten the burden, reduce potential social isolation, and prevent family burnout/caregiver role strain. ADRDA provides group support and family teaching and promotes research. Local groups provide a social outlet for sharing grief and promote problem-solving with such matters as financial/legal

Refer for family counseling or to appropriate ethical committee as indicated.

advice, home care, etc. NFCA also provides programs for educating caregivers/healthcare providers and a quarterly publication.

Differing opinions regarding client care/placement can result in conflict requiring professional mediation.

NURSING DIAGNOSIS	HOME MAINTENANCE MANAGEMENT, impaired/HEALTH MAINTENANCE, altered
May Be Related to:	Progressively impaired cognitive functioning
	Complete or partial lack of gross and/or fine motor skills
	Significant alteration in communication skills
	Ineffective individual/family coping
	Insufficient family organization or planning
	Unfamiliarity with resources; inadequate support systems
Possibly Evidenced by:	Overtaxed family members (e.g., exhausted, anxious)
	Household members express difficulty and request help in maintaining home safely and comfortably
	Home surroundings appear disorderly/unsafe
	Reported or observed inability to take responsibility for meeting basic health practices
	Reported or observed lack of equipment, financial, or other resources, impairment of personal support system
Desired Outcomes/Evaluation Criteria— Family/Caregiver(s) Will:	Verbalize ability to cope adequately with existing situation.
	Identify factors related to difficulty in maintaining a safe environment for the client.
	Assume responsibility for and initiate changes supporting client safety and healthcare goals.
	Demonstrate appropriate, effective use of resources (e.g., respite/day care, homemakers, support groups).

ACTIONS/INTERVENTIONS	RATIONALE

Independent

Evaluate level of cognitive/emotional/physical functioning (level of independence).

Identifies strengths, areas of need, and how much responsibility the client may be expected to assume. (Refer to ND: Self Care deficit.)

Assess environment, noting unsafe factors and ability of client to care for self.

Determines what changes need to be made to accommodate disabilities. (Refer to ND: Injury/Trauma, risk for).

Assist client to develop plan for keeping track of/dealing with health needs.

Schedule can be helpful to maintain system for managing routine healthcare services.

Identify support systems available to client/SO (e.g., other family members, friends).

Planning and constant care is necessary to maintain this client at home. If family system is unavailable/unaware, client needs (e.g., nutrition, dental care, eye exams) can be neglected. Primary caregiver can benefit from sharing responsibilities/constant care with others. (Refer to ND: Caregiver Role Strain.)

Evaluate coping abilities, effectiveness, commitment of caregiver(s)/support persons.

Progressive debilitation taxes caregiver(s) and may alter ability to meet client/own needs. (Refer to ND: Family Coping, ineffective: compromised/disabling.)

Collaborative

Identify alternate care sources (such as sitter/day-care facility), senior care services (e.g., homemaking, cleaning, handyman).

As client's condition worsens, SO may need additional help from several sources or may eventually be unable to maintain client at home.

Refer to supportive services as needed.

Medical and social services consultant may be needed to develop ongoing plan/identify resources as needs change.

Identify in home healthcare options, e.g., medical, dental, diagnostic services.

Delivery of healthcare needs "on site" may prevent exacerbation of confusion, increase cooperation, and provide more accurate picture of client's status.

NURSING DIAGNOSIS	CAREGIVER ROLE STRAIN, risk for
Risk Factors May Include:	Illness severity of the care receiver; duration of caregiving required, complexity/amount of caregiving tasks
	Caregiver is female; spouse
	Care receiver exhibits deviant, bizarre behavior
	Family/caregiver isolation; lack of respite and recreation
Possibly Evidenced by:	[Not applicable; presence of signs/symptoms establishes in *actual* diagnosis.]
Desired Outcomes/Evaluation Criteria— Caregiver Will:	Identify individual risk factors and appropriate interventions.
	Demonstrate/initiate behaviors or lifestyle changes to prevent development of impaired function.
	Use available resources appropriately.
	Report satisfaction with plan and support available.

ACTIONS/INTERVENTIONS	RATIONALE

Independent

Note physical/mental condition, therapeutic regimen of care receiver.

Determines individual needs for planning care. Identifies strengths and how much responsibility the client may be expected to assume as well as disabilities requiring accommodation.

Determine caregiver's level of responsibility and involvement in care as well as the anticipated length of care. Use assessment tool such as Burden Interview to further determine caregiver's abilities, when appropriate.

Progressive debilitation taxes caregiver and may alter ability to meet client/own needs. (Refer to ND: Family Coping, ineffective: compromised/disabling.)

Identify strengths of caregiver and care receiver.

Helps to use positive aspects of each individual to the best of abilities in daily activities.

Discuss caregiver's view and concerns about situation.

Allows ventilation and clarification of concerns, promoting understanding.

Determine available supports and resources currently used.

Provides information regarding adequacy of supports/current needs.

Facilitate family conference to share information and develop plan for involvement in care activities as appropriate.

When others are involved in care, the risk of one person becoming overloaded is lessened.

Identify additional resources to include financial, legal, respite care.

These areas of concern can add to burden of caregiving if not adequately resolved.

Identify equipment needs/resources, adaptive aids.

Enhances independence and safety of the care receiver.

Provide information and/or demonstrate techniques for dealing with acting-out/violent or disoriented behavior.

This helps caregiver to maintain sense of control and competency. Enhances safety for caregiver and care receiver.

Stress importance of self-nurturing (e.g., pursuing self-development interests, personal needs, hobbies, and social activities).

Taking time for self can lessen risk of "burnout"/being overwhelmed by situation.

Assist caregiver to plan for changes that may be necessary for the care receiver (e.g., eventual placement in long-term care facility).

Planning for this eventuality is important for the time when burden of care becomes too great.

Collaborative

Refer to alternate-care sources (e.g., sitter/day-care facility), senior care services (e.g., meals-on-wheels/respite care) home-care agency.

As client's condition worsens, SO may need additional help from several sources to maintain client at home, even on a part-time basis.

Refer to supportive services as needed.

Medical case manager or social services consultant may be needed to develop ongoing plan to meet changing needs of client and SO/family.

NURSING DIAGNOSIS

Risk Factors May Include:

RELOCATION STRESS SYNDROME, risk for

Little or no preparation for transfer to hospital/long-term setting

Changes in daily routine

	Sensory impairment, physical deterioration
	Separation from support systems
Possibly Evidenced by:	[Not applicable; presence of signs/symptoms establishes an *actual* diagnosis.]
Desired Outcomes/Evaluation Criteria— Client Will:	Experience minimal disruption of usual activities.
	Display limited increase in agitation.
Family/Caregiver Will:	Be aware of potential impact of changes on client.
	Plan for/coordinate move as situation permits.
	Recognize need to provide stability for client during adaptation period.

ACTIONS/INTERVENTIONS	RATIONALE
Independent	
Discuss ramifications of move to new surroundings.	Discussing pros and cons of this decision helps those involved to reach an informed decision and feel better about/plan for the future.
Encourage visitation to facility prior to planned move.	Familiarizes family and client with new options to enable them to make informed decision.
Provide clear, honest information about actions/events.	Decreases "surprises." Assists in maintaining trust and orientation. When the client knows the truth about what is happening, coping may be enhanced.
Determine clients' usual schedule of activities and incorporate into agency routine. Identify activities for SO/family participation (e.g., personal care, mealtime, exercise program).	Consistency provides reassurance and may lessen confusion and enhance cooperation. Admission to a new facility disrupts client's routine and can intensify behavioral problems, especially in the person with cognitive dysfunctions. Presence of SO provides reassurance and may reduce sense of isolation.
Place client in private room as appropriate.	Provides opportunity to control environment and protect others from client's disruptive behavior.
Note behavior, presence of suspiciousness/paranoia, irritability, defensiveness. Compare with SO's description of customary responses.	Increased stress, physical discomfort/pain, and fatigue may temporarily exacerbate mental deterioration (cognitive inaccessibility) and further impair communication (social inaccessibility). This represents a *catastrophic* episode that can escalate into a panic state and violence.
Deal with aggressive behavior by imposing firm limits; provide "time-out" as appropriate.	Calm acceptance can reduce fear and aggressive response. This defuses situation and gives the client time to regain emotional and behavioral control.

DEMENTIA DUE TO HIV DISEASE

DSM-IV
DEMENTIAS DUE TO OTHER MEDICAL CONDITIONS
294.1 DEMENTIA DUE TO HIV DISEASE (CODE 042 ON AXIS III)

Dementia is impairment of short- and long-term memory, abstract thinking, and judgment with personality changes, severe enough to interfere with work, normal social activities, and relationships.

Human immunodeficiency virus (HIV) has been shown to affect the brain directly by crossing the blood-brain barrier on two types of immune cells—monocytes and macrophages. Cells within the central nervous system (CNS) have been found to have express CD4 receptor sites for HIV entry into cells. Although several hypotheses have been proposed, it is not known exactly by what mechanism neurological dysfunction occurs. Neuropsychiatric symptoms may range from barely perceptible changes in a person's normal psychological presentation to acute delirium to profound dementia. Because of the associated immune dysfunction, secondary brain infections may cause further damage.

Studies have shown CNS abnormalities in a large percentage of clients, with 3 people in 10 who are HIV-symptomatic exhibiting symptoms of dementia. Recent studies suggest symptoms can occur prior to an acquired immunodeficiency syndrome (AIDS) diagnosis, as they are the first clinical symptoms of progression.

CLIENT ASSESSMENT DATA BASE

Activity/Rest

Low energy level, constant fatigue
Insomnia, change in sleep patterns
Yawning frequently
Wakefulness at night

Ego Integrity

Emotional lability (e.g., irritability, anxiety, agitation, combativeness, and panic attacks)
Reports feeling like he or she is losing his or her mind
Feelings of powerlessness, worthlessness

Elimination

Constipation/diarrhea
Increasing frequency of incontinence

Food/Fluid

Decreased interest in food
Apraxia (inability to carry out motor functions of chewing and swallowing despite intact sensory function)
Agnosia (failure to recognize foods despite intact sensory function); may report change in taste/smell
Weight loss

Hygiene

Unable to do simple/difficult tasks of activities of daily living (ADL)
Deficits in many/all personal care areas
No concern for hygiene; disheleved, unkempt appearance

Neurosensory

Changes in mental status, forgetfulness, poor concentration/decreased alertness, apathy; impaired impulse control (loss of mental acuity/ability to problem-solve)

Unrealistic expectations, free-floating anxiety, paranoid ideation

Organic psychosis (hallucinations, delusions)

Psychomotor retardation/slowed responses, decreased grip strength, decreased pinprick sensation, ataxic gait

Impaired sensation or sense of position

Numbness, tingling of feet (paresthesias)

Deterioration in handwriting, decreased verbal comprehension, aphasia, mutism

Seizure activity; falls/accidental fractures

Antisocial personalities (drug users)

Pain/Discomfort

Headache

Pain in lower extremities, burning in feet

Guarding behavior (posturing, withdrawal), request not to be touched

Safety

Decline in general strength; muscle tremors, sense of lack of balance; spastic weakness, changes in gait/ataxia, hemiparesis

Bruises, burns/lesions

Not completing tasks (e.g., not turning off stove/burning food)

Needle marks on skin (injection drug use)

Sexuality

Decreased interest in sexual activity; withdrawal from others (intimacy)

Decreased ability/inability to obtain arousal

Unsafe sexual practices related to drug abuse

Social Interactions

Disinterest in friends/social interaction; loss of social responsiveness; withdrawal

Labile personality, increased anger

Slurred speech/aphasia, mutism (late)

Disorganized activities

Chaotic lives owing to drug use (e.g., homelessness, unemployment)

DIAGNOSTIC STUDIES

Choice of studies depends on individual situation to rule out conditions with symptoms mimicking HIV dementia, especially depression.

Weschsler Adult Intelligence Scale (WAIS-R): Used to screen for the presence of HIV-induced brain damage; a low score may indicate memory loss or sensorimotor deficit (may be influenced by depression, anxiety, and hostile states).

Minnesota Multiphasic Personality Inventory (MMPI): Identifies degree of depression, presence of personality disorders.

Picture Drawing: Differentiates depression from dementia (depressed person can draw, demented person cannot).

Tumor Necrosis Factor (TNF): Elevated levels may account for white matter pallor.

Mental Status Examinations (e.g., Galveston Orientation and Amnesia Scale [GOAT]; Neurobehavioral Rating Scale [NRS, Freeman]; Self-Rating Depression Scale; Cognitive Evaluation): Identify specific deficits.

CBC: May show anemia, affecting cerebral oxygenation/mentation.

Blood Chemistries: Rule out metabolic causes (e.g., diabetes mellitus, hypoglycemia, hypothyroid) and electrolyte deficiencies.

B$_{12}$: Identifies diminished levels (affects synaptic responses and biochemical interactions).

Albumin: Provides a measure of nutritional status.

Arterial Blood Gases (ABGs): Rule out/determine contribution of hypoxia on mentation.

Serology Rapid Plasma Reagin (RPR)/Screens: May reveal infection by STD, requiring treatment.

Alcohol/Drug Screen: Rules out acute drug intoxication, drug or alcohol withdrawal.

CT/MRI/Positron Emission Tomography (PET): Determine changes in brain mass (lesions or atrophy) and activity (expect to find cerebral atrophy mainly in the subcortical regions, white matter pallor, and ventricular enlargement).

Lumbar Puncture: Rule out tumors, identify CNS infections; may show increased protein (60%), glucose, elevated white blood count (WBC) (which may reflect cytomegalovirus [CMV]); with culture/sensitivity done to identify/rule out specific infective agents/treatment options.

NURSING PRIORITIES

1. Promote socially acceptable responses, limit inappropriate behavior.
2. Prevent injury/complications.
3. Support SO/family involvement in care.
4. Provide information about condition, prognosis, and treatment.

DISCHARGE GOALS

1. Maximal level of independent functioning achieved.
2. Injury prevented/minimized, complications resolved.
3. SO/family effectively participating in care.
4. Condition, prognosis, and therapeutic regimen understood at level of ability.
5. Plan in place to meet needs after discharge.

NURSING DIAGNOSIS	CONFUSION acute/chronic
May Be Related to:	Direct CNS infection by HIV, disseminated systemic opportunistic infection, hypoxemia, brain malignancies, and/or CVA/hemorrhage; vasculitis
	Alteration of drug metabolism/excretion, accumulation of toxic elements; severe electrolyte imbalance
	Sleep deprivation
Possibly Evidenced by:	Fluctuation in cognition; progressive/long-standing cognitive impairment
	Fluctuation or no change in level of consciousness
	Increased agitation, restlessness
	Altered interpretation/response to stimuli; misperceptions
	Changes in sleep/wake cycle
	Clinical evidence of organic impairment

ACTIONS/INTERVENTIONS	RATIONALE
Independent	
Assess mental and neurological status using appropriate tools (e.g., Neurobehavioral Rating Scale [Freeman]). Note changes in orientation, response to stimuli, ability to problem-solve, anxiety, altered sleep patterns, hallucinations, paranoid ideation. Repeat serial/periodic evaluation at least every 2 to 4 months.	Establishes functional level at time of admission. Serial evaluations alert the nurse to changes in status that may be associated with failure of prophylaxis, progression of HIV dementia, exacerbation of CNS infection/opportunistic disease, environmental/psychological stressors, or side effects of drug therapy.
Consider effects of emotional distress (e.g., anxiety, grief, anger, depression).	May contribute to reduced alertness, confusion, withdrawal, hypoactivity and require further evaluation and intervention.
Monitor medication regimen and usage.	Actions and interactions of various medications and prolonged drug half-life/altered excretion results in cumulative effects, potentiating risk of toxic reactions. Some drugs may have adverse side effects (e.g., Haldol can seriously impair motor function in clients with AIDS dementia complex) necessitating a change in therapy.
Note signs of acute CNS infection (e.g., headache, nuchal rigidity, vomiting, fever, changes in motor function).	CNS symptoms associated with disseminated meningitis/encephalitis may range from subtle personality changes to confusion, irritability, drowsiness, stupor, seizures, and dementia. Sudden onset of motor changes may indicate polyradiculopathy and need for immediate medical response.
Approach client in a slow, calm manner.	Hurried approaches can startle/threaten the confused client who misinterprets or feels threatened by imaginary people and/or situations.
Maintain a pleasant environment, with appropriate auditory, visual, and cognitive stimuli.	Providing normal environmental stimuli can help in maintaining some sense of reality orientation.
Decrease noise, especially at night.	Promotes sleep, reducing cognitive symptoms and sleep deprivation.
Maintain safe environment: e.g., excess furniture out of the way, call bell within client's reach, bed in low position/rails up or bed against wall and padding on	Decreases the possibility of client injury.

floor, restriction of smoking (unless monitored by caregiver/SO), seizure precautions, soft restraints if indicated.

Provide information about care/answer questions simply and honestly without negating hope. Repeat explanations as needed and supplement with written materials as appropriate.

This can reduce anxiety and fear of unknown, may enhance client's/SO's understanding and involvement/cooperation in treatment; and maintain hope in the context of the individual situation.

Provide cues for reorientation (e.g., radio, television, calendars, clocks, room with an outside view). Use client's name; identify yourself.

Frequent reorientation to place, time, and person may be necessary, especially during fever/acute CNS involvement.

Maintain consistent personnel and structured schedules matching home routines as appropriate.

Sense of continuity may help limit confusion and reduce associated anxiety.

Suggest use of databooks, lists, alarm watch/pill box, other devices to keep track of activities and care needs.

These techniques help client to manage problems of forgetfulness.

Encourage client to do as much as he or she can (e.g., dress and groom daily, sit in chair, see friends).

Can help to maintain sense of normalcy and mental abilities for longer period.

Allow adequate time to complete ADLs, provide step-by-step directions for activities, as appropriate. Encourage family/SO to socialize and provide reorientation with current news, family events.

Familiar contacts are often helpful in maintaining reality orientation, especially if client is hallucinating.

Reduce provocative/noxious stimuli. Maintain bed rest in quiet room with subdued light, if indicated.

If the client is prone to agitation, violent behavior, or seizures, reducing external stimuli may be helpful. **Note:** A darkened room can create unusual shadows that are hard for client to identify and may increase confusion.

Provide/encourage physical and verbal interactions within client's level of tolerance.

Touch/gentle stroking and a soft voice can have a calming effect, helping to reduce anxiety. However, touch needs to be used with caution depending on response of client.

Redirect attention, set limits on maladaptive/ abusive behavior, avoid open-ended choices.

Provides sense of security/stability in an otherwise confusing situation.

Provide support for SO/family. Encourage discussion of concerns/fears.

Bizarre behavior/deterioration of abilities may be very frightening for loved ones and makes management of care/dealing with situation difficult. SO may feel a loss of control as stress, anxiety, burnout, and anticipatory grieving impair usual coping abilities.

Determine presence of Advance Directives/ Durable Medical Power of Attorney.

Clarifes client's wishes and establishes who is responsible for decision-making when client is cognitively impaired.

Discuss causes/future expectations and treatment if dementia is diagnosed. Use concrete terms.

Obtaining information that ZDV/protease inhibitors improve(s) cognition by dropping the viral load can provide hope and control for losses.

Explore options to meet long-term needs (e.g., home/ respite-care resources, extended-care facilities).

Progressive/unresolved dementia can exhaust SO/family abilities to care for client, necessitating outside placement.

147

Collaborative

ACTIONS/INTERVENTIONS	RATIONALE
Assist with/monitor diagnostic studies (e.g., MRI/CT scan, spinal tap) and laboratory studies as indicated (e.g., BUN/Cr, electrolytes, ABGs).	Choice of tests/studies depends on clinical manifestations and index of suspicion, as changes in mental status may reflect a variety of causative factors (e.g., CMV meningitis/encephalitis, drug toxicity, electrolyte imbalances, and altered organ function).
Administer medications as indicated:	
ZDV	Shown to improve neurological and mental functioning.
Amphotericin B (Fungizone);	Antifungal is useful in treatment of cryptococcosis meningitis.
Antibiotics (e.g., erythromycin);	May be effective against CMV.
Antipsychotics (e.g., haloperidol [Haldol]); and/or antianxietyagents (e.g., lorazepam [Ativan]);	Cautious use may help with problems of sleeplessness, emotional lability, hallucinations, suspiciousness, and agitation.
Dextroamphetamine (Dexedrine); methylphenidate (Ritalin).	These stimulants may improve mood and intellectual functioning.
Provide controlled environment/behavioral management.	Team approach may be required to protect client when mental impairment (e.g., delusions, loss of cognition) threatens client safety.
Refer to counseling as indicated.	May help client gain control in presence of thought disturbances or psychotic symptomatology.

NURSING DIAGNOSIS	ANXIETY (specify level)
May Be Related to:	Threat to self-concept; unmet needs
	Perceived threat or change in health status; threat of death
	Interpersonal transmission/contagion
Possibly Evidenced by:	Reports feeling scared, shaky, having increased tension, apprehension, "I feel like I'm going crazy"
	Increased somatic complaints; increased wariness
	Extraneous movements, tremors
Desired Outcomes/Evaluation Criteria—Client Will:	Verbalize awareness of feelings.
	Identify healthy ways to deal with anxiety and underlying causative factors.
	Use support systems effectively.
	Experience reduction in frequency and duration of episodes of anxiety.
	Direct energies to maintaining optimal level of functioning.

ACTIONS/INTERVENTIONS	RATIONALE

Independent

Assure client of confidentiality within limits of situation.	Provides client reassurance and the opportunity to problem-solve anticipated situations.

Establish a therapeutic relationship, conveying empathy and caring.

Promotes openness and opportunity for client to talk freely about concerns and fears.

Ascertain client's perception of the threat represented by the situation.

The client may be aware of cognitive changes, thus increasing the sense of anxiety. The potential for suicide may be worsened if client perceives the situation as hopeless.

Encourage client to acknowledge and express feelings.

Although an underlying medical cause for cognitive impairment may be present, the symptoms can increase anxiety.

Permit expressions of anger, fear, despair without confrontation. Give information that feelings are normal and are to be appropriately expressed.

Acceptance of feelings allows client to begin to deal with situation.

Assist the client to develop own awareness of verbal and nonverbal behaviors.

Being aware of self-behaviors brings increased understanding of responses of others.

Identify coping skills the individual is using. Review additional strategies when repertoire is limited.

Helps the client identify coping techniques and draw on past and current styles that may be helpful in the situation.

Maintain frequent contact with client. Talk with and touch client. Limit use of isolation clothing/masks, restrictive environment.

This assures the client that he or she is not alone or rejected. Conveys respect for and acceptance of the person, fostering trust. Avoiding unnecessary use of "protective clothing/ restrictions" promotes positive social contact and general sense of normalcy.

Identify and encourage client interaction with support systems. Encourage verbalization/ interaction with family/SO.

Reduces feeling of isolation. If family support systems are not available, outside sources can be contacted (e.g., local AIDS task force).

Provide accurate, consistent information regarding prognosis. Encourage cooperation with medical evaluation to rule out conditions requiring medical intervention.

Can reduce anxiety and enable client to make decisions/choices based on realities. Some causative factors for cognitive impairment are treatable/reversible.

Explain procedures, providing opportunity for questions. Stay with client during procedures and consultations.

Accurate information allows the client a sense of control. Client may be calmer when he or she understands procedure and expectations.

Review medication regimen for evidence of interactions between OTC and prescribed medications.

Certain drug interactions can induce anxiety.

Be alert to signs of denial/depression (e.g., withdrawal; angry, inappropriate remarks). Determine presence of suicidal ideation and assess potential on a scale of 1–10.

Client may use defense mechanism of denial and continue to hope that diagnosis is inaccurate. Feelings of guilt and spiritual distress may cause the client to become withdrawn. The individual may believe that suicide is a viable alternative.

Include SO as indicated when major decisions are to be made.

Ensures a support system for the client and allows the SO the chance to participate in client's life. Furthermore, SO may hold Durable Power of Attorney and be legally responsible for assisting in or making care decisions.
Note: If client, family, and SO are in conflict, separate care consultations and visiting times may be needed.

Collaborative

Monitor results of diagnostic studies.

Identification/treatment of underlying conditions (e.g., opportunistic infections, chemical

Administer antianxiety medications with caution. Begin with low doses and increase slowly.

Refer for ongoing individual/family psychiatric therapy as indicated. Identify available resources/support groups.

imbalances, or lymphomas) may limit progression/reverse cognitive impairment and corresponding anxiety.

Although these medications may be useful in individual situations, they may have increased untoward effects because these clients are sensitive to side effects.

May require further assistance in dealing with diagnosis/prognosis, especially when suicidal thoughts are present.

NURSING DIAGNOSIS	SLEEP PATTERN disturbance
May Be Related to:	Psychological stress (e.g., anxiety, depression)
	HIV neurological impairment (neurotransmitter impairment)
	Inactivity/changes in activity patterns
Possibly Evidenced by:	Verbalization of not feeling rested
	Difficulty falling asleep; frequent awakening
	Increasing irritability, disorientation, restlessness, or lethargy
Desired Outcomes/Evaluation Criteria—Client Will:	Identify appropriate interventions to promote sleep.
	Report improved sleep pattern, sense of being rested.

ACTION/INTERVENTIONS	RATIONALE

Independent

Identify factors contributing to insomnia and problem-solve solutions.	Chronic pain of neuropathy and cough associated with pneumonias and other URIs, medication interactions can interfere with sleep.
Evaluate use of caffeine and alcohol.	Overindulgence in these substances reduces REM sleep.
Reduce environmental stimulation. Provide soft music or "white noise," as appropriate.	Reduces sensory stimulation; soft music/white noise can block out disturbing sounds. If Stage IV sleep is not reached, there is increased risk of psychological symptoms.
Provide evening snack, warm milk, back rub, comfortable environmental temperature, and straighten linens.	Promotes relaxation. L-Tryptophan (found in milk) is believed to induce drowsiness.
Reduce fluid intake after 5 PM.	Prevents wakefulness related to sensation of bladder fullness and episodes of incontinence.

Administer pain medications when indicated (e.g., 30–60 minutes before bedtime).

Alleviating pain can help client to relax, fall asleep more quickly, and sleep better.

Collaborative

Administer medications as needed, such as amitriptyline (Elavil).

May reduce depression, pain of peripheral neuropathy, and promote sleep.

NURSING DIAGNOSIS	INJURY/TRAUMA, risk for
Risk Factors May Include:	Weakness, balancing difficulties, reduced tactile sensation
	Cognitive deficits, inability to recognize/identify danger in environment
	Smoking unattended
	Seizure activity
Possibly Evidenced by:	[Not applicable; presence of signs/symptoms establishes an *actual* diagnosis.]
Desired Outcomes/Evaluation Criteria— Client Will:	Remain safe, without injury to person or damage to environment.
Client/Caregiver Will:	Recognize potential risks in the environment.
	Identify and implement steps to correct/compensate for individual factors.

ACTIONS/INTERVENTIONS	RATIONALE

Independent

Assess degree of impairment in cognitive and functional abilities. Assist client/SO to identify risks and potential hazards.

Increases awareness of dangers and provides opportunity to implement anticipatory interventions.

Assist client/SO to plan for activities and safety measures to be considered (e.g., direct monitoring of cigarette use, and use of cane/walker for ambulation, seizure precautions).

Involving client in planning may reduce frustration, while increasing client sense of control and self-worth.

Inspect skin during self-care activities. Encourage client/SO to monitor skin periodically.

Presence of ecchymoses, lacerations, rashes, etc. may require treatment as well as signal need for closer monitoring/protective interventions.

Investigate availability of/evaluate client's ability to use home emergency call system.

Allows for periodic monitoring and prompt response as needed, enhancing safety in home setting.

Provide for protective environment when indicated, someone to stay with client on a full-time basis, use of restraints, admission to long-term care facility.

Near end-stage the client may no longer be able to recognize safety factors and may wander. **Note:** This is not likely to be a prolonged period of time for the client with HIV dementia.

NURSING DIAGNOSIS	FAMILY COPING, ineffective: compromised/disabling/CAREGIVER ROLE STRAIN
May Be Related to:	Situational conflict (parent-adult-child conflict, adult/child returning home with terminal illness; financial difficulties/insufficient resources)
	Disruptive/bizarre behavior of client
	Unpredictable illness course or instability in the care receiver's health, caregiver health impairment
	Individual helplessness/grief about watching loved one deteriorate
	Sense of shame surrounding a diagnosis of AIDS (regardless of how contracted)
	Prolonged disease/disability progression that exhausts the supportive capacity of SO
	Highly ambivalent family relationship
	Difficulty with acceptance/adaptation to client's sexual orientation/lifestyle/behaviors previous to caregiving situation
Possibly Evidenced by:	Family becoming embarrassed and socially immobilized
	Family feeling stress or nervousness in relationship with the care receiver; conflict around issues of providing care
	Lack of resources/inability to provide level of care indicated; difficult decisions with legal/financial considerations
	Caregiver worry about care receiver's health/emotional state, possibility of outside placement, concern
	Feelings of loss because care receiver is like a different person compared with before caregiving began
Desired Outcomes/Evaluation Criteria— Family/Caregiver Will:	Identify/verbalize resources within themselves to deal with the situation.
	Verbalize realistic understanding/expectations of client.
	Demonstrate positive coping behaviors in dealing with situation.
	Use outside support systems effectively.

ACTIONS/INTERVENTIONS	RATIONALE
Independent	
Review past life experiences, role changes, and coping skills.	Provides an opportunity to identify skills that may help individuals cope with grief of current situation more effectively.

Encourage unlimited visitation as tolerated by client.	Contact with family forms a base of reality and can provide a reassuring freedom from loneliness. Recurrent contact helps family members realize and accept situation.
Provide time/listen with regard to concerns/anxieties.	The self-sacrificing, painful nature of the care required in this disease necessitates constant support for SOs to deal effectively with the multifaceted problems arising during the course of this illness and to ease the process of adaptation and grieving.
Determine family's/SO's ability to care for client at home; reevaluate periodically.	Behaviors like hoarding, clinging, unjust accusations, angry outbursts, etc. can precipitate family/caregiver burnout and interfere with ability to provide effective care.
Include SOs in teaching and planning for home care.	Can ease the burden of home management and increase adaptation. Comfortable and familiar lifestyle at home is helpful in preserving the affected individual's need for belonging.
Focus on specific problems as they occur, the "here and now."	Disease progression follows no set pattern. Furthermore, premature focus on "what ifs" such as development of incontinence or possibility of LTC placement can impair the ability to cope with present issues.
Establish priorities.	Helps to create a sense of order and facilitates problem-solving.
Be realistic and honest in all matters.	Decreases stress that surrounds false hopes (e.g., that individual may regain past level of functioning from advertised or unproven medication/herbal preparations).
Help caregiver/family understand the importance of maintaining psychosocial functioning.	Embarrassing behavior, the demands of care, etc. may cause withdrawal from social contact.
Discuss possibility of isolation. Reinforce need for support system.	The belief that a single individual can meet all the needs of the client, increases the potential for physical/mental illness (caregiver role strain).
Provide positive feedback for efforts.	Reassures individuals that they are doing as well as they can and encourages continued efforts.
Support concerns generated by consideration/ decision to place in extended-care facility.	Constant care requirements may be more than can be managed by SO. Support is needed for this difficult, guilt-producing decision, which may create a financial burden as well as family disruption/dissension.
Discuss ways for family/SO to remain involved in care if placement is made.	Remaining involved in care enhances relationship, well-being of client, and sense of control in difficult situation.

Collaborative

Refer to local resources such as adult day care (if available), respite care, homemaker services, AIDS support organizations.	Coping with this individual is a full-time, frustrating task. Respite/day care may lighten the burden, reduce potential social isolation, and prevent family/caregiver burnout. AIDS organizations provide group support and family

153

teaching, and promote research. Local groups provide a social outlet for sharing grief and promote problem-solving with such matters as financial/legal advice, home care, etc.

Refer to CPs: Dementia of the Alzheimer's Type; Major Depression regarding issues of self-care, urinary elimination, nutrition, sensory-perceptual alterations, health maintenance, home maintenance management, etc.

CHAPTER 6

SUBSTANCE-RELATED DISORDERS

ALCOHOL-RELATED DISORDERS

DSM-IV
ALCOHOL-INDUCED DISORDERS
303.00 Alcohol intoxication
291.81 Alcohol withdrawal
291.89 Alcohol-induced mood disorder
291.89 Alcohol-induced anxiety disorder
292.81 Intoxication delirium

Alcohol is a CNS depressant drug that is used socially in our society for many reasons (e.g., to enhance the flavor of food, to encourage relaxation and conviviality, for feelings of celebration, and as a sacred ritual in some religious ceremonies). Therapeutically, it is the major ingredient in many OTC/prescription medications. It can be harmless, enjoyable, and sometimes beneficial when used responsibly and in moderation. Like other mind-altering drugs, however, it has the potential for abuse and, in fact, is the most widely abused drug in the United States (research suggests 5% to 10% of the adult population) and is potentially fatal. Frequently, the client in a residential care setting has been using alcohol in conjunction with other drugs. It is believed that alcohol is often used by clients who have other mental illnesses to assuage the pain they feel. The term "dual diagnosis" is used to mean an association between the use/abuse of drugs (including alcohol) and other psychiatric diagnoses. It may be difficult to determine cause and effect in any given situation to determine an accurate diagnosis. However, it is important to recognize when both conditions are present so that the often-overwhelming problems of treatment are instituted for both conditions.

This plan of care addresses acute intoxication/withdrawal and is to be used in conjunction with CP: Substance Dependence/Abuse Rehabilitation.

ETIOLOGICAL THEORIES

Psychodynamics

The individual remains fixed in a lower level of development, with retarded ego and weak superego. The person retains a highly dependent nature, with characteristics of poor impulse control, low frustration tolerance, and low self-esteem.

Biological

Enzymes, genes, brain chemistry, and hormones create and contribute to an individual's response to alcohol. The two types of alcohol-related disorders are (1) familial, which is largely inherited, and (2) acquired. A childhood history of attention-deficit disorder or conduct disorder also increases a child's risk of becoming alcoholic. Certain physiological changes also may cause addiction to alcohol, or alcoholism.

Family Dynamics

One in 12–15 persons has serious problems from drinking. In a dysfunctional family system, alcohol may be viewed as the primary method of relieving stress. Children of alcoholics are 4 times more likely to develop alcoholism than children of nonalcoholics. The child has negative role models and learns to respond to stressful situations in like manner. The use of alcohol is cultural, and many factors influence one's decision to drink, how much, and how often. Denial of the illness can be a major barrier to identification and treatment of alcoholism and alcohol abuse.

CLIENT ASSESSMENT DATA BASE

Data depend on the duration/extent of alcohol use, concurrent use of other drugs, degree of organ involvement, and presence of other psychiatric conditions.

Activity/Rest

Difficulty sleeping, not feeling well rested

Circulation

Peripheral pulses weak, irregular, or rapid
Hypertension common in early withdrawal stage but may become labile/progress to hypotension
Tachycardia common during acute withdrawal

Ego Integrity

Feelings of guilt/shame; defensiveness about drinking
Denial, rationalization
Reports of multiple stressors; problems with relationships
Multiple stressors/losses (relationships, employment, financial)
Use of substances to deal with life stressors, boredom, etc.

Elimination

Diarrhea
Bowel sounds varied (may reflect gastric complications [e.g., gastric hemorrhage])

Food/Fluid

Nausea/vomiting, food tolerance
Muscle wasting, dry/dull hair, swollen salivary glands, inflamed buccal cavity, capillary fragility (malnutrition)
Generalized tissue edema may be noted (protein deficiencies)
Gastric distension; ascites, liver enlargement (seen in cirrhosis)

Neurosensory

"Internal shakes"
Headache, dizziness, blurred vision, "blackouts"
Psychopathology such as paranoid schizophrenia, major depression (may indicate dual diagnosis)

Level of Consciousness/Orientation: Confusion, stupor, hyperactivity, distorted thought processes, slurred/incoherent speech

Memory loss/confabulation

Affect/Mood/Behavior: May be fearful, anxious, easily startled, inappropriate, silly, euphoric, irritable, physically/verbally abusive, depressed, and/or paranoid

Hallucinations: Visual, tactile, olfactory, and auditory (e.g., picking items out of air or responding verbally to unseen person/voices)

Nystagmus (associated with cranial nerve palsy)

Pupil constriction (may indicate CNS depression)

Arcus senilis, a ringlike opacity of the cornea (normal in aging populations, suggests alcohol-related changes in younger clients)

Fine motor tremors of face, tongue, and hands; seizure activity (commonly grand mal)

Gait unsteady/ataxia (may be due to thiamine deficiency or cerebellar degeneration [Wernicke's encephalopathy])

Pain/Discomfort

May report constant upper abdominal pain and tenderness radiating to the back (pancreatic inflammation)

Respiration

History of tobacco use, recurrent/chronic respiratory problems

Tachypnea (hyperactive state of alcohol withdrawal)

Cheyne-Stokes respirations or respiratory depression

Breath Sounds: Diminished/adventitious sounds (suggests pulmonary complications [e.g., respiratory depression, pneumonia])

Safety

History of recurrent accidents, such as falls, fractures, lacerations, burns, blackouts, or automobile accidents

Skin: Flushed face/palms of hands, scars, ecchymotic areas, cigarette burns on fingers, spider nevi (impaired portal circulation); fissures at corners of mouth (vitamin deficiency)

Fractures, healed or new (signs of recent/recurrent trauma)

Temperature elevation (dehydration and sympathetic stimulation); flushing/diaphoresis (suggests presence of infection)

Suicidal ideation/attempts (some research suggests alcoholic suicide attempts are 30% higher than national average for general population)

Social Interactions

Frequent sick days off work/school, fighting with others, arrests (disorderly conduct, motor vehicle violations [DUIs])

Denial that alcohol intake has any significant effect on the present condition/situation

Dysfunctional family system of origin; problems in current relationships

Mood changes affecting interactions with others

Teaching/Learning

History of alcohol and/or other drug use/abuse (including tobacco)

Ignorance and/or denial of addiction to alcohol or inability to cut down or stop drinking despite repeated efforts

Large amount of alcohol consumed in last 24–48 hours, previous periods of abstinence/withdrawal

Previous hospitalizations for alcoholism/alcohol-related diseases (e.g., cirrhosis, esophageal varices)

Family history of alcoholism/substance use

DIAGNOSTIC STUDIES

Blood Alcohol/Drug Levels: Alcohol level may/may not be severely elevated depending on amount consumed and length of time between consumption and testing. In addition to alcohol, numerous controlled/illicit substances may be identified in a polydrug screen (e.g., amphetamine, cocaine, morphine, Percodan, Quaalude).

CBC: Decreased (Hb/Hct) may reflect such problems as iron-deficiency anemia or acute/chronic GI bleeding. White blood cell count may be increased with infection or decreased, if immunosuppressed.

Glucose: Hyperglycemia/hypoglycemia may be present, related to pancreatitis, malnutrition, or depletion of liver glycogen stores.

Electrolytes: Hypokalemia and hypomagnesemia are common.

Liver Function Tests: CPK, LDH, AST, ALT, and amylase may be elevated, reflecting liver or pancreatic damage.

Nutritional Tests: Albumin is low and total protein decreased. Vitamin deficiencies are usually present, reflecting malnutrition/malabsorption.

Other Screening Studies (e.g., Hepatitis, HIV, TB): Dependent on general condition, individual risk factors, and care setting.

Urinalysis: Infection may be identified; ketones may be present related to breakdown of fatty acids in malnutrition (pseudodiabetic condition).

Chest X-Ray: May reveal right lower lobe pneumonia (malnutrition, depressed immune system, aspiration) or chronic lung disorders associated with tobacco use.

ECG: Dysrhythmias, cardiomyopathies, and/or ischemia may be present owing to direct effect of alcohol on the cardiac muscle and/or conduction system, as well as effects of electrolyte imbalance.

Addiction Severity Index (ASI): An assessment tool that produces a "problem severity profile" of the client, including chemical, medical, psychological, legal, family/social, and employment/support aspects, indicating areas of treatment needs.

NURSING PRIORITIES

1. Maintain physiological stability during withdrawal phase.
2. Promote client safety.
3. Provide appropriate referral and follow-up.
4. Encourage/support SO involvement in Intervention (confrontation) process.

DISCHARGE GOALS

1. Homeostasis achieved.
2. Complications prevented/resolved.
3. Sobriety being maintained on a day-to-day basis.
4. Ongoing participation in a rehabilitation program/attendance at group therapy (e.g., Alcoholics Anonymous).
5. Plan in place to meet needs after discharge.

   This plan of care is to be used in conjunction with CP: Substance Dependence/Abuse Rehabilitation.

NURSING DIAGNOSIS	BREATHING PATTERN, risk for ineffective
Risk Factors May Include:	Direct effect of alcohol toxicity on respiratory center and/or sedative drugs given to decrease alcohol withdrawal symptoms
	Tracheobronchial obstruction

	Presence of chronic respiratory problems, inflammatory process
	Decreased energy/fatigue
Possibly Evidenced by:	[Not applicable; presence of signs and symptoms establishes an *actual* diagnosis.]
Desired Outcomes Evaluation Criteria— Client Will:	Maintain effective respiratory pattern with respiratory rate within normal range, lungs clear, free of cyanosis and other signs/symptoms of hypoxia.

ACTIONS/INTERVENTIONS	RATIONALE
Independent	
Monitor respiratory rate/depth and pattern as indicated. Note periods of apnea, Cheyne-Stokes respirations.	Frequent assessment is important because toxicity levels may change rapidly. Hyperventilation is common during acute withdrawal phase. Kussmaul respirations are sometimes present because of acidotic state associated with vomiting and malnutrition. However, marked respiratory depression can occur because of CNS depressant effects of alcohol. This may be compounded by drugs used to control alcohol withdrawal symptoms.
Elevate head of bed.	Decreases possibility of aspiration; lowers diaphragm, enhancing lung inflation.
Encourage cough/deep breathing exercises and frequent position changes.	Facilitates lung expansion and mobilization of secretions to reduce risk of atelectasis/pneumonia.
Auscultate breath sounds. Note presence of adventitious sounds (e.g., rhonchi, wheezes).	Client is at risk for atelectasis related to hypoventilation and pneumonia. Right lower lobe pneumonia is common in alcohol-debilitated clients and is often due to aspiration. Chronic lung diseases are also common (e.g., emphysema, chronic bronchitis).
Have suction equipment, airway adjuncts available.	Sedative effects of alcohol/drugs potentiate risk of aspiration, relaxation of oropharyngeal muscles, and respiratory depression, requiring intervention to prevent respiratory arrest.
Collaborative	
Administer supplemental oxygen if necessary.	Hypoxia may occur with CNS/respiratory depression.
Review chest x-rays, pulse oximetry as available/indicated.	Monitors presence of secondary complications such as atelectasis/pneumonia; evaluates effectiveness of respiratory effort, identifies therapy needs.

159

NURSING DIAGNOSIS

NURSING DIAGNOSIS	**CARDIAC OUTPUT, risk for decreased**
Risk Factors May Include:	Direct effect of alcohol on the heart muscle
	Altered systemic vascular resistance
	Electrical alterations in rate, rhythm, conduction
Possibly Evidenced by:	[Not applicable; presence of signs and symptoms establishes an *actual* diagnosis.]
Desired Outcomes/Evaluation Criteria— Client Will:	Display vital signs within client's normal range; absence of/reduced frequency of dysrhythmias.
	Demonstrate an increase in activity tolerance.
	Verbalize understanding of the effect of alcohol on the heart.

ACTION/INTERVENTIONS	RATIONALE
Independent	
Monitor vital signs frequently during acute withdrawal.	Hypertension frequently occurs in acute withdrawal phase. Extreme hyperexcitability accompanied by catecholamine release and increased peripheral vascular resistance raises BP (and heart rate). However, BP may become labile/progress to hypotension. **Note:** Client may have underlying cardiovascular disease that is compounded by substance withdrawal.
Monitor cardiac rate/rhythm. Document irregularities/dysrhythmias.	Long-term alcohol abuse may result in cardiomyopathy/congestive heart failure. Tachycardia is common owing to sympathetic response to increased circulating catecholamines. Irregularities/dysrhythmias may develop with electrolyte shifts/imbalance. All of these may have an adverse effect on cardiac function/output.
Monitor body temperature.	Elevation may occur because of sympathetic stimulation, dehydration, and/or infections, causing vasodilation and compromising venous return/cardiac output.
Monitor intake/output. Note 24-hour fluid balance.	Preexisting dehydration, vomiting, fever, and diaphoresis may result in decreased circulating volume, which can compromise cardiovascular function. **Note:** Hydration is difficult to assess in the alcoholic because the usual indicators are not reliable, and overhydration is a risk in the presence of compromised cardiac function.
Be prepared for/assist in cardiopulmonary resuscitation.	Causes of death during acute withdrawal stages include cardiac dysrhythmias, respiratory depression/arrest, oversedation, excessive psychomotor activity, severe dehydration or overhydration, and massive infections. Mortality for unrecognized/untreated delirium tremens (DTs) may be as high as 15%–25%.

160

Collaborative

Monitor laboratory studies (e.g., serum electrolyte levels).

Electrolyte imbalance (e.g., potassium/magnesium) potentiates risk of cardiac dysrhythmias and CNS excitability.

Administer medications as indicated: e.g., clonidine (Catapres), atenolol (Tenormin);

Although the use of benzodiazepines is often sufficient to control hypertension during initial withdrawal from alcohol, some clients may require more specific therapy. **Note:** Atenolol and other beta-adrenergic blockers may speed up the withdrawal process and eliminate tremors, as well as lower heart rate, BP, and body temperature, reducing the need for benzodiazepines.

Potassium.

Corrects deficits that can result in life-threatening dysrhythmias.

NURSING DIAGNOSIS	INJURY, risk for (specify)
Risk Factors May Include:	Cessation of alcohol intake with varied autonomic nervous system responses to the suddenly altered state
	Involuntary clonic/tonic muscle activity (convulsions)
	Equilibrium/balancing difficulties, reduced muscle and hand/eye coordination
Possibly Evidenced by:	[Not applicable; presence of signs and symptoms establishes an *actual* diagnosis.]
Desired Outcomes/Evaluation Criteria— Client Will:	Demonstrate absence of untoward effects of withdrawal.
	Experience no physical injury.

ACTIONS/INTERVENTIONS

RATIONALE

Independent

Identify stage of alcohol withdrawal, symptoms: Stage I is associated with signs/symptoms of hyperactivity (e.g., tremors, sleeplessness, nausea/vomiting, diaphoresis, tachycardia, hypertension). Stage II is manifested by increased hyperactivity plus hallucinations and/or seizure activity. Stage III symptoms include delirium tremens (DTs) and extreme autonomic hyperactivity with profound confusion, anxiety, insomnia, fever.

Prompt recognition and intervention may halt progression of symptoms and enhance recovery/improve prognosis. In addition, recurrence/progression of symptoms indicates need for changes in drug therapy/more intense treatment.

Monitor/document seizure activity. Maintain patent airway. Provide environmental safety (e.g., padded side rails, bed in low position).

Grand mal seizures are most common and may be related to decreased magnesium levels, hypoglycemia, elevated blood alcohol, history of head trauma/preexisting seizure disorder. **Note:** In absence of previous history of other pathology causing seizure activity, seizures usually stop

161

	spontaneously, requiring only symptomatic treatment.
Check deep-tendon reflexes. Assess gait, if possible.	Reflexes may be depressed, absent, or hyperactive. Peripheral neuropathies are common, especially in malnourished clients. Ataxia (gait disturbance) is associated with Wernicke's syndrome (thiamine deficiency) and cerebellar degeneration.
Assist with ambulation and self-care activities as needed.	Prevents falls with resultant injury.
Provide for environmental safety when indicated. (Refer to ND: Sensory/Perceptual alteration [specify].)	May be required when equilibrium, hand/ eye coordination problems exist.

Collaborative

Administer IV/PO fluids with caution, as indicated.	Cautious replacement corrects dehydration and promotes renal clearance of toxins while reducing risk of overhydration.
Administer medications as indicated:	
Benzodiazepines such as: chlordiazepoxide (Librium), diazepam (Valium), clonazepam (Klonopin);	Commonly used to control neuronal hyperactivity that occurs as alcohol is detoxified. IV/PO administration is the route preferred, as intramuscular absorption is unpredictable. Muscle-relaxant qualities are particularly helpful to the client in controlling the "shakes," trembling, and ataxic quality of movements. Clients may initially require large doses to achieve desired effect, and then the drug(s) may be tapered and discontinued, usually within 96 hours. **Note:** These agents must be used cautiously in clients with hepatic disease, as the agents are metabolized by the liver.
Oxazepam (Serax);	Although less dramatic for control of withdrawal symptoms, this may be the drug of choice in a client with liver disease because of its shorter half-life.
Phenobarbital;	Useful in suppressing withdrawal symptoms and is an effective anticonvulsant. Use must be monitored to prevent exacerbation of respiratory depression.
Magnesium sulfate;	Reduces tremors and seizure activity by decreasing neuromuscular excitability.
Thiamine.	Thiamine deficiency (common in alcohol abuse) may lead to neuritis, Wernicke's syndrome, and/or Korsakoff's psychosis.

Nursing Diagnosis	**Sensory/Perceptual alterations (specify)**
May Be Related to:	Chemical alteration: Exogenous (e.g., alcohol consumption/sudden cessation) and endogenous (e.g., electrolyte imbalance, elevated ammonia and BUN)

Possibly Evidenced by:	Sleep deprivation
	Psychological stress (anxiety/fear)
	Disorientation in time, place, person, or situation
	Changes in usual response to stimuli; exaggerated emotional responses, change in behavior
	Bizarre thinking
	Restlessness, irritability, apprehension
Desired Outcomes/Evaluation Criteria— Client Will:	Regain/maintain usual level of cognition.
	Report absence of auditory/visual hallucinations.
	Identify external factors that affect sensory-perceptual abilities.

ACTIONS/INTERVENTIONS	RATIONALE
Independent	
Assess level of consciousness, ability to speak, response to stimuli/commands.	Speech may be garbled, confused, or slurred. Response to commands may reveal inability to concentrate, impaired judgment, or muscle coordination deficits.
Observe behavioral responses (e.g., hyperactivity, disorientation, confusion, sleeplessness, irritability).	Hyperactivity related to CNS disturbances may escalate rapidly. Sleeplessness is common because of loss of sedative effect gained from alcohol usually consumed prior to bedtime. Sleep deprivation may aggravate disorientation/confusion. Progression of symptoms may indicate impending hallucinations (Stage II) or DTs (Stage III).
Note onset of hallucinations. Document as auditory, visual, and/or tactile.	Auditory hallucinations are reported to be more frightening/threatening to client. Visual hallucinations occur more at night and often include insects, animals, or faces of friends/enemies. Clients are frequently observed picking the air; yelling may occur if client is calling for help from perceived threat (usually seen in Stage III).
Provide quiet environment. Speak in calm, quiet voice. Regulate lighting as indicated. Turn off radio/TV during sleep.	Reduces external stimuli during hyperactive stage. Client may become more delirious when surroundings cannot be seen, although some respond better to quiet, darkened room.
Provide care by same personnel whenever possible.	Promotes recognition of caregivers and a sense of consistency that may reduce fear.
Reorient frequently to person, place, time, and surrounding environment as indicated.	May reduce confusion/misinterpretation of external stimuli.
Avoid bedside discussion about client or topics unrelated to the client that do not include the client.	Client may hear and misinterpret conversation, which can aggravate hallucinations.

163

Provide environment safety (e.g., place bed in low position, leave doors in full open or closed position, observe frequently, place call light/bell within reach, remove articles that can harm client).

Client may have distorted sense of reality, be fearful, or be suicidal, requiring protection from self-harm.

Collaborative

Provide seclusion, restraints as necessary.

Clients with excessive psychomotor activity, severe hallucinations, violent behavior, and/or suicidal gestures may respond better to seclusion. Restraints are usually ineffective and add to client's agitation but occasionally may be required for short periods to prevent self-harm.

Monitor laboratory studies (e.g., electrolytes, magnesium levels, liver function studies, ammonia, BUN, glucose, ABGs).

Changes in organ function may precipitate or potentiate sensory-perceptual deficits. Electrolyte imbalance is common. Liver function is often impaired in the chronic alcoholic, and ammonia intoxication can occur if the liver is unable to convert ammonia to urea. Ketoacidosis is sometimes present without glycosuria; however, hyperglycemia or hypoglycemia may occur, suggesting pancreatitis or impaired gluconeogenesis in the liver. Hypoxemia and hypercarbia are common manifestations in chronic alcoholics who are also heavy smokers.

Administer medications as indicated, e.g.:

Antianxiety agents (Refer to ND: Anxiety [severe/panic]/Fear);

Reduces hyperactivity, promoting relaxation/sleep. Drugs that have little effect on dreaming may be desired to allow dream recovery (REM rebound) to occur, which has been suppressed by alcohol use.

Thiamine; vitamins C & B complex, multivitamins; Stresstabs.

Vitamins may be depleted because of insufficient intake and malabsorption. Vitamin deficiency (especially thiamine) is associated with ataxia, loss of eye movement and pupillary response, palpitations, postural hypotension, and exertional dyspnea.

NURSING DIAGNOSIS	**NUTRITION: altered, less than body requirements**
May Be Related to:	Poor dietary intake (replaced by alcohol consumption)
	Effects of alcohol on organs involved in digestion (e.g., stomach, pancreas, liver); interference with absorption and metabolism of nutrients and amino acids; and increased loss of vitamins in the urine
Possibly Evidenced by:	Reports of inadequate food intake, altered taste sensation, lack of interest in food, abdominal pain
	Body weight 20% or more under ideal

Pale conjunctiva and mucous membranes; sore, inflamed buccal cavity/cheilosis

Poor muscle tone, skin turgor

Hyperactive bowel sounds, diarrhea

Third spacing of circulating blood volume (e.g., edema of extremities, ascites)

Presence of neuropathies

Laboratory evidence of decreased red cell count (anemias), vitamin deficiencies, reduced serum albumin level, or electrolyte imbalance

Desired Outcomes/Evaluation Criteria—Client Will:

Verbalize understanding of effects of alcohol ingestion and reduced dietary intake on nutritional status and general well-being.

Demonstrate behaviors, lifestyle changes to regain/maintain appropriate weight.

Maintain stable weight or progressive weight gain toward goal with normalization of laboratory values and absence of signs of malnutrition.

ACTIONS/INTERVENTIONS	RATIONALE
Independent	
Evaluate presence/quality of bowel sounds. Note abdominal distension, tenderness.	Irritation of gastric mucosa is common and may result in epigastric pain, nausea, and hyperactive bowel sounds. More serious effects of GI system may occur secondary to cirrhosis and hepatitis.
Note presence of nausea/vomiting, diarrhea.	Nausea and vomiting are often among the first signs of alcohol withdrawal and may interfere with achieving adequate nutritional intake.
Assess ability to feed self.	Tremors, altered mentation, or hallucinations may interfere with ingestion of nutrients and indicate need for assistance.
Provide small, easily digested, frequent meals/snacks, and advance as tolerated.	May limit gastric distress and enhance intake and toleration of nutrients. As appetite and ability to tolerate food increase, diet should be adjusted to provide the necessary calories and nutrition for cellular repair and restoration of energy.
Collaborative	
Review laboratory tests (e.g., AST, ALT, LDH, serum albumin/prealbumin, transferrin).	Assesses liver function, adequacy of nutritional intake; influences choice of diet and need for/effectiveness of supplemental therapy.
Refer to dietitian/nutritional support team.	Useful in establishing and coordinating individual nutritional regimen.
Provide diet high in protein with at least half of calories obtained from carbohydrates.	Stabilizes blood sugar, thereby reducing risk of hypoglycemia, while providing for energy needs and cellular regeneration.

Administer medications as indicated, e.g.:

Antacids, antiemetics, antidiarrheal;

Vitamins,
thiamine.

Institute/maintain NPO status as indicated.

Reduces gastric irritation and limits effects of sympathetic stimulation.
Replace losses. **Note:** All clients should receive thiamine and vitamins, because deficiencies (clinical or subclinical) exist in most, if not all, clients with chronic alcoholism.
Provides gastrointestinal rest to reduce harmful effects of gastric/pancreatic stimulation in presence of GI bleeding or excessive vomiting.

NURSING DIAGNOSIS	ANXIETY [severe/panic]/FEAR
May Be Related to:	Cessation of alcohol intake/physiological withdrawal
	Situational crisis (hospitalization)
	Threat to self-concept, perceived threat of death
Possibly Evidenced by:	Feelings of inadequacy, shame, self-disgust, and remorse
	Increased helplessness/hopelessness with loss of control of own life
	Increased tension, apprehension
	Fear of unspecified consequences; identifying object of fear
Desired Outcomes/Evaluation Criteria—Client Will:	Verbalize reduction of fear and anxiety to an acceptable and manageable level.
	Express sense of regaining some control of situation/life.
	Demonstrate problem-solving skills and use resources effectively.

ACTIONS/INTERVENTIONS

RATIONALE

Independent

Identify cause of anxiety, involving client in the process. Explain that alcohol withdrawal increases anxiety and uneasiness. Reassess level of anxiety on an ongoing basis.

Develop a trusting relationship through frequent contact, being honest and nonjudgmental. Project an accepting attitude about alcoholism.

Inform client what you plan to do and why. Include client in planning process and provide choices when possible.

Clients in acute phase of withdrawal may be unable to identify and/or accept what is happening. Anxiety may be physiologically or environmentally caused. Continued alcohol toxicity will be manifested by increased anxiety and agitation as effects of medications wear off.

Provides client with a sense of humanness, helping to decrease paranoia and distrust. Client will be able to detect biased or condescending attitude of caregivers.

Enhances sense of trust, and explanation may increase cooperation/reduce anxiety. Provides sense of control over self in circumstances where

Reorient frequently. (Refer to ND: Sensory/ Perceptual alterations [specify].)

Client may experience periods of confusion, resulting in increased anxiety.

Collaborative

Administer medications as indicated, e.g.:
    Benzodiazepines: chlordiazepoxide (Librium), diazepam (Valium);

Antianxiety agents are given during acute withdrawal to help client relax, be less hyperactive, and feel more in control.

    Barbiturates: phenobarbital, or possibly secobarbital (Seconal), pentobarbital (Nembutal).

These drugs suppress alcohol withdrawal but need to be used with caution as they are respiratory depressants and REM sleep cycle inhibitors.

Arrange Intervention (confrontation) in controlled group setting.

The process of Intervention, wherein SOs/family members, supported by staff, provide information about how the client's drinking and behavior have affected each one of them, helps the client to acknowledge that drinking is a problem and has resulted in current situational crisis.

Provide consultation for referral to recovery/ rehabilitation program for ongoing treatment as soon as medically stable (e.g., oriented to reality).

Client is more likely to contract for treatment while still hurting and experiencing fear and anxiety from last drinking episode. Motivation decreases as well-being increases and person again feels able to control the problem. Direct contact with available treatment resources provides realistic picture of help. Decreases time for client to "think about it"/change mind or restructure and strengthen denial systems.

SAMPLE CLINICAL PATHWAY:
Alcohol Withdrawal Program ELOS: 7 days Behavioral Unit (3 days medical subacute as indicated)

ND and categories of care	Time dimension	Outcomes/actions	Time dimension	Outcomes/actions	Time dimension	Outcomes/actions
Risk for injury R/T varied autonomic and sensory responses	Day 1	Verbalize understanding of unit policies, procedures, and safety concerns relative to individual needs	Day 3	Vital signs stable I & O balanced	Day 7	Be free of injury resulting from ETOH withdrawal
	Day 4	Cooperate with therapeutic regimen	Day 4	Display marked decrease in objective symptoms		Display no objective symptoms of withdrawal
Referrals	Day 1	RN-NP or MD If indicated: Internist Cardiologist Neurologist				
Diagnostic studies	Day 1	BA level Drug screen (urine & blood) If indicated: CXR Pulse oximetry ECG	Day 2	SMA 20 Serum Mg, amylase RPR UA	Day 4	Repeat selected studies as indicated
Additional assessments	Day 1	VS, temp, respiratory status/breath sounds q4h	Day 2–3	VS q8h if stable	Day 4–7	VS qd
	Day 1–2	I & O q8h	Day 3–4	I & O qd		
	Day 1–4	Motor activity, body language, verbalizations, need for/type of restraint				
	Ongoing Stage I	Withdrawal symptoms: Tremors, N/V, hypertension, tachycardia, diaphoresis, sleeplessness				
	Stage II	Increased hyperactivity, hallucinations, seizure activity				

SUBSTANCE-RELATED DISORDERS: Alcohol-Related Disorders (Sample Clinical Pathway)

Medications
Allergies: ___

Stage III — Extreme autonomic hyperactivity, profound confusion, anxiety, fever

Day 1	Librium 200 mg PO; 25–50 mg PRN
Day 1–4	Thiamine 100 mg IM
Day 2	Librium 160 mg PO; 25 mg PRN
Day 3	Librium 120 mg PO; 15 mg PRN
Day 4	Librium 80 mg PO; 10 mg PRN
Day 5	Librium 40 mg PO; 5 mg PRN
Day 6	Librium 5 mg bid—PRN

Actions/Therapies

Day 1	Orient to room/unit, schedule, procedures
Day 5	Bed rest 12h if in withdrawal; Position change, HOB elevated; C, DB exercises if on bed rest
Day 1–2	Assist with ambulation, self-care as needed; Encourage fluids if free of N/V
Ongoing	Provide environmental safety measures, seizure precautions as indicated; Reorient as needed
Day 3–7	Encourage activity as tolerated
Day 5	Discuss need for ongoing therapy goals/availability of AA program
Day 7	Schedule followup visits if indicated

Ineffective individual coping R/T personal vulnerability, situational crisis, inadequate coping methods

Day 1–7	Participate in developmental/evaluation of treatment plan
Day 3	Verbalize understanding of relationship of ETOH abuse to current situation
Day 2–7	Interact in group sessions
Day 6	Identify/make contact with potential resources, support groups
Day 7	Plan in place to meet needs post discharge; Participating in ongoing program/support group

Referrals

Day 1	Psychiatrist
Day 2–7	Group sessions
Day 5	Community classes: Assertiveness training; Stress management

Additional assessments

Day 1	Understanding of current situation; Drinking pattern, previous withdrawal, other drug use, attitudes toward substance use
Day 2–3	Previous coping strategies/consequences; Perception of effect of drug use on life, employment, legal issues

170

ND and categories of care	Time dimension	Outcomes/actions	Time dimension	Outcomes/actions	Time dimension	Outcomes/actions
Additional assessments—continued		History of violence		Congruency of actions based on insight		Identify community resources for self/family
	Day 1–2	Relationships with others: personal, work/school Readiness for group activities	Day 3–7		Day 5–6	
Medications	Day 5–7	Naltrexone 50 mg/d if indicated				Review medication dose, frequency, side effects Provide written instructions for therapeutic program
Actions/Therapies	Day 1	Discuss physical effects on ETOH abuse	Day 2–5	Identify goals for change Discuss alternative solutions	Day 7	
	Day 1–2	Instruct in relaxation techniques	Day 7	Provide positive feedback for efforts		
	Day 1–7	Support client's taking responsibility for own recovery Provide consistent approach/ expectations for behavior Set limits/confront inappropriate behaviors	Day 2–7	Support during confrontation by peer group Encourage verbalization of feelings, personal reflection		
	Day 2	Review consequences of ETOH abuse	Day 3–7	Discuss human behavior and interactions with others/transactional analysis (TA)		
Altered nutrition: less than body requirements R/T poor intake, effects of ETOH on digestive system, and hypermetabolic response to withdrawal	Day 2–7	Select foods appropriately to meet individual dietary needs	Day 4	Verbalize understanding of effects of ETOH abuse and reduced dietary intake on nutritional status	Day 7	Display stable weight or initial weight gain as appropriate, and with laboratory results WNL

Category	Time	Intervention	Time	Intervention	Time	Intervention
Referrals	Day 1 & PRN	Dietitian				
Diagnostic studies	Day 1	CBC, liver function studies	Day 2–7	Fingerstick glucose PRN	Day 7	Weight
	Day 1	Serum albumin, transferrin				
Additional assessments	Day 1	Weight, skin turgor, condition of mucous membranes, muscle tone				
	Day 1–2	Bowel sounds, characteristics of stools				
	Day 1–7	Appetite, dietary intake				
Medications	Day 1–7	Antacid AC & HS	Day 2–7	Multivitamin tab/qd		
	Day 1–7	Imodium 2 mg PRN				
Actions/Therapies	Day 1–2	Review individual nutritional needs	Day 2–7	Discuss principles of nutrition, foods for maintenance of wellness		
	Day 1	Provide liquid/bland diet as tolerated	Day 4	Advance diet as tolerated to high-protein, high-carbohydrate diet		
	Day 1–7	Encourage small, frequent easily digested, nutritious meals/snacks				
		Encourage good oral hygiene PC & HS				

Adapted from Townsend, MC: Psychiatric Mental Health Nursing, ed 2. FA Davis, Philadelphia, 1996.

STIMULANTS (AMPHETAMINES, COCAINE, CAFFEINE, AND NICOTINE) AND INHALANT-RELATED DISORDERS

DSM-IV
AMPHETAMINE-INDUCED DISORDERS
292.81 Intoxication delirium
292.89 Amphetamine intoxication
292.0 Amphetamine withdrawal
292.11 Psychotic disorders with delusions
292.12 Psychotic disorders with hallucinations
CAFFEINE-INDUCED DISORDERS
305.90 Caffeine intoxication
292.89 Caffeine-induced anxiety disorder
292.89 Caffeine-induced sleep disorder
COCAINE-INDUCED DISORDERS
292.89 Cocaine intoxication
292.0 Cocaine withdrawal
292.81 Intoxication delirium
INHALANT-INDUCED DISORDERS
292.89 Inhalant intoxication
292.81 Inhalant intoxication delirium
292.84 Inhalant-induced mood disorder
292.89 Inhalant-induced anxiety disorder
NICOTINE-INDUCED DISORDER
292.0 Nicotine withdrawal

(For additional listings, consult *DSM-IV*.)

Stimulants are natural and manufactured drugs that speed up the nervous system. They can be swallowed, injected, inhaled, or smoked. These substances are identified by the behavioral stimulation and psychomotor agitation that they induce. They differ widely in their molecular structures and in their mechanisms of action. The most prevalent and widely used stimulants are caffeine and nicotine. Caffeine is readily available as a common ingredient in coffee, tea, colas, and chocolate. Nicotine is a primary substance in tobacco products. These are generally accepted as a part of our culture, are not usually seen in overdose situations, and are included here for information only. Other more potent stimulants (e.g., cocaine, amphetamines, and nonamphetamine stimulants) are regulated by the Controlled Substance Act. They are available for therapeutic purposes by prescription but are also widely available on the illicit drug market. The potential for overdose and even death is high.

Inhalant substances such as gasoline, glue, paint/paint thinners, spray paints, cleaning compounds, and correction fluid, to name a few, are not classified as stimulants; however, the intoxicating effects of these products and their therapeutic interventions are similar and therefore addressed here.

This plan of care addresses acute intoxication/withdrawal and is to be used in conjunction with CP: Substance Dependence/Abuse Rehabilitation.

ETIOLOGICAL THEORIES

Psychodynamics

Individuals who abuse substances fail to complete tasks of separation-individuation, resulting in underdeveloped egos. The person retains a highly dependent nature, with characteristics of poor impulse control, low frustration tolerance, and low self-esteem, low social conformity, neurotocism, and introversion. The superego is weak, resulting in absence of guilt feelings for behavior. Underlying psychiatric status must be assessed, as these individuals may use stimulants for varying self-medication reasons (dual diagnosis).

Biological

An apparent genetic link is involved in the development of substance use disorders. However, the statistics are currently inconclusive regarding abuse of stimulant drugs.

Family Dynamics

Predisposition to substance use disorders occurs in a dysfunctional family system. There is often one parent who is absent or who is an overpowering tyrant and/or one parent who is weak and ineffectual. Substance abuse may be evident as the primary method of relieving stress. The child has negative role models and learns to respond to stressful situations in like manner.

CLIENT ASSESSMENT DATA BASE

The client may present with intoxication or in various stages of withdrawal, affecting data gathered. Data depend on stage of withdrawal, concurrent use of alcohol/other drugs, or contaminants in drug "cut."

Activity/Rest

Insomnia; hypersomnia; nightmares
Anxiety
Hyperactivity, increased alertness, or falling asleep during activities; lethargy (inhalants)
Inability to tolerate or to correct chronic fatigue (depression and/or loneliness may be a factor)
General muscle weakness, incoordination, unsteady gait (inhalants)

Circulation

BP usually elevated; may be hypotensive
Tachycardia, irregular pulse
Diaphoresis

Ego Integrity

Need to feel elated, sociable, happy with self, desire to prove self-worth, improve self-concept; craving for excitement
Compulsion regarding substance use, or denial of powerlessness over the substance (use of drug for celebration or crisis, believing drug can be used in regulated quantities, often resulting in binge use); may think of recovery process as notion of willpower, subject to impulse control
Absence of guilt feelings for behavior
Underdeveloped ego; highly dependent nature, with characteristics of poor impulse control, low frustration tolerance, and low self-esteem; reckless/rebellious behavior, weak superego
May be seen or view self as susceptible to influence by others, having an inability to say "no"
Feelings of helplessness, hopelessness, powerlessness
Emotional status: Anxious, evasive, irritable, may be angry/hostile, belligerent

Food/Fluid

Nausea/vomiting, anorexia
Weight loss; thin, cachectic appearance
Compulsiveness with food (especially sugars)

Neurosensory

Emotional/psychological symptoms (e.g., elation, grandiosity, loquacity [excessive talkativeness], hypervigilance)

Numbness in hands and feet

Twitching, jerking in face, neck, arms, hands (dyskinesias; dystonias)

Dizziness

Pupillary dilation with slowed reaction to light; blurred vision or diplopia; nystagmus, lack of convergence (inhalants)

Tremors, convulsions, coma

Delirium with tactile and olfactory hallucinations, as well as hallucinations of insects or vermin crawling in/under the skin (formication); labile affect, violent or aggressive behavior, symptoms of a paranoid delusional disorder (amphetamine or similarly acting substances)

Fixed delusional system of a persecutory nature, lasting weeks to a year or more

Psychosis (can occur with a 1-time high dose of amphetamine [especially with IV administration] or with long-term use at moderate or high dose)

Ideas of reference

Aggressiveness, hostility, violence, quick response to anger; psychomotor agitation/hyperactivity

Hypersensitive to sound, light, touch

Stereotyped compulsive motor behavior (e.g., sorting, taking things apart and putting them back together, moving mouth from side to side)

Psychomotor retardation, depressed reflexes, unsteady gait (inhalants)

Anxiety; impaired judgment and perception

Apathy, stupor, coma, or euphoria (inhalants)

Pain/Discomfort

Bone/chest pan

Respiration

Tachypnea, coughing

Nasal rhinitis (chronic cocaine use)

Chronic/recurrent bronchiolitis; pneumonia

Pulmonary hemorrhage

Safety

History of accidents; exposure to STDs, including HIV

Acute allergic/anaphylactic reaction (response to contaminants in drug cut)

Elevated temperature; fever/chills, diaphoresis

Evidence of trauma (e.g., bruises, lacerations, burns); nasal damage (if drug is snorted)

Assaultive behavior (inhalants)

Sexuality

Diminished/enhanced sexual desire; disinhibition regarding sexual behavior (promiscuity/prostitution)

Increased likelihood of pregnancy/abortion

Social Interactions

Impairment in relationship, social, or occupational functioning; encounters with the legal system; expulsion from school

Dysfunctional family system (family of origin)

Teaching/Learning

Predominant age range of 21 to 44 years (stimulants), teenage population (inhalants)

Learning difficulties (e.g., attention-deficit hyperactivity disorder)

Family history of substance abuse (especially alcohol)

Concurrent use of alcohol/other drugs (compounds symptoms/reactions)

Pattern of habitual use of the particular drug or pathological abuse, with inability to reduce or to stop use, occurring for at least 1 month

Intoxication throughout the day, sometimes with daily involvement

During-Period of Abstinence: Drug hunger, delayed reemergence of withdrawal symptoms (reemergence may occur at 3 months, between 9 and 12 months, and perhaps as late as 18 months after abstinence)

Previous hospitalizations or having been in residential treatment program for substance use/dual diagnosis

Health beliefs about use of drugs (e.g., "Diet pills are OK to use to lose weight.")

Attendance at recovery groups (e.g., Narcotics/Alcoholics Anonymous or other drug-specific recovery groups)

DIAGNOSTIC STUDIES

Blood and Urine Drug Screens: To identify presence/type of drug(s) being used

Tests for Hepatitis and HIV: May be routine in known IV drug users or when client has identified risk factors.

Other Screening Studies: Depend on general condition, individual risk factors, and care setting.

Addiction Severity Index (ASI): Produces a "problem severity profile," which indicates areas of treatment needs.

NURSING PRIORITIES

1. Maintain physiological stability.
2. Promote safety and security.
3. Prevent complications.
4. Support client's acceptance of reality of situation.
5. Promote family involvement in Intervention/treatment process.

DISCHARGE GOALS

1. Homeostasis maintained.
2. Complications prevented/resolved.
3. Client is dealing with situation realistically/planning for the future.
4. Abstinence from drug(s) maintained on a day-to-day basis.
5. Attending rehabilitation program/therapy group.
6. Plan in place to meet needs after discharge.

NURSING DIAGNOSIS	CARDIAC OUTPUT, risk for decreased
Risk Factors May Include:	Drug (e.g., cocaine) effect on myocardium (dependent on drug purity/quantity used)
	Preexisting myocardiopathy (with or without previous prolonged drug abuse)
	Alterations in electrical rate/rhythm/conduction

Possibly Evidenced by:	[Not applicable; presence of signs/symptoms establishes an *actual* diagnosis.]
Desired Outcomes/Evaluation Criteria— Client Will:	Report absence of chest pain.
	Demonstrate adequate cardiac output free of signs of dysrhythmias, shock.

ACTIONS/INTERVENTIONS	RATIONALE
Independent	
Monitor BP.	BP fluctuations can be extreme, with both hypertension and hypotension affecting cardiac output.
Monitor cardiac rate and rhythm. Document dysrhythmias.	Ventricular dysrhythmias/cardiac arrest may occur at any time, especially with toxic levels of certain drugs (e.g., cocaine, "crack," "ice," and amphetamine cogeners).
Investigate reports of chest pain, indigestion/heartburn.	Incidence of myocardial infarction is increased in cocaine users.
Have emergency equipment/medications available.	Prompt treatment of dysrhythmias may prevent cardiac arrest.
Collaborative	
Administer supplemental oxygen as needed.	Tachycardia and other cardiac dyshythmias may be improved/decreased with increased oxygen delivery to tissues.
Administer medications as indicated, e.g.,	
propranolol (Inderal);	Beta-adrenergic blockers can reduce cardiac O_2 demand by blocking catecholamine-induced increases in heart rate, BP, and force of myocardial contraction.
Antidysrhythmics.	May be needed to abort life-threatening dysrhythmia/maintain cardiac function.
Transfer to medical setting as appropriate.	May be necessary to provide closer observation and more aggressive interventions.

NURSING DIAGNOSIS	VIOLENCE, risk for, directed at self/others
Risk Factors May Include:	Toxic reaction to drug, withdrawal from drug
	Panic state, profound depression/suicidal behavior
	Organic brain syndrome
[Possible Indicators:]	Overt and aggressive acts
	Increased motor activity
	Possession of destructive means

Desired Outcomes/Evaluation Criteria—Client Will:	Suspicion of others, paranoid ideation, delusions, and hallucinations
	Expressed intent directly/indirectly
	Acknowledge fearfulness and realities of situation.
	Verbalize understanding of behavior and precipitating factors.
	Demonstrate self-control as evidenced by use of problem-solving skills in situations that usually precipitate violence.

ACTIONS/INTERVENTIONS	RATIONALE

Independent

Obtain information specific to pattern of drug use over past month, what drugs have been used together, in addition to immunization history, allergies, medications used for other purposes.	Initial factual history can reveal information essential to treatment needs. Where person obtained drug could assist in investigating possible "cut" with other drugs.
Decrease stimuli; provide quiet in own room or place in stimulus-reduction room with supervision.	Reduces reactivity, enhances calm feelings. Observation enhances client safety, allowing for timely intervention.
Remove potentially harmful objects from environment.	Reduces opportunity for harmful behaviors. **Note:** Client may be suicidal when/if rebound CNS depression occurs secondary to stimulant withdrawal.
Explain consistent rules of unit (e.g., no violence, no threats).	Secure environment enhances sense of safety, which can decrease perceived threat. Enhances opportunity for client to learn ways to cope with aggressive feelings before reacting.
Maintain high staff profile in situations in which potential violence can occur.	May prevent onset of violence and allows quick response if violence does occur.
Provide opportunities for verbal expression of aggressive feelings in acceptable ways.	Encouragement of new avenue of expression helps client learn new coping skills.
Assist client in identifying what provokes anger.	Awareness of reaction is the first step in learning change.
Provide outlets for expression that involve physical activity (e.g., walking, stationary bicycle).	Physical activity in protected environment can lessen aggressive drive.
Discuss consequences of aggressive behavior.	Learning choices helps client gain control of situation and self.
Be alert to violence potential (e.g., increased pacing, verbalization of delusional persecutory content, hypervigilance regarding specific persons in the milieu, gesturing aggressively, threatening others verbally or physically).	Recognizing potential and helping client gain control can be more effective before violent outbreak.
Isolate client immediately if he or she becomes violent, using adequate number of staff trained in assaultive management. Maintain calm, nonpunitive attitude.	Client will feel safer if others take control until internal locus of control can be regained. An attitude of acceptance is important while refusing

177

Negotiate conditions for coming out of isolation/ "quiet time" when the client is calm, based on agreement of social appropriateness.

Build trust: follow through on commitments/ agreements, maintain consistent staff and frequent brief contact with client.

to tolerate the violent behavior. **Note:** Use of seclusion and restraints may exacerbate hyperactivity.

Clear expectations help client feel secure about own control.

Trust is essential to working with all clients. Brief contacts can prevent overstimulation.

Collaborative

Administer medications as indicated, e.g.:

Chlorpromazine (Thorazine), haloperidol (Haldol);

Short-term use of antipsychotics during acute intoxication/psychosis helps client gain self-control; promotes sedation/rest when agitated, assaultive, overstimulated. **Note:** Thorazine may cause postural hypotension, and Haldol may provoke acute extrapyramidal reaction, requiring additional evaluation/medication.

Diazepam (Valium), chlordiazepoxide (Librium).

Occasionally useful for treatment of acute cocaine intoxication. Either drug is useful for preventing delirium tremens when substance use is combined with alcohol.

NURSING DIAGNOSIS	SENSORY/PERCEPTUAL alterations (specify)
May Be Related to:	Chemical alteration: exogenous (CNS stimulants or depressants, mind-altering drugs)
	Altered sensory reception, transmission, and/or integration: altered status of sense organs
Possibly Evidenced by:	Bizarre thinking, anxiety/panic
	Preoccupation with/appears to be responding to internal stimuli from hallucinatory experiences (e.g., assumes "listening pose," laughs and talks to self, stops in midsentence and listens, "picks" at self and clothing, tries to "get away from bugs")
	Changes in sensory acuity, decreased pain perception
Desired Outcomes/Evaluation Criteria— Client Will:	Distinguish reality from altered perceptions.
	State awareness that hallucinations may result from substance use.

ACTIONS/INTERVENTIONS	RATIONALE

Independent

Notice client's preoccupation, responses, gesturing, social skills.	Helps assess whether or not client is hallucinating without overstimulating verbally.

178

Assist client in checking perceptions verbally, provide reality information.	Can calm the client and provide reassurance of safety and that formication (illusion of insects crawling on the body) or other misperceptions are not occurring.
Acknowledge client's emotional state; letting client know safety will be maintained.	Empathetic response can diminish intensity of fear.
Explore ways of calming client. Encourage use of relaxation techniques (e.g., deep-breathing exercises, focusing on caregiver).	Relaxation can promote positive outlook, distracting from negativity and enhancing clarity of perception. **Note:** Visualization/guided imagery techniques and touch may increase agitation/hallucinations and are usually not recommended.
Be aware that altered sensation and perception may cause injury (e.g., be alert for client burning self with cigarette, excessive scratching at skin to rid self of bugs or drug [which may feel as though it is inside the skin], accidentally harming self through poor judgment or misperceptions). (Refer to ND: Violence, risk for, directed at self/others.)	Amphetamine use causes impaired judgment, increasing risk of injury/self-harm. Overdose of many stimulants causes frightening hallucinations, often of large insects crawling on skin.
Inform client (if calm enough) of temporary nature of hallucinations that have resulted from stimulant use.	Learning cause, effect, and possible temporary nature of misperceptions may reduce fear, anxiety, and negativity. This may inject hope and positive attitude.

NURSING DIAGNOSIS	FEAR/ANXIETY [specify level]
May Be Related to:	Paranoid delusions associated with stimulant use
Possibly Evidenced by:	Feelings/beliefs that others are conspiring against or are about to attack/kill client
Desired Outcomes/Evaluation Criteria—Client Will:	Recognize frightening feelings before preoccupying self with acting on fears.
	Discuss reality base of persecutory fears with staff.
	Report fear/anxiety reduced to manageable level.
	Demonstrate appropriate range of feelings and appear relaxed.

ACTIONS/INTERVENTIONS	RATIONALE

Independent

Establish consistent staff assignment and stress importance of being reliable, honest, genuine, prompt.	Builds trust and rapport, which are necessary for overcoming fear.
Acknowledge awareness of client's feelings (e.g., fear, terror, feeling overwhelmed, panic, anxiety, confusion).	Empathy can assist client to tolerate/deal with own feelings.
Be concrete, clear in communication. Assess client's readiness for humor and/or touch.	Fear negatively influences one's ability to attend to and interpret stimuli. Fear is serious to the

179

perceiver and must be respected. Laughter and touch can be misinterpreted/increase anxiety.

Encourage verbalization of fears/anxieties.	Ventilating feelings to trusted staff can lessen intensity of fearfulness. This provides opportunity to clarify misunderstandings and comforts client.
Assist client in reality-checking fears. Use gentle confrontation.	Client can reduce fear if he or she understands difference between reality and delusions. Should be used cautiously, as reality-checking a delusional system puts trust at risk.

NURSING DIAGNOSIS	**NUTRITION: altered, less than body requirements**
May Be Related to:	Anorexia (stimulant use)
	Insufficient/inappropriate use of financial resources
Possibly Evidenced by:	Reported/observed inadequate intake
	Lack of interest in food; weight loss
	Poor muscle tone
	Signs/laboratory evidence of vitamin deficiencies
Desired Outcomes/Evaluation Criteria— Client Will:	Demonstrate progressive weight gain toward goal.
	Verbalize understanding of causative factors and individual nutritional needs.
	Identify appropriate dietary choices, lifestyle changes to regain/maintain desired weight.

ACTIONS/INTERVENTIONS	RATIONALE

Independent

Ascertain intake pattern over past several weeks.	Stimulants cause decreased appetite and impaired judgment regarding nutritional needs.
Discuss needs/likes/dislikes about food choices.	Will be more likely to maintain desired intake if individual preferences are considered.
Anticipate hyperphagia and weigh every other day.	Overeating may be a consequence of stimulant withdrawal and may result in sudden/ inappropriate weight gain.
Provide meals in a relaxed, nonstimulating environment.	Stimulus reduction aids relaxation and ability to focus on eating.
Encourage frequent nutritional snacks, small nutritious meals.	Small amounts of food frequently can prevent/reduce GI distress.

Collaborative

Obtain/review routine diagnostic studies (e.g., CBC; serum protein, albumin, vitamin levels; UA).	Assessment of nutritional state is necessary to treat preexisting deficiencies and rule out anemia, dehydration, or ketosis.

Consult with dietitian.

Useful in establishing individual nutritional needs/dietary program.

Administer multivitamins as indicted.

Supplementation enhances correction of deficiencies.

NURSING DIAGNOSIS	INFECTION, risk for
Risk Factors May Include:	IV-drug-use techniques; impurities of injected drugs
	Localized trauma; nasal septum damage (snorting cocaine)
	Malnutrition; altered immune state
Possibly Evidenced by:	[Not applicable, presence of signs and symptoms establishes an *actual* diagnosis.]
Desired Outcome/Evaluation Criteria—Client Will:	Verbalize understanding of individual risk factors.
	Identify interventions to prevent/reduce risk factors.
	Demonstrate lifestyle changes to promote safe environment.
	Achieve timely healing of infectious process if present and be afebrile.

ACTIONS/INTERVENTIONS	RATIONALE

Independent

Obtain information specific to pattern of drug use over past month, immunization history, allergies, specific medications used for other purposes.	Helps identify risk factors, can reveal information essential to need for further evaluation/treatment.
Assess skin integrity and character. Assist as needed with body and oral hygiene; provide clean clothes, properly fitting shoes.	Maintaining skin integrity requires cleanliness. If sores are present, they may need care to prevent infection.
Use blood/body fluid precautions as appropriate.	Protects caregivers from possible contamination by infectious disease/viruses (e.g., hepatitis, HIV).
Monitor vital signs. Assess level of consciousness.	Abnormal signs, including fever, can indicate presence of infection. Cerebral complications (e.g., meningitis, brain abscess) may occur, affecting mentation. **Note:** Fever is also a symptom of toxic CNS effect.
Review physical assessment regularly.	Can reveal daily changes and problematic areas. Physical assessment provides recognition of pathology and identifies areas for providing information for health promotion and problem prevention.
Investigate recurrent cough; note characteristics of sputum. Auscultate breath sounds.	These clients are at increased risk for development of pulmonary infections.

181

Observe for nasal stuffiness, pain, bleeding, abnormal mucus production.

Cocaine snorting can cause erosion of the nasal septum, requiring additional therapy/interventions.

Investigate reports of acute/chronic deep bone pain, tenderness, guarding with movement, regional muscle spasm.

Occasionally, osteomyelitis may develop because of hematogenous spread of bacteria, most often affecting lumbar vertebrae.

Ascertain health status of family members/SO(s) currently in contact with client.

May have exposed client to diseases such as colds, tuberculosis, hepatitis, HIV, which could be problematic for client.

Collaborative

Review laboratory studies (e.g., UA, CBC, Biochem screen, RPR, ESR, ELISA/Western Blot test).

May identify complications of injection drug use such as hepatitis, nephritis, tetanus, vasculitis, septicemia, subacute bacterial endocarditis, embolic phenomena, malaria. Toxic allergic reactions may result from other substances in the cut, and immunological abnormalities may occur because of repeated antigenic stimulation. **Note:** Injection drug users are at high risk for contamination with HIV and hepatitis viruses.

NURSING DIAGNOSIS	SLEEP PATTERN disturbance
May Be Related To:	CNS sensory alterations: External factor (stimulant use), internal factor (psychological stress)
Possibly Evidenced By:	Altered sleep cycle; initial signs of insomnia, and then hypersomnia
	Constant alertness; racing thoughts that prevent rest
	Denial of need to sleep or report of inability to stay awake
Desired Outcomes/Evaluation Criteria—Client Will:	Sleep 6–8 hours at night.
	Rest minimally, appropriately, during the day.
	Verbalize feeling rested when awakens.

ACTIONS/INTERVENTIONS	RATIONALE

Independent

Establish sleep cycle in which client sleeps at night, is awake during day with only brief rest periods as needed.

Adequate rest and sleep can improve emotional state; restoration of regular pattern is a priority in a sleep-deprived stimulant user.

Decrease stimuli and enhance relaxation prior to bedtime; encourage use of presleep routines (e.g., hot bath, warm milk, stretching).

Client may need calming to attempt rest.

Provide opportunities for fresh air, mild exercise, noncaffeinated beverages, and provide quiet environment as client can tolerate.

Promotes drowsiness/desire for sleep.

DEPRESSANTS (BARBITURATES, NONBARBITURATES, HYPNOTICS AND ANXIOLYTICS, OPIOIDS)

DSM-IV

SEDATIVE-, HYPNOTIC-, OR ANXIOLYTIC-INDUCED DISORDERS
292,89 Sedative, hypnotic, or anxiolytic intoxication
292.0 Sedative, hypnotic, or anxiolytic withdrawal
292.81 Intoxication delirium
292. 84 Induced mood disorder
OPIOID-RELATED DISORDERS
292.89 Opioid intoxication
292.81 Intoxication delirium
292.0 Opioid withdrawal

(For further listings, consult *DSM-IV.*)

CNS depressants are drugs that slow down the central nervous system. They are usually divided into four types: barbiturates, antianxiety agents, sedative-hypnotics, and narcotics (opioids such as morphine, heroin).

CNS depressants prescribed for symptoms of anxiety, depression, and sleep disturbances are among the most widely used and abused drugs. These drugs are very likely to be abused when the underlying conditions remain untreated. Sometimes these drugs are used in conjunction with stimulants, with the user developing a pattern of taking a stimulant to be "up," then needing the depressant drug to "come down."

Several principles apply to all CNS depressants: (1) The effects are interactive and cumulative with one another and with the behavioral state of the user; (2) there is no specific antagonist that will block the action of these drugs; (3) low doses produce an initial excitatory response; (4) they are capable of producing physiological and psychological dependency; and (5) cross-tolerance and cross-dependence may exist between various CNS depressants. Although the margin of safety of these drugs is great, they have a characteristic syndrome of withdrawal that can be very severe.

This plan of care addresses acute intoxication/withdrawal and is to be used in conjunction with CP: Substance Dependence/Abuse Rehabilitation.

ETIOLOGICAL THEORIES

Psychodynamics

Individuals who abuse substances fail to complete tasks of separation-individuation, resulting in underdeveloped egos. The person has a highly dependent nature, with characteristics of poor impulse control, low frustration tolerance, and low self-esteem. The superego is weak, resulting in absence of guilt feelings. Underlying psychiatric status must be assessed, as these individuals may use stimulants for varying self-medication reasons.

Psychostructural factors (e.g., personality) are seen as significant. The defect is believed to precede the addiction, with the ego structure breaking down and the substance being used as a maladaptive coping mechanism. Characteristics that have been identified include impulsivity, negative self-concept, weak ego, low social conformity, neuroticism, and introversion.

Biological

A genetic link is thought to be involved in the development of substance use disorders. Although statistics are currently inconclusive, hereditary factors are generally accepted to be a factor in the abuse of substances.

Family Dynamics

There is an apparent predisposition to substance abuse disorders in the dysfunctional family system. Factors such as the absence of a parent or a parent who is an overpowering tyrant or weak and ineffectual, and the use of substances as the primary method of relieving stress, appear to contribute to this dysfunction. These role models have a negative influence, and the child learns to handle stress in like manner. However, parents may be average, normal individuals with children who succumb to overwhelming peer pressure and become involved with drugs. Cultural factors such as acceptance of the use of alcohol and other drugs may also influence the individual's choice.

CLIENT ASSESSMENT DATA BASE

Data depend on stage of withdrawal and concurrent use of alcohol/other drugs.

Activity/Rest

General malaise
Interference with sleep pattern, insomnia (withdrawal)
Lethargy, drowsiness, somnolence
Yawning

Circulation

Pulse usually slowed; tachycardia (suggests withdrawal syndrome); irregular pulse (atrial
    fibrillation, ventricular dysrhythmias)
Hypotension

Ego Integrity

Substance use for stress management
Feelings of helplessness, hopelessness, powerlessness
Underdeveloped ego; highly dependent nature, with characteristics of poor impulse
    control, low frustration tolerance, and low self-esteem
Weak superego, with absence of guilt feelings
Psychostructural factors (e.g., personality) are seen as significant with substance use/abuse
    (maladaptive coping mechanisms)

Elimination

Diarrhea, occasionally constipation

Food/Fluid

Nausea/vomiting

Neurosensory

Twitching
Mental Status: Confusion, concentration, and memory problems; impaired judgment with
    some affective change; alterations in consciousness may exist, from extreme agitation
    to coma; slurred speech
Behavior: Mood swings, lack of motivation, aggression, combativeness (related to general
    "disinhibiting" effect of the drug, loss of impulse control), dysphoric mood
    (withdrawal)
Temporary psychosis with acute onset of auditory hallucinations and paranoid delusions
    (unexplained neuropsychiatric presentation may be indicative of drug use)
Psychomotor activity may be increased
Hypersensitivity (e.g., anxiety, tremors, hypotension, irritability, restlessness, and seizure
    activity)

Pupils small/pinpoint constriction (opiates), dilated (barbiturates); reaction to light slowed; horizontal gaze, nystagmus, lack of convergence
Gait unsteady/staggering, loss of coordination, positive Romberg's sign

Pain/Discomfort

Headache, abdominal pain/severe cramping
Muscle aches
Deep muscle/bone pain (methadone abusers)

Respiration

Continuous rhinorrhea, excessive lacrimation, sneezing
Respiratory depression (overdose)
Increased respiratory rate (withdrawal syndrome)

Safety

Hot/cold flashes; diaphoresis
Thermoregulation instability with hyperpyrexia, hypothermia possible
Skin: Piloerection ("gooseflesh"); puncture wounds on arms, hands, legs, under tongue, indicating injection drug use

Social Interactions

Dysfunctional family of origin system
Dysfunctional patterns of interaction with family/others

Teaching/Learning

Preexisting physical/psychological conditions
Family history of substance use/abuse
History of chronic condition/disease process
Concurrent use of other drugs, including alcohol

DIAGNOSTIC STUDIES

Drug Screen: Identifies drug(s) being used.
STD Screening: To determine presence of HIV, hepatitis B, etc.
Other Screening Studies: Depend on general condition, individual risk factors, and care setting.
Addiction Severity Index (ASI): Produces a problem-severity profile, which indicates areas of treatment needs.

NURSING PRIORITIES

1. Achieve physiological stability.
2. Protect client from injury.
3. Provide appropriate referral and follow-up.
4. Promote family involvement in the withdrawal/rehabilitation process.

DISCHARGE GOALS

1. Homeostasis achieved.
2. Complications prevented/resolved.
3. Abstinence from drug(s) initiated/maintained on a day-to-day basis.
4. Attends rehabilitation program, group therapy (e.g., Narcotics Anonymous).
5. Plan in place to meet needs after discharge.

NURSING DIAGNOSIS	TRAUMA/SUFFOCATION/POISONING, risk for
Risk Factors May Include:	CNS depression (effect of overdose)
	CNS agitation (effect of abrupt withdrawal)
	Hypersensitivity to the drug(s)
	Psychological stress (narrowed perceptual fields seen with anxiety)
Possibly Evidenced by:	[Not applicable; presence of signs and symptoms establishes an *actual* diagnosis.]
Desired Outcomes/Evaluation Criteria—Client Will:	Verbalize understanding of risks of taking drugs.
	Refrain from acting on hallucinations/impaired judgment.
	Complete withdrawal without injury to self/development of complications.

ACTIONS/INTERVENTIONS	RATIONALE

Independent

Talk with client/SO regarding when person was last seen well; noting history/duration of health problems, sleep patterns, and prescriptions used.	Determines degree and approximate time frame for impairment, with sleep disruption often the first observable sign of problem. Ongoing health problems (e.g., chronic pain conditions) potentiate substance use. Prescription information provides clues to identify drug(s) and amount taken.
Identify drug(s) taken, when taken, and route used, if possible.	Helpful to identify interventions for specific drug. Determining drug(s) taken may be difficult without blood/urine testing as the client may not feel free to tell because of embarrassment or for legal reasons, or may not know what has been ingested.
Assess level of consciousness (e.g., agitated, stuporous, lethargic, confused, or comatose). Note pinpoint pupils.	May indicate degree of intoxication and level of intervention required. Constricted pupils are a classic sign of opioid (heroin) use.
Evaluate for evidence of head trauma.	This is important to note for differential diagnosis, to prevent inappropriate treatment/interventions.
Determine when food was last eaten. Note reports of nausea.	Presence of food in stomach may slow absorption of drug(s) into the bloodstream; however, if level of consciousness is depressed, presence of food in stomach increases the risk of vomiting and aspiration.
Monitor temperature as indicated. Observe for signs of dehydration.	Hypothermia may be seen in intoxication, whereas hyperpyrexia may occur with withdrawal or indicate infectious process. **Note:** Dehydration often accompanies hyperpyrexia, requiring additional intervention/fluid replacement.

Monitor BP, pulse, respirations.

Changes in these signs depend on drug taken (e.g., Valium may be evidenced by hypotension, tachycardia).

Provide quiet, lighted room (e.g., an isolation room with simple furniture).

Reduces internal or external stimuli, which may lead to injury as depressant effect lessens.

Observe client at all times; use staff or family members as available.

Client with varying levels of consciousness should not be left alone because of the danger of accidental injury.

Reorient to surroundings and circumstances as needed.

Maintaining contact provides reassurance, reduces anxiety when sensorium clears.

Note presence of tremors.

Involuntary movements of one or more parts of the body may result from abrupt removal of drug.

Provide seizure precautions (e.g., padded side rails, bed in low position, airway adjunct/ suction at bedside).

These precautions can prevent injury if convulsions occur during withdrawal.

Note changes in behavior indicative of psychosis (e.g., distorted reality, altered mood, impaired language and memory).

Drug intoxication can precipitate an alteration in perceptions/psychotic behavior.

Assess emotional state, noting psychiatric history and suicide gestures/attempts. Note use/abuse of other substances.

Patterns of drug use will indicate likelihood of intentional or accidental overdose. Substance abuse/suicidal attempts may be symptom of, or response to, underlying psychiatric illness or to hallucinations caused by sensitivity to drug.

Determine history/characteristics of hallucinations.

May be auditory, visual, or tactile and be very frightening. May also trigger suicidal/homicidal behavior.

Institute suicide precautions, as indicated.

May need environmental restraints to protect client until own coping abilities improve and internal locus of control is attained/regained.

Collaborative

Administer medication per current treatment/ protocol, e.g.:

Phenobarbital;

Prolonged effect provides smoother sedation with "high" of more rapidly acting drugs. Also has an anticonvulsant effect.

Methadone;

Replaces heroin or other narcotic analgesics in detoxification program, reducing/minimizing withdrawal symptoms.

Clonidine (Catapres);

Can suppress/reverse symptoms of opioid withdrawal and has lesser likelihood of abuse than methadone. Drug may be used instead of or in combination with methadone during detoxification. **Note:** May be contraindicated for some clients because of high degree of sedation and hypotension.

Buprenorphine (Buprenex).

Current research suggests low doses of this drug may block opioid-withdrawal symptoms.

Assist with barbiturate detoxification program.	Reintoxication should be done before drug withdrawal is attempted. This establishes an independent estimate of prior drug use and provides a baseline on which to begin the detox schedule. Reintoxication is done so the drug can be withdrawn on a strict schedule and should begin as soon as there are signs of intoxication (e.g., nystagmus, slurred speech, ataxia on backward and forward tandem gait).
Involve in Intervention (confrontation) and/or therapy as indicated.	Client will need ongoing assistance to acknowledge and maintain drug-free existence.
Transfer to medical setting as indicated.	Severe CNS depression/deterioration of condition (physiological instability) requires more aggressive intervention than that generally provided in psychiatric setting.

NURSING DIAGNOSIS	BREATHING PATTERN, risk for ineffective/GAS EXCHANGE, risk for impaired
Risk Factors May Include:	Neuromuscular impairment
	Decreased energy/fatigue
	Inflammatory process
	Decreased lung expansion
Possibly Evidenced by:	[Not applicable; presence of signs/symptoms establishes an *actual* diagnosis.]
Desired Outcomes/Evaluation Criteria—Client Will:	Maintain normal/effective breathing pattern with absence of cyanosis or other symptoms of respiratory distress

ACTIONS/INTERVENTIONS	RATIONALE

Independent

Monitor respiratory rate/depth/rhythm and breath sounds.	Sedative/depressant effects on CNS may result in loss of airway patency and/or respiratory depression. Prompt treatment is necessary to prevent respiratory arrest. **Note:** Acute pulmonary edema is a common complication in heroin overdose/intoxication.
Have suction equipment/airway adjuncts available.	Sedative effects of drugs, increased salivation, and vomiting potentiate risk of aspiration. Relaxation of oropharyngeal muscles and respiratory depression requires prompt intervention to prevent respiratory compromise/arrest.

Collaborative

Review chest x-ray.	Common complications of depressant (opiate) abuse include pneumonia, aspiration pneumonitis, lung abscess, and atelectasis, which will require specific treatment.
Monitor pulse oximetry, when indicated.	Chronic addiction may result in decreased vital capacity and pulmonary diffusion affecting gas exchange. Presence of septic pulmonary emboli or pulmonary fibrosis (from talc granulomatosis occurring in injection drug abuse) may further compromise respiratory function.
Provide supplemental oxygen.	May be necessary to improve oxygen intake in presence of respiratory depression.
Administer medications, as indicated, e.g.,	
Naloxone (Narcan), nalmefene (Revex); and transfer to medical setting	Narcotic antagonists can reverse the effects of respiratory depression in opioid intoxication. **Note:** Narcan may trigger acute withdrawal syndrome, requiring more aggressive intervention. Revex has a longer half-life (approximately 11 hours) and is less likely to cause reemergence effects.

NURSING DIAGNOSIS	**INFECTION, risk for**
Risk Factors May Include:	Injection drug use techniques, impurities in injected drugs
	Localized trauma
	Malnutrition; altered immune state
Possibly Evidenced by:	[Not applicable; presence of signs/symptoms establishes an *actual* diagnosis.]
Desired Outcomes/Evaluation Criteria— Client Will:	Verbalize understanding of and demonstrate lifestyle changes to reduce risk factor(s).
	Achieve timely healing of infectious process, if present, and be afebrile.

ACTIONS/INTERVENTIONS	RATIONALE

Independent

Refer to CP: Stimulants, ND: Infection, risk for, for interventions specific to this nursing diagnosis.

189

HALLUCINOGEN-, PHENCYCLIDINE-, AND CANNABIS-RELATED DISORDERS

DSM-IV
HALLUCINOGEN-RELATED/INDUCED DISORDERS
292.89 Hallucinogen intoxication
292.81 Intoxication delirium
292.89 Hallucinogen persisting perception disorder (flashbacks)
292.89 Hallucinogen-induced anxiety disorder
292.84 Hallucinogen-induced mood disorder
PHENCYCLIDINE (OR PHENCYCLIDINE-LIKE)/INDUCED DISORDERS
292.89 Phencyclidine intoxication
292.81 Intoxication delirium
292.11 Induced psychotic disorder with delusions
292.12 Induced psychotic disorder with hallucinations
CANNABIS-RELATED/INDUCED DISORDERS
292.89 Cannabis intoxication
292.81 Intoxication delirium
292.89 Cannabis-induced anxiety disorder

Hallucinogenic substances can distort an individual's perception of reality, altering sensory perception, and inducing hallucinations. For this reason, these substances are referred to as "mind expanding." They are highly unpredictable in the effects they may induce each time they are used, and adverse reactions, including "flashbacks," can recur at any time, even without current use of the drug. Hallucinogens have been used as part of religious ceremonies and at social gatherings by Native Americans for more than 2000 years. Therapeutic uses for LSD have been proposed; however, more research is required. At this time, no real evidence speaks to the safety and efficacy of LSD in humans.

Of the drugs that produce mood and perceptual changes varying from sensory illusions to hallucinations, the most popular and well-known are ergot and related compounds (LSD, morning glory seeds), phenyl alkylamines (mescaline, "STP," and MDMA or "Ecstasy"), and indole alkaloids (DMT).

A separate classification of drugs includes phencyclidine (PCP, "angel dust," HOG) and similarly acting compounds such as ketamine (Ketalar) and the thiophene analogue of phencyclidine (TCP). Although these drugs have an entirely different chemical structure, they can have similar hallucinogenic effects and therefore are included here.

Additionally, cannabis (marijuana, hashish, synthetic THC) also produces an altered state of awareness accompanied by feelings of relaxation and mild euphoria and is often used in conjunction with other substances.

This plan of care addresses acute intoxication/withdrawal and is to be used in conjunction with CP: Substance Dependence/Abuse Rehabilitation.

ETIOLOGICAL THEORIES

Psychodynamics

Individuals who abuse substances fail to complete tasks of separation-individuation, resulting in underdeveloped egos. The person is thought to have a highly dependent nature, with characteristics of poor impulse control, low frustration tolerance, and low self-esteem. The superego is weak, resulting in absence of guilt feelings for behavior.

Certain personality traits may play an important part in the development and maintenance of dependence. Characteristics that have been identified include impulsivity, negative self-concept, weak ego, low social conformity, neuroticism, and introversion. Substance abuse has also been associated with antisocial personality and depressive response styles.

Biological

A genetic link is thought to be involved in the development of substance abuse disorders. Although statistics are currently inconclusive, hereditary factors are generally accepted to be a factor in the abuse of substances. Research is currently being done into the role biochemical factors play in the problems of substance abuse.

Family Dynamics

A predisposition to substance use disorders is found in the dysfunctional family system. Often one parent is absent or is an overpowering tyrant, and/or another parent is weak and ineffectual. Substance abuse may be evident as the primary method of relieving stress. The child has negative role models and learns to respond to stressful situations in like manner. However, parents may be average, normal individuals with children who succumb to overwhelming peer pressure and become involved with drugs.

In the family the effects of modeling, imitation, and identification on behavior can be observed from early childhood onward. Peer influence may exert a great deal of influence also. Cultural factors may help to establish patterns of substance use by attitudes of acceptance of such use as a part of daily or recreational life.

CLIENT ASSESSMENT DATA BASE

Factors that can affect the kind of reaction (positive or negative) experienced by the hallucinogen user include individual circadian rhythms (fatigue), previous drug-taking experience, personality, mood, and expectations. Concurrent use of alcohol/other drugs can compound symptoms/reactions. One's educational level can also cause different perceptions.

Activity/Rest

Insomnia, fatigue
Disturbances of sleep/wakefulness
Hyperactivity (LSD, mescaline, PCP)

Circulation

Diastolic BP decreased (cannabis, high-dose PCP)
Hypertension, hypertensive crisis (low- to moderate-dose PCP)
Tachycardia/palpitations; possible dysrhythmias (high-dose PCP)

Ego Integrity

Euphoria, anxiety, suspiciousness, paranoia (PCP psychosis)
Substance abuse as the primary method of coping
Highly dependent nature, with characteristics of poor impulse control, low frustration
     tolerance, low self-concept; depersonalization, weak superego, possibly resulting in
     absence of guilt feelings for behavior or self-reproach, excessive guilt, fearfulness
Moods reflect depression or anxiety
Preoccupation with the idea that brain is destroyed and/or will not return to a normal state

Food/Fluid

Increased appetite (cannabis)
Nausea/vomiting, increased salivation

Neurosensory

Blurred vision, altered depth perception
Dizziness, headache (LSD)

Flashback (spontaneous transitory recurrence of a drug-induced experience [LSD] in a drug-free state) often associated with fatigue, emotional stress, and other drug use (especially alcohol, marijuana)

"Bad trips" (self-limiting and confined to period of intoxication)

LSD: Three kinds: (1) bad body trip (e.g., "my body is purple"), (2) bad environment trip (e.g., visual distortions so real the person thinks he or she is going crazy), (3) bad mind trip (e.g., unexpected subconscious material bursts forth into consciousness, as in, "I'm responsible for my mother's death.")

PCP: Aggravates any underlying psychopathology

Cannabis: Rare; however, when occurs, panic attacks are usually seen

Pupillary dilation, catatonic staring (LSD, PCP, mescaline); vertical and horizontal nystagmus, lack of convergence (PCP)

Muscle incoordination/tremors, spasms, or increased muscle strength may be noted with PCP (the anesthetic effect deadens pain perception), deep-tendon reflexes increased (low- to moderate-dose PCP) or depressed (high-dose PCP), opisthotonos (body-arching spasm)

Level of Consciousness: Usually responsive; coma may occur (especially if intracranial hemorrhage occurs with PCP); slurred speech, mutism

Mental Status: Perceptual changes, e.g., sensation of slowed time, perceptions enhanced (colors richer, music more profound, smells and tastes heightened), synesthesia (merging of senses, colors are "heard" or sounds are "seen"), changes in body image, hallucinations (usually visual), depersonalization

Delirium with clouded state of consciousness (sensory misperception, disorientation, memory impairment, difficulty in sustaining attention, disordered stream of thought, psychomotor activity); delusions, illusions, hallucinations (rare with cannabis intoxication); may occur within 24 hours after use or following recovery days after PCP taken

Delusions occurring in a normal state of consciousness; may persist beyond 24 hours after cessation of hallucinogen use (persecutory delusions can follow cannabis use immediately or may occur during the course of cannabis intoxication)

Mood: Euphoria/dysphoria; anxiety, emotional lability, apathy, grandiosity

Behavioral Findings: May include assaultiveness, bizarre behavior, impulsivity, unpredictability, belligerence, impaired judgment, paranoid ideation, panic attacks

Seizure activity (high-dose PCP)

Pain/Discomfort

Decreased awareness of pain

Sudden intense chest pain or persistent chest discomfort (if drug is smoked)

Respiration

Decreased rate/depth of respiration (PCP, heavy cannabis use)

Rhonchi, gurgling sounds

Safety

Participation in high-risk behaviors

History of accidental injuries

Diaphoresis

Conjunctival redness/infection (cannabis)

Assaultive behavior (PCP psychosis), risk to self (impaired judgment/acting on altered perceptions)

Temperature elevated

Social Interactions

Sense of "happy sociability," friendliness (intoxication)

Dysfunctional family system—an overbearing, tyrannical, absent, or weak and ineffectual parent

Overwhelming peer pressure leading to drug involvement

Impaired social or occupational functioning may be seen with drug use/tolerance (fights, loss of friends, absence from work, loss of job, or legal difficulties)

Teaching/Learning

Concurrent use of other drugs, including alcohol

Family history of substance abuse

DIAGNOSTIC STUDIES

Drug Screen/Urinalysis: To identify drug(s) being used.

Other Screening Studies (e.g., Hepatitis, HIV, TB): Depend on general conditions, individual risk factors, and care setting.

Addictive Severity Index (ASI): To assess substance abuse and determine treatment needs.

NURSING PRIORITIES

1. Protect client/others from injury.
2. Promote physiological/psychological stability.
3. Provide appropriate referral and follow-up.
4. Support client/family in Intervention (confrontation) process for decision to stop using drugs.

DISCHARGE GOALS

1. Homeostasis achieved.
2. Complications prevented/resolved.
3. Abstinence from drug(s) maintained on a day-to-day basis.
4. Participation in drug rehabilitation program.
5. Plan in place to meet needs after discharge.

NURSING DIAGNOSIS	VIOLENCE, risk for, directed at self/others
Risk Factors May Include:	Chemical alteration, exogenous (CNS stimulants/mind-altering drug), toxic reactions to drug(s)
	Organic brain syndrome (drug anesthetizes mind and body)
	Psychological state (narrowed perceptual field)
[Possible Indicators:]	Synesthesias, hallucinations, illusions, visual/auditory distortions; panic state; suspiciousness of others, paranoid ideation, delusions
	Hostile, threatening verbalizations; exaggerated emotional response; increased motor activity, pacing, excitement, irritability, agitation
	Change in behavior pattern; unpredictable behavior; increasing anxiety, fear, and feelings of loss of control
	Overt and aggressive acts; self-destructive behavior
	Decreased response to pain

Desired Outcomes/Evaluation Criteria— Client Will:	Demonstrate self-control, as evidenced by relaxed posture, free of violent behavior.
	Acknowledge reality of situation and understanding of relationship of behavior to drug use.
	Participate in treatment program.

ACTIONS/INTERVENTIONS	RATIONALE

Independent

Place in darkened, quiet, nonthreatening environment with a nonintrusive observer.	Lowered stimulation decreases the likelihood of confusion and fear; thus, there is less chance of violent behavior. Use of an observer promotes safety. **Note:** PCP users seek help only after the situation has gotten out of hand, and it is therefore important to take safe action immediately.
Speak in a soft, nonthreatening voice. Use "Talk-downs" when LSD has been taken. If technique is tried with other drugs (particularly PCP) and agitation increases, stop immediately.	Nonthreatening communication may have a calming effect. However, "Talk-downs" (the use of orientation, support, and reassuring words/touch) may be deleterious in the presence of PCP intoxication, resulting in an increase in the client's agitation level.
Observe for escalating anxiety, fear, irritability, and agitation.	May indicate potential for progression to violent behavior. **Note:** Client is not in complete control of self because of drug use.
Accept and deal with client's anger without reacting on an emotional basis.	Responding emotionally on a personal level is not constructive and may escalate reactions.
Provide protection within the environment via constant observation and removal of objects that may be used to hurt self or others.	Reduces risk of injury to client and/or staff. Client may not feel pain and may not be able to follow directions because of use of the drug.
Observe behavior without administering medications.	A period of drug-free observation should precede any decision to administer medications (e.g., antianxiety agents), so that a clear clinical picture can develop. In addition, because it is not known what other drugs may also have been taken, it is not generally advisable to add another drug.

Collaborative

Administer medications as necessary, e.g.: diazepam (Valium);	Used to reduce muscle spasms and/or restlessness in PCP user.
haloperidol (Haldol).	Preferred to control psychosis and assaultive behavior.
Avoid use of phenothiazine neuroleptics.	Drugs such as chlorpromazine (Thorazine) are generally avoided because of the possibility of potentiating PCP anticholinergic effects.
Apply restraints, if needed, and document reason(s) for use.	Restraints should be avoided in a frightened, hallucinating client but may be necessary because of potential injury to self or others, or when other

194

dangerous drugs have been taken. PCP users are unpredictable, so it is best to err on the side of safety (using restraints with sufficient documentation) rather than to risk injury.

NURSING DIAGNOSIS	TRAUMA/SUFFOCATION/POISONING, risk for
Risk Factors May Include:	Internal factors, host: psychological perception (hallucinations); clouded sensorium and impaired judgment; fear
	Muscle incoordination; reduced hand/eye coordination
	Decreased response to/perception of pain, reduced temperature/tactile sensation
	Clonic movements, muscle rigidity (may precede or occur with generalized seizure activity)
	Interactive conditions between individual and environment that impose a risk to the defensive and adaptive resources of the individual (e.g., placing hand in open flame, "flying out of window"); unfamiliar environment
Possibly Evidenced by:	[Not applicable; presence of signs/symptoms establishes an *actual* diagnosis.]
Desired Outcomes/Evaluation Criteria— Client Will:	Verbalize understanding of factors (e.g., drug use) that contribute to possibility of injury and take steps to correct situation.
	Initiate behaviors and lifestyle changes necessary to minimize and/or prevent injury.
	Maintain/achieve physiological stability as evidenced by patent airway and adequate respiratory/cardiac function.

ACTIONS/INTERVENTIONS	RATIONALE

Independent

Ascertain what drugs have been taken.	Necessary for appropriate intervention/anticipation of needs. Lethal overdoses of hallucinogenic drugs (except for MDA, PCP) are rare; however, caution must be taken because adulterants such as sedatives, hypnotics, anticholinergics, and strychnine are often used for "cutting" the drug. **Note:** Two reasons one might not know what drug was taken are (1) the individual lies for legal concerns or may feel embarrassed and (2) the person who sold the drugs to the client either did not know what was in them or lied to the client. In either case, the

Anticipate some form of unpredictability and be prepared for the unexpected, including physiological as well as psychological emergencies.

nurse needs to listen to the client but be aware that the information the client gives may not be accurate.

These drugs are dangerous and lead to bizarre thinking/harmful behavior.

Maintain client under close observation. Note precursors that might indicate increasing agitation (e.g., body tension, rising voice tone, quickening of movements). (Refer to ND: Violence, risk for.)

These drugs alter thinking, and many are anesthetic; therefore, the client may hurt self because of bizarre thinking (e.g., attempt to jump out window or escape from restraints).

Remove objects that may be used to hurt self or others.

Provides protection within the environment.

Provide a hockey/bicycle helmet as indicated.

If client is banging head against hard objects, a helmet can decrease the potential for/severity of injury.

Monitor vital signs, respiratory rate/depth and rhythm.

Decreased diastolic BP (cannabis) or hypertensive crisis (PCP) may develop. Bradypnea/respiratory arrest may also occur, especially with PCP or heavy cannabis use.

Assess gag/swallow response and character of respirations.

Hypersalivation and vomiting, especially in the presence of ineffective cough and/or loss of muscle tone, may result in occlusion of airway, crowing/gurgling/choked respirations, leading to respiratory arrest.

Position client on side, or with head to the side, as indicated.

Facilitates drainage of vomitus and buildup of saliva and prevents aspiration in sedated/comatose client.

Encourage fluid intake frequently, if client can swallow safely.

Increased hydration keeps secretions loose and easier to expectorate and enhances renal clearance of drugs.

Have emergency equipment (including airway adjunct/suction) and medications available.

Toxic effects of several of these drugs on the heart and respiratory system may result in cardiac/respiratory arrest, requiring prompt intervention to prevent death.

Collaborative

Administer medications, e.g., diazepem (Valium) as indicated.

May be useful to reduce agitation and hyperactivity once drug(s) used is identified.

Apply restraints with caution when used.

May prevent injury to self or others. However, restraints should be avoided, if possible, in a frightened, hallucinating client, as they can increase agitation.

Transfer to acute medical setting as indicated.

Provides closer monitoring and more aggressive therapy (e.g., IV fluids with ammonium chloride or ascorbic acid for forced diuresis and acidifying of urine to enhance renal clearance of PCP). **Note:** Drug effects are dose related: >5 mg = low dose; >10 mg = high dose; >20 mg can lead to hypertensive crisis, coma, and death because of respiratory/cardiac failure.

NURSING DIAGNOSIS	TISSUE PERFUSION, risk for altered cerebral
Risk Factors May Include:	Alterations in blood flow (hypertensive crisis)
Possibly Evidenced by:	[Not applicable; presence of signs and symptoms establishes an *actual* diagnosis.]
Desired Outcomes/Evaluation Criteria— Client Will:	Regain/maintain usual level of consciousness free of adverse neurological symptoms/complications.

ACTIONS/INTERVENTIONS	RATIONALE

Independent

Elevate head of bed; keep client's head in midline position.	Enhances venous drainage, thereby reducing risk of vascular congestion that increases intracranial pressure, with possibility of hemorrhage in PCP intoxication.
Observe for pupillary or vital sign changes, decreased level of consciousness and/or motor function.	Provides for early detection and intervention to minimize intracranial pressure/injury.
Encourage rest and quiet. Reduce environmental stimuli.	Promotes relaxation and may help lower blood pressure.
Monitor BP.	Evaluates need for/effectiveness of interventions.

Collaborative

Administer antihypertensive medications, e.g., diazoxide (Hyperstat), hydralazine (Apresoline).	Effective in lowering blood pressure to prevent hypertensive crisis, which can be associated with PCP intoxication.

NURSING DIAGNOSIS	THOUGHT PROCESSES, altered
May Be Related to:	Physiological changes (use of hallucinogenic substance)
	Impaired judgment with loss of memory
Possibly Evidenced by:	Inaccurate interpretation of environment, memory impairment, bizarre thinking, disorientation
	Inability to make decisions; unpredictable behavior
	Cognitive dissonance; distractibility
	Inappropriate/nonreality-based thinking
	Sleep deprivation
	Inability to communicate needs/desires effectively (mutism or confusion)
Desired Outcomes/Evaluation Criteria— Client Will:	Exhibit return of cognition/memory and ability to function.

197

Communicate effectively.

Report absence of visual/auditory distortions.

Verbalize understanding that the drug is the cause of/contributes to alteration in perception.

ACTIONS/INTERVENTIONS	RATIONALE
Independent	
Observe the client closely; do not leave him or her unattended; make sure restraints are secure when used. Remove objects from the environment that client could use to harm self and/or others. (Refer to ND: Violence, risk for.)	PCP is an anesthetic that alters thinking, and client may hurt self by attempting to jump out window, jump in front of cars, escape from restraints, etc. Removal of potentially harmful objects provides for protection and safety.
Anticipate some form of unpredictable behavior and be prepared for the unexpected.	Use of hallucinogens can lead to bizarre thinking/harmful responses.
Tell client that current thoughts and feelings are a result of the drug, when appropriate.	This information may be helpful to the client who can accept it; however, it may cause agitation.
Allow client to sleep whenever possible.	Sleep cycle is disturbed, and client will need sleep after being agitated and expending excessive amounts of energy. Sleeping also provides time for drug(s) to clear system.
Observe for behavioral indicators of psychosis (e.g., delusions, hallucinations).	Overdose may precipitate a psychotic episode that will clear within hours to days. If psychosis remains, this may indicate precipitation of preexisting condition (e.g., schizophrenia).
Note altered speech ability/patterns. Refer to loss of speech as temporary.	Mutism and confusion may occur, and information may reassure client that problem is drug-induced and that it will improve with time. **Note:** "Talk-down" approach may agitate the client and should be used with caution.
Anticipate client's needs and allow more time for client to respond to any necessary questions and/or comments.	This may reduce need to communicate in presence of confusion/interference with memory. Adequate time allows full expression. **Note:** Be aware that touching and/or physical closeness may increase anxiety and agitation.
Collaborative	
Administer medications as indicated, e.g., diazepam (Valium), chlordiazepoxide (Librium).	Chronic PCP users in whom psychiatric conditions develop/coexist may require further treatment for the thought disorder or depressive illness. The response may be very slow because of the persistence of PCP in the body tissues, sometimes for a period of several months or more.

NURSING DIAGNOSIS	ANXIETY [specify level]/FEAR
May Be Related to:	Situational crisis; threat to/change in health status; perceived threat of death

Possibly Evidenced by:	Inexperience or unfamiliarity with the effect of drug(s) (e.g., PCP, LSD)
	Impaired thought processes; sensory impairment
	Assumptions of "losing my mind, losing control"; verbalized concern about unknown consequences/outcomes
	Sympathetic stimulation (e.g., cardiovascular excitation, superficial vasoconstriction, pupil dilation, vomiting/diarrhea, restlessness, trembling)
	Preoccupation with feelings of impending doom; apprehension
	Attack behavior
Desired Outcomes/Evaluation Criteria—Client Will:	Verbalize awareness/cause of feelings of anxiety. Report anxiety reduced to a manageable level.
	Appear relaxed, resting/sleeping appropriately.
	Identify the fear and verbalize feelings of control of self and situation.

ACTIONS/INTERVENTIONS	RATIONALE
Independent	
Assess level of anxiety on an ongoing basis.	Increased anxiety may lead to agitation and violent behavior, as client is not in complete control of actions/responses.
Place in darkened, quiet, nonthreatening environment with a nonintrusive observer.	Lowered stimulation decreases the likelihood of confusion and fear. Observer is used for safety (with other personnel available to help if needed).
Orient client to surroundings, time, and who is with him or her. Speak in soft voice, in a nonthreatening manner.	Knowing where one is can increase the feeling of security when experiencing a "bad trip."
Use "Talk-down" with caution, telling the client that the ingested drug is the cause of feelings of anxiety, the effects are only temporary, and permanent damage should not occur.	Information that provides reassurance can be the single most important therapeutic intervention. "Talk-downs" are effective with persons who have taken LSD or similar substances. If the client can realize that the perceptions are drug-related, then an increase in control can take place. However, in some situations (e.g., PCP), "Talk-downs" can result in an increase in fear and agitation.
Encourage verbal expression of changes in perception that are occurring.	Can be used for assessment and provides guidance on direction for support.
Collaborative	
Administer sedatives if necessary, e.g., diazepam (Valium), chlordiazepoxide (Librium).	These are drugs of choice to be used in extreme cases to calm client. **Note:** Medications are often discouraged because bad trips are usually self-limiting, and time is the best remedy for treating the negative effects.

199

NURSING DIAGNOSIS	SELF CARE deficit
May Be Related to:	Perceptual/cognitive impairment
	Therapeutic management (restraints)
Possibly Evidenced by:	Inability to meet own physical needs
Desired Outcomes/Evaluation Criteria— Client Will:	Resume/perform self-care activities within level of own ability.
	Verbalize commitment to lifestyle changes to meet self-care needs.

ACTIONS/INTERVENTIONS

Independent

Provide care as needed.

Involve client in formulation of plan of care, as possible.

Work with client's present abilities. Do not pressure to perform beyond capabilities.

Provide and promote privacy within limits of safety needs.

Collaborative

Include client in team meeting/staffing as indicated. Problem-solve particulars of self-care needs.

RATIONALE

Client may be agitated and care will need to be postponed until control is regained.

Enables client to participate at level of ability and enhances sense of control. **Note:** PCP user often cannot interact without becoming agitated.

Failure can produce discouragement, depression, and agitation.

Acknowledges human need, important to enhance self-esteem.

Multidisciplinary approach with involvement of everyone who is caring for the client, along with the client, increases probability of plan being effective/successful.

SUBSTANCE DEPENDENCE/ABUSE REHABILITATION

DSM-IV
ALCOHOL USE DISORDERS
303.90 Alcohol dependence
305.00 Alcohol abuse
AMPHETAMINE (OR AMPHETAMINE-LIKE) USE DISORDERS
304.40 Amphetamine dependence
305.70 Amphetamine abuse
CANNABIS USE DISORDERS
304.30 Cannabis dependence
305.20 Cannabis abuse
COCAINE USE DISORDERS
304.20 Cocaine dependence
305.60 Cocaine abuse
HALLUCINOGEN USE DISORDERS
304.60 Hallucinogen dependence
305.30 Hallucinogen abuse
INHALANT USE DISORDERS
304.60 Inhalant dependence
305.90 Inhalant abuse
NICOTINE USE DISORDERS
305.10 Nicotine dependence
OPIOID USE DISORDERS
304.00 Opioid dependence
305.50 Opioid abuse
PHENCYCLIDINE USE DISORDERS
304.90 Phencyclidine dependence
305.90 Phencyclidine abuse
SEDATIVE, HYPNOTIC, OR ANXIOLYTIC SUBSTANCE USE DISORDERS
304.10 Sedative, hypnotic, or anxiolytic dependence
305.40 Sedative, hypnotic, or anxiolytic abuse
POLYSUBSTANCE USE DISORDER
304.80 Polysubstance dependence
(For other listings, consult *DSM-IV* manual.)

Many drugs and volatile substances are subject to abuse (as noted in previous plans of care). This disorder is a continuum of phases incorporating a cluster of cognitive, behavioral, and physiological symptoms that include loss of control over use of the substance and a continued use of the substance despite adverse consequences. A number of factors have been implicated in the predisposition to abuse a substance (e.g., biological, biochemical, psychological [including developmental], personality, sociocultural and conditioning, and cultural and ethnic influences). However, no single theory adequately explains the etiology of this problem.

This plan of care addresses issues of dependence and is to be used in conjunction with plans of care relative to acute intoxification/withdrawal from specific substance(s).

CLIENT ASSESSMENT DATA BASE

Refer to appropriate acute plan of care regarding involved substance(s).

DIAGNOSTIC STUDIES

Drug (including-alcohol) Screen: Identifies drug(s) being used.
Addiction Severity Index (ASI) Assessment Tool: Produces a "problem severity profile" of

201

the patient, including chemical, medical, psychological, legal, family/social and employment/support aspects, indicating areas of treatment needs.

Other Screening Studies (e.g., Hepatitis, HIV, TB): Depend on general condition, individual risk factors, and care setting.

NURSING PRIORITIES

1. Provide support for decision to stop substance use.
2. Strengthen individual coping skills.
3. Facilitate learning of new ways to reduce anxiety.
4. Promote family involvement in rehabilitation program.
5. Facilitate family growth/development.
6. Provide information about condition, prognosis, and treatment needs.

DISCHARGE GOALS

1. Responsibility for own life and behavior assumed.
2. Plan to maintain substance-free life formulated.
3. Family relationships/enabling issues being addressed.
4. Treatment program successfully begun.
5. Condition, prognosis, and therapeutic regimen understood.

NURSING DIAGNOSIS	DENIAL ineffective
May Be Related to:	Personal vulnerability; fear; difficulty handling new situation
	Learned response patterns; cultural factors, personal/family value systems
Possibly Evidenced by:	Delay in seeking, or refusal of, healthcare attention to the detriment of health/life
	Does not perceive personal relevance of symptoms or danger, or admit impact of condition on life pattern; projection of blame/responsibility for problems
	Use of manipulation to avoid responsibility for self
Desired Outcomes/Evaluation Criteria— Client Will:	Verbalize awareness of relationship of substance abuse to current situation.
	Engage in therapeutic program.
	Verbalize acceptance of responsibility for own behavior.

ACTIONS/INTERVENTIONS	RATIONALE

Independent

Ascertain by what name client would like to be addressed.	Shows courtesy and respect, giving the client a sense of orientation and control.
Convey attitude of acceptance of client, separating individual from unacceptable behavior.	Promotes feelings of dignity and self-worth.

202

Ascertain reason for beginning abstinence, involvement in therapy.

Provides insight into client's willingness to commit to long-term behavioral change and whether client even believes that he or she *can* change. **Note:** If treatment is court-ordered, client may just be "doing time" until case is resolved and therefore may not be fully committed to the program. (Denial is one of the strongest and most resistant symptoms of substance abuse.)

Review definition of drug dependence and categories of symptoms (e.g., patterns of use, impairment caused by use, tolerance to substance).

This information helps client make decisions regarding acceptance of problem and treatment choices.

Answer questions honestly and provide factual information. Keep all promises.

Creates trust, which is the basis of the therapeutic relationship.

Provide information about addictive use versus experimental, occasional use; biochemical/genetic disorder theory (genetic predisposition); use activated by environment; pharmacology of stimulant; compulsive desire as a lifelong occurrence.

Progression of use continuum in the addict is from experimental/recreational to addictive use. Comprehending this process is important in combating denial. Education may relieve client of guilt and blame and may help awareness of recurring addictive characteristics.

Discuss current life situation and impact of substance use.

First step in decreasing use of denial is for client to see the relationship between substance use and peer group. Use confrontation with caring. personal problems.

Confront and examine denial/rationalization in peer group. Use confrontation with caring.

Because denial is the major defense mechanism in addictive disease, confrontation by peers can help the client accept the reality of adverse consequences of behaviors and that drug use is a major problem. Caring attitude preserves self-concept and helps decrease defensive response.

Provide information regarding effects of addiction on mood/personality.

Individuals often mistake effects of addiction on mood/personality for its cause and use this to justify or excuse drug use.

Confront use of anger, rationalization, or projection.

Anger is often a response of defensiveness, and pointing this out to the client can help him or her to accept feelings underlying anger. These defense mechanisms prolong the stage of denial that problems exist in client's life because of substance use.

Remain nonjudgmental. Be alert to changes in behavior (e.g., restlessness, increased tension).

Confrontation can lead to increased agitation, which may compromise safety of client/staff.

Provide positive feedback for expressing awareness of denial in self/others.

Necessary to enhance self-esteem and to reinforce insight into behavior.

Maintain firm expectation that client attend recovery support/therapy groups regularly.

Attendance is related to admitting need for help, to working with denial, and for maintenance of a long-term drug-free existence.

Encourage and support client's taking responsibility for own recovery (e.g., development of alternative behaviors to drug urge/use). Assist client to learn own responsibility for recovering.

Denial can be replaced with responsible action when client accepts the reality of own responsibility.

NURSING DIAGNOSIS	COPING, INDIVIDUAL, ineffective
May Be Related to:	Personal vulnerability
	Negative role modeling; inadequate support systems
	Previous ineffective/inadequate coping skills with substitution of drug(s)
Possibly Evidenced by:	Altered social patterns/participation
	Impaired adaptive behavior and problem-solving skills
	Decreased ability to handle stress of illness/hospitalization
	Financial affairs in disarray; employment difficulties (e.g., losing time on job/not maintaining steady employment, poor work performance, on-the-job injuries)
	Verbalization of inability to cope/ask for help
Desired Outcomes/Evaluation Criteria— Client Will:	Identify ineffective coping behavior/ consequences, including use of substances as a method of coping.
	Use effective coping skills/problem-solving.
	Initiate necessary lifestyle changes.

ACTIONS/INTERVENTIONS	RATIONALE
Independent	
Review program rules, philosophy, expectations.	Having information provides opportunity for client to cooperate and function as member of group/milieu, enhancing sense of control and sense of success.
Determine understanding of current situation and previous/other methods of coping with life's problems.	Provides information about degree of denial; acceptance of personal responsibility/commitment to change; identifies coping skills that may be used in present situation.
Set limits and confront client's efforts to get caregiver to grant special privileges, making excuses for not following through on behaviors agreed on and attempting to continue drug use.	Client has learned manipulative behavior throughout life and needs to learn a new way of getting needs met. Following through on consequences of failure to maintain limits can help the client to change ineffective behaviors.
Be aware of staff attitudes, feelings, and enabling behaviors.	Lack of understanding, judgmental/enabling behaviors can result in inaccurate data collection and nontherapeutic approaches.
Encourage verbalization of feelings, fears, anxieties.	May help client begin to come to terms with long-unresolved issues.
Explore alternative coping strategies.	Client may have little or no knowledge of adaptive responses to stress and needs to learn other

Assist client to learn/encourage use of relaxation skills, guided imagery, visualizations.	options for managing time, feelings, and relationships without drugs.
	Helps client to relax, develop new ways to deal with stress, enhances problem-solving.
Structure diversional activity that relates to recovery (e.g., social activity within support group), wherein issues of being chemically free are examined.	Discovery of alternative methods of coping with drug hunger can remind client that addiction is a lifelong process and opportunity for changing patterns is available.
Use peer support to examine ways of coping with drug hunger.	Self-help groups are valuable for learning and promoting abstinence in each member, using understanding and support, and peer pressure.
Encourage involvement in therapeutic writing. Have client begin to write autobiography.	Therapeutic writing can enhance participation in treatment; serving as a release for grief, anger, and stress; provides a useful tool for monitoring client's safety; and can be used to evaluate client's progress. Autobiographical activity provides an opportunity for the client to remember and identify sequence of events in his or her life that relate to current situation.
Discuss client's plans for living without drugs.	Provides opportunity to develop/refine plans. Devising a comprehensive strategy for avoiding relapses helps move client into maintenance phase of behavioral change.

Collaborative

Administer medications as indicated, e.g.: disulfiram (Antabuse);	This drug can be helpful in maintaining abstinence from alcohol while other therapy is undertaken. By inhibiting alcohol oxidation, the drug leads to an accumulation of acetaldehyde with a highly unpleasant reaction if alcohol is consumed (or even absorbed through the skin via colognes or shaving preparations).
acamprosate;	Helps to prevent relapses in alcoholism by lowering the activity of receptors for the excitatory neurotransmitter glutamate. This agent may become the drug of choice as it does not make the user sick if alcohol is consumed; it has no sedative, anti-anxiety, musle relaxant, or antidepressant properties, and produces no withdrawal symptoms.
methadone (Dolophine);	This drug is thought to blunt the craving for/diminish the effects of opioids and is used to assist in withdrawal and long-term maintenance problems. It can allow the individual to maintain daily activities and ultimately withdraw from drug use.
naltrexone (Revia), Nalmefene (Revex).	Used to suppress craving for opioids and may help prevent relapse in the client abusing alcohol. Current research suggests that naltrexone suppresses urge to continue drinking by interfering with alcohol-induced release of endorphins. **Note:** Nalmefene has fewer side effects than naltrexone.

205

Encourage involvement with self-help resources (e.g., Alcoholics/Narcotics Anonymous).	Puts client in direct contact with support systems necessary for managing sobriety/drug-free life as meetings are available at many different times and places in most communities.

NURSING DIAGNOSIS	POWERLESSNESS
May Be Related to:	Substance addiction with/without periods of abstinence
	Episodic compulsive indulgence; attempts at recovery
	Lifestyle of helplessness
Possibly Evidenced by:	Ineffective recovery attempts; statements of inability to stop behavior/requests for help
	Continuous/constant thinking about drug and/or obtaining drug
	Alteration in personal, occupational, and social life
Desired Outcomes/Evaluation Criteria— Client Will:	Admit inability to control drug habit, recognize powerlessness over addiction.
	Verbalize acceptance of need for treatment and awareness that willpower alone cannot control abstinence.
	Engage in peer support.
	Demonstrate active participation in program.
	Regain and maintain healthy state with a drug-free lifestyle.

ACTIONS/INTERVENTIONS	RATIONALE
Independent	
Use crisis intervention techniques to initiate behavioral changes:	Client is more amenable to acceptance of need for treatment at this time.
Assist client to recognize problem exists; discuss in a caring, nonjudgmental manner how drug has interfered with life.	In the *precontemplation phase*, the client has not yet identified that drug use is problematic. While client is hurting, it is easier to admit substance use has created negative consequences.
Involve client in development of treatment plan using problem-solving process in which client identifies goals for change and agrees to desired outcomes.	During the *contemplation phase*, the client realizes a problem exists and is thinking about a change in behavior. The client is committed to the outcomes when the decision-making process involves solutions that are promulgated by the individual. Brainstorming helps creatively identify possibilities and provides sense of control. During the *preparation phase*, minor action may be taken as individual organizes resources for definitive change.
Discuss alternative solutions.	

Assist in selecting most appropriate alternative.

As possibilities are discussed, the most useful solution becomes clear.

Support decision and implementation of selected solutions.

Helps the client to persevere in process of change. During the *action phase*, the client engages in a sustained effort to maintain sobriety, and mechanisms are put in place to support abstinence.

Explore support in peer group. Encourage sharing about drug hunger, situations that increase the desire to indulge, ways that substance has influenced life.

Client may need assistance in expressing self, speaking about powerlessness, and admitting need for help, to face up to problem and begin resolution.

Assist client to learn ways to enhance health and structure healthy diversion from drug use (e.g., maintaining a balanced diet; getting adequate rest; exercising [e.g., walking, jogging, long-distance running]; and acupuncture, biofeedback, deep meditative techniques).

Learning to empower self in constructive areas can strengthen ability to maintain recovery. These activities help restore natural biochemical balance, aid detoxification, and manage stress, anxiety, use of free time, increasing self-confidence and thereby improving self-esteem. **Note:** Exercise promotes release of endorphins, creating a feeling of well-being.

Provide information regarding understanding of human behavior and interactions with others (e.g., transactional analysis).

Understanding these concepts can help the client begin to deal with past problems/losses and prevent repeating ineffective coping behaviors and self-fulling prophecies.

Assist client in self-examination of spirituality, faith.

Although not necessary to recovery, surrendering to and faith in a power greater than oneself has been found to be effective for many individuals in substance recovery; may decrease sense of powerlessness.

Instruct in and role-play assertive communication skills.

Effective in assisting in ability to refuse use, to stop relationships with users and dealers, to build healthy relationships, and regain control of own life.

Provide treatment information on an ongoing basis.

Helps client know what to expect and creates opportunity for client to be a part of what is happening and make informed choices about participation/outcomes.

Collaborative

Refer to/assist with making contact with programs for ongoing treatment needs (e.g., partial hospitalization drug treatment programs, Narcotics/Alcoholics Anonymous, peer support group).

Continuing treatment is essential to positive outcome. Follow-through may be easier once initial contact has been made.

NURSING DIAGNOSIS	**NUTRITION: altered, less than body requirements**
May Be Related to:	Insufficient dietary intake to meet metabolic needs for psychological, physiological, or economic reasons

Possibly Evidenced by:	Weight loss; weight below norm for height/body build; decreased subcutaneous fat/muscle mass
	Reported altered taste sensation; lack of interest in food
	Poor muscle tone
	Sore, inflamed buccal cavity
	Laboratory evidence of protein/vitamin deficiencies
Desired Outcomes/Evaluation Criteria— Client Will:	Demonstrate progressive weight gain toward goal, with normalization of laboratory values and free of signs of malnutrition.
	Verbalize understanding of effects of substance abuse and reduced dietary intake on nutritional status.
	Demonstrate behaviors, lifestyle changes to regain and maintain appropriate weight.

ACTIONS/INTERVENTIONS	RATIONALE
Independent	
Assess height, weight, age, body build, strength, activity level. Note condition of oral cavity.	Provides information about individual on which to base caloric needs/dietary plan. Type of diet/foods may be affected by condition of mucous membranes and teeth.
Obtain anthropometric measurements (e.g., triceps skinfold).	Calculates subcutaneous fat and muscle mass to aid in determining dietary needs.
Note total daily calorie intake; maintain a diary of intake, as well as times and patterns of eating.	Information about client's dietary pattern will help identify nutritional needs/deficiencies.
Evaluate energy expenditure (e.g., pacing or sedentary), and establish an individualized exercise program.	Activity level affects nutritional needs. Exercise enhances muscle tone, may stimulate appetite.
Provide opportunity to choose foods/snacks to meet dietary plan.	Enhances participation/sense of control, may promote resolution of nutritional deficiencies, and helps evaluate client learning of dietary teaching.
Recommend monitoring weight weekly.	Provides information regarding effectiveness of dietary plan.
Collaborative	
Consult with dietitian.	Useful in establishing individual dietary needs/plan and provides additional resource for learning.
Review laboratory studies, as indicated (e.g., glucose, serum albumin/prealbumin, electrolytes).	Identifies anemias, electrolyte imbalances, other abnormalities that may be present, requiring specific therapy.
Refer for dental consultation as necessary.	Teeth are essential to good nutritional intake and dental hygiene/care is often a neglected area in this population.

NURSING DIAGNOSIS	SELF ESTEEM, chronic low
May Be Related to:	Social stigma attached to substance abuse, expectation that one control behavior
	Negative role models; abuse/neglect, dysfunctional family system
	Life choices perpetuating failure; situational crisis with loss of control over life events
	Biochemical body change (e.g., withdrawal from alcohol/other drugs)
Possibly Evidenced by:	Self-negating verbalization, expressions of shame/guilt
	Evaluation of self as unable to deal with events; confusion about self, purpose or direction in life
	Rationalizing away/rejecting positive feedback, exaggerating negative feedback about self
Desired Outcomes/Evaluation Criteria— Client Will:	Identify feelings and underlying dynamics for negative perception of self.
	Verbalize acceptance of self as is and an increased sense of self-worth.
	Set goals and participate in realistic planning for lifestyle changes necessary to live without drugs.

ACTIONS/INTERVENTIONS	RATIONALE

Independent

Provide opportunity for and encourage verbalization/discussion of individual situation.	Client often has difficulty expressing self and has even more difficulty accepting the degree of importance substance has assumed in life and its relationship to present situation.
Assess mental status. Note presence of other psychiatric disorders (dual diagnosis).	Many clients use substances in an attempt to obtain relief from depression or anxiety, which may predate use and/or be the result of substance use. Approximately 60% of substance-dependent clients have underlying psychological problems, and treatment for both is imperative to maintain abstinence.
Spend time with client. Discuss client's behavior/use of substance nonjudgmentally.	The nurse's presence conveys acceptance of the client as a worthwhile person. Discussion provides opportunity for insight into the problems substance abuse has created for the client.
Provide information for positive actions and encourage client to accept this input.	Failure and lack of self-esteem have been problems for this client, who needs to learn to accept self as an individual with positive attributes.
Observe family interactions/SO dynamics and level of support.	Substance abuse is a family problem, and how the members act and react to the client's behavior affects the course of the disease and how the client sees self. Many unconsciously become "enablers,"

helping the individual to cover up the consequences of the abuse. (Refer to ND: Family Process, altered: alcoholism.)

Encourage expression of feelings of guilt, shame, and anger.	The client often has lost self-respect and believes that the situation is hopeless. Expression of these feelings helps the client begin to accept responsibility for self and take steps to make changes.
Help the client acknowledge that substance use is the problem and that problems can be dealt with without the use of drugs. Confront the use of defenses (e.g., denial, projection, rationalization).	When drugs can no longer be blamed for the problems that exist, the client can begin to deal with the problems and live without substance use. Confrontation helps the client accept the reality of the problems as they exist.
Ask the client to list and review past accomplishments and positive happenings.	There are things in everyone's life that have been successful. Often when self-concept is low, it is difficult to remember these successes or to view them as successes.
Use techniques of role rehearsal.	Assists client to practice developing skills to cope with new role as a person who no longer uses or needs drugs to handle life's problems.

Collaborative

Involve client in group therapy.	Group sharing helps encourage verbalization, as other members of group are in various stages of abstinence from drugs and can address the client's concerns/denial. The client can gain new skills, hope, and a sense of family/community from group participation.
Formulate plan to treat other mental illness problems. (Refer to appropriate CP as indicated.)	Clients who seek relief for other mental health problems through drugs will continue to do so once discharged. The substance use and mental health problems need to be treated together to maximize abstinence potential.
Administer antipsychotic medications as necessary.	Prolonged/profound psychosis following LSD or PCP use can be treated with these drugs, as this condition may be the result of an underlying functional psychosis that has now emerged. **Note:** Avoid the use of phenothiazines, as they may decrease seizure threshold and cause hypotension in the presence of LSD/PCP.

NURSING DIAGNOSIS	**FAMILY PROCESS, *altered:* alcoholism [substance abuse]**
May Be Related to:	Abuse of substance(s); resistance to treatment
	Family history of substance abuse
	Addictive personality
	Inadequate coping skills, lack of problem-solving skills

Possibly Evidenced by:	Anxiety, anger/suppressed rage; shame and embarrassment
	Emotional isolation/loneliness; vulnerability; repressed emotions
	Disturbed family dynamics; closed communication systems, ineffective spousal communication and marital problems
	Altered role function/disruption of family roles
	Manipulation; dependency; criticizing; rationalization/denial of problems
	Enabling to maintain drinking (substance abuse); refusal to get help/inability to accept and receive help appropriately
Desired Outcomes/Evaluation Criteria— Family Will:	Verbalize understanding of dynamics of enabling behaviors.
	Participate in individual family programs.
	Identify ineffective coping behaviors and consequences.
	Initiate and plan for necessary lifestyle changes.
	Take action to change self-destructive behaviors/alter behaviors that contribute to partner's/SO's addiction.

ACTIONS/INTERVENTIONS	RATIONALE
Independent	
Review family history; explore roles of family members, circumstances involving drug use, strengths, areas of growth.	Determines areas for focus, potential for change.
Explore how the SO has coped with the client's habit (e.g., denial, repression, rationalization, hurt, loneliness, projection).	The person who enables also suffers from the same feelings as the client and uses ineffective methods for dealing with the situation, necessitating help in learning new/effective coping skills.
Determine understanding of current situation and previous methods of coping with life's problems.	Provides information on which to base present plan of care.
Assess current level of functioning of family members.	Affects individual's ability to cope with situation.
Determine extent of enabling behaviors being evidenced by family members; explore with each individual and client.	Enabling is doing for the client what he or she needs to do for self (rescuing). People want to be helpful and do not want to feel powerless to help their loved one to stop substance use and change the behavior that is so destructive. However, the substance abuser often relies on others to cover up own inability to cope with daily responsibilities.
Provide information about enabling behavior, addictive disease characteristics for both the user and nonuser.	Awareness and knowledge of behaviors (e.g., avoiding and shielding, taking over responsibilities, rationalizing, and subserving) provide opportunity for individuals to begin the process of change.

211

Identify and discuss sabotage behaviors of family members.	Even though family member(s) may verbalize a desire for the individual to become substance-free, the reality of interactive dynamics is that they may unconsciously not want the individual to recover, as this would affect the family members' own role in the relationship. Additionally, they may receive sympathy/attention from others (secondary gain).
Encourage participation in therapeutic writing, e.g., journaling (narrative), guided or focused.	Serves as a release for feelings (e.g., anger, grief, stress); helps move individual(s) forward in treatment process.
Provide factual information to client and family about the effects of addictive behaviors on the family and what to expect after discharge.	Many clients/SOs are unaware of the nature of addiction. If client is using legally obtained drugs, he or she may believe this does not constitute abuse.
Encourage family members to be aware of their own feelings, look at the situation with perspective and objectivity. They can ask themselves: "Am I being conned? Am I acting out of fear, shame, guilt, or anger? Do I have a need to control?"	When the enabling family members become aware of their own actions that perpetuate the addict's problems, they need to decide to change themselves. If they change, the client can then face the consequences of own actions and may choose to get well.
Provide support for enabling partner(s). Encourage group work.	Families/SOs need support as much as the person who is addicted to produce change.
Assist the client's partner to become aware that client's abstinence and drug use are not the partner's responsibility.	Partners need to learn that user's habit may or may not change despite partner's involvement in treatment.
Help the recovering (former user) partner who is enabling to distinguish between destructive aspects of behavior and genuine motivation to aid the user.	Enabling behavior can be partner's attempts at personal survival.
Note how partner relates to the treatment team/staff.	Determines enabling style. A parallel exists between how partner relates to user and to staff, based on partner's feelings about self and situation.
Explore conflicting feelings the enabling partner may have about treatment (e.g., feelings similar to those of substance abuser [blend of anger, guilt, fear, exhaustion, embarrassment, loneliness, distrust, grief, and possibly relief]).	Useful in establishing the need for therapy for the partner. This individual's own identity may have been lost—she or he may fear self-disclosure to staff and may have difficulty giving up the dependent relationship.
Involve family in discharge referral plans.	Drug abuse is a family illness. Because the family has been so involved in dealing with the substance abuse behavior, family members need help adjusting to the new behavior of sobriety/abstinence. Incidence of recovery is almost doubled when the family is treated along with the client.
Be aware of staff's enabling behaviors and feelings about client and enabling partner(s).	Lack of understanding of enabling and codependence can result in nontherapeutic approaches to clients and their families.

Collaborative

Encourage involvement with self-help associations such as Alcoholics/Narcotics Anonymous, Al-Anon, Alateen, and professional family therapy.	Puts client/family in direct contact with support systems necessary for continued sobriety and assists with problem resolution.

NURSING DIAGNOSIS	SEXUAL dysfunction
May Be Related to:	Altered body function: neurological damage and debilitating effects of drug use (particularly alcohol and opiates)
Possibility Evidenced by:	Progressive interference with sexual functioning
	In men: A significant degree of testicular atrophy is noted (testes are smaller and softer than normal), gynecomastia (breast enlargement), impotence/decreased sperm counts
	In women: Loss of body hair; thin, soft skin, and spider angioma (elevated estrogen); amenorrhea/increase in miscarriages
Desired Outcomes/Evaluation Criteria—Client Will:	Verbally acknowledge effects of drug use on sexual functioning/reproduction.
	Identify interventions to correct/overcome individual situation.

ACTIONS/INTERVENTIONS	RATIONALE
Independent	
Ascertain client's beliefs and expectations. Have client describe problem in own words.	Determines level of knowledge; identifies misperceptions, learning needs.
Encourage and accept individual expressions of concern.	Most people find it difficult to talk about this sensitive subject and may not ask directly for information.
Provide education opportunity (e.g., pamphlets, consultation from appropriate persons) for client to learn effects of drug on sexual functioning.	Much of denial and hesitancy to seek treatment may be decreased with sufficient and appropriate information.
Provide information about individual's condition.	Sexual functioning may have been affected by drug (alcohol) intake or physiological and/or psychological factors (such as stress). Information will assist client to understand own situation and identify actions to be taken.
Provide information about effects of substance use on the reproductive system/fetus (e.g., increased risk of premature birth, brain damage, and fetal malformation). Assess drinking/drug history of pregnant client.	Awareness of the negative effects of alcohol/other drugs on reproduction may motivate client to stop using drug(s). When client is pregnant, identification of potential problems aids in planning for future fetal needs/concerns.
Discuss prognosis for sexual dysfunction (e.g., impotence/low sexual desire).	In about 50% of cases, impotence is reversed with abstinence from drug(s); in 25%, the return to normal functioning is delayed; in approximately 25% impotence remains.
Collaborative	
Refer for sexual counseling, if indicated.	Couple may need additional assistance to resolve more severe problems/situations. Client may have difficult adjusting, if drug has improved sexual experience (heroin decreases dyspareunia in women/premature ejaculation in men).

213

Furthermore, the client may have engaged enjoyably in bizarre, erotic sexual behavior while under the influence of stimulant drug(s); client may have found no substitute for the drug, may have driven a partner away, and may have no motivation to adjust to sexual experience without drugs.

Review results of sonogram, if client is pregnant.

Assesses fetal growth and development to identify possibility of fetal alcohol syndrome (FAS) and future needs.

NURSING DIAGNOSIS	KNOWLEDGE deficit [LEARNING NEED] regarding condition, prognosis, treatment, self care and discharge needs
May Be Related to:	Lack of information; information misinterpretation
	Cognitive limitations/interference with learning (other mental illness problems/organic brain syndrome); lack of recall
Possibly Evidenced by:	Statements of concern; questions/misconceptions
	Inaccurate follow-through of instructions/development of preventable complications
	Continued use in spite of complications/"bad trips"
Desired Outcomes/Evaluation Criteria— Client Will:	Verbalize understanding of own condition/disease process, prognosis, and treatment plan.
	Identify/initiate necessary lifestyle changes to remain drug-free.
	Participate in treatment program.

ACTIONS/INTERVENTIONS	RATIONALE

Independent

Be aware of and deal with anxiety of client and family members.	Anxiety can interfere with ability to hear and assimilate information.
Provide an active role for the client/SO in the learning process (e.g., discussions, group participation, role-playing).	Learning is enhanced when persons are actively involved.
Provide written and verbal information as indicated. Include list of articles and books related to client/family needs and encourage reading and discussing what they learn.	Helps client/SO make informed choices about future. Bibliotherapy can be a useful addition to other therapeutic approaches.
Assess client's knowledge of own situation (e.g., disease, complications, and needed changes in lifestyle).	Assists in planning for long-range changes necessary for maintaining sobriety/drug-free status. Client may have street knowledge of the drug but be ignorant of medical facts.

Time activities to individual needs.

Facilitates learning, as information is more readily assimilated when pacing is considered.

Review condition and prognosis/future expectations.

Provides knowledge base on which client can make informed choices.

Discuss relationship of drug use to current situation.

Often client has misperception (denial) of real reason for admission to the psychiatric (medical) setting.

Discuss effects of drug(s) used, e.g., PCP is deposited in body fat and may reactivate (flashbacks) even after long interval of abstinence; alcohol use may result in mental deterioration, liver involvement/damage; cocaine can damage postcapillary vessels, increase platelet aggregation, promote thromboses and infarction of skin/internal organs, cause localized atrophie blanche of sclerodermatous lesions.

Information will help client understand possible long-term effects of drug use.

Discuss potential for reemergence of withdrawal symptoms from stimulant abuse as early as 3 months or as late as 9–12 months after discontinuing drug use.

Even though symptoms of intoxication may have passed, client may manifest denial, drug hunger, and periods of "flare-up," in which a delayed recurrence of withdrawal symptoms occurs (e.g., anxiety, depression, irritability, sleep disturbance, compulsiveness with food [especially sugars]).

Inform client of effects of disulfiram (Antabuse) in combination with alcohol intake and importance of avoiding use of alcohol-containing products (e.g., foods/candy, cough syrups, mouthwash, aftershave/cologne).

Interaction of alcohol and Antabuse results in nausea and hypotension, which may produce fatal shock. Clients taking Antabuse are sensitive to alcohol on a continuum, with some being able to drink while taking the drug and others having a reaction with only slight exposure to alcohol. Reactions also appear to be dose-related.

Review specific aftercare needs (e.g., PCP user should drink cranberry juice and continue use of ascorbic acid); alcohol abuser with liver damage should refrain from drugs/anesthetics or use of household cleaning products detoxified in the liver.

Promotes individualized care related to specific situation. Cranberry juice and ascorbic acid enhance clearance of PCP from the system. Substances that have the potential for liver damage are more dangerous in the client with impaired liver function.

Discuss variety of helpful organizations and programs that are available for assistance/referral.

Long-term support is necessary to maintain optimal recovery. Psychosocial needs, as well as other issues, may require addressing.

SAMPLE CLINICAL PATHWAY
Recovery from Addiction ELOS: 8 weeks Outpatient Program

ND and categories of care	Time dimension	Outcomes/actions	Time dimension	Outcomes/actions	Time dimension	Outcomes/actions
Denial/Ineffective Individual Coping R/T personal vulnerability, inadequate coping skills and learned responses	Day 1	Commit to program attendance and abstinence	Week 3	Identify effective coping strategies Engage in problem-solving Initiate lifestyle changes	Week 6	Initiate contact with community resources specific to own goals/needs
	Week 1	Verbalize awareness of relationship of substance use to current situation				
	Week 2	List ineffective coping behaviors Identify necessary lifestyle changes	Week 4	Demonstrate new coping behaviors Identify feelings and underlying dynamics for negative perception of self/abilities	Week 7	Verbalize acceptance of self as is and an increased sense of self-worth
Referrals	Day 1–2	All members of treatment team			Week 8	Arrangements made to continue peer support post discharge Participating in community program
Diagnostic studies	Day 1	Drug screen (blood and urine) Other studies based on individual need				
Additional Assessment	Day 1–2	Routine evaluations: Mental status Psychosocial Functional/Safety Nutritional Physical exam				
Medication	Day 1– ongoing	Antabuse/Trexan, Dolophin (as indicated) Antipsychotic (as indicated)				

Actions/therapies (G = group session; I = Individual)

Time		Intervention
Day 1		Orient to program
		Explain expectations/limits
		Provide reading list
Day 1– ongoing		Confront denial/inappropriate behavior
Day 2		Instruct in relaxation techniques
Week 1	G:	Ohlms Disease Concept/Theories of Addiction
Week 2	G:	Alcohol/Cocaine/Crack
	I:	Coping Strategies
Week 3	G:	Progression of disease
Week 4	G:	Relapse Prevention
	G:	Feelings
Week 5	G:	Enabling Behaviors
Week 6	G:	The 12-Steps/Community Resources
	I:	Wrapup/Post Treatment Maintenance Program
Week 7	G:	Forgiveness
	I:	Individual issues (if dual diagnosis)
Week 8	G:	Drug Interactions/AIDS
	G:	Managing a New Lifestyle

Powerlessness R/T substance addiction, episodic compulsive indulgence, lifestyle of helplessness

Time	Goal
Week 1	Verbalize acceptance of need for treatment
Week 2	Begin active participation in group
	Admit inability to control drug habit
Week 3	Engage in peer support
	Surrender to powerlessness over addiction
Week 4	Acknowledge own responsibility for change
Week 5	Verbalize awareness that willpower alone cannot control abstinence
Week 6	Recognize reality of losses in life including those associated with giving up use of substance
Week 7	Plan in place to meet needs postdischarge

Actions/therapies

Time		Intervention
Week 1	G:	Anger/Resentment
	I:	Treatment Plan/Individual Goals
Week 2	G:	Delusional Memory System
ongoing		Dual diagnosis (if indicated)
Week 3	G:	Shame
	I:	Locus of Control
Week 4	I:	Discharge/Future Plans
Week 5	G:	Spirituality
	I:	Personal Issues
Week 6	G:	Grief and loss
Week 7	G:	Healthy/Drug-Free Lifestyle

RECOVERY FROM ADDICTION ELOS: 8 WEEKS OUTPATIENT PROGRAM–*continued*

ND and categories of care	Time dimension	Outcomes/ actions	Time dimension	Outcomes/ actions	Time dimension	Outcomes/ actions
Altered Family Process: Substance Abuse R/T history of substance abuse, addictive personality, lack of problem-solving skills	Week 1	Commit to regular participation in program	Week 3	Verbalize awareness of family interaction patterns	Week 6	Take action to change destructive behaviors contributing to addiction
	Week 2	Express feelings freely and appropriately	Week 4	Identify healthy lifestyle changes	Week 7	Plan ways to improve communication between members
			Week 5	Verbalize understanding of dynamics of enabling behaviors	Week 8	Provide support for affected members to handle own life
Actions/therapies	Week 1 G:	Family Disease Concept	Week 3 G:	Family Roles/Rules	Week 6 G:	Multifamily Process group
	Week 2 G:	Multifamily Process Group	Week 4 G:	Multifamily Process Group	Week 7 G:	Communications
			Week 5 G:	"Codependency"-enabling	Week 8 G:	Multifamily Process Group

CHAPTER 7

SCHIZOPHRENIA AND OTHER PSYCHOTIC DISORDERS

SCHIZOPHRENIA

DSM-IV
SCHIZOPHRENIA
295.30 Paranoid type
295.10 Disorganized type
295.20 Catatonic type
295.90 Undifferentiated type
295.60 Residual type
(Refer to *DSM-IV* for other listings.)

Schizophrenia describes psychotic state that at some time is characterized by apathy, avolition, asociality, affective blunting, and alogia. The client has alterations in thoughts, percepts, mood, and behavior. Subjective experiences of disordered thought are manifested in disturbances of concept formation that sometimes lead to misinterpretations of reality, delusions (particularly delusions of influence and ideas of reference), and hallucinations. Mood changes include ambivalence, constriction or inappropriateness of feeling, and loss of empathy with others. Behavior may be withdrawn, regressive, or bizarre (Shader, 1994).

ETIOLOGICAL THEORIES

Psychodynamics

Psychosis is the result of a weak ego. The development of the ego has been inhibited by a symbiotic parent/child relationship. Because the ego is weak, the use of ego defense mechanisms in times of extreme anxiety is maladaptive, and behaviors are often representations of the id segment of the personality.

Biological

Certain genetic factors may be involved in the susceptibility to develop some forms of this psychotic disorder. Individuals are at higher risk for the disorder if there is a familial pattern of involvement (parents, siblings, other relatives). Schizophrenia has been determined to be a sporadic illness (which means genes cannot currently be followed from generation to generation). It is an autosomal dominant trait. However, most scientists agree that what is inherited is a vulnerability or predisposition, which may be due to an enzyme defect or some

219

other biochemical abnormality, a subtle neurological deficit, or some other factor or combination of factors. This predisposition, in combination with environmental factors, results in development of the disease. Some research implies that these disorders may be a birth defect, occurring in the hippocampus region of the brain. The studies show a disordering of the pyramidal cells in the brains of schizophrenics, while the cells in the brains of nonschizophrenic individuals appear to be arranged in an orderly fashion. Ventricular brain ratio (VBR) or disproportionately small brain (or specific areas of the brain) may be inherited and/or congenital. The cause can be a virus, lack of oxygen, birth trauma, severe maternal malnutrition, or cellular damage resulting from an RhD immune response (mother negative/fetus positive).

A biochemical theory suggests the involvement of elevated levels of the neurotransmitter dopamine, which is thought to produce the symptoms of overactivity and fragmentation of associations that are commonly observed in psychoses.

Although overall occurrence is relatively equal between males and females, resources report a predominant male bias with two-thirds of young adults with serious mental illnesses being male. Boys react more strongly than girls to stress and conflicts in the family home, and are more vulnerable to infantile autism. A significantly larger number of males than females exhibit obsessive and suicidal behaviors, fetishism, and schizophrenia. Schizophrenia develops earlier in males, and they respond less well to treatment and have less chance of recovery and return to normal life than females. The incidence in females may have more familial origins. The different brain organization of men and women, and the effect of sex hormones on brain growth are likely to result in subtle differences that define the "scope and range of sex differences in the incidence, clinical presentation, and course of specific psychiatric diseases" (Moir & Jessel, 1991).

Family Dynamics

Family systems theory describes the development of schizophrenia as it evolves out of a dysfunctional family system. Conflict between spouses drives one parent to become attached to the child. This overinvestment in the child redirects the focus of anxiety in the family, and a more stable condition results. A symbiotic relationship develops between parent and child; the child remains totally dependent on the parent into adulthood and is unable to respond to the demands of adult functioning.

Interpersonal theory relates that the psychotic person is the product of a parent/child relationship fraught with intense anxiety. The child receives confusing and conflicting messages from the parent and is unable to establish trust. High levels of anxiety are maintained, and the child's concept of self is one of ambiguity. A retreat into psychosis offers relief from anxiety and security from intimate relatedness. Some research indicates that clients who live with families high in expressed emotion (e.g., hostility, criticism, disappointment, overprotectiveness, and overinvolvement) show more frequent relapses than clients who live with families who are low in expressed emotion.

Current research of genetic and biological influences suggests that these family interactions are more likely to be contributing factors to rather than the cause of the disorder.

CLIENT ASSESSMENT DATA BASE

General

Activity/Rest

Interruption of sleep by hallucinations and delusional thoughts, early awakening, insomnia, and hyperactivity (e.g., pacing)

Hygiene

Poor personal hygiene, unkempt/disheveled appearance

220

Neurosensory

History of alteration in functioning for at least 6 months, including an active phase of at least 2 weeks in which psychotic symptoms were evident

Family reports of psychological symptoms (primarily in thought and perception) and deterioration from previous level of adaptive functioning

Mental Status:

  Thought: Delusions, loose association

  Perception: Hallucinations, illusions

  Affect: Blunted, flat, inappropriate, incongruous, or silly

  Volition: Cannot self-initiate or participate in goal-oriented activity

  Capacity to Relate to Environment: Mental/emotional withdrawal and isolation (autism) and/or psychomotor activity ranging from marked reduction to stereotypic, purposeless activity

  Speech: Frequently incoherent, echolalia may be noted/alogia (inability to speak) may occur

  Delusions:

   Disorganized type—Fragmentary delusions or hallucinations (disorganized, unthematized [without theme] content) common; systematized delusions absent

   Paranoid type—One or more systematized delusions with prominent persecutory or grandiose content; delusional jealousy may occur

   Undifferentiated type—Delusions prominent

  Behaviors: Grimaces, mannerisms, hypochondriacal complaints, extreme social withdrawal, and other odd behaviors

  Negativism: Resistance to all directions or attempts to move without apparent motive

  Rigidity: Rigid posture maintained despite attempts to move client

  Excitement: Purposeless motor activity not caused by external stimuli

  Posturing: Voluntarily assuming inappropriate or bizarre posture

  Emotions: Unfocused anxiety, anger, argumentativeness, and violence

Teaching/Learning

May have had previous acute episodes with impairment ranging from none to severe deterioration requiring institutionalization

Onset of symptoms most commonly occurring between the late teens and mid-30s

Correlations with family history of psychiatric illness; lower socioeconomic groups, higher stressors; premorbid personality described as suspicious, introverted, withdrawn, or eccentric

Disorganized

Neurosensory

Speech disorganized, communication consistently incoherent

Behavior regressive/primitive, incoherent, and grossly disorganized

Psychomotor: Stupor, markedly decreased reactivity to milieu, and/or reduced spontaneity of movement/activity or mutism

Affect: Incoherent, flat, incongruent, silly

Social Interactions

Extreme social impairment/withdrawal; odd mannersisms

Poor premorbid personality

Teaching/Learning

Chronic course with no significant remissions

Catatonic

(Although common several decades ago, incidence has decreased markedly with the advent of antipsychotic medications.)

Activity/Rest

Marked psychomotor retardation or excessive/purposeless motor activity
Exhaustion (extreme agitation)

Food/Fluid

Weight below norms; other signs of malnutrition

Neurosensory

Marked psychomotor disturbance (e.g., stupor, rigidity, mutism or excitement, negativism, waxy flexibility, and/or posturing)
Speech: Echolalia or echopraxia

Safety

Possible violence to self/others (during catatonic stupor or excitement)

Teaching/Learning

Possible hypochondriacal complaints or oddities of behavior

Paranoid

(Absence of symptoms characteristic of disorganized and catatonic types.)

Neurosensory

Systematized delusions and/or auditory hallucinations of a persecutory or grandiose nature, usually related to a single theme

Safety

Easily agitated, assaultive, and violent (if delusions are acted on)
Impairment in functioning (may be minimal), with gross disorganization of behavior (relatively rare)

Social Interactions

Significant impairment may be noted in social/marital areas
Affective responsiveness may be preserved but often with a stilted, formal quality or extreme intensity in interpersonal interactions

Sexuality

May express doubts about gender identity (e.g., fear of being thought of as, or approached by, a homosexual)

Teaching/Learning

Other family members may have history of paranoid problems

Undifferentiated

(This category is used when illness does not meet the criteria for the other specific types of schizophrenias, illness meets the criteria for more than one, or course of the last episode is unknown.)

Neurosensory

Prominent delusions/hallucinations, incoherence, and grossly disorganized behaviors

Residual

Neurosensory

Inappropriate affect

Social Interactions

Social withdrawal, eccentric behavior

Teaching/Learning

History of at least one episode of schizophrenia in which psychotic symptoms were evident, but the current clinical picture presents no psychotic symptoms

DIAGNOSTIC STUDIES

(Usually done to rule out physical illness, which may cause reversible symptoms such as: toxic/deficiency states, infections, neurological disease, endocrine/metabolic disorders.)

CT Scan: May show subtle abnormalities of brain structures in some schizophrenics (e.g., atrophy of temporal lobes); enlarged ventricles with increased ventricle-brain ratio may correlate with degree of symptoms displayed.

Positron Emission Tomography (PET) Scan: Measures the metabolic activity of specific areas of the brain and may reveal low metabolic activity in the frontal lobes, especially in the prefrontal area of the cerebral cortex.

MRI: Provides a three-dimensional image of the brain; may reveal smaller than average frontal lobes, atrophy of left temporal lobe (specifically anterior hippocampus, parahippocampogyrus, and superior temporal gyrus).

Regional Cerebral Blood Flow (RCBF): Maps blood flow and implies the intensity of activity in various brain regions.

Brain Electrical Activity Mapping (BEAM): Shows brain wave responses to various stimuli with delayed and decreased response noted, particularly in left temporal lobe and associated limbic system.

Addiction Severity Index (ASI): Determines problems of addiction (substance abuse), which may be associated with mental illness, and indicates areas of treatment need.

Psychological Testing (e.g., MMPI): Reveals impairment in one or more areas. **Note:** Paranoid type usually shows little or no impairment.

NURSING PRIORITIES

1. Promote appropriate interaction between client and environment.
2. Enhance physiological stability/health maintenance.
3. Provide protection; ensure safety needs.
4. Encourage family/significant other(s) to become involved in activities to promote independent, satisfying lives.

DISCHARGE CRITERIA

1. Physiological well-being maintained with appropriate balance between rest and activity.
2. Demonstrates increasing/highest level of emotional responsiveness possible.
3. Interacts socially without decompensation.
4. Family displays effective coping skills and appropriate use of resources.
5. Plan in place to meet needs after discharge.

NURSING DIAGNOSIS	THOUGHT PROCESSES, altered
May Be Related to:	Disintegration of thinking processes; impaired judgment
	Psychological conflicts; disintegrated ego boundaries (confusion with environment)
	Sleep disturbance
	Ambivalence and concomitant dependence (part of need-fear dilemma interferes with ability to self-initiate fulfilling diversional activities)
Possibly Evidenced by:	Presence of delusional system (may be grandiose, persecutory, of reference, of control, somatic, accusatory); commands, obsessions
	Symbolic and concrete associations; blocking ideas of reference
	Inaccurate interpretation of environment; cognitive dissonance; impaired ability to make decisions
	Simple hyperactivity and constant motor activity (ritualistic acts, stereotyped behavior) to withdrawal and psychomotor retardation
	Interrupted sleep patterns
Desired Outcomes/Evaluation Criteria—Client Will:	Recognize changes in thinking/behavior.
	Identify delusions and increase capacity to cope effectively with them by elimination of pathological thinking.
	Maintain reality orientation.
	Establish interpersonal relationships.

ACTIONS/INTERVENTIONS	RATIONALE
Independent	
Determine severity of client's altered thought processes, noting form (dereistic, autistic, symbolic, loose and/or concrete associations, blocking); content (somatic delusions, delusions of grandeur/persecution, ideas of reference); and flow (flight of ideas, retardation).	Identification of symbolic/primitive nature of thinking/communications promotes understanding of the individual client's thought processes and enables planning of appropriate interventions.

224

Establish a therapeutic nurse-client relationship.	Provides an emotionally safe milieu that enables interpersonal interaction and decreases autism.
Use therapeutic communications (e.g., reflection, paraphrasing) to intervene effectively.	Therapeutic communications are clear, concise, open, consistent, and require use of self. This reduces autistic thinking.
Structure communications to reflect consideration of client's socioeconomic, educational, and cultural history/values.	Lack of consideration of these factors can cause misdiagnosis/inaccurate interpretation (otherwise normal thinking viewed as pathological).
Express desire to understand client's thinking by clarifying what is unclear, focusing on the feeling rather than the content, endeavoring to understand (in spite of the client's unclearness), listening carefully, and regulating the flow of the thinking as needed (Active-listening).	Client is often unable to organize thoughts (easily distracted, cannot grasp concepts or wholeness but focuses on minutiae), and flow of thoughts is often characterized as racing, wandering, or retarded. Active-listening identifies patterns of client's thoughts and facilitates understanding. Expression of desire to understand conveys caring and increases client's feelings of self-worth.
Reinforce congruent thinking. Refuse to argue/ agree with disintegrated thoughts. Present reality and demonstrate motivation to understand client (model patience).	Provides opportunity for the client to control aggressive behavior. Decreases altered (disintegrated, delusional) thinking as client's thoughts compensate in response to presentation of reality.
Share appropriate thinking and set limits (cognitive therapy) if client tries to respond impulsively to altered thinking.	Enhances self-esteem and promotes safety for the client and others. Cognitive therapy is directed specifically at thinking patterns that have developed (e.g., illogical associations are made between events that most of us would not believe to be connected). Aim is to modify apparently fixed beliefs, faulty interpretations, and automatic thoughts, and by relating them to "normal experience" to reduce some of the fear attached to them.
Assess rest/sleep pattern by observing capacity to fall asleep, quality of sleep. Graph sleep chart as indicated until acceptable pattern is established.	Delusions, hallucinations, etc. may interfere with client's sleep pattern. Fears may alter ability to fall asleep. Sleep deprivation can produce behaviors such as withdrawal, confusion, disturbance of perception. Sleep chart identifies abnormal patterns and is useful in evaluating effectiveness of interventions.
Structure appropriate times for rest and sleep; adjust work/rest activity patterns as needed.	Consistency in scheduling reduces fears/insecurities, which may be interfering with sleep. Sleep is enhanced by balancing activity (physical, occupational) with rest/sleep.
Help client identify/learn techniques that promote rest/sleep (e.g., quiet activities, soothing music, before bedtime, regular hour for going to bed, drinking warm milk).	Enhances client's ability to optimize rest/sleep, maximizing ability to think clearly.
Assess presence/degree of factors affecting client's capacity for diversional activities.	Presence of hallucinations/delusions; situational factors such as long-term hospitalization (characterized by monotony, sensory deprivation); psychological factors such as decreased volition; physical factors such as immobility contribute to deficits in diversional activity.

Monitor medication regimen, observing for therapeutic effect and side effects (e.g., anticholinergic [dry mouth, etc.], sedation, orthostatic hypotension, photosensitivity, hormonal effects, reduction of seizure threshold, extrapyramidal symptoms, and fatigue/weakness with sore throat or signs of infection [agranulocytosis]).

Enables identification of the minimal effective dose to reduce psychotic symptoms with the fewest adverse effects. Prevention of side effects/timely intervention may enhance cooperation with drug regimen. Identification of the onset of serious side effects, such as neuroleptic malignant syndrome, provides for appropriate interventions to avoid permanent damage.

Collaborative

Administer medications as indicated, e.g.:
  Antipsychotics:
    Phenothiazines, such as
    chlorpromazine (Thorazine),
    thioridazine (Mellaril),
    fluphenazine (Prolixin),
    perphenazine (Trilafon);
    Thioxanthenes, such as
    chlorprothixene (Taractan),
    thiothixene (Navane);
    Butyrophenones, such as
    haloperidol (Haldol);
    Dibenzoxazepines, such as
    loxapine (Loxitane);

Used to reduce psychotic symptoms. May be given orally or by injection. For long-term maintenance therapy, a depot neuroleptic such as Prolixin may be the drug of choice to maintain medication adherence and prevent relapse in problematic clients. When given at bedtime, the sedative effects of psychotropic medication can enhance quality of sleep and reduce hypotensive side effects.

  Atypical antipsychotics:
    clozapine (Clozaril);

Useful in treating clients resistant to other medications or in the presence of unacceptable side effects. Clozapine causes no muscular rigidity and is associated with a relatively low rate of akathisia (feeling of restlessness, urgent need for movement). May not be used as first-line therapy because of a lowered seizure threshold or a 1%–2% potential for agranulocytosis, necessitating weekly blood testing for the duration of treatment. **Note:** Combination therapy, e.g., clozapine and a neuroleptic, such as fluphenazine or haloperidol, may be useful for some clients.

    olanzapine (Zyprexa);

Becoming a first-line drug choice as it specifically targets D_4 dopamine receptors, which may be present in unusually high numbers in clients with schizophrenia. Drug seems well tolerated, with many side effects appearing to be dose-related and no known drug interactions that affect plasma level or compromise efficacy.

    Risperidone (Risperdal);

Effective therapeutic agent has been associated with few uncomfortable or serious side effects, especially agranulocytosis.

  Antiparkinsonism drugs:
  Anticholinergics, such as
  trihexyphenidyl HCl (Artane), benztropine
    mesylate (Cogentin), procyclidine HCl
    (Kemadrin), biperiden HCl (Akineton);

Used to relieve drug-induced extrapyramidal reactions and treat all other forms of parkinsonism. They block action of acetylcholine, thereby reducing excitation of the basal ganglia.

  Antihistamines, such as
    diphenhydramine (Benadryl);

Suppress cholinergic activity and prolong the action of dopamine by inhibiting its reuptake and storage.

  Miscellaneous agents, such as
    amantadine (Symmetrel).

These agents release dopamine from presynaptic nerve endings in basal ganglia.

NURSING DIAGNOSIS	SENSORY/PERCEPTUAL alterations (specify)
May Be Related to:	Panic levels of anxiety
	Disturbance in thought, perception, affect, sense of self, volition, relationship to environment
	Psychomotor behavior
Possibly Evidenced by:	Illusions, delusions, and hallucinations
	Disorientation
	Changes in usual response to stimuli
Desired Outcomes/Evaluation Criteria— Client Will:	Identify self in relationship to environment.
	Recognize reality and dismiss internal voices.
	Demonstrate improved cognitive, perceptual, affective, and psychomotor abilities.

ACTIONS/INTERVENTIONS	RATIONALE

Independent

Assess the presence/severity of alterations in client's perceptions. Note possible causative/contributing factors (e.g., anxiety, substance abuse, fever, trauma, or other organic illnesses/conditions).	Provides information about client's behavior potentials regarding ADLs, sleep patterns, potential for violence (command hallucinations, homicide, suicide), nonverbal and verbal behaviors (content, form, style, flow).
Spend time with client, listening with regard and providing support for changes client is making.	Continued, consistent support/acceptance will reduce anxiety and fears and enable client to decrease altered perceptions.
Provide a safe environment by not arguing with or ridiculing the client.	Altered perceptions are frightening to the client and indicate loss of control. Because of lack of insight, client views altered perceptions as reality. Arguing only leads to defensiveness and a regressive struggle with the client.
Orient to reality by communicating effectively (clear, concise); reinforcing reality of client's altered perceptions; and clarifying time, place, and person.	Client's distortion of reality is a defense against actual reality, which is more frightening. Reality orientation assists client to correctly interpret stimuli within the milieu.
Set limits on client's impulsive response to altered perceptions. Remain with the client and provide distraction when possible.	Client who is perceiving the environment incorrectly lacks internal controls to prevent impulsive response to misperceptions. Often client feels more in control if nurse remains in room. Distraction (music, TV, games) may also support client to regain capacity to control response to altered perceptions.
Be honest in expressing fears, especially if potential for violence is perceived. (Refer to ND: Violence, risk for, directed at self/others.)	Informing client when behaviors are frightening and providing anticipatory guidance (by verbalizing actions) focuses attention on reality and helps reduce anxiety.

Collaborative

Provide external controls (quiet room, seclusion, restraints); inform client of intent to use touch, as indicated.

External limits and controls must be provided to protect client and others until client regains control internally and is able to ignore altered perceptions.

NURSING DIAGNOSIS	COMMUNICATION, impaired verbal
May Be Related to:	Psychological barriers, psychosis
	Autistic and delusional thinking
	Alterations in perception
Possibly Evidenced by:	Inability to verbalize rationally
	Verbal expressions, such as neologisms, echolalia, associative/looseness, paralogic language
	Nonverbal expressions, such as echopraxia, stereotypic behaviors (bizarre gesturing, facial expressions, and posturing)
Desired Outcomes/Evaluation Criteria— Client Will:	Verbalize or indicate an understanding of communication problems.
	Employ strategies to communicate effectively both verbally and nonverbally.
	Establish means of communication in which needs can be understood.

ACTIONS/INTERVENTIONS	RATIONALE

Independent

Evaluate degree/type of communication impairment.	Degree of impairment of verbal/nonverbal communications (loose associations, neologisms, echolalia, and echopraxia) will affect client's ability to interact with staff and others and to participate in care.
Demonstrate a listening attitude within the nurse-client relationship.	Enables the nurse to listen carefully, observe the client, and anticipate and watch certain patterns of client's communication that may emerge.
Acknowledge client's difficulty in communicating.	Recognition of client's difficulty in expressing ideas and feelings demonstrates empathy, lessening anxiety and enabling client to concentrate on communicating.
Provide a nonthreatening environment/safe forum for client's communications.	Atmosphere in which a person feels free to express self without fear of criticism helps to meet safety needs, increasing trust and providing assurance for tolerance and validation of appropriate negative communications.
Accept use of alternative communications, such as drawing, singing, dancing, mime.	Increases client's feelings of security, provides avenues for expressing needs.

228

Avoid arguing or agreeing with inaccurate communications; simply offer reality view in nonjudgmental style (communicate your lack of understanding to client).

Arguing is nontherapeutic and may cause the client to become defensive. Agreeing with the client's expression of inaccurate communication reinforces misinterpretation of reality.

Use therapeutic communication skills, such as paraphrasing, reflecting, clarification.

Client's flow of communications (too fast/too slow) may require regulation. These techniques assist with reality orientation, thereby minimizing misinterpretation and facilitating accurate communications.

Be open and honest in therapeutic use of verbal and nonverbal communications.

Client has increased sensitivity to nonverbal messages. Honesty increases sense of trust, a loss of which is at the base of the client's problem. Openness and genuineness in expression of feelings provide a role model for client.

Use a supportive approach to client by communicating desire to understand (ask client to help you do so).

Recognizes that client's past experiences have created distrust, which produces attempt to maintain distance by being vague and unclear in sending messages.

Identify the symbolic, primitive nature of the client's speech/communications.

Recognition of the symbolism of the client's primitive speech and thinking enables the nurse to better understand the client's feelings. Without this recognition, the actual communications may be vague and disorganized, indicating client's inability to focus and perceive clearly.

Note cultural beliefs (e.g., talking to dead relatives) that may be accepted as normal within the client's frame of reference.

Cultural attitudes need to be considered to avoid confusion with pathological condition.

NURSING DIAGNOSIS	**COPING, INDIVIDUAL, ineffective**
May Be Related to:	Personal vulnerability; inadequate support system(s)
	Unrealistic perceptions
	Inadequate coping methods
	Disintegration of thought processes
Possibly Evidenced by:	Impaired judgment, cognition, and perception
	Diminished problem-solving/decision-making capacities
	Poor self-concept
	Chronic anxiety and depression
	Inability to perform role expectations
	Alteration in social participation
Desired Outcomes/Evaluation Criteria—Client Will:	Identify ineffective coping behaviors and consequences.

229

Demonstrate understanding of and begin to use appropriate, constructive, effective methods for coping.

Display behavior congruent with verbalization of feelings.

ACTIONS/INTERVENTIONS	RATIONALE
Independent	
Determine the presence/degree of impairment of client's coping abilities.	Provides information about perceived and actual coping ability, life change units, anxiety level, stresses (internal, external), developmental level of functioning, use of defense mechanisms, and problem-solving ability.
Assist client to identify/discuss thoughts, perceptions, and feelings.	Client is able to view how perceptions/thinking/affect is processed and to strengthen reality orientation and coping skills.
Encourage client to express areas of concern. Support formulation of realistic goals and learning of appropriate problem-solving techniques.	This disorder first manifests itself at an early age, before the client has had an opportunity to learn effective coping skills. In a trusting relationship (a climate of acceptance), the client can begin to learn these skills, without fear of judgment.
Encourage client to identify precipitants that led to ineffective coping, when possible.	Knowledge of stressors that have precipitated deteriorated coping ability enables client to recognize and deal with these factors before problems occur.
Explore how client's perceptions are validated prior to drawing conclusions.	With support, client has the opportunity to learn to validate perceptions before selecting ineffective/inappropriate coping methods (such as acting-out behavior).
Assist client to recognize and develop appropriate/effective coping skills.	Increased/more flexible problem-solving or coping behaviors prevent decompensation (distorted reality, delusional system).

NURSING DIAGNOSIS	**SELF ESTEEM, chronic low/ROLE PERFORMANCE, altered/PERSONAL IDENTITY disturbance**
May Be Related to:	Disintegrated thought processes (perception, cognition, affect)
	Loose/disintegration of ego boundaries
	Perceived threats to the self
	Disintegration of behavior, affect
Possibly Evidenced by:	Expressions of worthlessness, negative feelings about self

Impaired judgment, cognition, and perception; protective delusional systems; disturbed sense of self (depersonalization and delusions of control)

Role performance deterioration in family, social, and work areas

Inadequate development of self-esteem and hopefulness

Ambivalence and autism (interfering with acceptance of self and meaning of own existence)

Desired Outcomes/Evaluation Criteria—Client Will:

Demonstrate enhanced sense of self by decreasing episodes of depersonalization and delusions.

Verbalize feelings of value/worthwhileness and view self as competent and socially acceptable (by self and others).

Develop appropriate plans for improvement of role performance that promote highest possible level of adaptive functioning.

Demonstrate self-directedness by expressing own needs and desires and making effective decisions.

Participate in activities with others.

ACTIONS/INTERVENTIONS	RATIONALE
Independent	
Assess the degree of disturbance in client's self-concept.	Documents own and others' perceptions, client's goals, significant losses/changes. Provides basis for determination of therapy needs and evaluation of progress.
Spend time with client; listen with positive regard and acceptance.	Conveys empathy, acceptance, support, which enhances client's self-esteem. Personal identity is strengthened as client identifies with the nurse and experiences therapeutic caring within the relationship.
Encourage client to verbalize areas of concern/feelings.	Self-esteem is improved by increased insight into feelings. Insight is gained as client verbalizes/identifies feelings (e.g., inadequacy, worthlessness, rejection, loneliness).
Help client identify how negative feelings decrease self-esteem.	Negative feelings can lead to severe anxiety and/or suspiciousness. Increased awareness/perception of factors that cause negative feelings can help client recognize how negative feelings cause deterioration.
Encourage client to recognize positive characteristics related to self.	Discussion of positive aspects of the self-system, such as social skills, work abilities, education, talents, and appearance, can reinforce client's feelings of being a worthwhile/competent person.

231

Review personal appearance and things client can do to enhance hygiene/grooming. (Refer to ND: Self Care deficit [specify].)	Positive personal appearance enhances body image and self-respect.
Encourage client to participate in appropriate activities/exercise program.	Enhances capacity for interpersonal relationships (both 1:1 and in small groups). Activities that use the five senses increase the sense of self. Physical exercise promotes positive sense of well-being.
Assess client's capacity to tolerate use of touch.	Careful use of touch can help client reestablish body boundaries (if the experience can be tolerated).
Provide positive reinforcement for client's abilities/efforts.	Positive feedback increases self-esteem, provides encouragement, and promotes a sense of self-direction.
Determine current level of role performance and note causative/contributing factors that affect it.	Factors such as inadequate knowledge, role conflict, alteration of self/others' perceptions of role, and change in usual patterns of responsibility can affect the client's physical and psychological capacity for effective role performance.
Assist the client to adapt to changing role performance by working with client/significant other(s) to develop strategies for dealing with disturbances in role and enhancing expectations of coping effectively.	The client's eventual level of performance may be positively influenced by a support system that is responsive and caring.
Help client set realistic goals for managing life and performing own ADLs.	Client needs to be productive and benefits from being given the responsibility for own life and direction within limits of ability.
Assess the current sense of personal identity, considering if client acknowledges sense of self. (Observe how client addresses self (e.g., may refer to self in third person). Also consider if client expresses feelings of unreadiness, merging with people/objects.	Identifies individual needs, appropriate interventions. Inability to identify self poses a major problem that can interfere with person's interactions with others.
Analyze the presence/severity of factors that alter personal identity (e.g., paranoia, blunted affect).	Disintegrated ego boundaries can cause a weakened sense of self. Clients often express fears of merging and thereby losing personal identity.
Assess presence/severity of factors that affect client's religious/spiritual orientation. Note presence of religiosity.	Disintegrated behaviors create such factors as displaced anger toward God, expression of concern with meaning of life/death/values (may be expressed as delusions, hallucinations). These concerns may negatively affect the individual's sense of self-worth. Client may use religious beliefs as a defense against fears.
Use therapeutic communication skills to support client's verbalization of sense of self and to discover its relationship to meaning of existence.	Therapeutic communications, such as Active-listening, summarizing, reflection, can support client to find own solutions.
Facilitate early discharge for client when hospitalization has been required.	Clients can increase their sense of self by early return to own milieu surrounded by personal possessions.

Collaborative

Administer appropriate tests (e.g., ask client to draw a stick figure of self, Body Image Aberration, Physical Anhedonia Scale).	These tests demonstrate client's view, the client's concept of self, and their correlation to many variables.

Refer to resources such as occupational therapist/ movement therapy/Outdoor Education Program; others.

Provides activities that promote feelings of self-worth and accomplishment during involvement with partial hospitalization program. Partial hospitalization may facilitate transition from hospital setting to community.

Initiate involvement in/refer to religious activities and resources as desired or appropriate. Note over-involvement in religious activity.

Spiritual resources such as a pattern of prayer, a sense of faith, or membership in an organized religious group may enhance the development of client's coping resources, sense of acceptance/self-worth. Strong attachment to an ideology (religiosity) may be used in an attempt to control feelings of anxiety.

NURSING DIAGNOSIS	**ANXIETY [specify level]/FEAR**
May Be Related to:	Disintegration of thought processes
	Perception and affect occurring in response to overwhelming feelings of losing control; threat to self-concept
	Change in environment, role functioning, interaction patterns
	Extremes in psychomotor activity (occurring with chronicity or severity)
Possibly Evidenced by:	Inappropriate/regressed or absent responses; poor eye contact
	Increased perception of danger; focus on self
	Decreased problem-solving ability
	Fear of perceived loss of control or approval from significant other(s); inappropriate response to such feelings; hurting self or others
	Psychomotor disturbances varying from excited motor behavior to immobility
Desired Outcomes/Evaluation Criteria— Client Will:	Respond appropriately to feelings of overwhelming anxiety (fears, loss of control, feelings of rejection) by decreasing regressive behaviors (disintegrated thinking/perception affect).
	Communicate anxious feelings openly in an acceptable manner.
	Orient to reality as evidenced by interpreting milieu correctly.
	Verbalize no perceived danger in interactions with others.

ACTIONS/INTERVENTIONS	RATIONALE

Independent

Note the level of the client's anxiety, considering severity, unfulfilled needs, misperceptions,

The weakened ego of schizophrenia causes a decreased capacity to distinguish reality and a

233

present use of defense mechanisms, and coping skills.

Assess the degree and reality of the fears currently perceived by the client.

Establish trust through a patient, supportive, caring, and accepting relationship.

Encourage the client to verbalize fears.

Assist client to identify/communicate sources of anxiety and areas of concern.

Monitor for drug effectiveness/side effects.

Demonstrate/encourage use of effective, constructive strategies for coping with anxiety (e.g., relaxation and thought-stopping techniques, meditation, and physical exercise). Use role-modeling, positive reinforcement.

Remain with the client and clarify reality.

Involve client in planning treatment.

diminished capacity to problem-solve. This can and coping skills.result in a heightened sense of helplessness and anxiety.

The client's experience of fear may contribute to decreased coping capacity and increased anxiety/fear.

Trust, which is difficult for schizophrenic clients, is the basis of a therapeutic nurse-client relationship. The mutuality of the 1:1 experience enables clients to work through their fears and to identify appropriate methods for problem-solving by role-modeling within the relationship.

Verbalization of frightening perceptions (fears) reduces withdrawal and/or potential for violence (projection of aggressive impulses).

Anxiety can arise from misperceived threats to self, unfulfilled needs, and perceived losses (of control/approval). Disintegration of thinking, perception, and affect may be reduced as client verbalizes frightening feelings.

Prevention of medication side effects can reduce frightening physiological experiences that can escalate anxiety.

Maladaptive coping needs to be examined with emphasis on ineffectiveness of outcomes. Reduces secondary gain and enables client to learn more adaptive/effective decision-making, problem-solving, coping skills. (Refer to NDs: Communication, impaired verbal; Sensory/Perceptual alterations.)

Assists the client to achieve effective coping. The presence of a trusted individual can help client feel protected from external dangers and maintain contact with reality.

Participation in treatment increases client's sense of control and provides opportunity to practice problem-solving skills.

NURSING DIAGNOSIS	SOCIAL ISOLATION
May Be Related to:	Disturbed thought processes that result in mistrust of others/delusional thinking
	Environmental deprivation, institutionalization (as a result of long-term hospitalization)
Possibly Evidenced by:	Difficulty in establishing relationships with others; social withdrawal/isolation of self
	Expressions of feelings of rejection

Desired Outcomes/Evaluation Criteria—Client Will:	Dealing with problems using anger/hostility and violence
	Verbalize willingness to be involved with others.
	Participate in activities/programs with others.
	Develop 1:1 trust-based relationship.

ACTIONS/INTERVENTIONS	RATIONALE

Independent

Assess presence/degree of isolation by listening to client's comments about loneliness.	Mistrust can lead to difficulty in establishing relationships, and client may have withdrawn from close contacts with others.
Spend time with client. Make brief, short interactions that communicate interest, concern, and caring.	Establishes a trusting relationship. Consistent, brief, honest contact with the nurse can help the client begin to reestablish trusting interactions with others.
Plan appropriate times for activities (by limiting withdrawal, varying daily routine only as tolerated).	Consistency in 1:1 relationship and sameness of milieu are required initially to enable client to decrease withdrawn behavior. Motivation is stimulated by the humanistic sharing of a 1:1 experience.
Assist client to participate in diversional activities and limited/planned interaction situations with others in group meeting/unit party, etc.	With toleration of 1:1 relationship and strengthened ego boundaries, client will be able to increase socialization and enter small-group situations. Brief encounters can help the client to become more comfortable around others and provide an opportunity to try out new social skills.
Identify support systems available to the client (e.g., family, friends, coworkers).	Support is an important part of the client's rehabilitation, providing a network to assist in social recovery.
Assess family relationships, communication patterns, knowledge of client condition.	Problems within family (poor social/relationship skills, high expressed emotion) may interfere with client's progress and indicate need for family therapy.
Note client's sense of self-worth and belief about individual identity/role within milieu and setting.	When client feels good about self and own value, family interactions with others are enhanced. (Refer to NDs: Self Esteem, chronic low/Role Performance, altered/Personal Identity disturbance.)

NURSING DIAGNOSIS	PHYSICAL MOBILITY, risk for impaired
Risk Factors May Include:	Disintegration of thought and behavior
	Perceptual impairment; sensory overload/deprivation

	Psychomotor retardation; diminished muscle strength; impaired coordination and limited range of motion/total immobility
	Psychomotor activity (occurring with chronicity or severity) varying from excited motor behavior to immobility
Possibly Evidenced by:	[Not applicable; presence of signs and symptoms establishes an *actual* diagnosis.]
Desired Outcomes/Evaluation Criteria— Client Will:	Maintain optimal mobility and muscle strength.
	Demonstrate awareness of the environment (psychomotor behavior) and capacity to regulate psychomotor activity.
	Engage in physical activities.

ACTIONS/INTERVENTIONS	RATIONALE

Independent

Determine the level of impairment (rate from complete independence to dependence with social withdrawal) in relation to preillness capacity, considering age, meaning (motivation, desire, tolerance), onset, duration, coordination, range of motion, muscle strength, and control. Measure capacity for activity by observing endurance (attention span, psychomotor response, appropriateness of participation).	Provides information to determine the amount of nursing assistance required and client potentials. Note the presence/severity of factors that affect the client's level of mobility, such as psychotic functioning, control needs, sensory overload/deprivation. These factors need to be considered in planning nursing care, as they can affect client's ability to perform activities.
Encourage client to identify need for/plan resumption of activities/exercise.	As psychotic functioning decreases, the capacity to relate to milieu/others and to self-initiate increases. Involving client in scheduling activities provides client with sense of independence (control over environment).
Determine current activity level appropriate for client by assessing attention span, capacity to tolerate others in milieu.	Presence of psychotic features can cause mental/emotional withdrawal or agitation.
Structure appropriate times for exercise/activity (turning/moving unaffected body parts); monitor environmental stimuli such as radio, TV, visitors.	Movement reduces physiological deterioration. Environmental stimulation can be used to maintain/promote sensory-perceptual capacity.
Schedule adequate periods of rest/sleep. Monitor client's response and set limits as needed.	Establishing a regular sleep pattern helps client become rested, reducing fatigue, and may improve ability to think. When client is able to think more clearly, participation in treatment program may be enhanced.

NURSING DIAGNOSIS	**VIOLENCE, risk for directed at self/others**
Risk Factors May Include:	Disintegrated thought processes stemming from ambivalence and autistic thinking, hallucinations, delusions

[Possible Indicators:]	Lack of development of trust and appropriate interpersonal relationships
	Disintegrated behaviors
	Perception of environmental and other stimuli/cues as threatening
	Physical aggression to self; irrational, threatening, or assaultive behavior
	Religiosity
Desired Outcomes/Evaluation Criteria— Client Will:	Demonstrate self-control, as evidenced by relaxed posture, nonviolent behavior.
	Resolve conflicts and/or cope with anxiety without the use of threats or assaultive behavior (to self or others).
	Participate in care and meet own needs in an assertive manner.

ACTIONS/INTERVENTIONS	RATIONALE

Independent

Assess the presence/degree of client's potential for violence (toward self or others) on a 1–10 scale. Determine suicidal/homicidal intent, indications of loss of control over behavior (actual or perceived), hostile verbal/nonverbal behaviors, risk factors, and prior/present coping skills.	Information essential for planning nursing care and documents degree of intent (may be no. 1 nursing priority if score is high). Prior history of violent behavior increases risk for violence, as would factors such as command hallucinations.
Provide safe, quiet environment; tell client "you are safe."	Keeping environmental stimuli to a minimum and providing reassurance will help prevent agitation.
Be careful in offering a pat on the shoulder/hug, etc.	Touch may be misinterpreted as an aggressive gesture.
Encourage verbalizations of feelings and promote acceptable verbal outlet(s) for expression, e.g., yelling in room, pounding pillows.	Ventilation of feelings may reduce need for inappropriate physical action.
Assist client to identify situations that trigger anxiety/aggressive behaviors.	Promotes understanding of relationship between severe anxiety and situations that result in destructive feelings leading to aggressive actions.
Explore implications and consequences of handling these situations with aggression.	Helps client realize the possibility and importance of thinking through a situation before acting.
Help client define alternatives to aggressive behaviors. Initially engage in solitary physical activities, instead of group. Monitor competitive activities; use with caution.	Enables client to learn to handle situations in a socially acceptable manner. Appropriate outlets will allow for release of hostility. Anxiety and fear may escalate during activities in which the client perceives self in competition with others and can trigger violent behavior.
Set limits, stating in a clear, specific, firm manner what is acceptable/unacceptable. Use demands only when situation requires.	Being clear and remaining calm increase chance that client will cooperate, lessening potential for violence. Having few but important limits enhances chances of having them observed.

237

Be alert to signs of impending violent behavior: increase in psychomotor activity; intensity of affect; verbalization of delusional thinking, especially threatening expressions; frightening hallucinations.

Promotes timely interventions as therapeutic techniques are more effective before behavior becomes violent.

Accept verbal hostility without retaliation or defense. Be aware of own response to client behavior (e.g., anger/fear).

Behavior is not usually directed at nurse personally, and responding defensively will tend to exacerbate situations. Looking at meaning behind the words will be more productive. Awareness of own response allows nurse to express/deal with those feelings.

Isolate promptly in nonpunitive manner, using adequate help if violent behavior occurs. Hold client. Tell client to STOP behavior.

Removal to quiet environment reduces stimulation, can help calm client. Usually the individual is being self-critical and afraid of own hostility and does not need external criticism. Sufficient help will prevent injury to client/staff. Often holding client and/or saying "Stop" is enough to help client regain control.

Collaborative

Place in seclusion, and/or apply restraints as indicated, documenting reasons for action.

May be needed for short-term control until client regains control over self.

Administer medications as indicated. (Refer to ND: Thought Processes, altered.)

Used to reduce psychotic symptoms, decrease delusional thinking, and assist client to regain control of self.

NURSING DIAGNOSIS	SELF CARE deficit (specify)
May Be Related to:	Perceptual and cognitive impairment
	Immobility resulting from social withdrawal, isolation, and decreased psychomotor activity
	Autonomic nervous system side effects of psychotropic medications
Possibly Evidenced by:	Inability/difficulty feeding self, keeping body clean, dressing appropriately, and/or toileting self
	Bladder stasis/paralysis; urinary calculi formation
	Decreased bowel activity with constipation, fecal impaction, and/or paralytic ileus
Desired Outcomes/Evaluation Criteria— Client Will:	Perform self-care and ADLs at highest level of adaptive functioning possible.
	Recognize cues/maintain elimination patterns, preventing complications.
	Identify/use resources available for assistance.

ACTIONS/INTERVENTIONS

RATIONALE

Independent

Determine current vs. preillness level of self-care (specify levels 0–4) for feeding, bathing/hygiene, dressing/grooming, toileting.

Identifies potentials and determines degree of nursing care to be provided.

Assess presence/severity of factors that affect client's capacity for self-care (e.g., disintegrative perceptual/cognitive abilities, mobility status).

Impairment in these areas can alter client's ability/readiness for self-care.

Discuss personal appearance/grooming and encourage dressing in bright colors, attractive clothes. Give positive feedback for efforts.

Appearance affects how the client sees self. A run-down, disheveled appearance conveys a sense of low self-worth, whereas an attractive, well-put-together appearance conveys a positive sense of self to the client as well as to others.

Determine client's regular elimination patterns and compare with current pattern. Monitor oral intake. Note contributing factors (e.g., anxiety, decreased attention span, disorientation, reduced psychomotor activity, as well as use of psychotropic medications).

Identifies appropriate interventions, as patterns of elimination are individually influenced by physiological (including amount of intake), cultural, and psychological factors. These factors can affect toileting (e.g., client does not pay attention to cues; dehydration from inadequate intake results in lessened urinary output and contributes to constipation; anticholinergic effect of medication may result in urinary retention).

Encourage/provide diet high in fiber and at least 2 liters of fluid each day. Encourage/structure appropriate times for intake. (Refer to ND: Nutrition, altered, less/more than body requirements.)

A diet high in fiber and residue promotes bulk formation and at least 2 liters of fluid daily regulates stool consistency (facilitating bowel elimination) and renal function. Scheduling of intake provides for an accurate record and helps to ensure that adequate amounts are ingested.

Monitor mental status, vital signs, weight, skin turgor; presence of medication interactions/side effects.

Careful monitoring and early recognition of symptoms can prevent complications of inadequate fluid intake (e.g., orthostatic hypotension, reduced circulating volume which directly affects cerebral perfusion/mentation, increased risk of tissue breakdown).

Observe/record urinary output as appropriate. Note changes in color, odor, clarity. Encourage client to observe/report changes.

Bladder paralysis/retention can occur from psychotropic medications, increasing risk of infection. **Note:** Polyuria is a frequent side effect of psychotropics.

Provide regular intervals for toileting.

A schedule prevents accidents that can occur due to polyuria from psychotropic medication or decreased attentiveness to cues and psychomotor activity.

Increase daily activity level as client progresses.

Adequate exercise increases muscle tone; consistency in daily routine stimulates bowel elimination.

Collaborative

Plan with client for effective use of community resources, such as nutritional programs, sheltered workshops, group/transitional/apartment homes, home care services.

Assists client to develop an effective plan for hygienic/self-care needs and promotes maximum level of independence.

Administer laxatives/stool softeners, as indicated.

Used cautiously for brief period or as needed to enhance bowel function. **Note:** Overuse can promote dependency.

239

NURSING DIAGNOSIS	NUTRITION: altered, less/more than body requirements
May Be Related to:	Imbalance between energy needs and intake
	Disintegration of thought and perception
	Inability/refusal to eat
Possibly Evidenced by:	Delusions or hallucinations related to food intake
	Reported dysfunctional eating patterns (e.g., eating in response to internal cues other than hunger; increased appetite [side effect of some psychotropic medications])
	Weight loss/gain
	Sore, inflamed buccal cavity
Desired Outcomes/Evaluation Criteria—Client Will:	Maintain adequate/appropriate nutritional intake.
	Demonstrate progressive weight gain/loss toward agreed-upon goal.
	Identify behaviors/lifestyle changes to maintain appropriate weight.

ACTIONS/INTERVENTIONS	RATIONALE

Independent

ACTIONS/INTERVENTIONS	RATIONALE
Assess presence/severity of factors that create altered nutritional intake.	Factors such as psychotic thinking or excessive activity to prevent frightening thoughts may cause inability/refusal to eat.
Review dietary intake via 24-hour recall/diary noting eating pattern and activity level.	Provides accurate information for assessment of client's nutritional status and needs. Alterations in dietary intake (decreased/increased calories, salt, fats, sugars) can aid in correcting faulty eating patterns. Lack of knowledge of appropriate dietary needs, perception of food, and activity/exercise (immobility) results in improper caloric intake.
Encourage client to regulate caloric intake with activity/exercise program.	A balance between activity and caloric intake maintains weight loss/gain, improves nutritional status, and can enhance mental functioning.
Structure consistent times for eating and limit use of food for other than nutritional needs.	Positively reinforces client's appropriate eating behaviors. Limits behaviors (rituals, acting out) that allow client to withdraw/refuse meals or overeat. Secondary gains that may occur can be reduced by setting appropriate expectations.
Provide small, frequent feedings as indicated.	May enhance intake when psychotic thought/behavior interferes with eating.
Encourage client to choose own foods, when possible.	Individual is more likely to eat chosen food than what has been arbitrarily given to him or her, especially when paranoid thoughts of poisoning are present.

Assess presence/severity of factors that affect client's oral mucous membranes. Identify strategies to relieve to minimize irritation, such as rinsing with water, chewing sugarless gum/candy or glycerin-based cough drops, drinking lemonade, and mouth care before and after meals.

Altered nutrition can cause dehydration, edema, oral lesions, or altered salivation, which can adversely affect/restrict intake. With relief of dry mouth, client's anxiety is reduced and nutritional intake enhanced.

Collaborative

Arrange consultation with dietitian/nutritional team, as indicated.

May be necessary to establish/meet individual dietary needs.

NURSING DIAGNOSIS	FAMILY PROCESSES, altered/FAMILY COPING, ineffective: disabling
May Be Related to:	Ambivalent family system/relationships; change of roles
	Difficulty family members have in coping effectively with client's maladaptive behaviors
Possibly Evidenced by:	Deterioration in family functioning; ineffective family decision-making process
	Failure to adapt to change/deal with crisis in a constructive manner and meet needs of its members
	Difficulty in relating to each other for mutual growth/development; failure to send/receive clear messages.
	Extreme distortion regarding client's health problem, including extreme denial about its existence/severity or prolonged overconcern
	Client's expressions of despair at family's lack of reaction/involvement; neglectful relationships with client
Desired Outcomes/Evaluation Criteria— Family Will:	Express feelings appropriately, honestly, and openly.
	Demonstrate improvement in communications (clear), problem-solving, behavior control, and affective spheres of family functioning.
	Verbalize realistic perception of roles within limits of individual situation.
	Encourage and allow member who is ill to handle situation in own way.

ACTIONS/INTERVENTIONS	RATIONALE

Independent

Determine current and preillness level of family functioning. Note factors such as problem-solving

Provides information about client and family to assist in developing plan of care and choosing

skills, level of this interpersonal relationships, outside support systems, roles, boundaries, rules, and communications.

interventions. These factors affect the family's capacity for returning to precrisis level of adaptive functioning as well as set the tone/expectations for a favorable prognosis. **Note:** Some family members may demonstrate psychopathologies that may make their influence detrimental to the client.

Determine whether family is high in expressed emotion (e.g., criticism, disappointment, hostility, solicitude, extreme worry, overprotectiveness, or emotional over-involvement).

The emotional climate of the client's family has been shown to significantly affect the client's recovery. Relapse is associated with the expression of certain feelings in specific ways rather than emotional openness itself. Relapse occurs significantly more often in families with a high degree of expressed emotion (EE), especially criticism and hostility. **Note:** Some studies suggest EE may be more a response to the client's bizarre behavior, rather than a family trait, and may lessen as the condition persists and the family becomes used to the symptoms.

Provide opportunity for family members to discuss feelings, impact of disorder on family, and individual concerns.

Feelings of guilt, shame, isolation; loss of hopes/expectations regarding client; and concerns for personal and client safety have an impact on family's ability to manage crisis and support client. Chronic nature of condition, with a wide range of socially, emotionally, and intellectually disabling symptoms that come and go unpredictably, can exhaust family physically, emotionally, and financially. The disproportionate allocation of resources can create deep feelings of resentment and family conflict as time and energy are focused on the client to the possible exclusion of the needs of other family members, and monetary expenses may restrict the family members' ability to take vacations, go to college, or even consider retirement.

Assess readiness of family members/significant other(s) to participate in client's treatment.

Family theorists believe that the "identified patient" also represents disintegrated/enmeshed schizophrenogenic family system. Aftercare of client must include family/SO(s) to raise level of interpersonal functioning.

Provide honest information about the nature and seriousness of the disorder and enlist cooperation of family members to help client to remain in the community.

The family that already has maladaptive coping skills may have difficulty dealing with diagnosis and implications of a long-term illness. Client's behavior may be difficult and embarrassing for some families who have problematic coping skills or have a high profile in the community.

Promote family involvement with nurses/others to plan care and activities.

Involvement with others provides a role model for individuals to learn new behaviors/ways of handling stress, and problem-solving.

Help client/family/SO(s) to identify maladaptive behaviors and consequences. Support efforts for change.

Client's success in treatment depends on effective change of whole systems rather than treatment of client's behaviors as a separate entity.

Establish/encourage ongoing open communication within the family.

Promotes healthy interaction, allows for timely problem-solving, and maintains effective relationships.

Help family identify potential for growth of family system and individual members. Role-model positive behaviors during this process.

Family that has previously functioned well has skills to build on and can learn new ways of dealing with changed family structure and challenges of marginally functioning family member. The nurse can provide an example for learning new skills.

Assess readiness of the family/SO(s) to reintegrate client into system, such as family's ability to use assistance or to cope with crisis appropriately by adaptation or change.

Ability to tolerate and assist with management of client behavior affects client's reentry into the family system.

Collaborative

Promote family involvement in behavioral management programs. Discuss negative aspects of blame and ways to avoid its use.

Helps family members to realize that, although they can have a positive or negative influence on the course of the illness, they are doing the best they can in a difficult situation, and communication/problem-solving skills can be learned to reduce stress. Blaming themselves or the client is counterproductive, and it is more important to talk about individual responsibility.

Encourage family to participate in family education, therapy, community support groups.

Multiple stressors, labile nature of disorder, lack of definitive treatment options, or lack of resolution of condition increases likelihood of family conflict, disorganization, and even dissolution. Providing the family with information about the disorder; showing them how to help the client, without neglecting family members' needs; and better ways to communicate with one another and with the client; as well as training family to identify and solve problems as they arise—enhances family's coping abilities and may lessen the client's risk of relapse.

Promote involvement with mental health treatment team (e.g., mental health center, family physician/psychiatrist, psychiatric/public health nurse, social/vocational services, occupational/physical therapist), and respite care, when necessary.

When bizarre behavior is difficult for family to manage, assistance/support may enhance coping abilities, improve the situation, and provide opportunity for individual growth, thereby strengthening the family unit. Having the opportunity to take time away from the situation enhances the family's ability to manage the client's long-term illness.

Provide client/family/SO(s) with assistance to deal with current life situation (e.g., therapy [family/couples/1:1]; aftercare services including day-care centers, night hospitals, halfway houses, sheltered workshops, rehabilitation services).

Aftercare may include efforts to enlarge social spheres and increase client's/family's level of functioning, enhancing ability to manage long-term illness and enabling the client to remain in the community.

NURSING DIAGNOSIS	HEALTH MAINTENANCE altered/HOME MAINTENANCE MANAGEMENT, impaired
May Be Related to:	Impaired perception, cognition, communication skills, and individual coping skills
	Inadequate developmental task accomplishment; lack of knowledge
	Inability or lack of cooperation
	Lower socioeconomic group with limited resources
	Impaired or diminished family functioning
Possibly Evidenced by:	Mistrust, lack of autonomy, and disturbed capacity for relationship formation
	Impairment of personal support system (e.g., family conflict/disorganization)
	Decreased capacity to identify and mobilize adequate support systems and maintain a safe, growth-promoting immediate environment
Desired Outcomes/Evaluation Criteria— Client Will:	Maintain optimal health and family functioning through improved communications and coping skills.
	Return home and maintain optimal wellness with minimal complications.
	Identify and use resources effectively.

ACTIONS/INTERVENTIONS	RATIONALE
Independent	
Compare present and preillness level of home/ health maintenance. Consider deficits in communication, knowledge, decision-making, developmental tasks, and support systems and their effect on client's basic health practices.	Dysfunction in family (diminished problem-solving, poor financial management/inadequate resources, and ineffective support system; emotional impoverishment) and lack of motivation to participate in treatment can impair functioning.
Assist client/family to identify appropriate healthcare needs/practices (e.g., dental, physician/clinic, regular hygiene practices, as well as some social contacts).	Poor organizational capacity for ADLs and socialization as well as personal involvement can lead to neglect of these areas and provides opportunity for nurse to assess capacity for/compliance with home/health management needs.
Involve client/SO(s) in the development of a long-term plan for optimal home health management, encouraging identification/use of resources.	Involvement increases the potential for cooperation with the plan.
Collaborative	
Provide referrals to community resources (e.g., medical/dental clinics, transportation	Ineffective coping requires support/ teaching, which often necessitates referrals.

assistance, sheltered living center, legal services).

Legal assistance may be required to provide conservatorships and client advocacy.

NURSING DIAGNOSIS	SEXUAL dysfunction
May Be Related to:	Ego boundary disintegration; inability to distinguish between self and environment
	Weakened sexual identification; gender identity confusion, which interferes with normal sexual orientation formation
	Development of delusions around the primitive sexual orientation
	Lack of drive and energy, normal social inhibitions, and passivity
Possibly Evidenced by:	Uninhibited sexual behavior; involvement in multiple sexual liaisons
	Preoccupation with sex or gender identity
	Inability to find sexual partner
	Endocrine changes associated with antipsychotic drugs (e.g., ejaculatory inhibitions, impotence in men/amenorrhea in women, decreased libido)
Desired Outcomes/Evaluation Criteria— Client Will:	Strengthen ego boundaries to enable identification and acceptance of sexual orientation.
	Verbalize understanding of, identify, and report changes in body functions (if they occur) while taking antipsychotic medications.
	Demonstrate behavioral restraint in public.
	Identify and use individually effective birth control method.
	Practice safer sex.

ACTIONS/INTERVENTIONS

RATIONALE

Independent

Have client describe own perceptions of sexuality/ sexual functioning.

When concerns and perceptions are shared, it provides an opportunity to understand the client's point of view, identify individual needs, and clarify misconceptions.

Determine presence/degree of factors that alter sexuality/sexual functioning.

Ego boundary disintegration can cause regressive behavior (withdrawal, preoccupation with self), which interferes with the formation of attachments and creates gender identity confusion. Antipsychotic medications can cause endocrine changes (amenorrhea, lactation in women; and impotence, ejaculatory inhibition, gynecomastia in men).

245

Provide information regarding medications, their effects and regulation, and counseling/teaching about problem-solving (expressing feelings of loss and seeking alternate solutions).

Lack of sufficient knowledge may be a contributing factor to the dysfunction.

Encourage client to identify/report any alterations in sexuality/sexual functioning.

Timely intervention may prevent future disintegration of ego boundaries and further side effects of medications.

Counsel client about birth control, genetic implications of having children.

Severely ill clients have difficulty with relationships and do not make good partners or parents. Although higher-functioning clients may find marriage supportive, they need to be aware that each child has a 12%–15% chance of developing schizophrenia. Premarital expert eugenic counseling is extremely important.

Identify "safer sex" practices and discuss risk of contracting sexually transmitted diseases (STDs).

The lack of social inhibitions (multiple partners, unprotected sex) places these clients at risk for the possibility of contracting a sexually transmitted disease, and a poor level of functioning may result in neglect of treatment.

NURSING DIAGNOSIS	KNOWLEDGE deficit [LEARNING NEED] regarding condition, prognosis, and treatment needs/THERAPEUTIC REGIMEN: Individual, ineffective management of
May Be Related to:	Cognitive limitation (altered thought process/psychosis)
	Misinterpretation/inaccurate information; unfamiliarity with information resources
	Chronic nature of the disorder
Possibly Evidenced by:	Ambivalence and dependency strivings
	Inappropriate or exaggerated behaviors; need-fear dilemma and withdrawal (can lead to abrupt termination of therapy, medication)
	Inaccurate follow-through of instructions; appearance of side effects of psychotropic medications
	Recidivism
Desired Outcomes/Evaluation Criteria— Client/SO(s) Will:	Verbalize understanding of disorder and treatment.
	Participate in learning process/treatment regimen.
	Assume responsibility for own learning within individual abilities.

ACTIONS/INTERVENTIONS

RATIONALE

Independent

Determine the current level of knowledge about the disorder and its management.

Identifies areas of need and misperceptions. Communication skills such as validation of

Assess the presence/severity of factors that affect client's cognitive framework for decision-making about disorder and management, noting lack of recall, and ignorance of resources and their use.

perceptions can assist in assessment of accuracy of client's/SO(s) knowledge base and readiness to learn.

Factors such as disintegrated thinking, cognitive deficits, ambivalence, denial, and dependency needs can limit learning/block use of knowledge for management of disorder.

Instruct client/family about disorder, its signs and symptoms, management (medication, ADLs, vocational rehabilitation, socialization needs).

Provides information and can promote independent behaviors within client's ability.

Identify/review side effects of medications client is taking (e.g., sedation, postural hypotension, photosensitivity, hormonal effects, agranulocytosis, and extrapyramidal symptoms [tremors, akinesia/akathisia, dystonia, oculogyric crisis, and tardive dyskinesia]).

The anticholinergic effects of psychotropics (and antiparkinsonian drugs that may be given concomitantly to decrease the incidence of extrapyramidal effects of neuroleptics) alter autonomic nervous system functioning and may cause dry mouth (xerostomia), oral lesions, or hemorrhagic gingivitis. Most side effects occur within the first few weeks of treatment and subside with time. However, signs indicative of adverse reactions such as agranulocytosis (sore throat, fever, malaise), extrapyramidal symptoms, and tardive dyskinesia need immediate attention.

Encourage measures such as frequent mouth care, chewing sugarless gum or sucking on hard (sugarless) candy, and drinking lemonade.

Reduces oval cavity discomfort associated with effects of medication. **Note:** Omit gum/hard candy for aged client when danger of choking is present (e.g., phenothiazines alter the swallowing reflex).

Emphasize importance of immediate medical attention for onset of high fever and severe muscle stiffness and discontinuation of the medication until able to consult with healthcare provider.

Severe muscle stiffness and high fever are the hallmarks of neuroleptic malignant syndrome, which can usually be effectively treated before it becomes life threatening if it is detected early.

Have individuals verbalize/paraphrase knowledge gained.

Evaluates comprehension of information regarding disorder's characteristics and management needs and may reduce recidivism.

Assist the client to develop strategies for continuing treatment. Make contract with client to provide for actions to take when problems arise.

Understanding that feeling better is no indication for discontinuing medication, that no addiction can develop with continued treatment, and that providing for self-administration often enhances cooperation with therapeutic regimen.

Discuss importance of, and establish schedule for, follow-up/postdischarge care.

Monitoring of client's behavior (e.g., medication usage, socialization, vocation, exercise, and diet) helps to determine appropriateness of therapy, problem-solve identified needs, reduce risk of recidivism.

Identify appropriate therapies and community support systems to meet individual needs.

Promotes trusting relationships and encourages further cooperation with treatment plan. Adequate management plans and organizing social supports for the family enable these clients to remain in the community.

SAMPLE CLINICAL PATHWAY:
Client with Schizophrenic Psychosis ELOS: 14-day Residential Program

ND and categories of care	Time dimension	Outcomes/ actions	Time dimension	Outcomes/ actions	Time dimension	Outcomes/ actions
Altered Thought Processes; Sensory/perceptual alteration R/T disintegration of thinking processes and ego boundaries, psychological conflicts, anxiety (panic); disturbance in perception, affect	Day 3	Involved with primary therapist/staff member in a 1:1 relationship	Day 5

Day 7 | Acknowledge/recognize changes in thinking behavior

Demonstrate improved cognitive, perceptual, affective, and psychomotor abilities | Day 10

Day 14 | Identify self in relationship to environment

Verbalize understanding of therapeutic regimen and treatment needs |
Referrals	Day 1	Psychiatrist Primary therapist (Psychologist, Clinical nurse specialist)	Day 3	Music therapist Occupational therapist Recreational therapist	Day 14	Outpatient/ community program
Diagnostic studies	Day 1 Day 2	Drug screen Neuropsyche evaluation	Day 3–5	Scans: CT, MRI, PET, EEG (These may be ordered to examine structure and function of the brain.)		
Additional assessments	Day 1 Day 1–14	VS every shift Access for: Delusions, hallucinations, loose associations, inappropriate affect, excitement/stupor, panic anxiety, suspiciousness Effectiveness/side effects of medications	Day 2–14 Day 3–10	VS daily if stable Monitor sleep/ rest pattern, graph as indicated		

Category	Day	Action/Intervention	Day		Day	Outcome
Medications	Day 1–14	Antipsychotic medication scheduled and PRN (may need order for concentrate/injectable form); Antiparkinson medication PRN				
Action/therapies	Day 1–14	Orient to/reinforce reality; Engage in cognitive therapy	Day 5–14	Structure therapeutic communications reflecting client's background	Day 9–14	Identify ways to de-escalate anxiety
	Day 7–14	Set limits on behavior/response to altered thinking; Adjust activity patterns, allow time for rest/sleep and presleep routine	Day 7–14	Discuss correlation between increased anxiety and psychotic symptoms	Day 12–14	Discuss importance of taking medications regularly, even when feeling well; Review possible side effects of medications and when to see the doctor
	Day 2–5	Develop trust relationship			Day 14	Schedule followup appointments
Risk for Violence: self-directed or directed at others R/T disintegrated thought processes (hallucinations, delusions), lack of trust and appropriate interpersonal relationships	Day 1–14	Be free of harm (self or others)	Day 7	Identify precipitating factors of increasing anxiety/aggressive behavior	Day 10–14	Demonstrate self-control through relaxed posture and nonviolent behavior
	Day 5	Acknowledge realities of situation				
Referrals	Day 1	Hostility Management Team	Day 4–14	Need for unit restrictions		

Client with Schizophrenic Psychosis ELOS: 14-day Residential Program (continued)

ND and categories of care	Time dimension	Outcomes/actions	Time dimension	Outcomes/actions	Time dimension	Outcomes/actions
Additional assessments	Day 1–14	Assess for signs of impending violent behavior: increase in psychomotor activity; angry effect; verbalized persecutory delusions or frightening hallucinations Effectiveness of seclusion/restraint				
Medications	Day 1–14	PRN antipsychotic medications when signs of agitation begin				
Actions/therapies	Day 1–3	Restrict to unit; limit environmental stimuli	Day 3–8	Explore implications/consequences of aggression	Day 9–14	Define alternative to aggressive behaviors
	Day 1–14	Set clear/specific limits on behavior Provide seclusion/restrain (chemical or mechanical) as indicated		Relaxation therapy: music group, stress management, exercise program		
Self Care deficit/Health Maintenance Management R/T perceptual and cognitive impairment, inability or lack of cooperation (withdrawal/isolation)	Day 1–14	Accomplish basic needs with assistance of staff	Day 5–8	Perform ADLs within physical limitations within minimal prompts	Day 12–14	Identify and access appropriate resources
			Day 9–14	Take responsibility for self/needs	Day 14	Plan in place to meet needs postdischarge

Referrals	Dietitian	Day 1 and PRN	Dental (as indicated)	Day 5	Community Mental Health/Maintenance Group	Day 12
Diagnostic studies						
Additional assessments	Nutritional screen	Day 1	Individual support/resources (family, community)	Day 5	Appropriateness of postdischarge placement	Day 11
	Functional level, individual needs	Day 1/ongoing	Nutritional status; Bowel/bladder function (including I/O as indicated)	Day 7–8		
			Financial resources			
Medications	Laxative/stool softeners PRN	Day 2–6				
	Vitamins and nutritional supplements as indicated	Day 2–14				
Assessments	Perform/assist with ADLs	Day 1–4	Perform/assist with ADLs	Day 5–8	Provide prompts for ADLs; Review individual healthcare needs/wellness activities	Day 10–12
	Provide nutritional diet to meet individual health needs; Encourage health-promoting activities: e.g., oral care, adequate intake of food/fluid	Day 1–14	Provide nutritional diet to meet individual health needs	Day 8–14	Review community resources: Clinics/Providers, Transportation, Sheltered living, Financial/legal services	
					Schedule followup evaluations/appointments as indicated	Day 12–14

Adapted from Townsend, MC: Psychiatric Mental Health Nursing, ed 2. FA Davis, Philadelphia, 1996.

SCHIZOAFFECTIVE DISORDER

DSM-IV
295.70 Schizoaffective disorder

This disorder emphasizes the temporal relationship of schizophrenic and mood symptoms and is used for conditions that meet the criteria for both schizophrenia and a mood disorder with psychotic symptoms lasting a minimum of 1 month. The clinical features must occur within a single uninterrupted period of illness (for some, this may be years or even decades) that is judged to last until the individual is completely recovered for a significant period of time, free of any significant symptoms of the disorder. In comparison with schizophrenia, schizoaffective disorder occurs more commonly in women than in men.

ETIOLOGICAL THEORIES

Psychodynamics

Refer to CPs: Schizophrenia, Major Depression, and Bipolar Disorder.

Biological

Refer to CPs: Schizophrenia, Major Depression, and Bipolar Disorder.

Recent studies suggest that schizoaffective disorder is a distinct syndrome resulting from a high genetic liability to both mood disorders and schizophrenia.

Family Dynamics

Refer to CPs: Schizophrenia, Major Depression, and Bipolar Disorder.

CLIENT ASSESSMENT DATA BASE

Neurosensory

Depressed mood (at least 2 wks); manic or mixed mood (at least 1 wk)
Pronounced manic and depressive features intermingled with schizophrenic features
Delusions and hallucinations for at least 2 wks (in absence of prominent mood symptoms)
Difficulty following a moving object with the eyes

Teaching/Learning

May report previous episode(s) and remission free of significant symptoms; usually begins
    in early adulthood (generally earlier than mood disorders)
Absence of substance use or general medical conditions that could account for symptoms

DIAGNOSTIC STUDIES

Refer to CPs: Schizophrenia, Major Depression, and Bipolar Disorder.

NURSING PRIORITIES

1. Provide protective environment; prevent injury.
2. Assist with self-care.
3. Promote interaction with others.
4. Identify resources available for assistance.
5. Support family involvement in therapy.

DISCHARGE GOALS

1. Signs of physical agitation are abating and no physical injury occurs.
2. Improved sense of self-esteem, lessened depression, and elevated mood are noted.
3. Approaches and socializes appropriately with others, individually and in group activities.
4. Adequate nutritional intake is achieved/maintained.
5. Client/family displays effective coping skills and appropriate use of resources.
6. Plan in place to meet needs after discharge.

(Refer to CPs: Schizophrenia, Major Depression, and Bipolar Disorder for other NDs that apply, in addition to the following.)

NURSING DIAGNOSIS	VIOLENCE, risk for, directed at self/others
Risk Factors May Include:	Depressed mood; feelings of worthlessness; hopelessness
	Unsatisfactory parent/child relationship; feelings of abandonment by significant other(s)
	Anger turned inward/directed at the environment
	Punitive superego and irrational feelings of guilt
	Numerous failures (learned helplessness)
	Misinterpretation of reality
	Extreme hyperactivity
[Possible Indicators:]	History of previous suicide attempts; making direct/indirect statements indicating a desire to kill self/having a plan
	Hallucinations; delusional thinking
	Self-destructive behavior (hitting body parts against wall/furniture); destruction of inanimate objects
	Temper tantrums/aggressive behavior; increased agitation and lack of control over purposeless movements
	Vulnerable self-esteem
Desired Outcomes/Evaluation Criteria— Client Will:	Express improved sense of well-being/self-concept.
	Manage behavior and deal with anger appropriately.
	Demonstrate self-control without harm to self or others.

ACTIONS/INTERVENTIONS	RATIONALE
Independent	
Note direct statements of a desire to kill self; also note indirect actions indicating suicidal wish, (e.g., putting affairs in order, writing a will, giving	Direct and indirect indicators of suicidal intent need to be attended to and addressed as being potentially acted on.

253

away prized possessions; presence of hallucinations and delusional thinking; history of previous suicidal behavior/acts; statements of hopelessness regarding life situation).

Ask client directly if suicide has been considered/planned and if the means are available to carry out the plan.

The risk of suicide is greatly increased if the client has developed a plan, and particularly if means exist to execute the plan.

Provide a safe environment for client by removing potentially harmful objects from access (e.g., sharp objects; straps, belts, ties; glass items; smoking materials).

Provides protection while treatment is being undertaken to deal with existing situation. Client's rationality is impaired, she or he may harm self inadvertently.

Assign to quiet unit, if possible.

Unit milieu may be too distracting, increasing agitation and potential for loss of control.

Reduce environmental stimuli (e.g., private room, soft lighting, low noise level, and simple room decor).

In hyperactive state, client is extremely distractible, and responses to even the slightest stimuli are exaggerated.

Stay with the client/request client remain in staff view. Provide supervision as necessary.

Provides support and feelings of security as agitation grows and hyperactivity increases.

Formulate a short-term verbal contract with the client stating that he or she will not harm self during specified period of time. Renegotiate contract as necessary.

An attitude of acceptance of the client as a worthwhile individual is conveyed. Discussion of suicidal feelings with a trusted individual provides a degree of relief to the client. A contract gets the subject out in the open and places some of the responsibility for own safety on the client.

Ask client to agree to seek out staff member/friend if thoughts of suicide emerge.

The suicidal client is often very ambivalent about own feelings. Discussion of these feelings with a trusted individual may provide assistance before the client experiences a crisis situation.

Encourage verbalization of honest feelings. Explore and discuss symbols of hope client can identify in own life.

Because of elevated anxiety, client may need assistance to recognize presence of hope in life situations.

Promote expression of angry feelings within appropriate limits. Provide safe method(s) of hostility release. Help client identify true source of anger, and work on adaptive coping skills for continued use.

Depression and suicidal behaviors may be viewed as anger turned inward on the self, or anger may be expressed as hostile acting-out toward others. If this anger can be verbalized and/or released in a nonthreatening environment, the client may be able to resolve these feelings, regardless of the discomfort involved.

Orient client to reality, as required. Point out sensory/environmental misperceptions, taking care not to belittle client's fears or indicate disapproval of verbal expressions.

Elevated level of anxiety may contribute to distortions in reality. Client may need help distinguishing between reality and misperceptions of the environment.

Spend time with the client on a regular schedule and provide frequent intermittent checks as indicated in response to client needs.

Provides a feeling of safety and security, while also conveying the message, "I want to spend time with you because I think you are a worthwhile person."

Provide structured schedule of activities that includes established rest periods throughout the day.

Structured schedule provides feeling of security for the client. Additional rest promotes relaxation for the agitated client.

Provide physical activities as a substitute for purposeless hyperactivity (e.g., brisk walks, housekeeping chores, dance therapy, aerobics).

Physical exercise provides a safe and effective means of relieving pent-up tension.

Observe for effectiveness and evidence of adverse side effects of drug therapy (e.g., anticholinergic [dry mouth, blurred vision], extrapyramidal [tremors, rigidity, restlessness, weakness, facial spasms]).

Individual reactions to medications may vary, and early identification can assist with changes in dosage and/or drug choice, possibly preventing client from discontinuing drug therapy prematurely with potential loss of control.

Collaborative

Administer medication, as indicated:
    Neuroleptics, e.g., chlorpromazine (Thorazine);

Pharmacological interventions need to be directed at the presenting symptoms and used on a short-term basis. Antipsychotics may be effective in reducing the hyperactivity associated with mania. May be combined with lithium or antidepressants and then gradually withdrawn.

    Antidepressants, e.g., imipramine (Tofranil);

Allows the accumulation of the neurotransmitters norepinephrine and serotonin, potentiating their antidepressant effect. Useful after psychosis has cleared.

    Antimanics, e.g., lithium (Eskalith, Lithobid);

The exact mechanism of action of these drugs is unknown; however, they are thought to alter chemical transmitters in the CNS, reducing manic behavior.

    Antipsychotics, e.g.: clozapine (Clozaril), risperidone (Risperdal), olanzapine (Zyprexa).

Used for management of manifestations of psychosis. **Note:** Elderly clients tend to respond well to Risperdal.

Prepare for/assist with electroconvulsive therapy (ECT).

May be indicated to alter mood until neuroleptics or antidepressants become effective. **Note:** Some research suggests this is the most effective treatment for some clients.

Identify community resources including crisis center/hotline.

Support systems promote independence/provide help for dealing with suicidal thoughts/feelings. Having a concrete plan for seeking assistance during a crisis may discourage or prevent self-destructive behaviors.

NURSING DIAGNOSIS	SOCIAL ISOLATION
May Be Related to:	Developmental regression
	Depressed mood; feelings of worthlessness
	Egocentric behaviors (which offend others and discourage relationships)
	Delusional thinking
	Fear of failure
	Impaired cognition fostering negative view of self
	Unresolved grief

Possibly Evidenced by:	Sad, dull affect
	Absence of supportive significant other(s): family, friends, group
	Uncommunicative/withdrawn behavior; absence of eye contact; seeking to be alone
	Preoccupation with own thoughts; repetitive, meaningless actions
	Assuming fetal position; catatonic behaviors
Desired Outcomes/Evaluation Criteria— Client Will:	Verbalize willingness to be with others.
	Spend time voluntarily with others, seek out group activities.
	Develop 1:1 trust-based relationship.

ACTIONS/INTERVENTIONS

RATIONALE

Independent

ACTIONS/INTERVENTIONS	RATIONALE
Spend time with client. (This may mean sitting in silence for a while.)	Nurse's presence helps improve client's perception of self as a worthwhile person.
Develop a therapeutic nurse-client relationship through frequent, brief contacts and an accepting attitude. Show unconditional positive regard.	The nurse's presence, acceptance, and conveyance of positive regard enhance the client's feeling of self-worth and facilitate trust and interaction with others.
Encourage attendance in group activities, after client feels comfortable in the 1:1 relationship. Nurse may need to attend with client the first few times to offer support. Accept client's decision to remove self from group situation if anxiety becomes too great.	The presence of a trusted individual provides emotional security for the client. Moving slowly into a more threatening activity and accepting client's decision to leave promotes self-trust and sense of control.
Provide positive reinforcement for client's voluntary interactions with others.	Enhances self-esteem and encourages repetition of desirable behaviors.
Verbally acknowledge client's absence from any group activities.	Knowledge that absence was noticed may reinforce the client's feelings of importance and self-worth.
Assist client to learn assertiveness techniques.	Knowledge of the appropriate use of assertive techniques could improve client's relationships with others.
Devise a plan of therapeutic activities and provide client with a written time schedule.	The depressed client needs structure because of the impairment in decision-making/problem-solving ability. A structured schedule provides security until the client can function independently.
Help client learn skills that may be used to approach others in a socially acceptable manner. Practice these skills through role-play, beginning with simple assignments (e.g., introduce self in safe environment).	With practice, these skills become easier in real-life situations, and client feels more comfortable performing them.
Limit group activities, when client is agitated. Help client to establish 1 or 2 close relationships.	Client's ability to interact with others is impaired. More security is felt in a 1:1 relationship that is consistent over time.

256

NURSING DIAGNOSIS	**NUTRITION: altered, less than body requirements**
May Be Related to:	Energy expenditure in excess of calorie intake
	Refusal/inability to sit still long enough to eat meals
	Lack of attention to/recognition of hunger cues
Possibly Evidenced by:	Lack of interest in food; weight loss
	Pale conjunctiva and mucous membranes
	Poor muscle tone/skin turgor
	Amenorrhea
	Abnormal laboratory findings (e.g., anemias, electrolyte imbalances)
Desired Outcomes/Evaluation Criteria—Client Will:	Identify and formulate plan to meet individual dietary needs.
	Demonstrate adequate intake to maintain individual nutritional balance/provide desired weight gain.
	Display normalization of laboratory values and be free of signs of malnutrition.

ACTIONS/INTERVENTIONS	RATIONALE
Independent	
Determine individual daily caloric requirement, considering body structure, height, and activity and realistic weight gain.	Important for the provision of adequate nutrition.
Have juice and snacks available at all times.	Nutritious intake is required on a regular basis to compensate for increased caloric requirements caused by hyperactivity.
Provide high-protein, high-calorie, nutritious finger foods and drinks that can be consumed on the run.	Client may have difficulty sitting still long enough to eat a meal because of hyperactive state. It is more likely that the client will consume food and drinks that can be carried around and eaten with little effort.
Maintain accurate record of intake, output, and calorie count.	Necessary to make an accurate nutritional assessment, identify individual needs, and maintain client safety.
Recommend weighing on a regular schedule as individually appropriate.	Helpful in evaluating therapeutic needs and effectiveness of treatment plan.
Determine client's dietary likes and dislikes.	Client is more likely to eat foods that are particularly enjoyed.
Pace or walk with client as finger foods are taken. As agitation subsides, sit with client during meals. Offer support and encouragement.	Presence of a trusted individual may provide feeling of security and decrease agitation. Encouragement and positive reinforcement increase self-esteem and foster repetition of desired behaviors.

257

Help client learn the importance of adequate nutrition and fluid intake.

Client may have inadequate or inaccurate knowledge regarding the contribution of good nutrition to overall wellness.

Collaborative

Consult with dietitian as indicated.

Helpful in establishing individual needs/program and provides educational opportunity.

Administer vitamin and mineral supplements, as indicated.

To improve and/or restore nutritional well-being.

Monitor laboratory values and report status/significant nutritional changes.

Provides an objective assessment of therapeutic needs/effectiveness.

DELUSIONAL DISORDER

DSM-IV
297.1 Delusional disorder

SPECIFIC TYPE:

Erotomanic (delusions that another person of higher status is in love with the individual)
Grandiose (delusions of inflated worth, power, knowledge, identity, or special relationship
    to a deity or famous person)
Jealous (delusions that one's sexual partner is unfaithful)
Persecutory (delusions that one, or someone to whom one is close, is being malevolently
    treated in some way)
Somatic (delusions that one has some physical defect or general medical condition)
Mixed (delusions characteristic of more than one of the above types, but no one theme
    predominates)

ETIOLOGICAL THEORIES

Psychodynamics

Emotional development is delayed because of a lack of maternal stimulation/attention. The infant is deprived of a sense of security and fails to establish basic trust. A fragile ego results in severely impaired self-esteem, a sense of loss of control, fear, and severe anxiety. A suspicious attitude toward others is manifested and may continue throughout life. Projection is the most common mechanism used as a defense against feelings.

Biological

A relatively strong familial pattern of involvement appears to be associated with these disorders. Individuals whose family members manifest symptoms of these disorders are at greater risk for development than the general population. Twin studies have also suggested genetic involvement.

Family Dynamics

Some theorists believe that paranoid persons had parents who were distant, rigid, demanding, and perfectionistic, engendering rage, a sense of exaggerated self-importance, and mistrust in the individual. The clients become vulnerable as adults because of this early experience.

CLIENT ASSESSMENT DATA BASE

Refer to CP: Schizophrenia for physical symptoms.

Ego Integrity

May present with severe anxiety; inability to relax, exaggeration of difficulties, being easily
    agitated
Expresses feelings of inadequacy, worthlessness, lack of acceptance, and trust of others
Demonstrates difficulty in coping with stress, uses maladjusted coping mechanisms (e.g.,
    excessive use of projection and aggressive behavior, takes unnecessary precautions,
    avoids accepting blame)

Neurosensory

Nonbizarre delusional system of at least 1 month's duration
Experiencing emotions and behavior congruent with the content of belief system/fears that

259

either self or significant others are in danger, are being followed/conspired against, poisoned, infected; have a disease; are being deceived by one's spouse, cheated by others; are loving/being loved from a distance.
Exhibits controlled, cold, unemotional affect; guarded/evasive/distrustful behavior
Vigilant, looks for hidden motives; every person/event is under suspicion
Displays keen perception; will demonstrate impaired judgment about the perception
Delusions of reference or control that may incorporate the FBI, CIA, radio/TV
(Prominent auditory or visual hallucinations not usually present)

Safety

May display assaultive/violent behavior

Social Interactions

Significant impairment in social/marital functioning possibly noted; behavior in all other areas of life usually normal
Litigiousness common

Teaching/Learning

Onset most often in middle or late adult life
May have history of substance abuse/physical illness

DIAGNOSTIC STUDIES

Refer to CP: Schizophrenia.

NURSING PRIORITIES

1. Promote safe environment, safety of client/others.
2. Provide open, honest atmosphere in which client can begin to trust self/others.
3. Encourage client/family to focus on defining methods for coping with anxieties and life stressors.
4. Promote a sense of self-worth and increased self-esteem.

DISCHARGE GOALS

1. Copes with anxiety without the use of threats or assaultive behavior.
2. Recognizes reality; agrees to give up or live with the delusional system.
3. Client/family/SOs participate in therapy (e.g., behavioral, group).
4. Family/SO(s) provide emotional support for the client.
5. Plan in place to meet needs after discharge.

NURSING DIAGNOSIS	VIOLENCE, risk for, directed at self/others
Risk Factors May Include:	Perceived threats of danger
	Increased feelings of anxiety
[Possible Indicators:]	Acting out in an irrational manner
	Becoming threatening or assaultive in the face of perceived threat
Desired Outcomes/Evaluation Criteria—Client Will:	Verbalize awareness of delusional system.
	Resolve conflicts, coping with anxiety without the use of threats or assaultive behavior.

ACTIONS/INTERVENTIONS	RATIONALE

Independent

Note prior history of violent behavior when under stress.

Indicator of increased risk for recurrence of aggression/violent behavior.

Assist client to identify situations that trigger anxiety and aggressive behaviors.

Understanding relationship between severe anxiety and aggressive feelings can help client identify options to avoid violent behavior.

Explore implications and consequences of handling these situations with aggression.

Emphasizes importance of thinking through situations before acting.

Encourage to engage in solitary activity instead of group activities to being with.

Anxiety, fear, and suspiciousness may escalate if client is involved in competitive/group activities.

Be careful in offering a pat on the shoulder/hug, etc.

Gestures involving touch may be misinterpreted as aggressive by the suspicious person.

Assist client to define alternatives to aggressive behaviors. Engage in physical activities such as Ping-Pong, foosball. (Monitor competitive activities; use with caution.)

Enables client to learn to handle situations in a socially acceptable manner. Appropriate outlets will allow for release of hostility. **Note:** Competition can trigger violent behavior.

Encourage verbalizations of feelings and promote outlet for expression.

Ventilation of feelings reduces need for physical action.

Monitor level of anger (i.e., questioning, refusal, verbal release, intimidation, blow-up).

Helps determine seriousness of therapeutic need and affects choice of interventions.

Be alert to signs of impending violent behavior (e.g., increase in psychomotor activity, intensity of affect, verbalization of delusional thinking, especially threatening expressions).

Therapeutic interventions are more effective before behavior becomes violent.

Accept verbal hostility without retaliation or defense. Nurse (caregiver) needs to be aware of own response to client behavior (e.g., anger/fear).

Behavior is not usually directed at nurse personally, and responding defensively may exacerbate situation. Concentrating on meaning behind the words is more productive. Awareness of own response allows nurse to confront/deal with those feelings.

Institute de-escalation actions as indicated, e.g.:

Can prevent escalation of violent behaviors and potential injury to client/caregivers or bystanders. Reduces the possibility that client will feel confronted or blocked.

Distance self from client, at least 4 arm lengths, position self to one side; remain calm, stand or sit still, assume "open" posture with hands in sight;

Speak softly, call client by name, acknowledge client's feelings, express regret about situation, show empathy;

Communicates sense of respect, belief that individual can be trusted to control self, and that caregiver is available to assist client with resolution of situation. **Note:** Even though you are projecting an attitude of trust, it is important to expect the unexpected and be prepared.

Avoid pointing, touching, ordering, scolding, challenging, interrupting, arguing with, belittling, or intimidating client;

These actions may be viewed as threatening and may provoke client to violence.

Request permission to ask questions; try to discern triggering event and any underlying emotions, such as fear, anxiety, or humiliation; offering solutions/alternatives.

Involves client in problem-solving and gives client some control over situation.

Provide safe, quiet environment; tell client she or he is "safe."

Keeping environmental stimuli to a minimum will help reassure client and assist with prevention of agitation.

Isolate promptly in nonpunitive manner, using adequate help if violent behavior occurs. Hold client if necessary. Tell client to STOP behavior.

Removal to a quiet environment can help calm client. Sufficient help will prevent injury to client/staff. Usually the individual is being self-critical and afraid of hostility and does not need external criticisms. Saying "Stop" may be enough to allow client to regain control.

Collaborative

Administer medications, as indicated. (Refer to ND: Anxiety, severe.)

Antipsychotic/antianxiety drugs may decrease anxiety and delusional thinking, decreasing suspicious thoughts/aggressive behaviors and aiding client in maintaining control.

NURSING DIAGNOSIS	ANXIETY [severe]
May Be Related to:	Inability to trust (has not mastered tasks of trust vs. mistrust)
Possibly Evidenced by:	Rigid delusional system (provides relief from stress that justifies the delusion)
	Frightened of other people and own hostility
Desired Outcomes/Evaluation Criteria— Client Will:	Acknowledge delusion and deal with it appropriately.
	Define methods to decrease own anxiety level.
	Report anxiety is reduced to a manageable level.
	Demonstrate a relaxed manner.

ACTIONS/INTERVENTIONS	RATIONALE

Independent

Develop primary nurse/client relationship.

The continuity of a primary care relationship can provide the time necessary to form an alliance with the suspicious person.

Assist client to identify sources of anxiety and concerns.

Increases awareness of problems/contributing factors. Client needs to become aware of how behavior affects others and take responsibility for it.

Explore present patterns of coping with anxiety and how effective they have been (e.g., threatening harm and/or shouting at others, believing "they are out to get me/my family").

Increases awareness that aggressive acts may have destructive outcome.

Discuss alternatives to current ineffective behaviors.

Client has been using maladjusted coping; identifying effective, constructive strategies to handle fearful situations can be an impetus to change.

Encourage implementation of new strategies, giving feedback on effectiveness.

Reinforces acceptable behaviors.

Avoid confrontation of delusion.

Logic does not work, and forcing the client to give up the delusion increases anxiety.

Observe for side effects of medications: note changes in behavior/response to environment, level of consciousness, intellectual responses/thought control; reports of dry mouth, blurred vision. Monitor vital signs, intake/output, weight.

Adverse reactions such as extrapyramidal symptoms, tardive dyskinesia, orthostatic hypotension, decreased sensation of thirst, constipation, urinary retention, weight gain may occur; paradoxical exacerbations of psychotic symptoms may develop and may actually heighten anxiety, suspiciousness

Collaborative

Develop behavioral therapy program with input and agreement of client, family/SO, and therapeutic team.

Hypersensitivity to the actions of others has been learned and can be unlearned. Breaking this cycle assists in reducing sensitivity to criticism and improving client's social skills.

Administer medications as indicated, e.g., fluphenazine (Prolixin), haloperidol (Haldol).

Decreases anxiety and delusional thinking, which can increase ability to problem-solve. **Note:** Decreased sensation of thirst and sensitivity to sun/photophobia are side effects of antipsychotic drugs that require increased fluid intake and avoidance of prolonged exposure to sun.

NURSING DIAGNOSIS	**POWERLESSNESS**
May Be Related to:	Lifestyle of helplessness: Feelings of inadequacies, sense of severely impaired self-esteem
	Interpersonal interaction
Possibly Evidenced by:	Verbal expressions of having no control/influence over situation(s)
	Use of paranoid delusions, aggressive behavior to compensate for lack of control
	Expressions of recognition of damage paranoia has caused self and others
Desired Outcomes/Evaluation Criteria— Client Will:	State belief that outcome of situations causing concern can be significantly affected by own actions.
	Identify individual actions to effect control.
	Demonstrate necessary behaviors/lifestyle changes to maintain control without use of aggression.

ACTIONS/INTERVENTIONS

RATIONALE

Independent

Encourage client to do as much for self as able, providing choices when possible.

Permits/enables control of situation so suspicion can be reduced.

Assist client to identify when feelings of loss of control began and events/situations that led to feelings of powerlessness and aggressive acts.

Increases understanding of sources of stressful events and that aggression is an attempt to compensate for feeling powerless.

Review previous relationships/social contacts. If client is no longer involved in these relationships, have her or him describe what happened.

Knowledge can be gained of how the client establishes relationships and why they deteriorated or remained intact, providing insight to change own behavior and enhancing future relationships.

Discuss predelusional period and how events might precede panic state.

Helps client discern how much of delusion is real and how much relates to anxiety state.

Explore alternate ways to regain control without resorting to aggression. (Refer to ND: Violence, risk for.)

Provides knowledge of constructive coping mechanisms.

Give positive feedback when client demonstrates use of constructive alternatives.

Enhances self-esteem and reinforces acceptable behaviors.

NURSING DIAGNOSIS	THOUGHT PROCESSES, altered
May Be Related to:	Psychological conflicts
	Increasing anxiety and fear (characteristic of the suspicious person)
Possibly Evidenced by:	Interference with the ability to think clearly and logically, difficulties in the process and character of thought, fragmentation and autistic thinking, delusions
	Beliefs and behaviors of suspicion/violence
Desired Outcomes/Evaluation Criteria— Client Will:	Recognize changes in thinking/behavior, and relationship of paranoid ideation to current situation.
	Identify the meaning of the delusion.
	Deal with anxieties/fears as evidenced by more logical/reality-based thinking.

ACTIONS/INTERVENTIONS

RATIONALE

Independent

State reality matter-of-factly. Communicate in clear, concise terms with clearly stated rules what client can/cannot do.

The very suspicious/delusional client needs to have straight information that differentiates him or her from the seemingly dangerous surroundings. Knowledge of the rules can provide this person with a sense of control.

Provide outlet(s) for expression of thoughts in 1:1 or group settings.

In a trusting relationship, feelings can be freely expressed without fear of judgment.

Have a client keep a log of anxious feelings and accompanying thoughts. Review with client.

Guided writing exercises can be used, with caution, to help client identify precipitating events

Help client identify/discuss thoughts, perceptions, and own conclusions of reality.

Note impulsive behaviors and request client to stop. If client does not stop, evaluate basis of behavior and whether it is potentially harmful. (Refer to ND: Violence, risk for.)

Encourage client to identify when fears/suspicions began and events that led to these feelings.

Explore how perceptions are validated before drawing conclusions. Discuss successes and failures of these attempts.

Guide client in defining methods to deal with misperceptions without distortion of reality or using delusional system.

Encourage development of exercise programs. Instruct in use of appropriate relaxation techniques (e.g., breathing exercises, progressive relaxation activity).

Gradually involve client in learning activities, occupational/recreational/activity therapies. (Refer to ND: Self Esteem disturbance.)

and provide an opportunity to identify reality and change behavior. **Note:** Narrative writing is not recommended, as it may actually reinforce delusional system.

Increases comprehension of what client sees as problems and gives insight into how information is being processed.

These behaviors are often the result of psychotic thought/perceptual distortions and not willful actions.

Gaining knowledge of stressors that have precipitated deterioration in coping ability may help prevent recurrence of these behaviors.

Validation of perceptions may prevent drawing the wrong conclusion and acting-out behaviors.

Decreasing fears/anxieties and the client's repertoire of coping behaviors may prevent decompensation. (Refer to ND: Anxiety [severe].)

Can alleviate tension, promoting sense of well-being. **Note:** Use of guided imagery may exacerbate delusional thinking.

As thought processes improve, task mastery opportunities can enhance self-esteem and enable the client to feel good about accomplishments.

NURSING DIAGNOSIS	SELF ESTEEM disturbance
May Be Related to:	Underdeveloped ego, fixation in earlier level of development, inability to trust
	Lack of positive feedback
Possibly Evidenced by:	Delusional system (attempt to hurt or strike out at someone else to protect the self); self-destructive behavior
	Inability to accept positive reinforcement
	Not taking responsibility for self-care; nonparticipation in therapy
Desired Outcomes/Evaluation Criteria—Client Will:	Verbalize feelings of increased self-value/worth.
	Identify self as a person capable of problem-solving and functioning in society in a manner acceptable to self and others.
	Demonstrate adaptation to changes by active participation in treatment program.

ACTIONS/INTERVENTIONS	RATIONALE

Independent

Provide clear, consistent verbal/nonverbal communication. Be truthful and honest; follow through on commitments.

Helpful in establishing trust and reaffirms that the individual has value and worth.

Encourage client to verbalize feelings of inadequacies, worthlessness, fear of rejection/need for acceptance by others.

Must have insight into own feelings to begin to improve self-esteem.

Explore how these negative feelings could lead to severe anxiety and suspiciousness.

Increases awareness of internal factors that cause feelings of inadequacy and how these feelings lead to decompensation.

Encourage client to identify positive aspects about self related to social skills, work abilities, education, talents, and appearance.

Reinforces own feelings of being a worthwhile person capable of adaptive functioning.

Give positive feedback regarding abilities and how they can be used to increase self-esteem.

Provides encouragement and promotes a sense of self-direction.

Engage in activities, increasing socialization and interaction with others as tolerated.

Opportunity to interact with others reduces isolation, enhances feelings of self-worth, and promotes social skills.

NURSING DIAGNOSIS	**SOCIAL INTERACTION, impaired**
May Be Related to:	Disturbed thought processes, mistrust of others/delusional thinking
	Knowledge/skill deficit about ways to enhance mutuality
Possibly Evidenced by:	Discomfort in social situations, difficulty in establishing relationships with others
	Expressions of feelings of rejection, no sense of belonging; isolation of self/withdrawal
	Dealing with problems with anger/hostility and violence
Desired Outcomes/Evaluation Criteria—Client Will:	Verbalize willingness to be involved with others.
	Participate in activities/programs with others with lessened discomfort.

ACTIONS/INTERVENTIONS	RATIONALE

Independent

Establish 1:1 relationship, use Active-listening, and provide safe environment for self-disclosure.

Consistent, brief, honest contact can help the client initiate and master tasks associated with learning to trust others.

Determine degree of impairment, listening to client's

Mistrust can lead to difficulty establishing

comments about loneliness. Note sense of self-esteem. (Refer to ND: Self Esteem disturbance.)

relationships, and client may have withdrawn from close contacts with others.

Encourage client to verbalize feelings of discomfort about social situations and perceptions of reasons for problems.

Acknowledgement helps client to become aware of feelings and begin to deal with them.

Observe and describe social/interpersonal behaviors in objective terms.

Provides insight into how others view them and may serve as a beginning for change.

Identify support systems available to the client: family, friends, coworkers, etc.

Can be an important part in the client's rehabilitation by improving socialization and diminishing sense of isolation.

Assess family relationships, communication patterns, knowledge of client condition.

Problems within the family can preclude members providing adequate support/continuing relationship and may interfere with client's progress. (Refer to ND: Family Coping, ineffective: compromised/Family Processes, altered.)

Explore and role-play means of changing social interactions/behaviors. Provide positive feedback for efforts.

Provides safe environment to try out new behaviors. Encouragement enhances repetition and risk-taking.

NURSING DIAGNOSIS	FAMILY COPING, ineffective: compromised/FAMILY PROCESSES, altered
May Be Related to:	Temporary family disorganization/role changes
	Inadequate or incorrect information or understanding by a primary person
	Prolonged progression of condition that exhausts the supportive capacity of significant other(s)
Possibly Evidenced by:	Family system does not meet physical/emotional/spiritual needs of its members
	Inability to express/accept wide range of feelings within self and other family members
	Inappropriate or poorly communicated family rules, rituals, symbols
	Inappropriate boundary maintenance
	Significant person describes preoccupation with personal reactions, withdraws or enters into limited or temporary personal communication with client at time of need
Desired Outcomes/Evaluation Criteria— Family Will:	Identify/verbalize resources within itself to deal with the situation.
	Interact appropriately with the client.
	Provide opportunity for client to deal with situation in own way.
	Identify need for outside support and use appropriately.

267

ACTIONS/INTERVENTIONS	RATIONALE
Independent	
Identify individual factors that may contribute to difficulty of family in providing needed assistance to the client.	Each member of a family system has an effect on other members, and members of this family may be in constant conflict with each other.
Determine information available to and understood by family/significant other(s).	Lack of understanding of illness can lead to angry responses in family members, resulting in continuing conflict.
Discuss underlying reasons for client's behaviors (e.g., fear of loss of control, extreme sensitivity, use of projection and blame to avoid looking at own responsibility).	Promotes understanding of client and provides opportunity for changing ineffective responses to positive, growth-promoting behaviors.
Encourage and assist client/family to develop problem-solving skills.	This client's behavior creates conflict among family members, and learning to resolve issues in an open, nonjudgmental manner lessens angry responses, allowing for resolution of the conflict.
Help individuals to look at own behavior in relation to the client's.	Interaction among family members often enables the client to maintain suspicions and paranoid ideation, and when this behavior is acknowledged and dealt with, behavior can begin to change.
Collaborative	
Refer to appropriate resources such as marital/family therapy, psychotherapy, support groups.	Since conflict is so prevalent in this family, and divorce is common, long-term assistance may be needed to maintain relationships or achieve amicable parting.

CHAPTER 8

MOOD DISORDERS

MAJOR DEPRESSION/DYSTHYMIC DISORDER

DSM-IV
DEPRESSIVE DISORDERS
296.xx Major depressive disorder
296.2x Single episode
296.3x Recurrent
300.4 Dysthymic disorder
311 Depressive disorder NOS

A disturbance of mood, characterized by a full or partial depressive syndrome, or loss of interest or pleasure in usual activities and pastimes with evidence of interference in social/occupational functioning.

ETIOLOGICAL THEORIES

Psychodynamics

Psychoanalytical theory focuses on an early unsatisfactory parent/child relationship, with an unresolved grieving process. This results in the individual remaining fixed in the anger stage of the grieving process and turning it inward on the self. The ego remains weak, while the superego expands and becomes punitive.

Cognitive theory projects a belief that depression occurs as a result of impaired cognition, fostering a negative evaluation of self through disturbed thought processes. The individual is pessimistic and views self as inadequate and worthless and life as hopeless.

Learning theorists propose that depressive illness arises out of the individual's having experienced numerous failures (either real or perceived). A feeling of inability to succeed at any endeavor ensues. This "learned helplessness" is viewed as a predisposition to depressive illness. The behavioral model states that the cause of depression is in the person-behavior-environment interaction. Although people are seen as capable of exercising control over their behavior, they are not totally free of environmental influence.

Biological

A family history of major affective disorders may exist in individuals with depressive disorders. Recently it has been found that the disease has a genetic marker, as shown by numerous studies that support the involvement of heredity in depressive illness.

Biochemical factors (e.g., electrolyte imbalances) appear to play a role in depressive illness. An error in metabolism results in the transposition of sodium and potassium within the neuron. Another theory implicates the biogenic amines norepinephrine, dopamine, and serotonin. The levels of these chemicals are deficient in individuals with depressive disorders. Controversy remains as to whether these biochemical changes *cause* the depression or whether they are *caused by* the illness. In recent years, a common form of major depression called *seasonal affective disorder* (SAD) has been identified. Recurring each year, starting in fall or winter and ending in spring, the symptoms are largely typical of depression, with some atypical symptoms (excessive sleep, increased appetite, and weight gain). This disorder is believed to be caused by the decreased availability of sunlight and is related to circadian cycles, which are set by each individual's internal biological clock. Circadian cycles are more precisely adjusted and coordinated by the alternation of darkness and light.

Impaired seratonergic transmission has also been investigated as a cause of depression (indolamine hypothesis). It has been shown that multiple regions of the brain in depressed clients lack metabolic responsivity, suggesting a generalized subresponsivity of the serotonergic system. Additionally, current research suggests that infection with the Borna disease virus (BDV) may be linked to some cases of major depression and other severe mood disorders.

Family Dynamics

Object loss theory suggests that depressive illness occurs if the person is separated from or abandoned by a significant other during the first 6 months of life. The bonding process is thereby interrupted, and the child withdraws from people and the environment.

CLIENT ASSESSMENT DATA BASE

Activity/Rest

Fatigue, malaise, decreased energy level, lethargy

Sleep disturbances (e.g., insomnia) occur in 90% of cases—either anxiety insomnia (with difficulty falling asleep) or depressive insomnia (with early morning awakening, accompanied by painful ruminations); also hypersomnia (with restlessness and feeling unrefreshed, particularly in SAD)

May report feeling best early in the morning, then continually feeling worse as the day progresses (dysthymia); or the opposite may be true (especially in severe depression)

Ego Integrity

Feelings of worthlessness: self-derogatory statements, expressions of guilt, or exaggeration of minor inadequacies; may assume delusional proportions with presentations of unrealistic evidence of self-worth/intense focus on self (e.g., feeling oneself responsible for major tragedies and catastrophes or persecuted for a failure)

Morbid sadness; actual loss or life stressor perceived as a loss (e.g., retirement, job loss, divorce, illness, aging); may or may not see connection between perceived losses and onset of depression

Feelings of helplessness, hopelessness, powerlessness, pessimism, irritability, excessive anger

Elimination

Constipation and urinary retention may be present

Food/Fluid

Decreased/increased appetite accompanied by significant change in weight (average gain of 10 pounds in SAD)

Hygiene

Inattention to personal care needs, unkempt appearance

Possible body odor

Posture may be bent/slouched (defeated-looking)

Neurosensory

Dejected or sad mood, with loss of interest/enjoyment in usual activities

Depressed mood for most of day, for more days than not, for at least 2 years (dysthymia), or with intermittent symptom-free periods, for at least 2 months (recurrent)

Expressed sadness, dejection, not caring about anything, not seeing any future for self; tending to sigh and be tearful

Irritability, headache

Psychotic features with prominent delusions and/or hallucinations (major depression)

Psychomotor Retardation: May present either a "slow motion" picture, with slowed speech and latencies (long pauses before responding), decreased amount of speech, and slowed body movements; or agitation, featuring constant, rapid, purposeless movements (severe depression)

Thinking characterized by poor concentration and decreased memory, indecision, suicidal ideation

Safety

Thoughts of suicide/wanting to die possibly occurring frequently throughout the illness; may range in severity from indifference about the consequences of behavior (e.g., lack of cooperation with medical treatment, or dangerous driving), to wishing it were "over" or for death, to specific suicide plans and attempts

Sexuality

Disinterest in sexual activities, and/or impotence

Women affected almost twice as often as men, primarily during the childbearing years of late 20s to early 30s and again in the postmenopausal years of late 40s to early 50s

Social Interactions

Participation diminished, difficulty starting activities, withdrawal (e.g., housebound or remains in a single room/bed)

Teaching/Learning

Family history of depression; high rates of alcoholism/other drug abuse

DIAGNOSTIC STUDIES

(The several biochemical alterations in depression are not, by themselves, indicative of depression but, combined with clinical observation, may indicate best pharmacological response.)

Thyroid-Stimulating Hormone Response to Thyrotropin-Releasing Hormone: Decreased level suggests depression.

Dexamethasone-Suppression Test (DST) (an indirect marker of melancholia): Postdexamethasone cortisol levels exceeding 5 g/dl indicate abnormal/positive result and can be used to predict effectiveness of antidepressants.

EEG Sleep Profile: This shows reduced latency of rapid eye movement (REM) sleep.

CBC, Blood Glucose, Electrolytes, Renal/Liver Function Tests: These identify abnormalities contributing to or resulting from depression.

Other medical tests that may be included:

Platelet Monoamine Oxidase Activity (MAO): Increased.

Biogenic Amines (Especially Norepinephrine and Serotonin Levels): Decreased (clients with low serotonin levels are 10 times more likely to commit suicide within a year).

α-Acid Glycoprotein: Inhibitor of serotonin transporter is elevated.

Urinary 3-Methoxy-4-Hydroxyphenylglycol (MHPG): If low, indicates decreased norepinephrine output.

Cerebrospinal Fluid Level of 5-Hydroxytryptamine (5HIAA): Reduced.

Minnesota Multiphasic Personality Inventory (MMPI): Scale 2 consistently elevated.

Wechsler Adult Intelligence Scale-Revised (WAIS-R): Overall performance score significantly lower than verbal score.

Rorschach Test: Long reaction times, chromatic color responses diminished.

Thematic Apperception Test (TAT): Short, stereotyped responses/simple descriptions of cards.

Zung (or Similar) Depressive Scale (ADS): Self-report reflecting affective, psychic, somatic characteristics of depression.

NURSING PRIORITIES

1. Promote physical safety with special focus on suicide prevention.
2. Provide for client's basic needs, promoting highest possible level of independent functioning.
3. Provide experience/interactions that enhance self-esteem, sense of personal power.
4. Support client/family participation in follow-up care/community treatment.
5. Provide information about condition, prognosis, and treatment needs.

DISCHARGE GOALS

1. Suicidal ideation/self-violent behaviors absent.
2. Physiological stability achieved with responsibility for self demonstrated.
3. Client expressing feelings appropriately with some optimism and hope for the future.
4. Client/family participating in follow-up care/community treatment.
5. Condition, prognosis, and therapeutic regimen understood.
6. Plan in place to meet needs after discharge.

NURSING DIAGNOSIS	**VIOLENCE, risk for self-directed**
Risk Factors May Include:	Depressed mood
	Feelings of worthlessness and hopelessness
[Possible Indicators:]	Verbalization of suicidal ideation/plan or futility of trying (e.g., "What's the use?")
	Giving possessions away/making a will
	Sudden mood elevation/appearing more energized or displaying calmer, more peaceful manner
	Refusal/reluctance to sign a "no harm" contract
Desired Outcomes/Evaluation Criteria— Client Will:	Voluntarily comply with suicide precautions, sign "no harm" contract.
	Verbalize a decrease/absence of suicidal ideas.
	State 2 reasons for not harming self.
	Commit no acts of self-violence.

ACTIONS/INTERVENTIONS	RATIONALE

Independent

Identify degree of risk/potential for suicide through direct questions (e.g., "Have you thought about killing yourself?"). Assess seriousness of suicidal tendency, noting behaviors such as gestures, threats, giving away possessions, previous attempts, presence of hallucinations or delusions. (Use scale of 1–10 and prioritize care according to severity of threat, availability of means.)

Degree of hopelessness expressed by client is important indicator of severity of depression and suicide risk. Eight of 10 clients who state an intention to commit suicide do so. The more thought-out the plan, the higher the chances of completing it. The chances of suicide increase if there was a previous suicide attempt or if a family history of suicide and depression is present. Impulsive clients are more likely to attempt suicide without giving clues, including those with psychotic thinking who are especially at risk when hallucinations or delusions encourage self-harm. **Note:** Individuals with untreated depression have a suicide rate of 15%.

Reevaluate potential for suicide periodically at key times (e.g., during mood changes, at initiation of/ changes in medication regimen, when increasing withdrawal occurs, when discharge planning becomes active, before sending out on pass, before discharge from program).

Suicide risk is the greatest during the first few weeks following admission to treatment. More than half of suicides by hospitalized clients occur out of the hospital, while they are on leave or during an unauthorized absence. The highest risk is when the client has both suicidal ideation and sufficient energy with which to act (e.g., at the point when the client begins to feel better).

Implement suicide precautions. For example, explain to client that you are concerned for his or her safety and that you will be helping client to stay "safe."

Communicates caring and provides sense of protection.

Create a time-specific contract with client on what client and nurse will do to provide for client's safety. Renew contract as appropriate. Place a copy of the "contract," signed by client and staff, in the chart/ file and give a copy to the client to keep.

Documents actions taken to prevent suicide and client response. It also promotes communication and can help client realize that others care what happens. Short-term contracts encourage client to deal with the here-and-now and provide opportunity to reassess situation.

When hospitalized:

Provide close observation (1:1 or random checks every 10 to 15 minutes for most acute risk). Place in room close to nurse's station; do not assign to a single room. Accompany to off-ward activities if attendance is indicated. Ask client to stay in view of staff member at all times.

Being alert for suicidal and escape attempts facilitates being able to prevent or interrupt harmful behavior.

Be alert to use of hazardous equipment; remove hazardous personal items (e.g., scarves, belts, razor blades, scissors).

Provides environmental safety; removes objects that may prompt suicidal thoughts/attempts.

Check all items brought in to or by the client as indicated. Ask family and other visitors to avoid bringing hazardous items.

Suicidal clients may bring harmful items back from a pass or may ask family for items, with a suicide plan in mind.

Maintain special care in administration of medications.

Prevents the client from saving medication up to overdose or discarding and not taking medication.

Be alert when client is using bathroom.

Although decreasing the client's privacy may seem awkward, it is essential that the suicidal client be within caregiver's view at all times to prevent self-harm (e.g., hanging).

Make rounds at frequent, irregular intervals (especially at night, toward early morning, at change of shift, or other predictably busy times for staff).

Prevents staff surveillance from becoming predictable. To be aware of client's location is important, especially when staff is busy and least available/observant.

Routinely check environment for hazards. Provide for environmental safety (e.g., lock doors/windows when not supervised; block access to stairways, roof, and construction areas; monitor cleaning chemicals/repair supplies).

Minimizing opportunities for self-harm is an ongoing issue requiring constant attention and consideration of the unusual.

Review medical regimen, including electro-convulsive therapy (ECT), allowing client/family to ask questions and express feelings freely.

Antidepressant drugs may take 3 or more weeks to lift mood. In the meantime, other forms of therapy may be required to provide protection for the suicidal client. ECT is generally a second line of treatment, used if depression has not responded to pharmacological treatment and/or client continues to display suicidal ideation, sleeplessness, refusal to eat and drink. Client may fear ECT, and nurse needs to empathize with client's fears while supporting ECT as being a positive treatment alternative.

Be aware of staff attitudes toward the use of ECT, and avoid influencing client negatively.

When nurses/others have negative or ambivalent feelings toward this treatment, these feelings can be communicated to the client, causing confusion/reluctance to accept appropriate therapy.

Collaborative

Administer medications as indicated, e.g.: SSRIs: fluoxetine (Prozac), fluvoxamine (Luvox), paroxetine (Paxil), sertraline (Zoloft); tricyclics, e.g., amitriptyline (Elavil), desipramine (Norpramin), doxepin (Sinequan), imipramine (Tofranil); heterocyclics, e.g., amoxapine (Asendin), bupropion (Wellbutrin), maprotiline (Ludiomil), trazodone (Desyrel); monoamine oxidase inhibitors (MAOIs), e.g., phenelzine (Nardil), isocarboxazid (Marplan), tranylcypromine (Parnate).

Selective serotonic reuptake inhibitors and cyclic antidepressants are generally considered the safest and easiest to manage of the antidepressants and so are started first. If response is not noted in 4 to 6 weeks, an MAOI may be the drug of choice. These drugs act by blocking enzyme degradation of neurotransmitters (norepinephrine, serotonin). **Note:** Medications inhibiting reuptake of serotonin, or heterocyclic drugs (e.g., Wellbutrin), are usually preferred for treating depression in bipolar disorders, whereas tricyclics and MAOIs may increase possibility of switch to manic behavior. (Tricyclics use a "shotgun approach," whereas newer generations of drugs usually target a specific neurotransmitter. TCAs also can cause toxicity before therapeutic levels are achieved, and MAOIs can cause fatal central serotonin syndrome if administered within 2 weeks of SSRI therapy).

Evaluate cardiac status, obtain ECG as appropriate.

TCAs can increase cardiac conduction disturbances and cause dangerous interaction with antidysrhythmic medications.

Prepare for/assist with ECT as indicated.

ECT becomes essential and in some cases life saving when depression does not respond to other treatments and suicide is a major risk. (Of clients with major depression, 80% to 90% show marked improvement after ECT.)

NURSING DIAGNOSIS	GRIEVING, dysfunctional
May Be Related to:	Multiple life changes, actual/perceived loss including loss of physiopsychosocial well-being (poor nutrition, little or no exercise)
	Thwarted grieving response to a loss, lack of resolution of previous grieving response
	Absence of anticipatory grieving
Possibly Evidenced by:	Perception of areas in life as unfulfilled or as losses; denial of loss; expression of unresolved issues, guilt
	Crying/labile affect
	Interference with life functioning, alterations in concentration/pursuit of tasks, changes in eating habits, sleep/dream patterns, activity level, libido
Desired Outcomes/Evaluation Criteria— Client Will:	Demonstrate progress in dealing with stages of grief at own pace.
	Participate in work/self-care activities at level of ability.
	Verbalize a sense of progress toward resolution of the grief and hope for the future.

ACTIONS/INTERVENTIONS

RATIONALE

Independent

Assess losses that have occurred in the client's life. Discuss meaning these have had for the client.

Denial of the impact/importance of a loss may be contributing to severity of depression.

Determine cultural factors and ways individual has dealt with previous loss(es).

Cultural beliefs affect how people express and accept grieving processes.

Encourage verbalization of and assist in identification of feelings and relationship between feelings and event/stressor, when the event is known.

Verbalization of feelings in a nonthreatening environment can help client begin to deal with unrecognized/unresolved issues that may be contributing to depression. Helps client realize response (feeling) is connected to the stressor or precipitating event.

Discuss ways to identify and cope with underlying feelings (e.g., hurt, rejection, anger). Set limits regarding destructive behavior.

Begins to increase the client's repertoire of coping strategies. Learning that choices are available for behaving differently can often decrease the feeling of being stuck. "Storytelling" of how others have handled situations may be helpful, not only in providing potential solutions but also in giving the idea that the problem is manageable.

275

Identify normal stages of grief and acknowledge reality of associated feelings, e.g., guilt, anger, powerlessness.

Helps client understand normalcy of feelings and may alleviate some of the guilt generated by these feelings.

Assist client to identify need to address problem differently. Describe all aspects of the problem through the use of therapeutic communication skills.

Contracting for change begins with agreeing on "the problem." It helps the client to consider all aspects of the problem, to define clearly what the client is dealing with.

Help client recognize early symptoms of depression and plan ways to alleviate them. Help client formulate steps to take for outside support if symptoms continue.

Involves the client actively, reducing sense of powerlessness. Rehearsal promotes generalization of recently learned coping strategies to new situations and may help to minimize recurrence of depressive feelings.

Reinforce the positive aspects of being able to reach out for help.

Encourages the client to learn how to manage/take care of self. It is important that the client has support available should help be needed and that the client experience needing to reach out as positive, reflecting sense of empowerment and own self-worth.

NURSING DIAGNOSIS	ANXIETY [moderate to severe]/THOUGHT PROCESSES, altered
May Be Related to:	Psychological conflicts; unconscious conflict about essential values/goals of life
	Unmet needs
	Threat to self-concept
	Sleep deprivation
	Interpersonal transmission/contagion
Possibly Evidenced by:	Reports of nervousness or fearfulness, feelings of inadequacy
	Agitation, angry or tearful outbursts, rambling and discoordinated speech
	Restlessness, hand-rubbing or -wringing, tremulousness
	Poor memory and concentration, decreased ability to grasp ideas, inability to follow, impaired ability to make decisions, circumstantiality (unable to get to the point)
	Numerous, repetitious physical complaints without organic cause
	Ideas of reference, hallucinations/delusions
Desired Outcomes/Evaluation Criteria— Client Will:	Verbalize awareness of feelings of anxiety, changes in thinking/behavior.
	Identify ways to deal effectively with decision-making.

Converse appropriately with staff or in groups.

Attend to and complete tasks (ADLs, occupational therapy projects, etc.) of increasing length and difficulty.

Report anxiety is reduced to manageable level.

ACTIONS/INTERVENTIONS	RATIONALE
Independent	
Evaluate/reevaluate level of anxiety.	Approaches differ, depending on level of anxiety. (Refer to CP: Generalized Anxiety Disorder.)
Recognize and deal with own feelings in response to client's anxiety.	Anxiety is highly communicable. If the nurse becomes anxious (or impatient, irritable, etc.), this will be communicated and feed client's anxiety.
Listen nonjudgmentally to client's expressions; convey empathy; acknowledge or label feelings for client.	Helps client identify basis for anxious feelings, communicates acceptance, and assists in reducing current level of anxiety.
Use short, concrete communication. Assume calm, "in-control-of-things" manner. Let client know about safety and supportive attentions of the staff/facility.	Attention, concentration, and problem-solving are compromised by anxiety. Benign attention/monitoring by staff may be interpreted in a paranoid manner by the client.
Decrease environmental stimulation; remove to quiet area away from other clients. Suggest activity that may be relaxing (e.g., warm bath, back rub). Involve in a quiet activity when calmer.	Reduces anxiety-provoking stimuli and distractions. Helps client refocus away from anxiety.
Maintain a calm attitude and use physical touch, if acceptable to client.	May prove helpful if anxiety stems from delusions/hallucinations; touch can restore client to reality. Caution is required with suspicious clients who may interpret touch as aggression.
Defer problem-solving, assessment of precipitating factors until anxiety is reduced to a more manageable level.	Ability to problem-solve is compromised, and such requests may increase anxiety.
Analyze incident with client and staff to identify precipitating factors, early signs of building anxiety, previously helpful interventions.	Develops an individualized plan that will help decrease anxiety; establishes/reestablishes previous coping skill. Client needs to learn how to manage own anxiety by recognizing the signs and then acting to lower the anxiety.
Stay with client as indicated.	Promotes sense of safety and provides opportunity to focus on present and use techniques to alleviate anxious feelings.
Decrease decision-making for client by offering a choice between only 2 options (e.g., whether to have cereal or eggs, rather than a full menu).	Decreasing options lessens the amount of information to process and enhances decision-making. As ability to think through incoming information increases, more options can be added.
Choose for the client when necessary, based on knowledge of the client's interest and activity level, telling client how the choice was decided.	Judicious choosing for the client may decrease sense of inadequacy when client feels overwhelmed and may provide role-modeling of decision-making process.

277

Discourage use of caffeine.	Can produce anxiety-like symptoms, compounding clinical picture and client's perception of situation.
Assist client to learn relaxation/imagery exercises. Use tapes of relaxation exercises and calm music. Prompt client to use these techniques when becoming anxious.	Develops skills for coping with anxiety responses.
Engage in role-playing and encourage practice of stress relief techniques when client is not feeling anxious.	Enables client to use skill more effectively (automatically) as needed and helps individual handle problems/pressures as they occur.
Encourage creative activities and development of greater leisure skills.	Helps expand positive energy and attention. Enhances self-worth.
Encourage participation in regular exercise program, sporting activities, occupational/recreational therapy including brisk walls, jogging, punching bag, volleyball.	Participation in individually prescribed activities and large motor exercises provides safe, effective methods for discharging pent-up tensions, learning to trust self, and enhancing self-esteem. Exercise releases endorphins, enhancing sense of well-being. **Note:** Exercise therapy does not need to be aerobic or intensive to achieve desired effect.
Involve in group settings, encouraging and reinforcing appropriate participation. Redirect into activities, e.g., interaction with others, as indicated.	Increases opportunities for/reinforcement of desired, productive interaction style. Sharing with others decreases sense of being the only one. Client may learn new coping styles from stress of participation as well as from peers who have experienced similar stressors.
Deal with physical complaints in matter-of-fact style. Investigate appropriately if new; redirect if not new or validated. Do not ask how client is or feels. Help client recognize physical symptoms as anxiety signals when appropriate. Note history of mitral valve prolapse (MVP).	Detection of physical problems and prevention of discounting client's discomfort are important. Reduces reinforcement for focusing on self and symptoms while providing opportunity and reinforcement for other-directed, more appropriate interaction style. **Note:** Focus on physical complaints occurs in depressed persons in about 25% of cases. Palpitations resulting from MVP may increase anxiety to panic state and require medical evaluation/treatment.

Collaborative

Provide phototherapy as indicated.	Light therapy using white fluorescent lights (2500 to 10,000 lx) at a distance of 3 feet from the client for several hours a day has been found to improve mood within 2 to 4 days in presence of SAD. Treatment has few disadvantages, although relapse is common if therapy is discontinued. For this reason, light therapy may be combined with medication.

NURSING DIAGNOSIS	**PHYSICAL MOBILITY, impaired/SELF CARE deficit (specify)**
May Be Related to:	Disinterest or unconcern; lack of energy/inertia; psychomotor retardation
	Impaired self-concept; depression; severe anxiety

Possibly Evidenced by:	Impaired ability to make decisions, such as whether to get out of bed, what to wear/eat; disheveled appearance
	Reports of "I can't/don't want to" or "Wait until later" to perform self-care activities
	Requests for help in the absence of physical incapacity
	Inactivity
Desired Outcomes/Evaluation Criteria— Client Will:	Verbalize understanding of own situation and individual treatment regimen.
	Demonstrate resumption of activities, increased concern/attention to grooming and hygiene, and behaviors to begin to direct own life.
	Initiate/perform self-care and other activities independently.

ACTIONS/INTERVENTIONS	RATIONALE

Independent

Speak directly to client; respect individuality and personal space as appropriate.	Promotes sense of worthwhileness of the person.
Provide structured opportunities for client to make choices of care, (e.g., what to wear today, what activity to participate in).	Begins to establish own ability to make decisions and accept/deal with consequences.
Be aware of the amount of time client actually spends in bed/chair, especially clients who appear in a poor nutritional state.	Immobility places client at increased risk for skin lesions/decubitus, circulatory stasis, constipation, and infection.
Examine skin over bony prominences for redness (include heels) after client has been in bed/chair awhile.	Identifies compromised tissues receiving decreased circulation (because of prolonged pressure) and requiring prompt intervention.
Encourage/provide skin care with attention to cleanliness; gentle massage and lotion every 2–3 hours. Recommend change position every 2 hours, including bed to chair or to stroll "once around the day room." Progress to regular exercise program.	Until etiological factors are remedied (immobility and nutritional status) these actions help prevent skin breakdown by alleviating pressure and promoting circulation. Also stimulates peristalsis, enhancing elimination.
Set progressive activity goals with client.	Reduces risks of complication related to sedentary lifestyle/immobility. Activity can also release natural endorphins, which help elevate mood.
Monitor intake and output. Note color/ concentration of urine. Observe for complications of reduced fluid intake (e.g., dry mucous membranes and lips, poor skin turgor, constipation), and treat accordingly.	Direct indicators of individual needs/presence of problems. Poor hydration directly affects tissues (increasing risk of damage/breakdown in face of decreased mobility) and elimination.
Offer fluids frequently/leave small amounts of fluid within easy reach. Encourage intake of at least 1500–2000 ml/day.	Improves overall intake in depressed person to whom everything seems too difficult. Client may drink because it is available. Small amounts prevent guilt over things being "wasted" if all is

279

Note dietary intake/deficits. Increase roughage; provide fruit juices, stimulant beverages (hot or caffeine-containing, if tolerated).

Promotes general well-being, helps increase energy level, and promotes improved pattern of elimination. Fiber improves stool consistency and bowel function. Caffeine has a cholinergic effect, and some juices, such as prune, contain a by-product that stimulates intestinal mobility.

Perform/assist with needed self-care activities for client, as necessary. Note frequency of elimination pattern.

Ensures that needed activities are accomplished if client is unable/unwilling to perform alone. Promotes prompt intervention as indicated, reducing risk of complications (e.g., constipation).

Provide/obtain needed equipment, client's own supplies, clothing.

Availability may prompt performance; having one's own things enhances self-esteem, autonomy.

Choose one self-care activity and plan with client how to implement in a simple, concrete fashion.

Assists client toward self-care in a slow and achievable manner. Depressed clients feel overwhelmed, and it is important that success is experienced l task at a time.

Provide low-key reinforcement for improved functioning in this area.

Enhances self-esteem; low-key style avoids provoking discounting, self-derogation.

Give low-key reminder regarding need to perform a self-care activity.

Gentle prodding can be helpful to the client; however, reminders may be perceived as criticism and can feed into self-derogatory thinking.

Collaborative

Refer to occupational/recreational therapy involving motor activities (e.g., walking, working with clay, aerobic exercise, crafts, activities of daily living).

These activities help to discharge anger and aggression and relieve guilt, as well as build self-confidence and prepare client for return to previous occupation/leisure-time activities.

Encourage beautician/barber appointments, if services accessible.

Can enhance self-image, stimulate participation in self-care activities.

Administer stool softener/bulk preparation.

May be used to supplement dietary inadequacies/ soften stool until normal stool is established.

Provide glycerine suppository or laxative product according to protocol, if no bowel movement occurs.

Prevents impaction and helps to restore regular pattern.

NURSING DIAGNOSIS	NUTRITION: altered, less/more than body requirements
May Be Related to:	Inappropriate nutritional intake to meet metabolic needs
Possibly Evidenced by:	Lack of interest in eating/food or choosing nutritional foods; aversion to eating
	Dysfunctional eating pattern (e.g., eating in response to internal cues other than hunger)

Desired Outcomes/Evaluation Criteria—Client Will:

Recent weight loss, poor muscle tone, decreased subcutaneous fat/muscle mass; pale conjunctiva and mucous membranes; or weight gain

Sedentary activity level

Demonstrate progressive weight gain/loss toward goal.

Be free of signs of malnutrition with normalization of laboratory values.

Identify actions/lifestyle changes to regain and/or to maintain appropriate weight.

ACTIONS/INTERVENTIONS	RATIONALE
Independent	
Monitor/record amount and type of food eaten, calculate total calorie intake. Note how client perceives food and the act of eating.	Provides baseline data and documents change/progress toward goal.
Explain to client that malnutrition itself decreases energy levels and ability to think cohesively (e.g., decreased protein and vitamin B affect and may deepen depression).	May provide incentive to eat, increasing cooperation with regimen and intake of nutritious foods.
Determine calorie requirements based on physical factors and activity. Increase calorie intake as activity level increases.	Caloric requirements need to be adapted to provide sufficient energy to meet expenditures/maintain appropriate weight.
Monitor body weight, depending on the seriousness of the problem and the client's response to being weighed.	Provides information about therapeutic needs/effectiveness. **Note:** Increased appetite is one of the earliest responses to antidepressant use.
Avoid getting into a "power struggle" about these issues.	Focuses attention on food and weight, overemphasizing them (possibly providing secondary gain) rather than underlying dynamics.
Provide small meals and interval feedings, emphasizing nutritious choices (e.g., high protein/carbohydrates, increased fiber).	A full meal may look like an insurmountable challenge, especially for client who is depressed.
Identify and obtain foods client thinks would be interesting/appealing. Use family/friends as resources as indicated.	May enhance desire to eat and promote increased/balanced intake. Family can provide information about client's likes and dislikes, other helpful ideas to increase food intake.
Feed client, if indicated by physical condition and refusal/inability to eat.	Assisting client to eat can help to meet nutritional needs.
Collaborative	
Consult with dietitian as necessary.	Helpful in determining individual needs, alternate dietary therapy, reinforcing proper eating habits.
Monitor laboratory studies (e.g., serum albumin, prealbumin, glucose, electrolytes, nitrogen balance).	Detects deficiencies/imbalances, identifies therapeutic needs/effectiveness.
Provide tube feeding, as indicated.	May be necessary when client refuses or is unable to eat and client safety/condition requires.

NURSING DIAGNOSIS	SLEEP PATTERN disturbance
May Be Related to:	Biochemical alterations (decreased serotonin)
	Unresolved fears and anxieties
Possibly Evidenced by:	Difficulty in falling/remaining asleep, early morning awakening/awakening later then desired
	Reports of not feeling rested
	Hypersomnia, using sleep as an escape
Desired Outcomes/Evaluation Criteria— Client Will:	Identify interventions to promote/enhance sleep.
	Report falling asleep within 30 minutes of retiring and sleeping 4–6 hours before awakening.
	Verbalize having had a satisfactory night's sleep/feeling well rested.
	Refrain from using sleep as a means of escaping real feelings and fears.

ACTIONS/INTERVENTIONS	RATIONALE

Independent

Identify nature of sleep disturbance and variation from usual pattern (e.g., insomnia [difficulty falling asleep or may awaken early and be unable to return to sleep] or hypersomnia).	Patterns provide clues to help client and nurse to work together to solve the problem.
Assess what client does when awake and plan with client to change pattern as indicated.	Clients often awaken and ruminate about themselves in a hopeless/helpless manner. Having client set aside a period during the day to ruminate may extinguish this behavior at night.
Establish a realistic goal with client.	Some individuals have unrealistic ideas of a "normal" night's sleep.
Identify previous bedtime rituals that may have been interrupted by illness/hospitalization, and reestablish when possible.	Restoring familiar, successful rituals may allow the client to reestablish usual pattern.
Decrease afternoon and evening caffeine intake (coffee, tea, chocolate, colas).	Avoids stimulants, which may affect ability to fall/stay asleep.
Restrict evening fluids and have client void before retiring.	Reduces need to rise at night to void.
Provide light bedtime nourishment, such as milk, if client likes it and it is not otherwise contraindicated.	Milk (with L-tryptophan) is thought to be helpful in promoting sleep. Snack may prevent awakening during night because of hunger.
Encourage relaxation exercises to soft music prior to sleep.	Aids in release of tension and promotes falling asleep.
Reduce environmental stimuli (e.g., lights, noises, loudspeakers, etc.). Encourage use of white noise as appropriate.	Decreases distracting stimuli that may interfere with sleep.

Provide night lights, environmental control (room adequately warm or cool); appropriate nightwear/ bedding, including special blanket/pillow, which can be brought from home.

May prevent confusion upon awakening. Ensures personal comfort, promotes sleep, sense of security.

Schedule treatments, procedures, assessments, and medications during the daytime.

Prevents unnecessary interruption during sleep.

Increase daytime activity, including stimulating diversionary activities in daily schedule. Set limits on time spent in room, discourage returning to bed during the day.

Increased activity without overexertion promotes sleep. **Note:** If client must nap, morning napping disrupts sleep pattern less than afternoon naps.

Explore fears and feelings that sleep is helping to suppress.

Identifies these factors so they can be dealt with to enable client to progress with therapy.

Collaborative

Provide hypnotic or sedative only if other methods fail.

Products may suppress REM sleep, resulting in not feeling rested upon awakening.

Recommend use of/administer antidepressants or other medication with sedative side effects at bedtime when possible.

Decreases daytime drowsiness and aids sleeping at night.

NURSING DIAGNOSIS	**SOCIAL ISOLATION/SOCIAL INTERACTION, impaired**
May Be Related to:	Alterations in mental status/thought process (depressed mood)
	Inadequate personal resources; decreased energy/inertia
	Difficulty engaging in satisfying personal relationships
	Feelings of worthlessness/low self-concept; inadequacy in or absence of significant purpose in life
	Knowledge/skill deficit about social interactions
Possibly Evidenced by:	Verbalization/demonstration of awareness that interpersonal or social interactions do not have desired, satisfactory, or reinforcing outcomes
	Changes in patterns or interacting/communication (e.g., slowed speech, latencies, decreased amount of speech, muteness)
	Decreased involvement with others; expressed feelings of difference from others; dysfunctional interaction with peers, family, and/or others
	Refusing invitations/suggestions of social involvement; remaining in home/room/bed

283

Desired Outcomes/Evaluation Criteria— Client Will:	Attend/then participate in a specific number of activities per day/week.
	Participate in 1:1 interaction for specified number of minutes.
	Complete errands, initiate socialization activities a specific number of times per week.
	Reinstate 2 previously enjoyed activities involving others or develop new ones.
	Verbalize increased satisfaction with outcomes of social interactions.

ACTIONS/INTERVENTIONS	RATIONALE

Independent

ACTIONS/INTERVENTIONS	RATIONALE
Be consistent and on time in planned meetings with client.	Client will experience lateness as further evidence of decreased self-worth. In building trust, client needs to know that the nurse will follow through on previously agreed meetings/commitments.
Greet routinely, beginning with client's name and personal comment (e.g., appearance, clothing); share pertinent information from shift report, observations, etc. without concern for response by client.	Reinforces individuality, gets attention. Provides a "no-demand" acceptance, opportunity to interact if client chooses. Matter-of-fact manner prevents demand for client to provide a response when depressed feelings interfere.
Use touch, unless contraindicated.	Touch is a basic form of communication and can help client in interactions, demonstrate caring, and reinforce sense of self-worth.
Start conversation and "give" client a topic (e.g., unit or world event, OT project, etc.).	Initiating activity is often very difficult for client and having an assignment helps get the activity started.
Keep input fairly short and concrete. Ask only one question (about one thing) at a time. Avoid asking "yes-no" and "why" questions.	Requires less effort for client to attend to and retain. Promotes focus and requires that client put thinking into response. "Why" questions are often perceived as threatening/demanding of an answer.
Take adequate time; wait patiently for responses. Observe and give feedback regarding the feeling tone conveyed and interaction style observed.	Indicates interest, enhances self-esteem. Recognition of these feelings demonstrates empathy, sensitivity. Promotes understanding of how client is perceived by others, when discomfort and feelings of inadequacy have been experienced and provides opportunity for insight/change.
Emphasize attendance at routine unit activities as well as nondemanding activities (e.g., movies). Initially emphasize attendance rather than participation or enjoyment to be gained.	Starting with achievable goals gives client the ability to succeed and enhance self-esteem. Attendance precedes participation.
Contract with client (e.g., for nonsuicidal client, 1 hour of attendance at an activity is rewarded by 1 hour in room without being "pestered").	Involving client in decision-making increases sense of control over situation and may promote cooperation.
Gradually increase activity schedule. Involve with one other person or in quiet activity in day area.	Enhances changes of cooperation, diminishes threat, promotes progression of interaction.

284

Avoid taking client's difficulty in responding or negative/hostile responses personally.

Client will try to reinforce feeling of "worthlessness" by trying to create negative responses from others. Working with depressed client requires much patience and ability to recognize small goals as improvement.

Encourage visits by friends, relatives, other social contacts identified/located by family member.

Helps reestablish neglected, previously rewarding relationships.

Determine what the client's interests/activities were, and ask client to share those. Let client teach others about past skills by asking questions, indicating desire to learn about client's contributions to job and family. Obtain hobby equipment from home, if indicated.

Revitalizes memories from a time when client felt better, promoting client's individuality and sense of offering self to others. Encourages resumption of previously enjoyed activities, reduces sense of isolation, and increases sense of purpose.

Involve family and friends to escort/transport on outings and functional (shopping, business, obtaining belongings at home) or social activities (a brief meal, religious service, etc.).

Events such as these require little of client but increase social involvement and yield social reinforcement. Decreases sense of isolation from outside world.

Assist individual to assess own satisfaction with outcome(s) of interpersonal interactions. Avoid asking client if activities are "enjoyable" or "fun."

Helps client plan what is to be expected from interacting and how client can behave to realize those expectations. Involves the client in problem identification and helps to evaluate whether goals are realistic. **Note:** Cheerfulness may be interpreted as false.

Request feedback on outings and activities from both client and others involved (therapists, companions).

The goal is to increase involvement, and because client will likely report a less successful event than a more objective observer, input is important from both. The client can also hear others' perception of an event, which can serve to validate/add to the client's perception.

Use social skills training model to help client identify alternative strategies; role-play/rehearse new (more effective) behavior; obtain feedback and reinforcement; try new behavior in a "real situation."

Client may need to learn social skills and practice new behaviors. Improved social skills are more likely to have results that satisfy/reinforce interactions.

Use group situations for maximum impact/reinforcement (e.g., group therapy, OT, RT, etc.).

Group situations provide more opportunity for interactions, feedback, reinforcement.

Give positive reinforcement regarding attendance/performance (e.g., increased involvement in groups, demonstration of more effective social skills).

Client is unable to discount reinforcement and is thus reinforced for participation. Positive reinforcement increases the reward for trying the new tactics, encourages repetition of desired behaviors.

Assist client in identifying the natural reinforcers that occur with more effective interactions.

These reinforcers will increase the client's confidence and strengthen the behavior.

NURSING DIAGNOSIS	SEXUAL dysfunction/SEXUALITY PATTERNS, altered
May Be Related to:	Decreased energy and concern, apathy; loss of sexual desire
	Decreased self-esteem; values conflict

	Misinformation/misconceptions about sexual functioning/behavior
	Impaired relationship with SO; psychosocial abuse (e.g., harmful relationships)
Possibly Evidenced by:	Reported difficulties, limitations, or changes in sexual behaviors/activities (e.g., inability to achieve desired satisfaction, women may express a loss of interest; men may experience impotence and loss of libido)
	Actual/perceived limitation imposed by condition/therapy
	Alteration in relationship with partner
Desired Outcomes/Evaluation Criteria— Client Will:	Verbalize understanding of effect of depression on sexual functioning.
	Identify stressors that contribute to dysfunction and make changes as able.
	Resume sexual functioning at level desired/as agreed on by client and partner.

ACTIONS/INTERVENTIONS

RATIONALE

Independent

ACTIONS/INTERVENTIONS	RATIONALE
Review client's sexual history and degree of satisfaction prior to depression.	Establishes a baseline and elicits client's feelings about previous sexual satisfaction. **Note:** May need to discuss this when client is well into recovery, as feelings of self-worth are intertwined with feelings about sexual satisfaction.
Assist client to define expectations for sexual satisfaction and decide what can be done to attain these.	Planning can help the client identify more clearly what own desires are and whether they are reasonable/attainable.
Provide sex education as necessary. Include significant other/partner as appropriate.	Often sexual problems are partly ignorance and misconceptions about sexual facts, and knowledge can assist with problem resolution. **Note:** Client may need support to terminate abusive relationships/initiate involvement with others.
Review medication regimen; observe for side effects of drugs prescribed.	Many medications can affect libido, cause delayed or inability to achieve orgasm, impaired erectile capacity, delayed ejaculation, or impotence, putting a strain on a relationship and interfering with treatment. Evaluation of drug and individual response is important to ascertain whether drug is responsible for the problem.
Discuss appropriateness of delaying scheduled antidepressant dose until after coitus.	Increases likelihood that client will continue therapeutic regimen if it does not interfere with sexual performance.

Collaborative

ACTIONS/INTERVENTIONS	RATIONALE
Evaluate need for dose reduction, drug substitution, or combination therapy.	May help reduce unwanted side effects of medication.

Refer for further counseling/sex therapy as indicated.

May need additional or more in-depth assistance if problems are severe/unresolved as depression lifts.

NURSING DIAGNOSIS	FAMILY PROCESSES, altered
May Be Related to:	Situational crisis of illness of family member
	Developmental crisis (e.g., loss of family member/relationship)
Possibly Evidenced by:	Expressions of confusion; statements of difficulty coping with situation
	Family system not meeting needs of its members; difficulty accepting or receiving help appropriately
	Ineffective family decision-making process; failure to send and receive clear message.
Desired Outcomes/Evaluation Criteria—Family Will:	Express feelings freely and appropriately.
	Demonstrate individual involvement in problem-solving processes directed at appropriate solutions for the situation/crisis.
	Encourage and allow member who is ill to handle situation in own way, progressing toward independence.
	Identify/use community resources appropriately.

ACTIONS/INTERVENTIONS	RATIONALE

Independent

ACTIONS/INTERVENTIONS	RATIONALE
Assess degree of family dysfunction and current coping methods of individual members.	Identifies problems of individual family members, provides direction for intervention. Areas most affected are communication, marital adjustment and satisfaction, expressed emotion and problem-solving. **Note:** These families tend to have a greater degree of functional impairment than families dealing with other major mental illnesses.
Identify family developmental stage (e.g., newly married couple/divorced, children leaving home); components of family and client's role in the family constellation.	Developmental stage may be a factor in current situation and client's depression. Disruption of client's role may contribute to family disorganization/strain on other family members who have to step in and assume duties client usually takes care of.
Identify patterns of communication within the family. Are feelings freely expressed? Is blame or fault assigned? What is the process of decision-making in the family and who makes the decisions? What is the interaction between family members?	Dysfunctional communication (such as high levels of tension, negative expressions, self-preoccupation, diminished nonverbal patterns of support) contributes to feelings of inadequacy, rejection, and inability to cope on the part of the members of the family.
Acknowledge difficulties observed while giving permission to express feelings and discussing more effective methods of communication.	Reassures family that feelings are acceptable and can be dealt with appropriately.

287

Note the extent of feelings of powerlessness and lack of pleasure in daily life. Discuss effect on family members.	Client often displays hopelessness and anhedonia, which are very stressful and can be disruptive to family functioning. Promotes understanding that these feelings are part of the illness and enables family members to deal with own frustrations appropriately.
Provide information as necessary in verbal, written, and/or tape format as appropriate.	Provides opportunity for family members to review and incorporate new knowledge to assist in resolution of current situation.
Establish/discuss goals and expectations of family members/clients following discharge from care. Let individuals know the importance of "taking it slow" and not pressuring each other to change.	Realistic expectations of abilities of client to assume place in the family are crucial to continued recuperation. Family needs to understand that members need to continue to work on new style of communication and changing ways of dealing with conflict issues.

Collaborative

Involve in group, family and psychotherapy, as indicated.	Opportunity to hear others discuss shared problems and ways of handling can encourage family members to look at new ways of interacting. **Note:** Children living in this setting have as high as a 45% risk of developing affective disorders and may require focused therapy.
Provide information about resources available as needed (e.g., social services, homemaker assistance, counseling [e.g., marital, spiritual], visiting nurse services).	Assistance may be needed for family members to assimilate new skills and begin to make necessary lifestyle changes to promote wellness. There is a high rate of relapse for individuals dealing with major depression, and divorce rates are 9 times higher in the presence of greater expressed emotion than the national average.

NURSING DIAGNOSIS	**KNOWLEDGE deficit [LEARNING NEED] regarding diagnosis, prognosis, treatment and self care needs**
May Be Related to:	Lack of information about pathophysiology and treatment of depression
	Misconceptions about mental illness
Possibly Evidenced by:	Inaccurate statements about own situation and potential for recovery
	Lack of follow-through with treatment regimen
	Inappropriate behavior, apathy
Desired Outcomes/Evaluation Criteria— Client Will:	Exhibit increased interest, participating in learning process.
	Verbalize understanding of condition, prognosis, and therapeutic regimen.
	Assume responsibility for following through on treatment options.
	Identify/use resources appropriately.

ACTIONS/INTERVENTIONS	RATIONALE

Independent

Determine level of knowledge, mental/emotional readiness for learning.

May be first experience with illness/mental health system. Previous experience may or may not have provided accurate information. May be too depressed to access information accurately.

Provide information about depression/treatment as indicated. Give written as well as verbal information.

Provides opportunity for client to learn about own situation and enhances recall.

Provide information about drug therapy and potential side effects, e.g., anticholinergic effects, sedation, orthostatic hypotension of antidepressants; possibility of hypertensive crisis if individual consumes foods containing tyramine while taking MAOIs; dysrhythmias; photosensitivity; reduction of seizure threshold.

Client needs to know what to expect from drug trial. Knowledge can increase cooperation with drug regimen. Particularly, clients need to be aware that improvement may not occur for 4–6 weeks after drug therapy is begun, and that side effects will generally improve/disappear within 2 weeks.

Encourage frequent fluids, lip salve, ice chips, as indicated.

Provides relief of dry mouth caused by anticholinergic effect of drug therapy.

Suggest medication dosage be taken at bedtime, when appropriate.

Sedative effect may be helpful in promoting and maintaining sleep.

Discuss importance of monitoring blood pressure as indicated. Suggest client rise slowly from sitting/lying position.

Most common side effect of antidepressants is orthostatic hypotension, which can result in dizziness, injury following sudden position change.

Review diet restrictions (e.g., tyramine-free diet [avoid aged cheeses, fermented foods, wine/beer, liver, sour cream/yogurt, soy sauce, yeast products], limitation of caffeine).

Necessary to avoid interaction (hypertensive crisis) when MAOIs are used, and for 2 weeks following discontinuation of drug.

Discuss importance of healthy diet and regular exercise.

Important for general well-being. Additionally, bone mineral density of depressed clients may be significantly lower, requiring focused interventions.

Emphasize necessity to avoid driving or operating dangerous machinery during initiation/changes in medication regimen.

Side effects of drowsiness or dizziness are usually self-limiting but require adjustment in activities until resolved.

Encourage client to stop smoking, avoid alcohol intake.

Smoking increases metabolism of tricyclic medications, necessitating adjustment in dosage to achieve therapeutic effect. Alcohol potentiates CNS effects of antidepressants.

Instruct client to contact provider before taking other prescription or OTC medications and to notify other healthcare providers of drug regimen.

Many medications contain substances that, in combination with antidepressants, could precipitate a life-threatening crisis.

Discuss use of identification bracelet/card.

Provides information, if needed, in emergency situation to prevent sudden termination of medication, which could be detrimental.

Reinforce importance of not stopping drugs abruptly.

Sudden cessation of drugs can result in untoward effects (e.g., may aggravate condition, deepening depression, and cause withdrawal with nausea/vomiting and diarrhea).

Refer to resources/agencies (e.g., social services, homemaker/baby-sitting, support groups).

May be helpful to client for long-range planning for regaining/maintaining wellness.

289

NURSING DIAGNOSIS	INJURY, risk for [effects of ECT therapy]
Risk Factors May Include:	Electroconvulsive effects on the cardiovascular, respiratory, musculoskeletal, and nervous systems
	Pharmacological effects of anesthesia
Possibly Evidenced by:	[Not applicable; presence of signs and symptoms establishes an *actual* diagnosis.]
Desired Outcomes/Evaluation Criteria— Client Will:	Maintain physiological stability, free of injury/complications.

ACTIONS/INTERVENTIONS	RATIONALE
Independent	
Review medical testing (e.g., CBC, ECG, chest x-ray, urinalysis, and x-rays of lateral aspects of the spine) before procedure.	A complete medical workup can identify preexisting problems and the potential for problems, which should be reported to personnel involved with procedure.
Discuss what will be done (e.g., anesthesia, muscle relaxants, oxygenation, drugs used, who will be with the client, and how the client is likely to feel after ECT).	Knowledge can reduce anxiety and decrease fear response and is necessary for informed consent to procedure. Client will feel more secure knowing nurse will be there upon awakening. Awareness that confusion/memory loss are temporary helps alleviate associated fears.
Verify informed consent/signed permission form has been obtained.	Indicates that client agrees to procedure and received appropriate information.
Have client empty bladder, remove jewelry/hair decorations, eyeglasses/contacts, and dentures before treatment.	Reduces risk of injury/aspiration.
Orient client upon awakening after the treatment, and support client while immediate confusion clears.	Short-term memory may be affected, and client awakens confused. May be frightened by amnesia. Confusion increases with each treatment, knowledge that after-effects disappear will be reassuring.
Monitor vital signs every 15 minutes until stable.	Premedication, muscle relaxants, and anesthesia may produce dysrhythmias and respiratory depression, which need immediate intervention.
Have emergency equipment, suction, Ambu bag, etc. available.	Prompt treatment of respiratory depression/ airway obstruction can prevent/correct life-threatening complications.
Collaborative	
Restrict oral intake as indicated.	Reduces risk of vomiting/aspiration.
Provide supplemental oxygen as necessary.	Provides for optimum oxygenation during period of reduced ventilation.
Administer preprocedural medications as indicated (e.g., atropine sulfate).	Decreases secretions to prevent aspiration and increases heart rate to offset response to vagal stimulation caused by ECT.

BIPOLAR DISORDERS

DSM-IV

296.xx Bipolar I disorder
296.0x Single manic episode
296.40 Most recent episode hypomanic
296.4x Most recent episode manic
296.6x Most recent episode mixed
296.7 Most recent episode unspecified
296.5x Most recent episode depressed
296.89 Bipolar II disorder (recurrent major depressive episodes with hypomania)
301.13 Cyclothymic disorder
296.80 Bipolar disorder NOS

Bipolar disorders are characterized by recurrent mood swings of varying degree from depression to elation with intervening periods of normalcy. Milder mood swings such as cyclothymia may be manifested or viewed as everyday creativity rather than an illness requiring treatment. Hypomania can actually enhance artistic creativity and creative thinking/problem-solving.

This plan of care focuses on treatment of the manic phase. (**Note:** Bipolar II disorder is characterized by periods of depression and hypomania, but without manic episodes.) Refer to CP: Depressive Disorders for care of depressive episode.

ETIOLOGICAL THEORIES

Psychodynamics

Psychoanalytical theory explains the cyclic behaviors of mania and depression as a response to conditional love from the primary caregiver. The child is maintained in a dependent position, and ego development is disrupted. This gives way to the development of a punitive superego (anger turned inward or depression) or a strong id (uncontrollable impulsive behavior or mania). In the psychoanalytical model, mania is viewed as the mirror image of depression, a "denial of depression."

Biological

There is increasing evidence to indicate that genetics plays a strong role in the predisposition to bipolar disorder. Research suggests a combination of genes may create this predisposition. Incidence among relatives of affected individuals is higher than in the general population. Biochemically there appear to be increased levels of the biogenic amine norepinephrine in the brain, which may account for the increased activity of the manic individual.

Family Dynamics

Object loss theory suggests that depressive illness occurs if the person is separated from or abandoned by a significant other during the first 6 months of life. The bonding process is interrupted and the child withdraws from people and the environment. Rejection by parents in childhood or spending formative years with a family that sees life as hopeless and has a chronic expectation of failure makes it difficult for the individual to be optimistic. The mother may be distant and unloving, the father a less-powerful person, and the child expected to achieve high social and academic success.

CLIENT ASSESSMENT DATA BASE (MANIC EPISODE)

Activity/Rest

Disrupted sleep pattern or extended periods without sleep/decreased need for sleep (e.g., feels well rested with 3 hours of sleep)
Physically hyperactive, eventual exhaustion

Ego Integrity

Inflated/exalted self perception, with unrealistic self-confidence

Grandiosity may be expressed in a range from unrealistic planning and persistent offering of unsolicited advice (when no expertise exists) to grandiose delusions of a special relationship to important persons, including God, or persecution because of "specialness"

Humor attitude may be caustic/hostile

Food/Fluid

Weight loss often noted

Hygiene

Inattention to ADLs common

Grooming and clothing choices may be inappropriate, flamboyant, and bizarre; excessive use of makeup and jewelry

Neurosensory

Prevailing mood is remarkably expansive, "high," or irritable

Reports of activities that are disorganized and flamboyant or bizarre, denial of probable outcome, perception of mood as desirable and potential as limitless

Mental Status: Concentration/attention poor (responds to multiple irrelevant stimuli in the environment), leading to rapid changes in topics (flight of ideas) in conversation and inability to complete activities

Mood: labile, predominantly euphoric, but easily changed to anger or despair with slightest provocation; mood swings may be profound with intervening periods of normalcy

Delusions: paranoid and grandiose, psychotic phenomena (illusions/hallucinations)

Judgment: poor, irritability common

Speech: rapid and pressured (loquaciousness), with abrupt changes of topic; can progress to disorganized and incoherent

Psychomotor agitation

Safety

May demonstrate a degree of dangerousness to self and others; acting on misperceptions

Sexuality

Increased libido; behavior may be uninhibited

Social Interactions

May be described or viewed as very extroverted/sociable (numerous acquaintances)

History of overinvolvement with other people and with activities; ambitious, unrealistic planning; acts of poor judgment regarding social consequences (uncontrolled spending, reckless driving, problematic or unusual sexual behavior)

Marked impairment in social activities, relationship with others (lack of close relationships), school/occupational functioning, periodic changes in employment/frequent moves

Teaching/Learning

First full episode usually occurs between ages 15 and 24 years, with symptoms lasting at least 1 week

May have been hospitalized for previous episodes of manic behavior

Periodic alcohol or other drug abuse

DIAGNOSTIC STUDIES

Drug Screen: Rule out possibility that symptoms are drug-induced.
Electrolytes: Excess of sodium within the nerve cells may be noted.
Lithium Level: Done when client is receiving this medication to ensure therapeutic range between 0.5 and 1.5 mEq/liter.

NURSING PRIORITIES

1. Protect client/others from the consequences of hyperactive behavior.
2. Provide for client's basic needs.
3. Promote reality orientation, realistic problem-solving, and foster autonomy.
4. Support client/family participation in follow-up care/community treatment.

DISCHARGE GOALS

1. Remains free of injury with decreased occurrence of manic behavior(s).
2. Balance between activity and rest restored.
3. Meeting basic self-care needs.
4. Communicating logically and clearly.
5. Client/family participating in ongoing treatment and understands importance of drug therapy/monitoring.
6. Plan in place to meet needs after discharge.

NURSING DIAGNOSIS	TRAUMA, risk for/VIOLENCE, risk for directed at others
Risk Factors May Include:	Emotional difficulties; irritability and impulsive behavior; delusional thinking; angry response when ideas are refuted/wishes denied
	Manic excitement
	History of assaultive behavior
[Possible Indicators:]	Body language, increased motor activity
	Difficulty evaluating the consequences of own actions
	Overt and aggressive acts; hostile, threatening verbalizations
Desired Outcomes/Evaluation Criteria—Client Will:	Demonstrate self-control with decreased hyperactivity.
	Acknowledge why behavior occurs.
	Verbalize feelings (anger, etc.) in an appropriate manner.
	Use problem-solving techniques instead of violent behavior/threats or intimidation.

ACTIONS/INTERVENTIONS	RATIONALE

Independent

Decrease environmental stimuli, avoiding exposure to areas or situations of predictable high stimulation and removing stimulation from area if client becomes agitated.	Client may be unable to focus attention on only relevant stimuli and will be reacting/responding to all environmental stimuli.

293

Continually reevaluate client's ability to tolerate frustration and/or individual situations.

Facilitates early intervention and assists client to manage situation independently, if possible.

Provide safe environment, removing objects and rearranging room to prevent accidental/purposeful injury to self or others.

Grandiose thinking (e.g., "I am Superman") and hyperactive behavior can lead to destructive actions such as trying to run through the wall/into others.

Intervene when agitation begins to develop, with strategies such as being verbally direct, prompting more effective behavior, redirecting or removing from the provoking situation, voluntary "Time out" in room or a quiet place, physical control (e.g., holding).

Intervention at earliest sign of agitation can assist client in regaining control, preventing escalation to violence and allowing treatment in least restrictive manner.

Defer problem-solving regarding prevention of violence and information collection about precipitating or provoking stimuli until agitation/irritability is diminished (e.g., no "why," analytical questions).

Questions regarding prevention increase frustration because agitation decreases ability to analyze situation.

Communicate rationale for staff action in a concrete manner.

Agitated persons are unable to process complicated communication.

Allow client to enter areas of increased stimuli gradually when he or she is ready to leave "Time out" seclusion area.

Tolerance of environmental stimuli is reduced, and gradual reentry fosters coping ability.

Avoid arguing when client verbalizes unrealistic or grandiose ideas or "put-downs."

Prevents triggering agitation in predictably touchy areas.

Ignore/minimize attention given to undesired behaviors (e.g., bizarre dress, use of profanity), while setting limits on destructive actions.

Avoids giving reinforcement to these behaviors, while providing control for potentially dangerous activities.

Avoid unnecessary delay of gratification. Give concrete and nonjudgmental rationale if refusal is necessary.

In hyperactive state, client does not tolerate waiting or deal well with abstractions, and unnecessary delay can trigger aggressive behavior.

Offer alternatives when available ("I don't have any coffee. Would you like a glass of juice?")

Uses client's distractibility to help decrease the frustration of being refused.

Provide information regarding more independent and alternative problem-solving strategies when client is not labile or irritable.

Improves retention, as agitated person will not be able to recall or use strategies discussed.

Encourage client, during calm moments, to recognize antecedents/precipitants to agitation.

Promotes early recognition of developing problem, allowing client to plan for alternative responses and intervene in a timely fashion.

Assist client in identifying alternative behaviors that are acceptable to both client and staff. Role-play, if indicated. Intervene as necessary to protect client when behavior is provocative or offensive (Refer to ND: Social Interaction, impaired.)

Client will be more apt to follow through on alternatives if they are mutually acceptable. Practice in a nonagitated time helps client learn new behavior. Client may become physically violent with others when behavior is socially unacceptable/rejected.

Provide reinforcement/positive feedback when client attempts to handle frustrating incidents without violence.

Increases feeling of success and the likelihood of client repeating that behavior again.

Collaborative

Analyze any violent incidents with involved staff/observers, identifying antecedents or provoking situations, client indicators of increasing agitation, client response(s) to intervention attempted, etc.

Information is used to develop individualized and proactive interventions based on experience.

Administer medications, as indicated:

Antimanic drugs, e.g., lithium carbonate (Lithobid, Eskalith);

Anticonvulsants, e.g., clonazepam (Klonopin), carbamazepine (Tegretol), valproic acid (Depakene);

Calcium channel blockers, e.g., verapamil (Isoptin);

Antipsychotic drugs, e.g., chlorpromazine (Thorazine), haloperidol (Haldol).

Provide seclusion and/or restraint (according to agency policy).

Prepare for electroconvulsive therapy as indicated.

Lithium is the drug of choice for mania. It is indicated for alleviation of hyperactive symptoms. Have been found to be useful for the alleviation of manic symptoms.

Some clinicians have achieved satisfactory results with these drugs alone, or in combination with lithium.
Useful in decreasing the level of extreme hyperactivity and ameliorating accompanying thought disorder until therapeutic level of lithium can be achieved, or when lithium is ineffective.

May be required for brief period when other measures fail to protect client, staff, or others.

ECT may be required in presence of severe manic decompensation, when client does not tolerate/fails to respond to lithium or other drug treatments. (Refer to CP: Depression Disorders, ND: Injury, risk for.)

NURSING DIAGNOSIS	NUTRITION: altered, less than body requirements
May Be Related to:	Inadequate intake in relation to metabolic expenditures
Possibly Evidenced by:	Body weight 20% or more below ideal weight
	Observed inadequate intake
	Inattention to mealtimes; distraction from task of eating
	Laboratory evidence of nutritional deficits/imbalances
Desired Outcomes/Evaluation Criteria— Client Will:	Verbalize importance of adequate intake.
	Display increased attention to eating behaviors.
	Demonstrate weight gain toward goal.
	Display normalization of laboratory values reflecting improved nutritional status.

ACTIONS/INTERVENTIONS

RATIONALE

Independent

Monitor/record nutritional and fluid intake (including calorie count) and activity level on an ongoing basis.

Helps determine deficits/needs and progress toward goal.

Weigh routinely.

Provides information about therapeutic needs/effectiveness.

295

ACTIONS/INTERVENTIONS	RATIONALE
Offer meals in area with minimal distracting stimuli.	Promotes focus on task of eating and prevents distractions from interfering with food intake.
Walk or sit with client during meals/snack times.	Provides support and encouragement to eat adequate amounts of nutritious foods even if client is unable to sit through meal time.
Have snack foods and juices available at all times.	Nutritious intake is required on a regular basis to compensate for increased caloric requirements resulting from hyperactivity.
Provide opportunity to select foods when client is ready to deal with choices.	Can provide favored foods, sense of control, if alternatives do not add confusion.

Collaborative

Refer to dietitian.	Helpful in determining client's individual needs and most appropriate options to meet needs.
Offer high-protein high-carbohydrate diet. Provide interval feedings, using finger foods.	Maximizes nutritional intake and allows additional opportunity to "boost" dietary intake as client may eat foods that are easily picked up and/or carried around. **Note:** As mania subsides, caloric requirements decline, necessitating adjustment of diet based on client's weight, health status, and activity level.
Review laboratory studies as indicated (e.g., chemistry profile [including electrolytes] and urinalysis).	Indicates nutritional status, identifies therapeutic needs/effectiveness.
Administer supplemental vitamins and minerals.	Corrects dietary deficiencies, improving nutritional status.

NURSING DIAGNOSIS	SLEEP PATTERN disturbance
May Be Related to:	Psychological stress, lack of recognition of fatigue/need to sleep, hyperactivity
Possibly Evidenced by:	Denial of need to sleep
	Interrupted nighttime sleep, one or more nights without sleep
	Changes in behavior and performance, increasing irritability/restlessness
	Dark circles under eyes
Desired Outcome/Evaluation Criteria—	Recognize cues indicating fatigue/need for sleep.
Client Will:	Reestablish sleep pattern as individually appropriate.
	Report feeling well rested and appear relaxed.

ACTIONS/INTERVENTIONS	RATIONALE

Independent

Decrease environmental stimuli in room and common areas.	Manic client is unable to relax and decrease attention to stimuli, affecting ability to fall asleep. **Note:** May need private room, seclusion.

Restrict intake of caffeine (e.g., coffee, tea, cocoa, cola drinks).	May stimulate CNS, interfering with relaxation, ability to sleep.
Offer small snack/warm milk at bedtime or when awake during the night.	Inattention to personal needs may have led to a less than adequate intake, and hunger at night may distract from sleep. Also, L-tryptophan in milk may promote sleep.
Encourage engaging in physical activities/exercise during morning and afternoon. Restrict activity in the evening prior to bedtime.	Enhances sense of fatigue and promotes sleep/rest. Evening activity may actually stimulate client and interfere with/delay sleep.
Encourage routine bedtime activities, relaxation techniques.	Reinforces need for rest, "setting stage" for client to quiet mind and prepare for sleep.
Reroute to bed matter-of-factly, without providing the distraction of other activities.	Avoids stimuli that may stimulate client or provide irritability.

Collaborative

Administer medications as indicated, e.g.: Sedatives;	Careful use may assist in reestablishing sleep pattern.
Antipsychotics, e.g., olanzapine (Zyprexa).	Produces a calming effect, reducing hyperactivity and promoting rest/sleep.

NURSING DIAGNOSIS	SELF CARE DEFICIT: grooming/hygiene, management of personal belongings
May Be Related to:	Lack of concern; impulsivity; poor judgment
	Hyperactivity
Possibly Evidenced by:	Unkempt appearance, dirty, wearing inadequate and/or inappropriate clothing
	Giving away clothing, money, etc., spending or "charging" extravagantly
Desired Outcomes/Evaluation Criteria—Client Will:	Perform self-care activities within level of own ability.
	Use resources/assistance as needed.
	Take responsibility for/manage personal belongings appropriately.

ACTIONS/INTERVENTIONS	RATIONALE

Independent

Assess current level of functioning; reevaluate daily.	Provides information about changes in individual abilities necessary for planning/altering care.
Provide physical assistance, supervision and simple directions/reminders, encouragement and support, as needed.	Helps focus attention on task. Providing only required assistance fosters autonomous functioning.
Acquire needed supplies, including clothing, if not immediately available. Obtain client's own toiletries/clothing as soon as possible.	May not have own necessities if disorganized prior to hospitalization or hospitalized as an emergency measure. Having own supplies/clothing supports autonomy, self-esteem.

297

Limit the selection of clothing available, as indicated.	May be necessary during time of extreme hyperactivity and distractibility until client is able to refrain from bizarre dress and/or care for personal belongings.
Monitor ability to manage money and valuables as well as other personal effects.	May give possessions away, spend money extravagantly, or become involved in grandiose plans.
Intervene to protect client from own impulsivity and from exploitation, if indicated, decreasing restrictions as soon as possible.	Provides protection from deleterious consequences of impulsivity without compromising or undue restriction of civil/personal liberties or autonomous functioning.
Set goals to establish minimum standards for self-care as condition improves (e.g., take a bath every other day, brush teeth twice a day).	Promotes idea that client can begin to assume responsibility for self, enhances sense of self-worth.

NURSING DIAGNOSIS	SENSORY/PERCEPTUAL alterations [overload]
May Be Related to:	Decrease in sensory threshold; psychological stress (narrowed perceptual fields)
	Chemical alteration: endogenous
	Sleep deprivation
Possibly Evidenced by:	Increased distractibility and agitation (in areas/times of increased environmental stimuli); anxiety
	Disorientation; poor concentration; bizarre thinking; auditory/visual hallucinations
	Motor incoordination
Desired Outcomes/Evaluation Criteria— Client Will:	Verbalize awareness/causes of sensory overload.
	Demonstrate behaviors to reduce/manage sensory input (e.g., sits quietly, attends to simple tasks and completes them).
	Initiate and/or take "Time out" in quieter area when prompted.
	Attend and be appropriately involved in activities (e.g., unit meeting, groups).

ACTIONS/INTERVENTIONS	RATIONALE

Independent

| Orient to reality (e.g., identify primary caregiver, where room is). Keep communications simple. | May be disoriented/confused as a result of change of surroundings, multiple distractions. |
| Assist client in focusing on input or task (e.g., address by name; use short, 1-stage directions; provide a low-stimulus area for interview, meals, tasks). | Decreases distractions/choices that are available, helping to gain client's attention in presence of multiple distractions. |

Avoid looking at watch, taking notes, talking to others when focusing on client.

Causes distracting stimuli, adding to stimulation, which can increase hyperactivity.

Remove to area of lower environmental stimulus level if client shows increasing agitation or distractibility.

Reduces distractions, thereby reducing stimulation and diminishing hyperactive behavior.

Explain upcoming events, necessary treatments in advance, giving reasons and using simple terms.

Stimuli may be less overwhelming when client is prepared.

Limit invasion of personal space (e.g., touching clothing, items in room). Use physical touch judiciously.

Reduces stimuli, shows respect for client, who may view touch as threatening.

Observe/monitor for indicators of improved tolerance for multiple sensory stimuli; and increase exposure toward environment, people, activities accordingly.

Allows greatest possible participation in treatment milieu, personal freedom.

NURSING DIAGNOSIS	SOCIAL INTERACTION, impaired
May Be Related to:	Poor judgment; impulsivity; self focus/egocentricity
	Hyperactivity
Possibly Evidenced by:	Inappropriate behavior (e.g., interrupts; is intrusive, demanding, hypercritical and verbally caustic/hostile, provocative and/or teasing; does not respect others' personal space)
	Inappropriate and/or flamboyant social behavior with bizarre dress
	Problematic sexual behavior
Desired Outcomes/Evaluation Criteria— Client Will:	Listen/converse without consistent interruptions.
	Participate appropriately or constructively in 1:1, group, OT.
	Demonstrate social behavior and dress individually consistent with social norms of the client's peer group.
	Respect the privacy and personal property of others.

ACTIONS/INTERVENTIONS	RATIONALE

Independent

Observe for, gently confront manipulative behaviors (e.g., not taking responsibility for own actions, getting others to do things they normally would not do).

Grandiose behavior may be inappropriately used with client becoming demanding and overbearing, interfering with relationships with others. Clients who are manic are attuned to sources of conflict and may consciously or unconsciously escalate the conflict to refocus attention from self, thus putting others on the defensive.

Discuss consequences of client's behavior and ways in which client attempts to attribute them to others.

Redirect or suggest more appropriate behavior using low-key, matter-of-fact, nonjudgmental style.

Ask client to wait until a specified time and give rationale if gratification of a request is not possible.

Maintain a nondefensive response to criticism or suggestions regarding better ways to run things, such as the unit. Use suggestions when appropriate.

Act, as needed, to protect the client when behavior is provocative or offensive.

Offer feedback (positive as well as negative) regarding the impact of social behavior, in 1:1, OT, group therapy.

Help client identify positive aspects about self, recognize accomplishments, and feel good about them.

Problem-solve with client (when able) regarding more effective ways to achieve goals.

Client needs to accept responsibility for own behavior before adaptive change can occur.

Avoids triggering agitated/angry response. Helps reduce and control exaggerated/unrealistic thinking and behaviors.

When the client believes staff responses have reasons, refusals will provoke less agitation.

A low-key response can reduce the volatility of the situation. (This may be frustrating when the client is either outrageous or partly correct.)

When the client is not taking this responsibility, the nurse must be responsible for protecting the client's safety.

The manic client is "outward oriented" and responsive to reinforcement.

As self-esteem is increased, client will feel less need to manipulate others for own gratification.

When lability and poor concentration have improved, client will be able to focus and to control behavior enough to learn/"try out" new behaviors.

NURSING DIAGNOSIS	**SELF ESTEEM, chronic low**
May Be Related to:	Retarded ego development; unmet dependency needs; lack of positive feedback
	Unrealistic self-expectations; personal vulnerability
	Perceived lack of control in some aspect of life; experience of real or perceived failures
Possibly Evidenced by:	Demonstration of exaggerated expectations or sense of own abilities; grandiosity
	Unsatisfactory interpersonal relationships; imperious, demanding behavior; criticism of others
	Hypersensitivity to slights or criticism; excessively seeking reassurance
Desired Outcomes/Evaluation Criteria— Client Will:	Verbalize appropriate/realistic evaluation of own abilities.
	Identify feelings and methods for coping with underlying negative perception of self.
	Formulate realistic plans for recovery.
	Describe strategies for minimizing future impact of personal actions, which can contribute to control of illness.

ACTIONS/INTERVENTIONS	RATIONALE

Independent

Ask how client would like to be addressed. Avoid approaches that imply a different perception of the client's importance.

Grandiosity is thought actually to reflect low self-esteem.

Explain rationale for requests by staff, unit routine, etc. Maintain a nondefensive stance; strictly adhere to respectful/courteous approaches, matter-of-fact style, passive, friendly attitude.

Nursing approaches should reinforce patient dignity, worth. Understanding reasons enhances cooperation with regimen. Nondefensive stance promotes reasoned response, may reduce conflict.

Encourage verbalization and identification of feelings related to issues of chronicity, lack of control impacting self-concept.

Problem-solving begins with agreeing on "the problem."

Help client identify aspects in which control is possible in the therapeutic setting and encourage appropriate assertion of personal control/autonomy.

Allows client to "practice," provides experience of assuming control.

Provide choices of activities (e.g., when to bathe, food desired, participation in social interactions), when possible.

This strategy reduces the client's sense of powerlessness.

Assist client, as reasonable, to maintain personal privacy.

Provides sense of appreciation for the client's dignity.

Offer matter-of-fact feedback regarding unrealistic plans, self-evaluation; use 1:1, group, OT, etc.

Provides an opportunity to cast doubt on unrealistic self-evaluation in the context of accepting relationships. **Note:** These individuals may form therapeutic relationships easily as they are eager to please and appreciate attention. However, the interactions tend to remain shallow.

Identify and reinforce successes and gains made in 1:1, group, and OT settings.

Addressing issues of self-esteem allows the client to be positively reinforced for realistic successes.

Ascertain religious beliefs and spiritual concerns and discuss as indicated, avoiding reinforcing religiosity.

Grandiose behavior is often displayed in over-exaggerated activities related to religious beliefs. Although it is important to support spiritual needs, religiosity does not help client to deal with these needs in an appropriate manner.

Encourage client to view life after discharge and identify aspects over which control is possible. Identify how the client will demonstrate that control.

Role rehearsal helps return client to level of independent functioning. When individual is functioning well, sense of self-esteem is enhanced.

Frame relationship with healthcare provider after discharge as one of collaboration. Emphasize choices, decisions, personal control that will be possible.

Enhances the client's self-perception and sense of control in relation to "experts" promoting feelings of self-worth.

Help client identify a plan that will prevent/minimize severe recurrence of illness. Encourage identification of signs of recurrence and concrete response to symptoms (e.g., "If I go two nights without sleep, I will call my doctor.").

Establishes some concrete guidelines and a plan that will allow community-based care providers to intervene, perhaps preventing an acute episode.

301

Collaborative

Discuss community resources as appropriate, e.g., self-management group (such as National Depressive and Manic-Depressive Association, Recovery, Inc.), social services, spiritual advisor.

Additional resources can help client manage daily lives in the presence of highs and lows of this illness.

NURSING DIAGNOSIS	POISONING, risk for [lithium toxicity]
Risk Factors May Include:	Narrow therapeutic range of drug
	Client's ability (or lack of) to follow through with medication regimen
	Denial of need for information
Possibly Evidenced by:	[Not applicable; presence of signs and symptoms establishes an *actual* diagnosis.]
Desired Outcomes/Evaluation Criteria—Client Will:	List the symptoms of lithium toxicity and appropriate actions to take.
	Identify factors that cause lithium level to change and ways of avoiding this.

ACTIONS/INTERVENTIONS	RATIONALE

Independent

Observe for/review signs of impending drug toxicity (e.g., blurred vision, ataxia, tinnitus, persistent nausea/vomiting, and severe diarrhea). Differentiate from common side effects (e.g., mild nausea, loose stools, thirst/polyuria, metallic taste, headache, tremor).

As there is a very narrow margin between therapeutic and toxic levels, toxicity can occur quickly and requires immediate intervention. The common side effect of tremor may be lessened by use of low doses of propranolol (Inderal) or atenolol (Tenormin).

Assess current understanding, perceptions about medications. Evaluate ability to self-administer medication correctly.

Identifies misinformation/misconceptions about drug therapy and establishes learning needs and likelihood of successful medication routine.

Provide information regarding lithium, using a structured format and informational handout.

Structured client education is more effective. Handout provides a memory prompt.

Frame adherence to medication and follow-up treatment, attention to lifestyle as ways of assuming personal control.

Linking follow-up treatment to the client's goals for self-control may enhance feelings of self-esteem and continued participation in care.

Draw parallel to other kinds of chronic illness (e.g., diabetes, epilepsy).

Supports the need for ongoing care and normalcy of lifelong medication.

Stress importance of adequate sodium and fluid in diet.

Sodium and fluid are required for appropriate lithium excretion, which is necessary to the prevention of toxicity.

Discuss use of nonsteroidal, anti-inflammatory drugs (e.g., ibuprofen [Motrin, Advil, Nuprin]) or thiazide diuretics.

Use of NSAIDs and some diuretics can alter renal clearance of lithium, increasing blood levels and risk of toxicity. **Note:** Potassium-sparing diuretics (e.g., amiloride [Midamon] or triamterene [Dyrenium]) appear to have a higher level of safety in combination with lithium therapy.

302

Encourage involvement of family in regimen/monitoring.

Provide opportunity for client to demonstrate learning after initial class and at least once again before discharge. Clarify misconceptions, confusion about drug use/follow-up care.

Document information that has been given and how client/family demonstrate learning.

Collaborative

Monitor serum lithium levels at least twice a week upon initiation of drug therapy until serum levels are stable, then weekly to bimonthly, as indicated.

Provide a schedule for regular laboratory testing and follow-up appointments at discharge.

Enhances understanding of reason for/importance of drug therapy.

Determines success of client education/additional needs and helps to plan appropriate follow-up.

Provides continuity, communicates to other providers the level of client's/family's knowledge.

Narrow therapeutic range increases risk of developing toxicity. Early detection and prompt intervention may prevent serious complications.

Assists client to stay on medication and maintain improved state.

NURSING DIAGNOSIS	FAMILY PROCESSES, altered
May Be Related to:	Situational crises (illness, economic, change in roles)
	Euphoric mood and grandiose ideas/actions of client
	Manipulative behavior and limit-testing, client's refusal to accept responsibility for own actions
Possibly Evidenced by:	Statements of difficulty coping with situation
	Lack of adaptation to change or not dealing constructively with illness; ineffective family decision-making process
	Failure to send and to receive clear messages; inappropriate boundary maintenance
Desired Outcomes/Evaluation Criteria—Family Will:	Express feelings freely and appropriately.
	Demonstrate individual involvement in problem-solving processes directed at appropriate solutions.
	Verbalize understanding of illness, treatment regimen, and prognosis.
	Encourage and allow member who is ill to handle situation in own way, progressing toward independence.

ACTIONS/INTERVENTIONS	RATIONALE

Independent

Determine individual situation and feelings of individual family members (e.g., guilt, anger, powerlessness, despair, and alienation).

Living with a family member with bipolar illness engenders a multitude of feelings and problems that can affect interpersonal relationships/functioning and may result in dysfunctional responses/family disintegration.

303

Observe patterns of communication (e.g., Are feelings expressed freely? Who makes decisions? What is the interaction between family members?).

Provides clues to degree of problem being experienced by individual family members and coping skills being used to handle crisis of illness.

Identify boundaries of family members (e.g., Do members share family identity and have little sense of individuality, or do they seem emotionally distant?).

Degree of symbiotic involvement/distancing of family members affects ability to resolve problems related to behavior of identified patient.

Determine patterns of behavior displayed by client in relationships with others (e.g., manipulation of self-esteem of others, perceptiveness to vulnerability and conflict, projection of responsibility, progressive limit-testing, and alienation of family members).

These behaviors are typically used by the manic individual to manipulate others. These clients are sensitive to others' vulnerability and can intentionally escalate conflict, shifting responsibility from self to others and putting the other person on the defensive. Family members assume blame and continually try to keep peace at any cost. The client will test limits, constantly getting concessions from others and creating feelings of guilt and ambivalence. The result of these behaviors is alienation and high rate of divorce.

Assess role of client in family (e.g., nurturer, provider) and how illness affects the roles of other members.

When the role of the ill person is not filled, dissonance and family disintegration can occur. The spouse and children of the manic individual may not understand what is happening and react in an adversarial manner, escalating the conflicts that exist.

Identify other sources of conflict such as spiritual values/religious beliefs, financial issues.

Client's behavior has an impact on all areas of life, resulting in multiple conflicts that must be addressed to achieve stability.

Acknowledge difficulties observed while reinforcing that some degree of conflict is to be expected and can be used to promote growth.

Provides support for family members who may feel helpless to change the client and/or what is happening in his or her life.

Provide information (including books and articles) about behavior patterns and expected course of the illness. Encourage discussion of the acute episode with the client. Assist families to understand normal aspects of bipolar illness.

This knowledge may relieve guilt and promote family discussion of the problems and solutions. Family members tend to hide the illness of the client and excuse the manic's behavior with a variety of rationalizations. The use of bibliotherapy can enhance learning and the process of change.

Encourage family members to confront client's behavior.

Family may be afraid to discuss the behavior because of the client's volatile temper. Confrontation can promote insight into the dynamics of the illness and bring about a positive resolution of the family situation.

Instruct in use of stress management techniques (e.g., appropriate expression of feelings, use of relaxation exercises, imagery [when appropriate]).

Assists individuals to develop coping skills to deal with the client and difficult situations. Imagery may be counterproductive for the client when not in touch with reality.

Collaborative

Involve family members in planning of treatment regimen.

Agreement with goals and therapeutic regimen enhances commitment. Family support can be instrumental in client's success/failure.

Encourage participation of client and family members in support groups (such as, Families of Depressives and Depressive Support Group), psychological counseling/family therapy.

Refer to additional resources as appropriate (e.g., spiritual advisor, social services, legal counsel).

May provide additional assistance in dealing with daily life and incorporating lifestyle changes that may be helpful.

Manic behavior and grandiose behavior may have entangled client in situations that require specific assistance.

CHAPTER 9

ANXIETY DISORDERS

GENERALIZED ANXIETY DISORDER

DSM-IV
300.02 Generalized anxiety disorder

Although some degree of anxiety is normal in life's stresses, anxiety can be adaptive or maladaptive. Problems arise when the client has coping mechanisms that are inadequate to deal with the danger, which may be recognized or unrecognized. The essential feature of this inadequacy is unrealistic or excessive anxiety and worries about life circumstances. Anxiety disorders are the most common of all major groups of mental disorders in the United States, sharing comorbidity with major depression and substance abuse, increasing the client's risk of suicide.

ETIOLOGICAL THEORIES

Psychodynamics

The Freudian view involves conflict between demands of the id and superego, with the ego serving as mediator. Anxiety occurs when the ego is not strong enough to resolve the conflict. Sullivanian theory states that fear of disapproval from the mothering figure is the basis for anxiety. Conditional love results in a fragile ego and lack of self-confidence. The individual with anxiety disorder has low self-esteem, fears failure, and is easily threatened.

Dollard and Miller (1950) believe anxiety is a learned response based on an innate drive to avoid pain. Anxiety results from being faced with two competing drives or goals.

Cognitive theory suggests that there is a disturbance in the central mechanism of cognition or information processing with the consequent disturbance in feeling and behavior. Anxiety is maintained by this distorted thinking with mistaken or dysfunctional appraisal of a situation. The individual feels vulnerable, and the distorted thinking results in a negative outcome.

Biological

Although biological and neurophysiological influences in the etiology of anxiety disorders have been investigated, no relationship has yet been established. However, there does seem to be a genetic influence with a high family incidence.

The autonomic nervous system discharge that occurs in response to a frightening impulse and/or emotion is mediated by the limbic system, resulting in the peripheral effects of the autonomic nervous system seen in the presence of anxiety.

Some medical conditions have been associated with anxiety and panic disorders, such as abnormalities in the hypothalamic-pituitary-adrenal and hypothalamic-pituitary-thyroid axes, acute myocardial infarction, pheochromocytomas, substance intoxication and withdrawal, hypoglycemia, caffeine intoxication, mitral valve prolapse, and complex partial seizures.

Family Dynamics

The individual exhibiting dysfunctional behavior is seen as the representation of family system problems. The "identified patient" (IP) is carrying the problems of the other members of the family, which are seen as the result of the interrelationships (disequilibrium) between family members rather than as isolated individual problems.

It is recognized that multiple factors contribute to anxiety disorders.

CLIENT ASSESSMENT DATA BASE

Activity/Rest

Restlessness, pacing anxiously, or, if seated, restlessly moving extremities
Feeling "keyed up"/"on edge," unable to relax
Easily fatigued
Difficulty falling or staying asleep; restlessness, unsatisfying sleep

Circulation

Heart pounding or racing/palpitations; cold and clammy hands; hot or cold spells, sweating; flushing, pallor
High resting pulse, increased blood pressure

Ego Integrity

Excessive worry about a number of events/activities, occurring more days than not for at least 6 months
Complains vociferously about inner turmoil, has difficulty controlling worry
May demand help
Facial expression in keeping with level of anxiety felt (e.g., furrowed brow, strained face, eyelid twitch)
May report history of threat to either physical integrity (illness, inadequate food and housing, etc.) or self-concept (loss of significant other; assumption of new role)

Elimination

Frequent urination; diarrhea

Food/Fluid

Lack of interest in food, dysfunctional eating pattern (e.g., responding to internal cues other than hunger)
Dry mouth, upset stomach, discomfort in the pit of the stomach, lump in the throat

Neurosensory

Absence of other mental disorder, such as depressive disorder or schizophrenia
Motor tension: shakiness, jitteriness, jumpiness, trembling, muscle tension, easily startled
Dizziness, lightheadedness, tingling hands or feet
Apprehensive expectation: anxiety, worry, fear, rumination, anticipation of misfortune to self or others, inability to act differently (feeling stuck)
Excessive vigilance/hyperattentiveness resulting in distractibility, difficulty in concentrating or mind going blank, irritability, impatience
Free-floating anxiety usually chronic or persisting over weeks/months

Pain/Discomfort

Muscle aches, headaches

307

Respiratory

Increased respiratory rate, shortness of breath, smothering sensation

Sexuality

Women twice as likely to be affected as men

Social Interactions

Significant impairment in social/occupational functioning

Teaching/Learning

Age of onset usually 20s and 30s

DIAGNOSTIC STUDIES

Drug Screen: Rules out drugs as contribution to cause of symptoms.
Other diagnostic studies may be conducted to rule out physical disease as basis for individual symptoms (e.g., ECG for severe chest pain, echocardiogram for mitral valve prolapse; EEG to identify seizure activity; thyroid studies).

NURSING PRIORITIES

1. Assist client to recognize own anxiety.
2. Promote insight into anxiety and related factors.
3. Provide opportunity for learning new, adaptive coping responses.
4. Involve client and family in educational/support activities.

DISCHARGE GOALS

1. Feelings of anxiety recognized and handled appropriately.
2. Coping skills developed to manage anxiety-provoking situations.
3. Resources identified and used effectively.
4. Client/family participating in ongoing therapy program.
5. Plan in place to meet needs after discharge.

NURSING DIAGNOSIS	ANXIETY [severe]/POWERLESSNESS
May Be Related to:	Real or perceived threat to physical integrity or self-concept (may or may not be able to identify the threat)
	Unconscious conflict about essential values (beliefs) and goals of life; unmet needs
	Negative self-talk
Possibly Evidenced by:	Persistent feelings of apprehension and uneasiness (related to unidentified stressor or stimulus) that client has difficulty alleviating
	Sympathetic stimulation; restlessness; extraneous movements (foot shuffling, hand/arm fidgeting, rocking movements)
	Poor eye contact; focus on self

Desired Outcomes/Evaluation Criteria— Client Will:	Impaired functioning; verbal expressions of having no control or influence over situation, outcome, or self-care
	Free-floating anxiety
	Nonparticipation in care or decision-making when opportunities are provided
	Verbalize awareness of feelings of anxiety.
	Identify effective coping mechanisms to successfully deal with stress.
	Report anxiety is reduced to a manageable level.
	Demonstrate problem-solving skills/lifestyle changes as indicated for individual situation.

ACTIONS/INTERVENTIONS

RATIONALE

Independent

ACTIONS/INTERVENTIONS	RATIONALE
Establish and maintain a trusting relationship through the use of warmth, empathy, and respect. Provide adequate time for response. Communicate support of the client's self-expression.	The client may perceive the nurse as a threat, which may increase the client's anxiety. Attending behaviors can increase the degree of comfort the client experiences with the nurse.
Be aware of any negative or anxious feelings nurse may have because of client's conscious or unconscious resistance of nurse's helpful efforts.	Negative reactions to the client will block future progress. Anxiety is "contagious," and nurse needs to recognize and control own anxiety.
Identify behaviors of the client that produce anxiety in the nurse. Explore these behaviors with the client once relationship is established.	Promotes growth and change and helps client realize how own behavior affects others.
Use supportive confrontation as indicated.	Confrontation can be useful when client's progress is blocked but may heighten anxiety to a level that is detrimental to the therapy process. Therefore, it should be used with caution.
Have client identify and describe the sensations of emotional and physical feelings. Assist the client to link behavior and feelings. Validate all inferences and assumptions with the client.	To adopt new coping responses, the "5 R's" of anxiety reduction are used. The client first needs to **RECOGNIZE** anxiety and be aware of feelings, how they link to certain maladaptive coping responses, and own responsibility in learning to control behavior.
Help to explore conflictual issues by beginning with nonthreatening topics and progressing to more conflict-laden ones.	Anxious client does not think clearly, and beginning with simple topics promotes comfort level, increasing sense of success and progress.
Monitor the anxiety level of the nurse/client interaction on an ongoing basis.	Moderate anxiety may be productive for/motivate client, but too high a level of anxiety can interfere with the interaction and ability to attend to information.
Assist the client to identify the situations and interactions that immediately precede the anxiety. Suggest that the client keep an "anxiety notebook" that focuses on feelings and what is going on in the environment when anxious feelings begin.	After the client recognizes feelings of anxiety, examination of the development of the anxiety (e.g., what precipitates it, the strength of the stressor[s]) and what resources are available can help the client develop new coping skills.

309

Help client correlate cause-and-effect relationships between stressor and anxiety.

Therapeutic writing serves to decrease the anxiety while the client is learning about it, making it more tangible/controllable.

Gives more control over situation. Increases sense of power if client can identify cause of anxiety.

Note when reports of anxiety move from one concern to another (e.g., money, health, relationships), and help client recognize what is happening.

Feelings of anxiety can become "free-floating," becoming attached to one concern after another, and the client needs to recognize this so it can be dealt with.

Link the present experience with relevant ones from the past. Ask questions like, "Does that seem familiar to you? What does it remind you of from the past?"

Provides opportunity for client to make connections between these events and development of current anxiety, promoting insight and learning experience.

Explore how client dealt with anxiety in the past and what methods produced relief. Encourage use of adaptive coping responses that have worked in the past.

Increases confidence in own ability to deal with stress. The client is capable of learning new, adaptive coping responses by analyzing coping mechanisms used previously, identifying available resources, and accepting personal responsibility for change, effectively **REMOVING** the threat or stressors underlying the anxiety. (Refer to ND: Coping, Individual, ineffective.)

Include significant others as resources and social supports in helping client learn new coping responses.

Enhances ability to cope when one does not feel alone. In addition, because anxiety may have an interpersonal basis, involvement of SO(s) can enhance the client's relationship skills. **RELATIONSHIPS** can provide support, help, and reassurance, enabling the use of others as resources rather than using withdrawal to cope.

Ask client to remember times when she or he anticipated the worst and it did *not* happen. Focus attention on those situations.

May be useful to help client understand the dynamics of negative thinking and its relationship to feelings of anxiety.

Encourage and support more realistic thoughts, e.g., "I don't know for certain that (blank) will happen." "Whatever happens, I can manage." "I'll delay worrying for now and think about something calming."

Replacing negative thoughts with positive or calming thoughts can be helpful in stopping the cycle of negative thinking.

Keep the focus of responsibility for change on the client.

Increases feelings of self-control and self-esteem.

Expose client slowly to anxiety-provoking situations; use role-playing as appropriate.

RE-ENGAGEMENT allows the client time to identify/implement and practice new, adaptive coping responses and to become comfortable in using them.

Assist to reevaluate goals, modify behavior, use resources, and test out new coping responses.

Goals may have been too rigid and may have set up client for anxiety that could be avoided by change in behavior/responses.

Develop regular physical activity program.

Excess energy is discharged in a healthful manner through physical exercise. Biochemical effects of exercise therapy decrease feelings of anxiety.

Encourage client to use relaxation techniques (e.g., meditation, massage, breathing techniques, exercises, guided imagery, and biofeedback).

RELAXATION is the ultimate stress management technique because it brings about a decreased heart rate, lowers metabolism, and decreases respiration rate. The relaxation response is the physiological opposite of the anxiety response.

Collaborative

Administer medication as indicated, e.g., buspirone (BuSpar), benzodiazepines, e.g., alprazolam (Xanax), clonazepam (Klonopin), clorazepate (Tranxene), chloridiazepoxide (Librium), diazepam (Valium), oxazepam (Serax).

Anxiolytics provide relief from the immobilizing effects of anxiety. BZDs have few side effects, are generally well tolerated, have a fairly rapid rate of onset, and do not impair sleep. **Note:** When anxiety is associated with depression, anti-depressant agents alone may provide relief of symptoms. Unlike BZDs, BuSpar is nonaddicting, has a delayed onset of action (10 days–2 weeks), and must be taken on a regular basis (not PRN).

NURSING DIAGNOSIS	COPING, INDIVIDUAL, ineffective
May Be Related to:	Level of anxiety being experienced by client
	Inadequate coping methods
	Personal vulnerability; unmet expectations; inadequate support systems
	Little or no exercise
	Multiple stressors, repeated over period of time
Possibly Evidenced by:	Maladaptive coping skills; verbalization of inability to cope
	Chronic worry, emotional tension; muscular tension/headaches; chronic fatigue, insomnia
	Inability to problem-solve
	Alteration in societal participation
	High rate of accidents; overeating, excessive smoking, or drinking/drug use
Desired Outcomes/Evaluation Criteria— Client Will:	Identify ineffective coping behaviors and consequences.
	Express feelings appropriately.
	Identify options and use resources effectively.
	Use effective problem-solving techniques.

ACTIONS/INTERVENTIONS	RATIONALE

Independent

Assess current functional capacity, developmental level of functioning, and level of coping. Determine

Knowing how client's coping ability is affected by current events determines need for/type of defense mechanisms used (e.g., denial, repression, conversion, dissociation, reaction formation, undoing, displacement or projection).

Identify previous methods of coping with life problems.

Determine use of substances (e.g., alcohol, other drugs; smoking habits; eating patterns).

Observe and describe behavior in objective terms. Validate observations with client as possible. Note physical complaints.

Assess for premenstrual tension syndrome, when indicated.

Active-listen client concerns and identify perceptions of what is happening.

Confront client behaviors in context of trusting relationship, pointing out differences between words and actions, when appropriate.

Help client identify maladaptive effects of present coping mechanisms.

Provide information about different ways to deal with situations that promote anxious feelings (e.g., identification and appropriate expression of feelings and problem-solving skills).

Use role-play and rehearsal techniques as indicated.

Encourage and support client in evaluating lifestyle, noting activities and stresses of family, work, and social situations.

Have client identify short- and long-term goals that are attainable, prioritized according to individual client needs and realistic time requirements.

Recommend dividing tasks into manageable units. Let client know it is OK to say "No" to requests for additional work/other commitments.

Suggest simplifying work environment; interrupting stressful periods with breaks for relaxation.

Emphasize importance of structuring life to provide adequate exercise/sleep, diversional activities, and nutrition.

intervention. People tend to regress during illness/crisis and need acceptance and support to regain/improve coping ability.

How client has handled in the past problems is a reliable predictor of how current problems will be handled.

Substances are often used as coping mechanism to control anxiety and can interfere with client's ability to deal with current situation.

Provides accurate picture of client situation and avoids judgmental evaluations. Anxious people may have increased somatic concerns. (Refer to CP: Somatoform Disorders.)

Increased progesterone may cause increased anxiety for women during the luteal phase of the menstrual cycle.

Promotes sense of self-worth and value for beliefs and clarifies client view of situation.

Helps client to become aware of distortions of reality resulting from anxiety state.

Promotes understanding of relationship of what the individual does to undesired consequences.

Provides opportunity for client to learn new coping skills and incorporate these into own lifestyle.

Promotes practice of new skills in a nonthreatening environment.

Helps client to look at difficult areas that may contribute to anxiety and to make changes gradually without undue/debilitating anxiety.

Helps provide direction, enables evaluation of progress, promotes feelings of success as goals are attained. Unrealistic goals set client up for failure and reinforce feelings of powerlessness.

Focuses on achieving goals by small steps. Giving permission to refuse to take on more than client can handle frees individual from added stressors, increasing likelihood of success.

Enhances coping skills by reducing distractions, promoting sense of control, and allowing individual to return to task refreshed.

Structure provides feeling of security for the anxious client. Promotes a less stressful lifestyle, enhances feelings of general well-being and ability to cope.

Collaborative

Refer to outside resources (e.g., support groups, psychotherapy/counselor, spiritual advisor, sexual counseling) as indicated.

May need additional assistance or support to maintain improvement/control.

NURSING DIAGNOSIS	SOCIAL INTERACTION, impaired/SOCIAL ISOLATION
May Be Related to:	Use of unsuccessful social interaction behaviors
	Inadequate personal resources; absence of available significant others/peers
	Self-concept disturbance
	Altered mental status, hypervigilance
Possibly Evidenced by:	Verbalized/observed discomfort in social situations; dysfunctional interactions
	Expression of feelings of difference from others; preoccupation with own thoughts, irritability, impatience, difficulty in concentrating
	Sad, dull affect; uncommunicative, withdrawn behavior; absence of eye contact
Desired Outcomes/Evaluation Criteria— Client Will:	Recognize anxiety and identify factors involved with feelings of isolation/impaired social interactions.
	Participate in activities to enhance interactions with others.
	Give self positive reinforcement for changes that are achieved.

ACTIONS/INTERVENTIONS	RATIONALE

Independent

Listen to client comments regarding sense of isolation. Differentiate isolation from solitude and loneliness.	Provides information about individual concerns/problems of feelings of aloneness. Client may not be aware of difference between being alone by choice and feeling of being alone even when others are around.
Spend time with client, discussing areas of concern (e.g., reasons anxious feelings interfere with ability to be involved with others). Express positive regard for the client; Active-listen concerns.	Provides opportunity for learning ways to deal with feelings of anxiety in social situations. Communicates belief in client's self-worth and provides safe environment for self-disclosure.
Develop plan of action with client; look at available resources, risk-taking behaviors, appropriate self-care.	Involvement of client communicates sense of competence and ability to change behavior, even in presence of anxious feelings.
Assess client's use of coping skills and defense mechanisms.	Awareness of defenses individual is using provides for choice of changing behavior. Helps to develop skills that can be used to manage anxiety and promote social interaction.

Help client learn social skills and use role-playing for practice.

Encourage journal-keeping and daily recording of social interactions for review.

Provides for new ways to handle anxiety in interaction with others.

Helps client recognize the comfort/discomfort that is experienced and possible causes, providing insight that may reduce anxiety. Therapeutic writing is also useful in evaluating individual responses/coping behaviors. (Refer to ND: Coping, Individual, ineffective.)

Recommend that client share/discuss situation with peers/coworkers.

Helps others understand condition, reducing risk of misinterpretation and decreasing individual anxiety. Provides opportunity for client to hear own words, gain new perspective, and begin to problem-solve new ways of handling stressors.

Collaborative

Involve in classes/programs directed at resolution of problems (e.g., assertiveness training, group therapy, outdoor education program).

Developing positive social skills/behaviors provides opportunity for diminishing anxiety and promoting involvement with others.

NURSING DIAGNOSIS	SLEEP PATTERN disturbance
May Be Related to:	Psychological stress
	Repetitive thoughts
Possibly Evidenced by:	Reports of difficulty in falling asleep/awakening earlier or later than desired; not feeling rested
	Dark circles under eyes; frequent yawning
Desired Outcomes/Evaluation Criteria— Client Will:	Verbalize understanding of relationship of anxiety and sleep disturbance.
	Identify appropriate interventions to promote sleep.
	Report improvement in sleep pattern, increased sense of well-being, and feeling well-rested.

ACTIONS/INTERVENTIONS

RATIONALE

Independent

Determine type of sleep pattern disturbance present, including usual bedtime, rituals/routines, number of hours of sleep, time of arising, environmental needs, and how much of a problem it is to client.

Identification of individual situation and degree of interference with functioning determines need for/appropriate interventions.

Provide quiet environment, comfort measures (e.g., back rub, wash hands/face, bath), and sleep aids, such as warm milk. Restrict use of caffeine and alcohol before bedtime.

Promotes relaxation and cues for falling asleep. Stimulating effects of caffeine/alcohol interfere with ability to fall asleep.

Discuss use of relaxation techniques/thoughts, visualization.

Promotes reduction of anxious feelings, resulting in improved sleep/rest.

314

Suggest ways to handle waking/not sleeping (e.g., do not lie in bed and think, but get up and remain inactive, or do something boring).	Having a plan can reduce anxiety about not sleeping.
Involve client in exercise program, avoiding exercise within 2 hours of going to bed.	Increases fatigue, promotes sleep but avoids excessive stimulation from activity before bedtime.
Avoid use of sedatives, when possible.	Sedative drugs interfere with REM sleep and affect quality of rest. A rebound effect may lead to intense dreaming, nightmares, and more disturbed sleep.

Collaborative

Administer medications as indicated, e.g., zolpidem (Ambien).	Although drug is recommended for short-term use only, it may be beneficial until other therapeutic interventions are successful.

NURSING DIAGNOSIS	FAMILY COPING: ineffective, risk for compromised
Risk Factors May Include:	Inadequate or incorrect information or understanding by a primary person
	Temporary family disorganization and role changes
	Prolonged disability that exhausts the supportive capacity of significant other(s)
Possibly Evidenced by:	[Not applicable, presence of signs and symptoms establishes an *actual* diagnosis.]
Desired Outcomes/Evaluation Criteria— Family Will:	Identify resources within themselves to deal with situation.
	Interact appropriately with the client, providing support and assistance as needed.
	Recognize own needs for support, seek assistance, and use resources effectively.

ACTIONS/INTERVENTIONS	RATIONALE

Independent

Assess information available to and understood by family/SO(s).	Lack of understanding of client's behavior can lead to dysfunctional interactional patterns, which contribute to anxiety in family members.
Identify client's role in family and how the illness has changed the family organization (e.g., mother who does not maintain household, father who does not go to work).	Degree of disability suffered by the client that interferes with performance of usual family role can contribute to family stress/disorganization.
Note other factors besides illness (e.g., anxiety, personality disorders) that affect family members' ability to provide needed support.	Systems theory maintains that other members of the family also exhibit dysfunctional behavior, but the client is the "identified patient."

Discuss underlying reasons for client's behaviors.	Helps family understand and accept behaviors that may be difficult to handle.
Assist family and client to understand who "owns" the problem and who is responsible for resolution.	Promotes responsibility of knowing that whoever has the problem has to solve it. The individual can ask for help, but others do not rescue or try to solve it for the person.
Encourage development of problem-solving skills.	Helps family learn new ways to deal with conflicts and reduce anxiety-provoking situations.

Collaborative

Refer to appropriate resources as indicated (e.g., counseling, psychotherapy; financial, spiritual advisors).	May need additional assistance to maintain family integrity.

SAMPLE CLINICAL PATHWAY:
Generalized Anxiety Disorder ELOS: 6 sessions—Clinical Nurse Specialist, Private Practice

ND and categories of care	Time dimension	Outcomes/ actions	Time dimension	Outcomes/ actions	Time dimension	Outcomes/ actions
Anxiety (severe)/Powerlessness R/T real or perceived threat to physical integrity or self-concept, unconscious conflict about essential values/ beliefs and goals of life, unmet needs, negative self talk, inadequate coping methods	Session 1 Session 2	Verbalize awareness of feelings of anxiety Identify ineffective coping behaviors and consequences	Session 3 Session 3–6 Session 4–5	Identify effective coping mechanisms to successfully deal with stress Report anxiety reduced to manageable level Demonstrate effective problem-solving skills Initiate lifestyle changes as indicated	Session 5 Session 6	Express feelings freely Identify options and use resources effectively
Referrals	Session 1	Primary care provider, Psychologist/ Psychiatrist	Session 4	Spiritual advisor as appropriate	Session 6	Healthcare providers/ community resources based on individual need
Diagnostic Studies		(Based on individual need: Rule out physical illness, e.g., ECG, echocardiogram, thyroid levels, EEG, PMS evaluation, drug screen)				
Additional Assessment	Session 1 Session 1–6 Session 2–3	Psychosocial history Level of anxiety Review physical exam from care provider Verify status/results of medical screening evaluation (based on physical findings)			Session 3–6	Response to medication and side effects (if used) Review journal entries, identify concerns

continued

317

Generalized Anxiety Disorder ELOS: 6 sessions—Clinical Nurse Specialist, Private Practice (continued)

ND and categories of care	Time dimension	Outcomes/actions	Time dimension	Outcomes/actions	Time dimension	Outcomes/actions
Medication Allergies: ———	Session 2–6	Anxiolytic, antidepressant as indicated				
Action/therapies	Session 1	Establish nurse/client relationship Identify anxious feelings/triggers Active-listen concerns Identify stressful aspects of lifestyle/work Determine use of substances	Session 3	Correlate cause and effect relationship of anxious feelings Discuss possible modifications of environment Instruct in relaxation techniques Use supportive confrontation when necessary	Session 5	(Family session)
	Session 2	Explore conflictual issues Determine defense mechanisms used and previous methods of coping Begin process of cognitive restructuring Discuss exercise program Initiate journal keeping Instruct in use, expected effects, adverse reactions of medications if prescribed	Session 4	Keep focus of responsibility for change on client Discuss problem-solving process Role-play identified behavior changes	Session 6	[20 mins following family session] Review discharge plan, community resources. therapeutic regimen
Risk for Ineffective Family Coping—Risk factors: temporary family disorganization, role changes, prolonged disability exhausting supporting capacity of SOs	Session 5	Identify resources within members to deal with situation	Session 6	Interact appropriately with client providing support and assistance as needed		

Referrals		Family therapy/counseling, spiritual advisor, financial planner
	Session 6	
Additional assessments	Session 5	Information available to/understood by family members
Action/therapies	Session 5	Identify each member role in family and change in family organization due to illness
		Discuss and explain underlying reasons for behaviors
		Discuss who owns problem
		Identify ways to deal with changes in client/family interactions; helping skills
	Session 6 (first 30 min)	Review problem-solving skills
		Determine future expectations
		Role-play anticipated changes as indicated

PANIC DISORDER/PHOBIAS

DSM-IV
PANIC DISORDER/PHOBIAS
300.01 Panic disorder without agoraphobia
300.21 Panic disorder with agoraphobia
300.22 Agoraphobia without history of panic disorder
300.23 Social phobia
300.29 Specific phobia

Panic attack is a discrete period of intense fear or discomfort with onset spontaneous/ unpredictable or situationally bound, peaking within 10 minutes.

ETIOLOGICAL THEORIES

Psychodynamics

Phobic object may symbolize the underlying conflict, although there is not always a clear connection. Personal perceptions, life experiences, and cultural values color the meaning of the symbol for the client.

The freudian view is that anxiety feelings stem from loss of love and support from the mothering figure, which increases the client's dependency needs. The client combats the diffuse intolerable anxiety by an exaggerated use of displacement on a particular object or situation, which makes the anxiety more manageable.

Phobic partners may develop in the family; these are "helpers" who stand by and participate in maintaining phobic behavior, protecting phobic client from acute panic and anxiety. Participation of partner furthers the unconscious wish of phobic client to be taken care of and to be in control.

Biological

(Refer to CP: Generalized Anxiety Disorder.)

Temperament may be a factor in that some fears are innate. These fears represent a part of the overall characteristics with which one is born that influence how the individual responds to specific situations throughout his or her life. Research suggests irregularities in the synthesis and release of norepinephrine and/or hypersensitivity of receptors for neurotransmitters (including serotonin and gamma-aminobutyric acid [GABA]), or an interaction between norepinephrine transmitters. The trigger may lie in the locus coeruleus located in the brainstem. There also may be a genetic susceptibility to either an excess or deficiency of CO_2 levels and a sensitivity to lactate associated with the panic attack.

Family Dynamics

(Refer to CP: Generalized Anxiety Disorder.)

CLIENT ASSESSMENT DATA BASE

Circulation

Palpitations or tachycardia
Sweating, hot flashes, or chills

Ego Integrity

A persistent fear of some object/situation that poses no actual danger or in which the danger is magnified out of proportion to its seriousness; tries to avoid or escape contact with the feared object or situation

Degree of discomfort may vary from mild anxiety to incapacitation; may be unable to move, speak, or identify ways of decreasing anxiety or may begin running about aimlessly and shouting

May express a sensation of dread and a certain knowledge that death is at hand or may fear dying, going crazy, or doing something uncontrolled

Food/Fluid

Nausea/abdominal distress

Neurosensory

May exhibit one of three types of phobias:

Agoraphobia: Fears any situation in which individual may feel helpless or humiliated if a panic attack should occur and client cannot readily escape from public view

Specific/Simple Phobia: Fear involving specific objects such as spiders or snakes or situations such as heights, darkness, or closed spaces

Social Phobia: Fear of talking or writing in public and/or eating, blushing, urinating, etc.; fear of these behaviors resulting in public scorn

Preoccupied with bodily symptoms and feelings of terror

Feelings of faintness, dizziness, or lightheadedness; trembling/shaking; paresthesias (numbness or tingling sensations)

May experience brief periods of delusional thinking, hallucinations, inability to test reality

Depersonalization or derealization

Pain/Discomfort

Chest pain or discomfort

Respiratory

Shortness of breath (dyspnea); smothering sensations, choking; hyperventiliation, labored breathing

Sexuality

Occurs more frequently in women than in men

May avoid sexual involvement because of fear of arousal, particular sexual acts, and/or relationships

Social Interactions

More common among people who have experienced an early traumatic loss, such as the death of a parent

Manipulates environment and depends on others to avoid confrontation with the object or situation

Some constriction of life activities present

Teaching/Learning

Usually begins in late teens or early adulthood (panic attacks rare after age 65)

Attacks may be associated with magic or witchcraft

No history of a physical disorder (e.g., hyperthyroidism, hypoglycemia), although mitral valve prolapse is common

May report other disorders such as major depression, somatization disorder, schizophrenia, personality disorder

Increased rate of alcohol abuse

321

DIAGNOSTIC STUDIES

Drug Screen: Identifies drugs that may be used by client to reduce anxiety, rules out drugs that may produce symptoms.

Other diagnostic studies may be conducted to rule out physical disease as a basis for individual symptoms, e.g.:

EEG: To rule out epilepsy, other neurological disorders.

EKG: In the presence of severe chest pain to rule out cardiac conditions.

Thyroid Studies: To rule out hyperthyroidism.

NURSING PRIORITIES

1. Provide for physical safety.
2. Assist client to recognize onset of anxiety.
3. Help client learn alternative responses.
4. Assist with desensitization to phobic object/situation, if present.
5. Promote involvement of client/family in group or community support activities.

DISCHARGE GOALS

1. Stays in feared situation even when discomfort is experienced.
2. Identifies techniques to lower/keep fear at manageable level.
3. Confronts the phobia and is desensitized to the stimulus.
4. Demonstrates greater independence and an increasingly freer lifestyle.
5. Plan in place to meet needs after discharge.

(Refer to CP: Generalized Anxiety Disorder for needs/concerns in addition to the following NDs.)

NURSING DIAGNOSIS	FEAR
May Be Related to:	Unfounded morbid dread of a seemingly harmless object/situation (e.g., fear of being alone in public places, snakes, spiders, dark, heights, stormy weather [virtually any object/situation])
Possibly Evidenced by:	Physiological symptoms, mental/cognitive behaviors indicative of panic
	Withdrawal from or total avoidance of situations that place client in contact with feared object
Desired Outcomes/Evaluation Criteria—Client Will:	Acknowledge and discuss fears.
	Demonstrate understanding through use of effective coping behaviors and active participation in treatment regimen.
	Resume normal life activities.

ACTIONS/INTERVENTIONS	RATIONALE
Independent	
Encourage discussion of the phobia. Investigate sexual concerns, noting problems expressed (e.g., sex is a duty/obligation that is not enjoyed by the client).	Only when a difficulty is acknowledged can it be dealt with. **Note:** Phobic reaction to sex may indicate a problem of incest/sexual abuse.

Provide for client's safety (e.g., a secure environment, staying with the client, letting the client know the nurse will provide for safety).

In severe anxiety, client fears total disintegration and loss of control.

Suggest that the client substitute positive thoughts for negative ones.

Emotion connected to thought, and changing to a more positive thought can decrease the level of anxiety experienced. This also gives the client an alternative way of looking at the problem.

Discuss the process of thinking about the feared object/situation before it occurs.

Anticipation of a future phobic reaction allows client to deal with the physical manifestations of fear.

Encourage client to share the seemingly unnatural fears and feelings with others, especially the nurse therapist.

Clients are often reluctant to share feelings for fear of ridicule and may have repeatedly been told to ignore feelings. Once the client begins to acknowledge and talk about these fears, it becomes apparent that the feelings are manageable.

Share own experience with client as indicated after relationship has been established.

If nurse therapist has dealt successfully with phobia in own life, client may be encouraged by the fact that someone has overcome a similar problem. Use judiciously to avoid meeting own needs rather than focusing on the client's needs.

Encourage to stop, wait, and not rush out of feared situation as soon as experienced. Support use of relaxation exercises (e.g., breath control, muscle relaxation, self-hypnosis).

Client fears disorganization and loss of control of body and mind when exposed to the fear-producing stimulus. This fear leads to an avoidance response, and reality is never tested. If client waits out the beginnings of anxiety and decreases it with relaxation exercises, then she or he may be ready to continue confronting the fear.

Explore things that may lower fear level and keep it manageable (e.g., use of singing while dressing, practicing positive self-talk while in a fearful situation).

Provides the client with a sense of control over the fear. Distracts the client so that fear is not totally focused on and allowed to escalate.

Use desensitization approach, e.g.:

Systematic desensitization (gradual systematic exposure of the client to the feared situation under controlled conditions) allows the client to begin to overcome the fear, become desensitized to the fear. **Note:** Implosion or flooding (continuous, rapid presentation of the phobic stimulus) may show quicker results than systematic desensitization, but relapse is more common or client may become terrified and withdraw from therapy.

Expose client to a predetermined list of anxiety-provoking stimuli rated in hierarchy from the least frightening to the most frightening.

Experiencing fear in progressively more challenging but attainable steps allows client to realize that dangerous consequences will not occur. Helps extinguish conditioned avoidance response.

Pair each anxiety-producing stimulus (e.g., standing in an elevator) with arousal of another affect of an opposite quality (e.g., relaxation, exercise, biofeedback) strong enough to suppress anxiety.

Helps client to achieve physical and mental relaxation as the anxiety becomes less uncomfortable.

Help client to learn how to use these techniques when confronting an actual anxiety-provoking situation. Provide for practice sessions (e.g., role-play), deal with phobic reactions in real-life situations.

Client needs continued confrontation to gain control over fear. Practice helps the body become accustomed to the feeling of relaxation, enabling the individual to handle feared object/situation.

Encourage client to set increasingly more difficult goals.

Develops confidence and movement toward improved functioning and independence.

Collaborative

Administer antianxiety medications as indicated: benzodiazepines, e.g., alprazolam (Xanax), clonazepam (Klonopin), diazepam (Valium), lorazepam (Ativan), chlordiazepoxide (Librium), oxazepam (Serax).

Biological factors may be involved in phobic/panic reactions, and these medications (particularly Xanax) produce a rapid calming effect and may help client change behavior by keeping anxiety low during learning and desensitization sessions. Addictive tendencies of CNS depressants need to be weighed against benefit from the medication.

Involve in interoceptive exposure therapy as appropriate, with client holding breath, hyperventilating and inhaling CO_2, or receiving sodium lactate injections as indicated.

Alters client's response to internal sensations as client learns that the feelings associated with panic do not indicate impending disaster.

NURSING DIAGNOSIS	**ANXIETY [severe to panic]**
May Be Related to:	Unidentified stressor(s)
	Contact with feared object/situation
	Limitations placed on ritualistic behavior
Possibly Evidenced by:	Attacks of immobilizing apprehension
	Physical, mental, and cognitive behaviors indicative of panic
	Expressed feelings of terror and inability to cope
Desired Outcomes/Evaluation Criteria—Client Will:	Verbalize a reduction in anxiety to a manageable level.
	Use individually appropriate techniques to interrupt progression of anxiety to panic level.
	Demonstrate increasing tolerance to phobic object/situation.
	Identify and use resources effectively.

ACTIONS/INTERVENTIONS	RATIONALE

Independent

Establish and maintain a trusting relationship by listening to the client; displaying warmth, answering questions directly, offering unconditional acceptance; being available and respecting the client's use of personal space.

Therapeutic skills need to be directed toward putting the client at ease, because the nurse who is a stranger may pose a threat to the highly anxious client.

324

Be aware and in control of *own* feelings; explore the cause of own anxiety and use this understanding therapeutically.

The nurse's anxiety can be communicated to the client, which only adds to the client's sense of terror. Discussion of these feelings can provide a role model for the client and show a different way of dealing with them.

Provide simple, clear explanations and instructions.

During period of increased anxiety, client may have difficulty focusing on/comprehending communications.

Support the client's defenses initially.

The client uses defenses in an attempt to deal with an unconscious conflict, and giving up these defenses prematurely may cause increased anxiety.

Verbally acknowledge the reality of the pain of the client's present coping mechanism (panic) without focusing on the symptoms that are being expressed.

The symptoms that the client is experiencing relieve some of the intolerable anxiety felt by the client. If client is unable to release this tension, the anxiety will only increase, possibly causing client to lose control.

Provide feedback about behavior, stressors, and coping responses. Validate what you observe with the client.

Sets groundwork for dealing with anxiety when client is calmer. Includes client in plan of care, providing sense of control/self-worth.

Emphasize relationship between physical and emotional health, and reinforce that this is an area to be explored when client feels better.

Client needs to be aware of mind-body relationship and the physiological changes that cause discomfort.

Observe for increasing anxiety. Assume a calm manner, decrease environmental stimulation, and provide temporary isolation as indicated.

Early detection and intervention facilitate modifying client's behavior by changing the environment and the client's interaction with it, to minimize the spread of anxiety.

Assist client/family to recognize and modify situations that cause anxiety when precipitating factor can be identified. (**Note:** Simple phobias are usually specific and object-centered; this is not so with all phobic disorders.)

Recognition of causes/relationships provides opportunity to intervene before anxiety escalates or loss of control occurs.

Determine/discuss use of alcohol and other drugs.

May be used to reduce anxiety/avoid panic attacks and can lead to abuse. (Refer to Ch. 5, Substance-Related Disorders.)

Note diagnosis of mitral valve prolapse.

This cardiac abnormality affects between $\frac{1}{4}$ and $\frac{1}{2}$ of panic disorder clients. Heart palpitations resulting from the failure of the valve to close properly can increase anxiety and trigger panic attacks.

Determine use of caffeine-containing beverages.

These clients may be more sensitive to the anxiety-producing effects of caffeine, which may precipitate panic/anxiety attacks.

Suggest supportive physical measures, such as warm baths/whirlpool, massage.

Provides physical relaxation and helps client manage anxiety/maintain control.

Encourage interest in outside activity through the following actions:

Increases participation in life while decreasing the amount of time and energy available for maladaptive coping mechanisms.

Share an activity with the client;

This is emotionally supportive and reinforces socially acceptable behavior.

Provide for physical exercise/activity of some type within client toleration;

Uses energy in constructive ways. Endorphins (the body's naturally produced "narcotics") induce feelings of wellness/euphoria and are thought to be released during exercise. **Note:** Use exercise therapy with caution, as half of clients have increased anxiety with exercise.

Structure the client's day with a list of planned activities realistic to client's capabilities. Include others in providing client care and support.

Provides opportunity to experience success, which enhances self-esteem and increases self-confidence.

Identify signs/symptoms of escalating anxiety and appropriate responses (e.g., relaxation, stopping negative self-talk).

Helps client become proactive in interrupting progression of anxiety to panic. Enhances sense of control.

Assess suicidal ideation.

These individuals have an increased rate of suicide/suicide attempts. This is of particular concern when therapeutic treatment of major depression lifts client's mood to the point at which she or he can act on suicidal thoughts.

Discuss side effects of medications, noting reactions that may occur (e.g., drowsiness, ataxia, confusion, headache, slurred speech, lethargy, giddiness, dizziness, vertigo, and impaired visual accommodation).

Side effects of antianxiety medications may cause concern heightening anxiety and may require evaluation/treatment.

Involve in cognitive behavioral techniques such as rational-emotive therapy and self-instruction.

Cognitive restructuring corrects misconceptions and develops self-confidence.

Collaborative

Administer medication as indicated:
  Antianxiety agents, e.g., alprazolam (Xanax), lorazepam (Ativan), clonazepam (Klonopin);

Provides relief from the immobilizing effects of anxiety and promotes participation in ADLs and therapy program. Drug effects may be noted shortly after beginning therapy but problems with dependence/withdrawal symptoms may occur.

  Antidepressants, e.g., imipramine (Tofranil), desipramine (Norpramin); or selective serotonin reuptake inhibitors (SSRIs), e.g., fluoxetine (Prozac), sertraline (Zoloft);

May be used in conjunction with other drugs as antidepressants may require several weeks before positive effects are noted, and still may not alter client's *fear* of panic attacks. SSRIs have fewer/milder side effects and may be better tolerated by client. **Note:** Upwards of 50% of client's with panic disorder also have an episode of major depression. These drugs have also been found to be effective in treating panic attacks. Side effects may be

  Monoamine-oxidase inhibitors (MAOIs), e.g., phenelzine sulfate (Nardil);

temporary, and caution needs to be exercised about food that should not be consumed while receiving these drugs.

  Propranolol (Inderal);

Several antihypertensive agents such as this beta blocker have potent effects on the somatic manifestations of anxiety (e.g., palpitations, tremors, etc.), although they have less dramatic effects on the psychological component of anxiety.

  Anticonvulsants, e.g., valproate (Depakene), carbamazepine (Tegretol).

These drugs have a sedative effect on the CNS and are used to stabilize mood in some clients, especially when other drugs are ineffective.

Refer client/family to counseling, psychotherapy, or groups, as indicated.

May need additional assistance/long-term support to make lifestyle changes necessary to achieve maximum recovery.

OBSESSIVE-COMPULSIVE DISORDER

DSM-IV
300.3 Obsessive-compulsive disorder

An obsession is an intrusive/inappropriate repetitive thought, impulse, or image that the individual recognizes as a product of his or her own mind but is unable to control. A compulsion is a repetitive urge that the individual feels driven to perform and cannot resist without great difficulty (severe anxiety). Most common obsessions are repetitive thoughts about contamination, repeated doubts, a need to have things in a specific order, aggressive or horrific impulses, or sexual imagery. The individual usually attempts to ignore or suppress such thoughts or to neutralize them with some other thought or action (compulsion).

ETIOLOGICAL THEORIES

Psychodynamics

Freud placed origin for obsessive-compulsive characteristics in the anal stage of development. The child is mastering bowel and bladder control at this developmental stage and derives pleasure from controlling his or her own body and indirectly the actions of others.

Erikson's comparable stage for this disorder is autonomy versus shame and doubt. The child learns that to be neat and tidy and to handle bodily wastes properly gains parental approval and to be messy brings criticism and rejection.

The obsessional character develops the art of the need to obtain approval by being excessively tidy and controlled. Frequently the parents' standards are too high for the child to meet, and the child continually is frustrated in attempts to please parents.

The defensive mechanisms used in obsessive-compulsive behaviors are unconscious attempts by the client to protect the self from internal anxiety. The greater the anxiety, the more time and energy will be tied up in the completion of the client's rituals. First, the client uses regression, a return to earlier methods of handling anxiety. Second, the obsessive thoughts are either devoid of feeling or are attached to anxiety. Thus, isolation is used. Third, the client's overt attitude toward others is usually the opposite of the unconscious feelings. Thus, reaction formation is being used. Last, compulsive rituals are a symbolic way of undoing or resolving the underlying conflict.

Biological

Although biological and neurophysiological influences in the etiology of anxiety disorders have been investigated, no relationship has yet been established. The mind-body connection is well accepted, but it is difficult to establish whether the biological changes cause anxiety or the emotional state causes physiological manifestations. However, recent findings suggest that neurobiological disturbances may play a role in obsessive-compulsive disorder, with physiological and biochemical factors also playing significant roles.

Family Dynamics

The individual exhibiting dysfunctional behavior is seen as the representation of family system problems. The "identified patient" (IP) is carrying the problems of the other members of the family, which are seen as the result of the interrelationships (disequilibrium) between family members rather than as isolated individual problems.

Multiple factors contribute to anxiety disorders.

CLIENT ASSESSMENT DATA BASE

(Also refer to CPs: Generalized Anxiety Disorder; Panic Disorders/Phobias.)

327

Activity/Rest

Difficulty relaxing
Pleasurable activities causing anxiety

Ego Integrity

May be very controlled from within
Pre-onset stressors (e.g., family death, pregnancy/childbirth, sexual failures) may be
    present

Hygiene

Characteristic rituals may influence/include repetitive hand-washing, intensive cleanliness,
    activities of daily living (e.g., dressing and undressing a number of times, placing
    articles in a specific order)

Neurosensory

Obsessive thoughts may be destructive or delusional, with most frequent themes, including
    contamination/dirt, health/illness, orderliness or need for symmetry, aggression,
    morality/religion, sex (e.g., shameful/degrading acts)
Thinking processes are rigid, intellectual, and sharply focused toward tasks; may express
    belief that nonpurposeful and nondirected activity is unsafe and bad
Repetitive mental acts (e.g., praying, counting, repeating words silently)
Impaired problem-solving ability
Ritualistic speech often noted

Social Interactions

More frequent occurrence in upper-middle class, with higher levels of intellectual functioning
Interference with normal routines, occupational functioning, social activities/relationships
May focus on details but be unproductive in work situations because of narrow scope and
    rigidity of ideas

Teaching/Learning

Most often seen in adolescence and early adulthood (average age of onset is 20)

DIAGNOSTIC STUDIES

(Refer to CPs: Generalized Anxiety Disorder, Panic Disorder/Phobias.)

NURSING PRIORITIES

1. Assist client to recognize onset of anxiety.
2. Explore the meaning and purpose of the behavior with the client.
3. Assist client to limit ritualistic behaviors.
4. Help client learn alternative responses to stress.
5. Encourage family participation in therapy program.

DISCHARGE GOALS

1. Anxiety decreased to a manageable level.
2. Ritualistic behaviors managed/minimized.
3. Environmental and interpersonal stress decreased.
4. Client/family involved in support group/community programs.
5. Plan in place to meet needs after discharge.

(Refer to CP: Generalized Anxiety Disorder for needs/concerns in addition to the following NDs.)

NURSING DIAGNOSIS	ANXIETY [severe]
May Be Related to:	Earlier life conflicts (may be reflected in the nature of the repetitive actions and recurring thoughts)
Possibly Evidenced by:	Repetitive action (e.g., hand-washing)
	Recurring thoughts (e.g., dirt and germs)
	Decreased social and role functioning
Desired Outcomes/Evaluation Criteria—Client Will:	Verbalize understanding of significance of ritualistic behaviors and relationship to anxiety.
	Demonstrate ability to cope effectively with stressful situations without resorting to obsessive thoughts or compulsive behaviors.

ACTIONS/INTERVENTIONS

Independent

Establish relationship through use of empathy, warmth, and respect. Demonstrate interest in client as a person through use of attending behaviors.

Acknowledge behavior without focusing attention on it. Verbalize empathy toward client's experience rather than disapproval or criticism. Better to say, "I see you undress 3 times every morning. That must be tiring for you," rather than "Try to dress only 1 time today."

Use a relaxed manner with the client; keep the environment calm.

Assist client to learn stress management, (e.g., thought-stopping, relaxation exercises, imagery).

Identify what the client perceives as relaxing (e.g., warm bath, music). Engage in constructive activities such as quiet games that require concentration, as well as arts and crafts such as needlework, woodworking, ceramics, and painting.

Encourage participation in a regular exercise program.

Give positive reinforcement for noncompulsive behavior. Avoid reinforcing compulsive behavior. Help significant other(s) learn the value of not focusing on the ritualistic behaviors.

Assist client to find ways to set limits on own behaviors. At the same time allow adequate time during the daily routine for the ritual(s).

RATIONALE

Anything about which the client feels anxious will serve to increase the ritualistic behaviors. Establishing trust provides support and communicates that the nurse accepts the client as a person with the right to self-determination.

Lack of attention to ritualistic behaviors can diminish them. As anxiety is reduced, the need for the behaviors is reduced. Reflecting the client's feelings may reduce the intensity of the ritualistic behavior.

Any attempts to decrease stress will help the client to feel less anxious, which may reduce the intensity of the ritualistic behaviors.

Stress-management techniques can be used, instead of ritualistic behaviors, to break habitual pattern.

Planned activities allow the client less time for compulsive behavior and distract her or him in a manner that allows creativity and positive feedback.

Exercise therapy can help relieve anxiety. **Note:** Exercise does not need to be aerobic or intensive to achieve the desired effect.

This approach will prevent the client from obtaining secondary gains from the maladaptive behaviors.

Encourages client to problem-solve ways to limit own behaviors while recognizing that behaviors cannot be stopped by others without increasing

329

anxiety. If the time required for performing the ritual(s) is not considered in planning care, client will feel rushed and anxious while performing behaviors. A mistake in compulsive behavior is more likely to be made if client feels rushed, and the whole ritual will have to be started again, resulting in increased anxiety—possibly to an unmanageable level.

Limit the amount of time allotted for the performance of rituals. Encourage client to gradually decrease this time.

Provides initial control of maladaptive behaviors until client can enforce own limits and substitute more adaptive response(s) to stress.

Encourage client to explore the meaning and purpose of behaviors; to describe the feelings when the behaviors occur, intensify, or are interrelated; and to examine the precipitating factors to the performance of the rituals.

This exploration provides an opportunity to begin to understand the process and gain control over the obsessive-compulsive sequence. When opportunity for ritualistic behavior does not occur, the client fears that something bad will happen. Recognizing precipitating factors allows client to interrupt escalating anxiety.

Discuss home situation, include family/SO as appropriate. Involve in discharge plan.

Returning to unchanged home environment increases risk that client will resume compulsive behaviors.

Collaborative

Administer medications as indicated, e.g.:
Fluvoxamine (Luvox), clomipramine (Anafranil), fluoxetine (Prozac);

These drugs help balance serotonin levels, decreasing feelings of anxiety, reducing need for ritualistic behavior(s), and allowing client to learn of other methods of stress reduction. **Note:** Luvox is classified as a selective serotonin reuptake inhibitor and has fewer side effects than tricyclics. Clients who are refractory to antidepressants may require combination therapy (e.g., buspirone and fluoxetine or lithium and clomipramine).

Buspirone (BuSpar) and lithium (Eskalith);

Sertraline (Zoloft), venlafaxine (Effexor).

These drugs are being used investigationally with some success for the treatment of obsessive-compulsive behaviors.

NURSING DIAGNOSIS	SKIN/TISSUE INTEGRITY, impaired/risk for
May Be Related to:	Repetitive behaviors related to cleansing, such as hand-washing, brushing teeth, showering
Possibly Evidenced by (Actual):	Disruption of skin surfaces; destruction of skin layers/tissues (e.g., mucous membranes)
Desired Outcomes/Evaluation Criteria— Client Will:	Identify risk factors.
	Verbalize understanding of treatment/therapy regimen.
	Engage in behaviors/techniques to prevent skin/tissue breakdown.
	Demonstrate timely healing/improvement in condition of dermal layers.

ACTIONS/INTERVENTIONS	RATIONALE

Independent

Assess changes in skin/tissue (e.g., alterations in skin turgor, edema, dryness, altered circulation, and presence of infections).

Encourage use of mild soap and hand creams, while using methods previously described in ND: Anxiety [severe] to decrease repetitive behaviors.

Discuss measures client can take during/after cleaning behaviors (e.g., use of rubber gloves and application of antiseptic cream).

Repetitive behaviors, such as hand-washing with detergents or cleaning with caustic substances, can damage the skin and underlying tissues.

Helps to minimize tissue trauma until other forms of therapy reduce damaging behaviors.

Protects skin and tissues in the presence of constant hand-washing, use of caustic substances.

NURSING DIAGNOSIS	ROLE PERFORMANCE, risk for altered
Risk Factors May Include:	Psychological stress
	Health-illness problems
Possibly Evidenced by:	[Not applicable; presence of signs and symptoms establishes an *actual* diagnosis.]
Desired Outcomes/Evaluation Criteria—Client Will:	Identify conflicts within work/family situations.
	Talk with family/SO(s) about situation and changes that have occurred.
	Maintain/resume role-related responsibilities.

ACTIONS/INTERVENTIONS	RATIONALE

Independent

Determine client's role within family and extent to which illness-related thoughts and actions affect role relationships.

Discuss client's perceptions of role, how obsessive-compulsive behaviors affect role, and whether perceptions are realistic.

Identify conflicts that exist within the family system and specific relationships that are affected. Encourage family members to begin to discuss identified problem areas.

Explore options for changes or adjustments in role and practice behaviors using role-play.

Encourage participation by all family members in problem-solving process and plans for change.

Provide positive reinforcement for movement toward resuming role responsibilities and decreasing ritualistic behaviors.

Identifies areas of concern and provides accurate information to formulate plan of care.

Client may deny extent of effect that behaviors have on daily activities.

Knowing what stressors as well as what adaptive and maladaptive responses are occurring helps individuals begin the process of positive change.

Planning and rehearsal of potential role transitions can reduce anxiety.

Likelihood of positive change increases when family system is involved in resolution of situations arising from client's ritualistic behaviors.

Enhances self-esteem and promotes repetition of desired behaviors.

331

POSTTRAUMATIC STRESS DISORDER

DSM-IV
309.81 Posttraumatic stress disorder (specify acute, chronic, or delayed onset)
308.3 Acute stress disorder

An anxiety disorder resulting from exposure to a traumatic event in which the individual has experienced, witnessed, or been confronted with an event or events that involve actual or threatened death/serious injury or a threat to the physical integrity of the self or others. The individual's response involved intense fear, helplessness, or horror. (A thorough physical examination should be done to rule out neurological organic problems.) Additionally, a newly recognized phenomenon is the development of PTSD-like symptoms in some individuals who have been involved over a long period of time in the treatment of (or living with) clients with PTSD.

ETIOLOGICAL THEORIES

Psychodynamics

The client's ego has experienced a severe trauma, often perceived as a threat to physical integrity or self-concept. This results in severe anxiety, which is not controlled adequately by the ego and is manifested in symptomatic behavior. Because the ego is vulnerable, the superego may become punitive and cause the individual to assume guilt for traumatic occurrence; the id may assume dominance, resulting in impulsive, uncontrollable behavior.

Biological

(Refer to CP: Generalized Anxiety Disorder.)
Some studies have revealed abnormalities in the storage, release, and elimination of catecholamines affecting function of the brain in the region of the locus coeruleus, amygdala, and hippocampus. Hypersensitivity in the locus coeruleus may lead to "learned helplessness." The amygdala appears to be the storehouse for memories, while the hippocampus provides narrative coherence and a location in time and space. Hyperactivation in the amygdala may prevent the brain from making coherent sense of its memories resulting in the memories being stored as nightmares, flashbacks, and physical symptoms.

Research is exploring the possibility of a genetic vulnerability including the belief that neurological disturbances in the womb or during childhood may influence the development of PTSD.

Family Dynamics

(Refer to CP: Generalized Anxiety Disorder.)
Types of formal education, family life, and lifestyle are significant forecasters of PTSD. Below average or lack of success in education, negative parenting behaviors, and parental poverty have been identified as predictors for development of PTSD, as well as for peritraumatic dissociation.

Current research also suggests that the effects of severe trauma may last for generations, meaning someone else's traumatic experience can be internalized by another, intruding into the second individual's own mental life.

CLIENT ASSESSMENT DATA BASE

Activity/Rest

Sleep disturbances, recurrent intrusive dreams of the event, nightmares, difficulty in falling or staying asleep; hypersomnia (intrusive thoughts, flashbacks, and/or nightmares are the triad symptomatic of PTSD)
Easy fatigability, chronic fatigue

Circulation

Increased heart rate, palpitations; increased blood pressure
Hot/cold spells, excessive perspiration

Ego Integrity

Various degrees of anxiety with symptoms lasting days, weeks, or months (2 days to maximum of 4 weeks occurring within 4 weeks of traumatic event [acute stress disorder]; duration of symptoms less than 3 months [acute PTSD], more than 3 months [chronic PTSD], or onset at least 6 months after traumatic event [delayed])
Difficulty seeking assistance (e.g., medical, legal) or mobilizing personal resources (e.g., telling family members/friends of experience)
Feelings of guilt, helplessness, powerlessness, isolation
Feeling shame for own helplessness; demoralization
Sense of a bleak or foreshortened future (e.g., expects failing relationships, early death)

Neurosensory

Cognitive disruptions, difficulty concentrating and/or completing usual life tasks
Hypervigilence (result of inability to assimilate and integrate experiences)
Excessive fearfulness of objects and/or situations in the environment triggered by reminders or internal cues that resemble or symbolize the events; e.g., startle response to loud noises (someone who experienced combat trauma/bombing), breaking out in a sweat when riding an elevator (for someone who was raped in an elevator)
Persistent recollection (illusions, dissociative flashbacks, hallucinations) or talk of the event, despite attempts to forget; impaired/no recall of an important aspect of the trauma
Poor impulse control with unpredictable explosions of aggressive behavior or acting-out of feelings such as anger, resentment, malice, and ill will (in high dudgeon)
Mental Status: Change in usual behavior (moody, pessimistic, brooding, irritable); loss of self-confidence, depressed affect; feelings seem unreal, business of life no longer matters
Muscular tension, tremulousness, motor restlessness

Pain/Discomfort

Pain/physical discomfort of the injury may be exaggerated beyond expectation in relation to severity of injury

Respiratory

Increased respiratory rate, dyspnea

Safety

Angry outbursts, violent behavior toward environment/other individuals
Suicidal ideation, previous attempts

Sexuality

Loss of desire; avoidance of/dissatisfaction with relationships
Inability to achieve sexual satisfaction/orgasm; impotence

Social Interactions

Avoidance of people/places/activities that arouse recollections of the trauma, decreased responsiveness, psychic numbing, emotional detachment/estrangement from others; inability to trust
Markedly diminished interest/participation in significant activities, including work
Restricted range of affect, absence of emotional responsiveness (e.g., absence of loving feelings)

333

Teaching/Learning

Occurrence of PTSD often preceded or accompanied by physical illness/harm
Use/abuse of alcohol or other drugs

DIAGNOSTIC STUDIES

(Refer to CPs: Generalized Anxiety Disorder; Pain Disorders/Phobias.)

NURSING PRIORITIES

1. Provide safety for client/others.
2. Assist client to enhance self-esteem and regain sense of control over feelings/actions.
3. Encourage development of assertive, not aggressive, behaviors.
4. Promote understanding that the outcome of the present situation can be significantly affected by own actions.
5. Assist client/family to learn healthy ways to deal with/realistically adapt to changes and events that have occurred.

DISCHARGE GOALS

1. Self-image improved/enhanced.
2. Individual's feelings/reactions are acknowledged, expressed, and dealt with appropriately.
3. Physical complications treated/minimized.
4. Appropriate changes in lifestyle planned/made.
5. Plan in place to meet needs after discharge.

NURSING DIAGNOSIS	ANXIETY [severe to panic]/FEAR
May Be Related to:	Current memory of past traumatic life event, such as natural disasters, accidental/deliberate manmade disasters, and events such as rape, assault, or combat
	Threat to self-concept/death, change in environment
	Negative self-talk (preoccupation with trauma)
Possibly Evidenced by:	Increased tension/wariness; restlessness
	Sense of helplessness; apprehension, fearfulness, uncertainty/confusion
	Somatic complaints; sympathetic stimulation (e.g., palpitations, shortness of breath, diaphoresis, pupil dilation)
	Sense of impending doom; fright, terror, panic, and/or withdrawal
Desired Outcomes/Evaluation Criteria— Client Will:	Verbalize awareness of feelings of anxiety/sense of control over fearful stimuli.
	Identify healthy ways to manage feelings.
	Demonstrate ability to confront situation using problem-solving skills.
	Report/display reduction of physiological symptoms.

ACTIONS/INTERVENTIONS	RATIONALE

Independent

Assess degree of anxiety/fear present, associated behaviors, and reality of threat perceived by client.	Identifies needs for developing plan of care/interventions. Clearly understanding client's perception is pivotal to providing appropriate assistance in overcoming the fear.
Maintain and respect client's personal space boundaries (approximately 4-foot circle around client).	Entering client's personal space without permission/invitation could result in an overwhelming anxiety response, resulting in an overt act of violence. (**Note:** Clients with PTSD have an expanded sense of personal space.)
Develop trusting relationship with the client.	Trust is the basis of a therapeutic nurse/client relationship and enables them to work effectively together. Client may be slow to form a therapeutic alliance and may need to participate in group situations, hearing others relate their own experiences, before being able to speak out or begin to trust others. **Note:** Some clients may distrust/view therapist as an authority figure affecting progress of individual counseling.
Identify whether incident has reactivated preexisting or coexisting situations (physical/psychological).	Concerns/psychological issues will be recycled every time trauma is reexperienced and affect how the client views current situation.
Observe for and elicit information about physical injury, and assess symptoms such as numbness, headache, tightness in chest, nausea, and pounding heart.	Physical injuries may have occurred during incident/panic of recurrence, which may be masked by anxiety of current situation. These need to be identified and differentiated from anxiety symptoms so appropriate treatment can be given.
Note presence of chronic pain or pain symptoms in excess of degree of physical injury.	Psychological responses may magnify/exacerbate physical symptoms.
Evaluate social aspects of trauma/incident (e.g., disfigurement, chronic conditions, permanent disabilities).	Problems that occurred in the original trauma may have left visible reminders that have to be dealt with daily.
Identify psychological responses (e.g., anger, shock, acute anxiety [panic], confusion, denial). Note laughter, crying, calm or agitation, excited (hysterical) behavior, expressions of disbelief and/or self-blame. Record emotional changes.	Although these are normal responses at the time of the trauma, they will recycle again and again until they are adequately dealt with.
Determine degree of disorganization. Indicator of level of intervention that is required (e.g., may need to be hospitalized when disorganization is severe). Note signs of increasing anxiety (e.g., silence, stuttering, inability to sit still/pacing).	May indicate inability to handle current happenings (e.g., feelings or therapy, suggesting need of more intensive evaluation/intervention).
Identify development of phobic reactions to ordinary articles (e.g., knives), situations (e.g., strangers ringing doorbell, walking in crowds of people), occurrences (e.g., car backfires).	These may trigger feelings from original trauma and need to be dealt with sensitively, accepting reality of feelings and stressing ability to client to handle them. (Refer to CP: Panic Disorders/Phobias.)
Stay with client, maintaining a calm, confident manner. Speak in brief statements, using simple words.	Can help client to maintain control when anxiety is at a panic level.

335

Provide for nonthreatening, consistent environment/atmosphere.	Minimizes stimuli, reducing anxiety and calming the individual, and helps break the cycle of anxiety/fear.
Gradually increase activities/involvement with others.	As anxiety (panic) level is decreased, client can begin to tolerate interaction with others. Activity further releases tension in an acceptable manner. (Refer to ND: Violence, risk for, directed at self/others.)
Discuss with client perception of what is causing anxiety.	Increases ability to connect symptoms to subjective feeling of anxiety, providing opportunity for client to gain insight/control and make desired changes.
Assist client to correct any distortions being experienced. Share perceptions with client.	Perceptions based on reality will assist to decrease fearfulness. How the nurse views the situation may help client to see it differently.
Help client identify feelings being experienced and focus on ways to cope with them. Encourage client to keep a journal about feelings, precipitating factors, associated behaviors.	Increases awareness of affective component of anxiety and ways to control and manage it. Therapeutic writing can provide a release for anger, stress, and grief, and provide new insights.
Explore with client the manner in which the client has coped with anxious events before the trauma.	Helps client regain sense of control and recognize significance of trauma.
Engage client in learning new coping behaviors (e.g., progressive muscle relaxation, thought-stopping).	Replacing maladaptive behaviors can enhance ability to manage anxiety and deal with stress. Interrupting obsessive thinking allows client to use energy to address underlying anxiety, while continued rumination about the incident can actually retard recovery.
Give positive feedback when client demonstrates better ways to manage anxiety and is able to calmly and/or realistically appraise own situation.	Provides acknowledgement and reinforcement, encouraging use of new coping strategies. Enhances ability to deal with fearful feelings and gain control over situation, promoting future successes.

Collaborative

Administer medications as indicated, e.g.: Antidepressants: fluoxetine (Prozac), amoxapine (Asendin), doxepin (Sinequan), imipramine (Trofranil), MAO inhibitor phenelzine (Nardil);	Used to decrease anxiety, lift mood, aid in management of behavior, and ensure rest until client regains control of own self. Helpful in suppressing intrusive thoughts and explosive anger. **Note:** Research suggests selective serotonin reuptake inhibitors (SSRIs) such as Prozac are more beneficial than other antidepressants.
Beta Blockers, e.g., propranolol (Inderal);	Reduces restlessness and anxiety by depressing the sympathetic nervous system.
Valproic acid (Depakene), carbamazepine (Tegretol), or clonidine (Catapres);	May be used in combination with tricyclic anti-depressants or beta-adrenergic receptor antagonists to counter a lower threshold for arousal in the limbic system of the brain.
Benzodiazepines, e.g.: alprazolam (Xanax), clonazepam (Klonopin);	May be used in combination with Nardil or Prozac to relieve anxiety and insomnia. **Note:** Use with caution as some degree of unpredictable disinhibition may occur.

Antipyschotics, e.g.: phenothiazines: chlor-promazine (Thorazine).

Low doses may be used for the reduction of psychotic symptoms when loss of contact with reality occurs, usually for client's with especially disturbing flashbacks.

Provide additional therapies, e.g.: hypnosis; Eye Movement Desensitization/Reprocessing (EMD/R) or Thought Reprocessing Therapy as appropriate.

When used by trained therapists, these short-term methods of therapy are particularly effective with individuals who have been traumatized or who have problems with anxiety and depression. Systematic desensitization, reframing, and reinterpretation of memories may be achieved through hypnosis.

NURSING DIAGNOSIS	POWERLESSNESS
May Be Related to:	Interpersonal interaction (lack of control of traumatic event)
	Being overwhelmed by symptoms of anxiety (e.g., intrusive thoughts, flashbacks; physical manifestations)
	Lifestyle of helplessness/poor coping skills
Possibly Evidenced by:	Verbal expression of lack of control over present situation/future outcome; passivity and/or anger
	Reluctance to express true feelings
	Dependence on others
	Nonparticipation in care or decision-making when opportunities are provided
Desired Outcomes/Evaluation Criteria—Client Will:	Identify areas over which individual has control.
	Express sense of control over present situation/future outcome.
	Demonstrate involvement in care and planning for the future.

ACTIONS/INTERVENTIONS	RATIONALE

Independent

Identify present/past effective coping behaviors and reinforce use.	Awareness of past successes enhances self-confidence and increases options for current use, promoting a sense of control.
Note ethnic background, cultural/religious perceptions and beliefs about the occurrence (e.g., retribution from God).	Sense of own responsibility (blame) and guilt about not having done something to prevent incident or not having been "good enough" to deserve surviving are strong beliefs in individuals who are influenced by background and cultural factors.
Formulate plan of care with client, setting realistic goals for achievement.	Actively involves client, providing a measure of control over life situation.

Encourage client to identify factors under own control as well as those not within own ability to control.	Recognition of areas of control decreases sense of helplessness. Confronting issues outside of client's control may encourage acceptance of that which cannot be changed.
Assist client to identify precipitating factors when feelings of powerlessness and loss of control began.	Increases understanding of sources of stressful events that trigger these feelings.
Explore actions client can use during periods of stress (e.g., deep breathing, counting to 10, reviewing the situation, reframing).	Provides information to assist client with learning constructive ways to cope with feeling of powerlessness and to regain control. Reframing stressors/situation in other words or positive ideas can help client recognize and consider alternatives.
Give positive feedback when client uses constructive methods to regain control.	Acknowledgement and reinforcement encourage repetition of desirable behaviors.
Promote involvement in group therapy.	Provides an opportunity for client to learn new coping behaviors from peers who have experienced similar traumatic events/reactions in the past. **Note:** Often guilt and anger are not dissipated until client talks about own life with someone who has had similar experiences and can empathize with the client on a personal level.

Collaborative

Involve in assertiveness training as appropriate.	Learning to problem-solve in areas of social skills and anger control provides a sense of power to the individual for dealing with life in general.

NURSING DIAGNOSIS	**VIOLENCE [actual]/risk for, directed at self/others**
Related/Risk Factors May Include:	Intrusive memory of event causing a sudden acting out of a feeling as if the event were occurring; startle reaction
	Rage Reactions: Breaking through of rage that has been walled off, rage at the sense of helplessness/dependency or at those who were exempted from the trauma
May Be Evidenced by/[Possible Indicators]:	Increased motor activity (pacing, excitement, irritability, agitation)
	Argumentative, dissatisfied, overreactive, hypersensitive, provocative behaviors; hostile, threatening verbalizations
	Overt and aggressive acts; goal-directed destruction of objects in environment
	Self-destructive behavior (including substance abuse) and/or active, aggressive, or suicidal/homicidal acts
Desired Outcomes/Evaluation Criteria— Client Will:	Acknowledge realities of the situation and precipitating factors.

Verbalize awareness of positive ways to cope with feelings.

Demonstrate self-control as evidenced by relaxed posture/manner, use of problem-solving rather than threats or assaultive behavior to resolve conflicts and/or cope.

ACTIONS/INTERVENTIONS	RATIONALE

Independent

Evaluate for presence of self-destructive and/or suicidal/homicidal behaviors (e.g., mood/behavior changes, increasing withdrawal). Assess seriousness of threat (e.g., gestures, previous attempts). (Use scale of 1–10 and prioritize according to severity of threat, availability of means.)

Client may be in such despair or self-esteem may be so low that behaviors may be engaged in that are violent toward self/others with conscious or unconscious wish for suicide. (**Note:** If scale is high, this may be no. 1 nursing concern.)

Encourage client to identify and verbalize triggering stimuli, causative/contributing factors that lead to potential or actual violence by client.

Client needs to learn to recognize what precipitates anger and tension. Early recognition and prompt intervention may prevent occurrence of violence.

Negotiated contract with client regarding actions to be taken when feeling out of control.

Contracting to let nurse/significant person know when feeling overwhelmed helps the client obtain assistance as needed and maintain a sense of control. **Note:** Client may project accumulated anger at therapist.

Assist client to understand that feelings of anger may be appropriate in the situation but need to be expressed verbally or in an acceptable manner rather than acted on in a destructive way.

Learning to discharge anxiety and affect in a socially acceptable manner reduces likelihood of violent outbursts.

Monitor level of anger (e.g., questioning, refusal, verbal release, intimidation, blow-up).

Stage of anger affects choice of interventions.

Tell the client to STOP violent behaviors. Use environmental controls (such as providing a quiet place for client to go, holding the client) if behavior continues to escalate. Talk gently and quietly.

Saying "Stop" may be sufficient to assist client to regain control, but external controls may be required if client is unable to call up internal controls. **Note:** Physical holding can provide a sense of contact and caring that may help client regain control.

Institute de-escalation actions as indicated, e.g.:

These actions can prevent escalation of violent behaviors and prevent injury to client/caregivers or bystanders.

Distance self from client, by at least 4 armlengths, position self to one side; remain calm, stand or sit still, assume "open" posture with hands in sight.

Reduces possibility that client will feel confronted or blocked. Gives client some control over situation.

Speak softly, call client by name, acknowledge client's feelings, express regret about situation, show empathy;

Communicates sense of respect, belief that individual can be trusted to control self, and that caregiver is available to assist client with resolution of situation. **Note:** "Expect the unexpected" and be prepared for unanticipated movement.

Avoid pointing, touching, ordering, scolding, challenging, interrupting, arguing, belittling, or intimidating client;

Request permission to ask questions, try to discern triggering event and any underlying emotions, such as fear, anxiety, or humiliation; offer solutions/alternatives.

Give client as much control as possible in other areas of life, helping to identify more appropriate solutions and responses to tension and anxiety.

Involve in exercise program, in outdoor activity program (hiking, wall/rock climbing, etc.); encourage sporting activities (group or individual).

These actions may be viewed as threatening and may provoke client to violent actions.

Involves client in problem-solving and gives client some control over situation.

Learning new ways of responding to impulsive tendencies increases capacity for controlling impulses.

Relieves tension and increases sense of well-being, promotes self-confidence. When activity is geared to individual interests, participation and therapeutic benefits are enhanced. **Note:** Exercise therapy does not need to be aerobic or intensive to achieve desired effect.

Collaborative

Use seclusion or restraints until control is regained, as indicated.

Administer medications, as indicated, e.g., lithium carbonate (Eskalith).

Provides external control to prevent injury to client/staff/others.

Low-dose therapy may be used to limit mood swings and suppress explosive behavior.

NURSING DIAGNOSIS	COPING, INDIVIDUAL, ineffective
May Be Related to:	Personal vulnerability; unmet expectations; unrealistic perceptions
	Inadequate support systems/coping method(s)
	Multiple stressors, repeated over period of time; overwhelming threat to self
Possibly Evidenced by:	Verbalization of inability to cope or difficulty asking for help
	Muscular tension/headaches
	Emotional tension; chronic worry
Desired Outcomes/Evaluation Criteria— Client Will:	Identify ineffective coping behaviors and consequences.
	Verbalize awareness of own coping abilities.
	Express feelings appropriately.
	Identify options and use resources effectively.

ACTIONS/INTERVENTIONS

RATIONALE

Independent

Identify and discuss degree of dysfunctional coping (e.g., denial, rationalization), including use/abuse of chemical substances.

Identifies needs/depth of interventions required. Individuals display different levels of dysfunctional behavior in response to stress, and

340

Review consequences of behaviors, how relationships/functioning are affected.

Be aware of, and assist client to use ego strengths in a positive way, acknowledging ability to handle what is happening.

Permit free expression of feelings at client's own pace. Do not rush client through expressions of feelings too quickly; avoid reassuring inappropriately.

Encourage client to become aware and accepting of own feelings and reactions when identified.

Give "permission" to express/deal with anger at the assailant/situation in acceptable ways.

Keep discussion on practical and emotional level, rather than intellectualizing the experience.

Identify supportive persons available for the client.

often the choice of alcohol and/or other drugs is a way of deadening the psychic pain.

Helps client recognize negative impact of life and provides focus to begin addressing problems.

Often the firm statement of the nurse's conviction that the client can handle what is happening connects with the inner self-belief that is inherent in people.

Nonjudgmental listening to all feelings conveys acceptance of the worth of the client. Taking own time to talk about what has happened and allowing feelings to be fully expressed aids in the healing process. If rushed, client may believe pain and/or anguish is misunderstood. Statements such as "You don't understand" or "You weren't there" are a defense, a way of pushing others away.

There are no bad feelings, and accepting them as signals that need to be attended to and dealt with can help the client move toward resolution.

Being free to express anger appropriately allows it to be dissipated so that underlying feelings can be identified and dealt with, strengthening coping skills.

When feelings (the experience) are intellectualized, uncomfortable insights and/or awareness are avoided by the use of rationalization, blocking resolution of feelings and impairing coping abilities.

Having unconditional support from loving/caring others can assist the client to confront situation, cope with it, and move on to live more fully.

Collaborative

Provide for sensitive counselors/therapists who are especially trained in crisis management and the use of therapies such as psychotherapy (in conjunction with medications), implosive therapy, flooding, hypnosis, relaxation, Rolfing, memory work, or cognitive restructuring.

Refer to occupational therapy, vocational rehabilitation.

Although it is not necessary for the helping person to have experienced the same kind of trauma as the client's, sensitivity and listening skills are important to helping the client confront fears and learn new ways to cope with what has happened. Therapeutic use of desensitization techniques (flooding, implosive therapy) provides for extinction through exposure to the fear. Body work can alleviate muscle tension. Some techniques (Rolfing) help to bring blocked emotions to awareness as sensations of the traumatic event are reexperienced.

Assistance with new activities and learning new skills may be needed to help the client develop coping skills to reintegrate into the work setting. New activities/work skills, while generating some anxiety, will help with the process of desensitization and reduction/elimination of anxiety.

NURSING DIAGNOSIS	GRIEVING, dysfunctional
May Be Related to:	Actual/perceived object loss (loss of self as seen before the traumatic incident occurred, as well as other losses incurred in/after the incident)
	Loss of physiopsychosocial well-being
	Thwarted grieving response to a loss; absence of anticipatory grieving; lack of resolution of previous grieving response
Possibly Evidenced by:	Verbal expression of distress at loss; difficulty in expressing loss; expression of guilt
	Expression of unresolved issues; reliving of past experiences
	Denial of loss; anger, sadness, crying; labile affect
	Alterations in eating habits, sleep and dream patterns, activity level, libido
	Alterations in concentration and/or pursuit of tasks
Desired Outcomes/Evaluation Criteria— Client Will:	Demonstrate progress in dealing with/movement through stages of grief.
	Participate in work and self-care/activities of daily living as able.
	Verbalize a sense of progress toward resolution of the grief and hope for the future.

ACTIONS/INTERVENTIONS	RATIONALE

Independent

Note verbal/nonverbal expressions of guilt or self-blame.	"Survivor's guilt" affects most people who have survived trauma in which others have died, and client questions "Why was I spared?" or perhaps believes, "I am not worthy, and others were."
Acknowledge reality of feelings of guilt, and assist client to take steps toward resolution.	Acceptance of feelings and support of new coping skills allow for taking risk of new behaviors.
Reinforce that client made the best decision he or she could have made at the time.	Regardless of the choices made, the client survived the event(s). The client needs unconditional positive acceptance and validation of decisions in order to resolve feelings of guilt and begin to deal with grief.
Note signs and stage of grieving for self and/or others (e.g., denial, anger, bargaining, depression, acceptance).	Identification and understanding of stages of grief assist with choice of interventions, planning of care, and movement toward resolution.
Be aware of avoidance behaviors (e.g., anger, withdrawal).	Client has avoided dealing with the feelings, which has led to her or his current situation. Recognition at this time can help with beginning new approach to solving the problem(s). **Note:**

342

	Avoidance should not be confused with extinction, a progressive and often spontaneous alleviation of memory-induced pain; although both attempt to distance the client from the traumatic event(s), extinction is adaptive.
Provide information about normalcy of feelings/actions in relation to stages of grief.	Individual may believe it is unacceptable to have these feelings, and knowing they are normal can provide sense of relief.
Give "permission" for client to be depressed—"to be at this point at this time."	Provides opportunity for the client to accept self and feel satisfied with current progress.
Encourage verbalization without confrontation about realities.	Helps client to begin resolution and acceptance. Confrontation may convey lack of acceptance and actually impede progress.
Identify cultural factors and ways individual has dealt with previous loss(es). Point out individual strengths/positive coping skills.	Different cultures deal with loss in different ways, and it is important to allow client to deal with situation in own healthy way. How the client has dealt with losses in the past can be a reliable predictor of how current losses are being dealt with and how they may be dealt with in the future, effectively or ineffectively. Client may discount/sabotage own capabilities.
Reinforce use of previously effective coping skills.	Identification of helpful ways client is already dealing with problems allows client to feel positive about self.
Assist significant other(s) to cope with client's response.	Support and understanding of reasons for client's behavior provides opportunity for family to work with client in development of new coping skills to resolve grief.

Collaborative

Refer to other resources (e.g., peer/support group, counseling, psychotherapy, spiritual advisor).	May need additional help to resolve situation/concomitant problems.

NURSING DIAGNOSIS	**SLEEP PATTERN disturbance**
May Be Related to:	Psychological stress (anxiety, depression with recurring disruptive dreams)
Possibly Evidenced by:	Verbal reports of difficulty in falling asleep/not feeling well rested
	Insomnia that causes awakening
	Reports of sleep disturbances (e.g., nightmares, dreams of personal death, disaster-related dreams, flashbacks, intrusive/trauma images, fear of re-experiencing the event)
	Hypersomnia (as a way of avoiding behaviors, events, or situations that arouse recollections)

Desired Outcomes/Evaluation Criteria—Client Will:	Verbalize understanding of sleep disorder/problem.
	Identify behaviors to promote sleep.
	Sleep adequate/appropriate number of hours for individual needs.
	Report increased sense of well-being and feeling rested.

ACTIONS/INTERVENTIONS	RATIONALE

Independent

Assess sleep pattern disturbance by observation and reports from client and/or SOs.	Subjective and objective information provides assessment of individual problems and direction for interventions.
Identify causative and contributing factors (e.g., intrusive/repetitive thoughts, nightmares, severe anxiety level). Note use of caffeine and/or alcohol, other drugs.	These factors interfere with both the ability to fall asleep and the REM cycle of sleep, affecting quality of rest.
Provide a quiet environment; arrange to have uninterrupted sleep as much as possible.	Assists in establishing optimal sleep/rest routine.
Encourage client to develop behavior routine when insomnia is present (e.g., no napping after noon, having warm bath/milk before bed, relaxing thoughts, getting out of bed 10 minutes after awakening if unable to fall asleep again, limiting sleep to 7 hours each night).	Rituals help decrease anxiety and fear of facing a sleepless night. **Note:** L-tryptophan in milk is believed to induce sleep.

Collaborative

Administer sedative, hypnotic, or antianxiety drugs as indicated. (Refer to ND: Anxiety [severe to panic]/Fear.)	May require short-term drug therapy to decrease sense of exhaustion/fear and promote relaxation to enhance sleep. (These drugs should be used sparingly to avoid dependence and addiction.)

NURSING DIAGNOSIS	SOCIAL ISOLATION/SOCIAL INTERACTION, impaired
May Be Related to:	Reduced involvement with the external world; numbing of responsiveness to the environment/affective numbing; difficulty in establishing and/or maintaining relationships with others
	Feelings of guilt and shame/survivor's guilt
	Unacceptable social behaviors/values
Possibly Evidenced by:	Conflicts with family, significant others; withdrawal from and avoidance of others/absence of supportive others; expressed feelings of

344

rejection/alienation; observed discomfort in social situations/use of unsuccessful social interaction behaviors

Chronic loss of interest and energy for work and relationships

Sense of vulnerability over fear of loss of control of aggressive impulses

Sense of responsibility (guilt) for inciting event or failing to control it; rage at those exempted from loss or injury

Drug (alcohol) abuse

Desired Outcomes/Evaluation Criteria— Client Will:

Verbalize recognition of causes of impaired interactions/isolation.

Acknowledge willingness to be more involved with others.

Demonstrate involvement/participation in appropriate activities and programs.

ACTIONS/INTERVENTIONS	RATIONALE
Independent	
Assess degree of isolation. Note withdrawn behavior and use of denial. Ascertain client's perceptions of reasons for problems.	Indicates need for/choice of interventions. Withdrawing and denial can inhibit/sabotage participation in therapy.
Help client differentiate between isolation and loneliness/aloneness.	Time for the client to be alone is important to the maintenance of mental health, but the sadness created by isolation and loneliness needs different interventions.
Identify support systems available to client (e.g., family, friends, coworkers).	Involvement of significant others can help to build and/or reestablish support system and reintegrate client into a social network.
Explore with client and role-play ways of making changes in social interactions/behaviors.	Developing and practicing strategies promotes and enhances possibility of change.
Acknowledge any positive efforts client makes in establishing contact with others.	Positive reinforcement of movement toward others can decrease sense of isolation and encourage repetition of behaviors, enhancing socialization.
Collaborative	
Encourage client to continue and/or seek outside or outpatient therapy/peer group activities.	Will need ongoing support and encouragement to reestablish social connections and develop/ strengthen relationships.
Refer client for employment counseling, if indicated. (Refer to ND: Coping, Individual, ineffective.)	Interpersonal difficulties may have affected work relationships and performance, and client may need help to reintegrate into current job or relocate.

345

NURSING DIAGNOSIS	FAMILY PROCESSES, altered
May Be Related to:	Situational crises, e.g., trauma, disabling responses, change in roles, economic setbacks
	Failure to master developmental transitions
Possibly Evidenced by:	Expressions of confusion about what to do and that family is having difficulty coping with situation; difficulty accepting/receiving help appropriately
	Not adapting to change or dealing with traumatic experience constructively; ineffective family decision-making process
	Difficulty expressing individual and/or wide range of feelings
	Family system does not meet physical, emotional, or spiritual needs of its members
Desired Outcomes/Evaluation Criteria—Family Will:	Express feelings freely and appropriately.
	Verbalize understanding of trauma, treatment regimen, and prognosis.
	Demonstrate individual involvement in problem-solving processes directed at appropriate solutions for the situation.

ACTIONS/INTERVENTIONS	RATIONALE
Independent	
Determine family members' understanding of client's illness/PTSD.	Family members and SO(s) often do not recognize that client's present behavior is the result of trauma that has occurred.
Identify patterns of communications in the family, e.g.: Are feelings expressed clearly and freely? Do family members talk to one another? Are problems resolved equitably? What are interactions among/between members?	How family members communicate provides information about their ability to problem-solve, understand one another, cooperate in making decisions, and resolve problems resulting from trauma.
Encourage family members to verbalize feelings (including anger) about client's behavior.	SO/spouse may feel angry/unloved and believe client is rejecting, rather than recognizing behaviors as a sign of client's pain.
Acknowledge difficulties each member is experiencing while reinforcing that conflict is to be expected and can be used to promote growth.	Recognition of what the person is feeling/going through provides a sense of acceptance. Most people have the fantasy that once the conflict has been resolved, everything will be fine. Discussing conflict as an ongoing problem that can be resolved so all parties win can help family members begin to believe a new method of handling it can be learned.
Identify and encourage use of previously successful coping behaviors.	In the stress of current situation, family members tend to focus on negative behaviors, feel hopeless,

Encourage use of stress-management techniques, e.g., appropriate expression of feelings, relaxation exercises, guided imagery.

Present information about PTSD and provide opportunity to ask questions/discuss concerns.

Collaborative

Refer to other resources as indicated, e.g., support groups, spiritual advisor, psychological/family therapy, marital counseling.

and neglect looking at positive behaviors used in the past.

Reduction of stress enables individuals to begin to think more clearly/develop new behaviors to cope with client.

These materials can help family members learn more about client's condition and assist in resolution of current crisis.

Additional/ongoing support and/or therapy may be needed to help family resolve family crisis and look at potential for growth. Client problems affect others in family/relationships, and further counseling may help resolve issues of enabling behavior/communication problems.

NURSING DIAGNOSIS	SEXUAL dysfunction/SEXUALITY PATTERNS, altered
May Be Related to:	Biopsychosocial alteration of sexuality (stress of posttrauma response)
	Loss of sexual desire
	Impaired relationship with a significant other
Possibly Evidenced by:	Alterations in achieving sexual satisfaction/relationship with significant other
	Change of interest in self and others; preoccupation with self
	Irritation, lack of affection
Desired Outcomes/Evaluation Criteria—Client/Partner Will:	Verbalize understanding of reasons for sexual problems/changes that have occurred.
	Identify stresses involved in lifestyle that contribute to the dysfunction.
	Demonstrate improved communication and relationship skills.
	Participate in program designed to resume desired sexual activity.

ACTIONS/INTERVENTIONS	RATIONALE

Independent

Inquire in a direct manner if there has been a change in sexual functioning/if problems exist, preferably in a conjoint session.

Client may prefer to dwell on reliving details of trauma and may not complain about this area of life. SO may not recognize relation of trauma to marital discord/sexual problems, and being with the client provides an opportunity for them to

347

Determine intimate behavior/closeness between couple recently and in comparison to quality of sexual relationship before the trauma, when appropriate.	begin to talk realistically about what is happening. **Note:** Men typically have loss of sexual desire and occasional impotence; women often experience lack of sexual pleasure and anorgasmia.
	May reveal problems that have not been acknowledged previously by the couple. Client may deny existence of difficulties, excusing self as being "sick" or "needing time to recover from trauma."
Provide information about the effect anxiety and anger have on sexual desire/ability to perform.	When partner does not know this, it is easy to feel unloved and not cared about or believe mate is having an affair. With understanding/insight into cause(s), partner's anxiety may be relieved, and support and affection can be extended to the client.
Encourage expression of feelings and emotions (e.g., crying) openly and appropriately.	Client/partner may believe they are helping by being stoic and not expressing feelings of powerlessness, helplessness, fear, etc. to each other.
Help client who has been the victim of sexual assault and partner to understand relationship of reluctance to have mate touch/make sexual advances to the event that occurred.	Client may have difficulty recognizing and feel embarrassed by the fact that mate's advances are reminder(s) of the trauma. Partner may view client's reluctance as rejection by the client.
Discuss substance use and relationship to sexual difficulties.	Some clients use alcohol and other drugs to dull the pain of PTSD. These substances interfere with sexual functioning, causing diminished desire and inability to achieve and maintain an erection. **Note:** It is not known what effect chronic use of alcohol has on female sexual functioning.
Review relaxation skills. (Refer to ND: Coping, Individual, ineffective.)	Learning to relax assists with reduction of anxiety and allows client/partner to focus on learning skills to regain/enhance sexual functioning.

Collaborative

Refer to other resources as indicated (e.g., sex therapist).	Specific techniques may be used to assist the couple in regaining comfort level/ability to engage in nongenital/genital activity and intimacy.

NURSING DIAGNOSIS	**KNOWLEDGE deficit [LEARNING NEED] regarding situation, prognosis, and treatment needs**
May Be Related to:	Lack of exposure to/misinterpretation of information
	Unfamiliarity with information resources
	Lack of recall
Possibly Evidenced by:	Verbalization of the problem; statement of misconception
	Inaccurate follow-through of instruction

	Inappropriate or exaggerated behaviors (e.g., hysterical, hostile, agitated, apathetic)
Desired Outcomes/Evaluation Criteria— Client Will:	Participate in learning process.
	Assume responsibility for own learning and begin to look for information/ask questions.
	Identify stressful situations and specific action(s) to deal with them.
	Initiate necessary lifestyle changes and participate in treatment regimen.

ACTIONS/INTERVENTIONS	RATIONALE

Independent

ACTIONS/INTERVENTIONS	RATIONALE
Provide information about what reactions client may expect, and let client know these are common reactions. Phrase in neutral terms (e.g., "[blank] may or may not happen").	Knowing what to expect can reduce anxiety and help the client in learning new behaviors to handle stressful feelings/situations. Having information about the commonality of experiences helps the individual feel less alone/strange, aiding in acceptance of these feelings.
Assist client to identify factors that may have created a vulnerable situation and that he or she may have power to change to protect self in the future. Avoid making value judgments.	Separates issues of vulnerability from blame. Factors such as body stance, carelessness, and not paying attention to negative cues may provide opportunity for tragic consequences that could possibly have been avoided/minimized. However, any inference that client is responsible for the incident is not therapeutic.
Discuss contemplated changes in lifestyle and how they will contribute to recovery.	Client needs to be able to look at these changes, what will be accomplished, and determine whether they are realistic/necessary.
Assist client to learn stress-management techniques.	Relaxation is a useful coping skill for dealing with stress of recurrent fears/exaggerated stress response.
Discuss recognition of and ways to manage "anniversary reactions," letting client know normalcy of thoughts and feelings at this time.	Planning ahead and knowing some skills to handle this time can help to avoid severe regression.
Identify available community resources (e.g., support groups for client/family, social or veteran services, vocational/educational counseling).	These resources may be helpful to client/SO in establishing a satisfying and productive life.

349

CHAPTER 10

SOMATOFORM DISORDERS

SOMATOFORM DISORDERS

DSM-IV
300.81   Somatization disorder
300.11   Conversion disorder
300.7   Hypochondriasis
300.7   Body dysmorphic disorder
307.xx   Pain disorder
307.80   Associated with psychological factors
307.89   Associated with both psychological factors and a general medical condition
300.82   Undifferentiated somatoform disorder
300.82   Somatoform disorder NOS

Somatization refers to all those mechanisms by which anxiety is translated into physical illness or bodily complaints. The expression of physical symptoms suggests the presence of physiological disorder, but there are no demonstrable organic findings/known pathological mechanisms, or the symptoms are not fully explained by any physical disorder. That is, the symptoms are in excess of what would be expected from the history, physical examination, or laboratory findings. There does exist, however, positive evidence, or a strong presumption, that the symptoms are linked to psychological factors or conflicts. These disorders are more common in women than in men, with somatization disorder rare in men.

ETIOLOGICAL THEORIES
Psychodynamics

This disorder may represent an unconscious transformation of internal conflicts into physical symptoms that can be explained in terms of the ego's ability to control the sensory and motor apparatus, which may have specific meaning for the client.

Dependency is common in individuals with somatoform disorders, and fixation in an earlier level of development may be evident. Repression is the primary defense mechanism, as severe anxiety is repressed and manifested by the presence of physical symptoms.

Biological

Although biological and neurophysiological influences in the etiology of anxiety have been investigated, no relationship has yet been established. However, there does seem to be a genetic influence with a high family incidence.

The autonomic nervous system discharge that occurs in response to a frightening impulse and/or emotion is mediated by the limbic system, resulting in the peripheral effects of

350

the autonomic nervous system seen in the presence of anxiety. These manifestations of anxiety may be related to physiological abnormalities.

Family Dynamics

The family contributes to these conditions by initiating, reinforcing, and perpetuating the behavior patterns. The children learn (overtly or covertly) that physical complaints are acceptable ways of coping with stress and obtaining attention, care, and gratification of dependency needs. The client may gain attention and meet these needs by overdramatization of the symptoms, resulting in overinvolvement of other family members in enmeshed behavior patterns. In the beginning, the client may exaggerate minor symptoms to prove she or he is really ill when others ignore reports of illness.

CLIENT ASSESSMENT DATA BASE

Activity/Rest

Fatigue
General weakness

Circulation

Heart rate may be elevated if symptoms mimic those of cardiopulmonary disease (similar to those experienced during panic attack)

Ego Integrity

Preoccupation with imagined defect in appearance or markedly excessive concern with slight physical anomaly not better accounted for by another mental disorder (e.g., dissatisfaction with body shape/size in anorexia nervosa [body dysmorphic disorder])
Evidence of severe psychological stress preceding onset/exacerbation of the physical symptoms (e.g., death of a loved one [conversion])
Preoccupation with fear of having a serious disease (hypochondriasis)
Use of denial; evidence that presence of the symptoms alleviates or promotes avoidance of the psychological conflict
Feelings of anger, helplessness, powerlessness
Report of issues suggesting unconscious secondary gain (e.g., attention of others, financial reimbursement, change in role expectations/responsibilities)

Elimination

Urinary retention
Constipation, diarrhea

Food/Fluid

Two or more GI symptoms (e.g., nausea, vomiting, bloating, intolerance of several different foods, difficulty swallowing [somatization])
Changes in eating patterns (loss of appetite/excessive intake)
Weight loss/gain

Hygiene

May neglect and/or report inability to perform basic ADLs
Excessive concern/preoccupation with/or more imagined defects in appearance (body dysmorphic disorder)

Neurosensory

Mental Status Exam:
  Fearfulness; preoccupation with belief of having serious disease; anxiety (symptoms associated with moderate to severe level) or *la belle indifférence* (lack of concern about loss of physical functioning)
  Depressed mood
  Amnesia
  Communication patterns: ruminating about physical symptoms
May display loss of consciousness other than fainting (somatization)
Apparent loss of or alteration in voluntary motor or sensory functioning that suggests neurological disease (e.g., blindness, double vision, deafness, paralysis, anosmia, aphonia, episodic seizure activity, and coordination disturbances [especially common in conversion disorder])

Pain/Discomfort

Pain in 1 or more anatomical sites of at least 6 months' duration and of sufficient severity to warrant clinical attention (pain disorder); involving 4 different sites of function (e.g., head, abdomen, back, joints, chest, during urination/menstruation/sexual intercourse [somatization])
Excessive use of analgesics with minimal relief of pain

Respiration

Respiratory rate may be increased
Shortness of breath without exertion

Safety

May report suicidal ideations, inability to continue in current situation

Social Interactions

Observed/reported impairment in social, occupational, or other areas of functioning
Acute withdrawal from life activities, fear of being seen/scrutinized by others in public setting (body dysmorphic disorder)

Sexuality

One or more sexual/reproductive symptoms other than pain, e.g., decreased libido/sexual indifference, irregular menses/excessive menstrual bleeding, erectile/ejaculatory difficulties, pseudocyesis (false pregnancy), somatization

Teaching/Learning

Reports of physical symptoms of several years' duration beginning before the age of 30 (somatization)
History of a past experience with true serious organic disease, in self or close family member (hypochondriasis)
History of frequent visits to physicians (doctor shopping) to obtain relief/requests for surgery despite medical reassurance of absence of organic pathology or need for plastic surgery (e.g., facelift, liposuction)
Failure to improve despite multiple approaches/therapies
Expression of anger and frustration toward physicians for "inability to determine cause of physical symptoms"

DIAGNOSTIC STUDIES

Virtually any diagnostic procedure (including exploratory surgery) may be performed as deemed appropriate to rule out organic pathology in light of the physical symptom(s) presented by the client.

Urine and/or Serum Toxicology Screen: Determines evidence of substance use/abuse

NURSING PRIORITIES

1. Alleviate or minimize physical symptoms/chronic pain.
2. Promote client safety.
3. Resolve potentially dysfunctional areas of client/family dynamics.
4. Promote independence in self-care activities.
5. Provide information and support for lifestyle changes.

DISCHARGE GOALS

1. Relief obtained from admitting physical symptom(s).
2. Client/family recognizes relationship between psychological stressors and onset/exacerbation of physical symptoms(s).
3. Stress management techniques used appropriately to prevent the occurrence/exacerbation of the physical symptom(s).
4. Level of function/independence increased.
5. Plan in place to meet needs after discharge.

NURSING DIAGNOSIS	COPING, INDIVIDUAL, ineffective
May Be Related to:	Severe level of anxiety, repressed; personal vulnerability
	Unrealistic perceptions
	History of self or loved one having experienced a serious illness
	Retarded ego development; fixation in earlier level of development; unmet dependency needs
	Inadequate coping skills
Possibly Evidenced by:	Verbalized inability to cope/problem-solve
	High illness rate, multiple physical complaints that are not fully explained by a known general medical condition
	Decreased functioning in social/occupational settings
	Narcissistic tendencies, with total focus on self and physical symptoms; demanding behaviors
	History of "doctor-shopping"
	Inappropriate use of defense mechanisms (e.g., denial of correlation between physical symptoms and psychologic problems); refusal to attend therapeutic activities

Desired Outcomes/Evaluation Criteria— Client Will:	Verbalize need for change within dysfunctional system.
	Recognize correlation between physical symptoms and pyschological problems.
	Demonstrate adaptive coping strategies in the face of stressful situations, discontinuing use of physical symptoms as a response.
	Report reduction of/relief from physical complaints.

ACTIONS/INTERVENTIONS	RATIONALE

Independent

Review laboratory and diagnostic results with the client in simple, easy-to-understand terminology. Answer any questions that may have arisen from discussions with the physician.	Client has the right to knowledge about own care. Honest explanation may help client to understand psychological implications. Anxiety is high, so learning is difficult, thus, explanations need to be kept simple and concrete.
Show unconditional positive regard. Convey that you understand the symptom is real to the client, even though no organic pathology can be found.	Denial of the client's feelings is nontherapeutic and interfaces with establishment of a trusting nurse/client relationship.
Discuss possibility of and client's perceptions of behavior(s) as self-destructive. Determine suicidal risk as appropriate.	Limitations imposed by chronic "illness/ disabilities" prevent client from full participation in life activities. In conjunction, multiple conflicts (e.g., medical, financial, family, legal) increase the likelihood of feelings of depression, helplessness, and hopelessness, which may in turn lead to substance abuse, dependence on pharmacological agents, and/or suicidal ideation necessitating additional therapeutic interventions.
Be available to assist the client with basic dependency needs in the initial stages of the relationship. Recognize, however, that the client may be using maladaptive behaviors	To deny client this need at this time would result in an increased anxiety level and intensification of the physical condition to preserve the dependency role.
Gradually decrease response to time and assistance required by the client as the trusting relationship becomes established. Encourage independent behaviors and respond with positive reinforcement.	Positive reinforcement enhances self-esteem and encourages repetition of desirable behaviors. Doing things for oneself helps to develop independence and improves coping ability.
Encourage verbalizations of honest feelings, including feelings of anger within appropriate limits.	Verbalization of feelings in a nonthreatening environment may help the client come to terms with the unresolved issues.
Provide safe method of hostility release (e.g., pounding pillows). Help client to identify true source of anger and work on adaptive coping skills for use outside the therapeutic setting.	Presence of depression and/or suicidal behaviors may be viewed as anger turned inward on self. When this anger is vented in a nonthreatening environment, the client may resolve these feelings, regardless of the discomfort involved.
Withdraw attention if rumination about physical symptoms begins.	Lack of response to maladaptive behaviors may discourage their repetition.

Help client identify symbols of hope in own life through exploration and discussion.

Encourages client to focus on reasons for wanting to change life.

Explore past experiences with client and correlate appearance of physical symptoms with times of stress.

Until denial defense is eliminated, change required for improvement will not occur.

Discuss possible alternative coping behaviors client may use in response to stress (e.g., relaxation techniques, deep breathing; physical activities, such as jogging, aerobics, brisk walks, housekeeping chores, sex). Offer positive reinforcement for use of these alternatives.

Because of high level of anxiety, client may require assistance in problem-solving and the ability to recognize available alternatives. Positive reinforcement enhances self-esteem and encourages repetition of desirable coping behaviors. **Note:** Stimulating activities/discussions should be avoided in late evening hours to prevent increasing level of anxiety, which could interfere with sleep.

Discourage excessive sleep during the day, and encourage establishment of a routine pattern of sleep and activity with inclusion of customary bedtime rituals (e.g., warm baths, massage, warm/nonstimulating drinks or reduction of fluid intake, light snacks).

Daytime sleep may be used as a defense to deal with pain/stressors. Ritualistic patterns and a realistic balance of activity and rest induce relaxation, promote inducement of sleep at appropriate times, and decrease interruptions of sleep. Obtaining quality sleep enhances client's ability to deal with pain and develop new coping strategies.

Report/investigate any new physical complaints.

Although physical symptoms have been used as a way of coping by the client, the possibility of organic pathology must always be considered to prevent jeopardizing client safety/well-being.

Collaborative

Provide information and recommendations regarding condition to other healthcare providers. Avoid suggesting that "the problem is all in the client's mind."

Understanding the client's psychological needs and symptoms may promote a team approach for healthcare. Research suggests a regular schedule of brief medical appointments/examinations every 4–6 weeks at preset times (not on demand), with the avoidance of laboratory tests, surgeries, and hospitalizations (unless absolutely necessary) can enhance the client's sense of well-being and actually reduce annual medical costs.

Administer medications, if indicated:

Psychopharmacological treatment is usually not indicated unless anxiety/depression is prominent.

Antianxiety agents, e.g., diazepam (Valium), chlordiazepoxide (Librium), alprazolam (Xanax);

Antianxiety medications have a calming effect on the client, masking the feelings of anxiety, which may minimize physical response. Careful monitoring of use of antianxiety agents is important because of high addiction potential. **Note:** Sedative side effects may induce sleep during day, thereby interfering with client's sleep at night.

Antidepressants, e.g., amitriptyline (Elavil), imipramine (Tofranil), fluoxetine (Prozac), sertraline (Zoloft).

Antidepressant medication may elevate the mood as it increases level of energy and decreases feelings of fatigue. **Note:** Potential for suicide increases as energy level improves.

355

NURSING DIAGNOSIS	PAIN, chronic
May Be Related to:	Severe level of anxiety, repressed
	Low-self-esteem; unmet dependency needs
	History of self or loved one having experienced a serious illness
Possibly Evidenced by:	Multiple reports of severe/prolonged pain
	Guarded movement/protective behaviors; facial mask of pain; fear of reinjury
	Altered ability to continue previous activities; social withdrawal
	Changes in weight, sleep patterns
	History of seeking assistance from numerous healthcare professionals; demands for therapy/medication
Desired Outcomes/Evaluation Criteria— Client Will:	Acknowledge relationship between psychological problems and onset/exacerbation of pain.
	Demonstrate techniques to interrupt escalating anxiety/pain.
	Verbalize noticeable reduction/relief of pain.

ACTIONS/INTERVENTIONS	RATIONALE

Independent

Note and record duration and intensity of pain. Assess factors that precipitate onset of pain. Observe and report any new or different pattern of pain behavior to physician.	The correlation of these factors provides client with information to become aware of cause/effect relationship and to gain control of outcome. **Note:** Changes in pain necessitate evaluation to rule out development of organic pathology.
Convey to client your belief that the pain is indeed real, even though no organic pathology can be found.	Denying or belittling the client's feelings is nontherapeutic and interferes with the development of a trusting relationship.
Provide nursing comfort measures with a matter-of-fact approach that does not provide added attention to the pain behavior (e.g., back rub, warm bath, heating pad).	May serve to provide some temporary relief of pain for the client. Secondary gains from solicitous behavior may provide positive reinforcement and can actually prolong use of maladaptive behaviors.
Assist client with activities that distract from focus on self and pain.	Helps the client to focus on adaptive behavior patterns and serves as a transition to higher levels of therapy.
Use distractors to facilitate initiation of discussion of unresolved psychological issues (e.g., open expression of feelings such as guilt, fear about life events).	Unresolved psychological issues must be dealt with before maladaptive patterns can be eliminated.
Help client connect times of onset/exacerbation of pain with times of increased anxiety.	Client's ability to connect pain to times of increased anxiety helps to decrease denial and is the first step in resolution of the problem.

Identify specific situations that cause anxiety to rise, and demonstrate techniques to interrupt the pain response (e.g., visual or auditory distractions, guided imagery, breathing exercises, massage, application of heat or cold, relaxation techniques).

Use of techniques described may help to maintain anxiety at manageable level and prevent the pain from becoming disabling.

Provide positive reinforcement when client is not focusing on pain.

Positive reinforcement, in the form of the nurse's presence and attention, may encourage a continuation of these more adaptive behaviors by the client.

Collaborative

Review ongoing assessments by physician and laboratory/other diagnostic studies.

The possibility of organic pathology needs to be ruled out.

Administer medications as indicated, e.g.:
    Aspirin, ibuprofen (Motrin, Advil);

ASA and other nonsteroidal anti-inflammatory agents have minimal side effects and low addiction potential and are useful in treating episodic exacerbations of chronic pain.

Low-dose antidepressants, e.g., amitriptyline (Elavil), doxepin (Sinequan), phenelzine (Nardil);

Helps combat depression, may enhance sleep, reduce level of fatigue, and promote feelings of well-being.

Anticonvulsants, e.g., phenytoin (Dilantin), carbamazepine (Tegretol), clonazepam (Klonopin);

Studies suggest short-term use may be of some benefit in treating neuropathic and neuralgic pain while other therapeutic interventions are initiated.

Sedative medications at bedtime, e.g., triazolam (Halcion).

Level of repressed anxiety/physical symptoms may interfere with obtaining quality sleep, which has a negative impact on energy level and coping ability. Sedatives should not be used for longer than a 3-week period, as they eventually interfere with, rather than promote, sleep.

Refer to chronic pain clinic.

May be helpful to learn ways to manage residual pain on a long-term basis.

NURSING DIAGNOSIS	BODY IMAGE disturbance
May Be Related to:	Severe level of anxiety, repressed
	Low self-esteem; unmet dependency needs
Possibly Evidenced by:	Preoccupation with real or imagined change in bodily structure and/or function that is out of proportion to any actual abnormality that may exist
	Negative feelings about body/self
	Fear of negative reaction or rejection by others; change in social involvement
Desired Outcomes/Evaluation Criteria—Client Will:	Verbalize realistic perception of bodily condition.
	Express positive feelings about body.
	Function independently and interact socially without experiencing discomfort.

ACTIONS/INTERVENTIONS	RATIONALE

Independent

Ascertain client's perception of own body image. Acknowledge that disability is real to the client, even in the absence of evidence of organic pathology.

Information about the way in which the individual views self aids in choosing appropriate interventions. Denial of client's feelings is nontherapeutic and impedes the development of trust.

Help client to see that image is distorted and out of proportion to reality of actual change in structure and/or function. Correct inaccurate perceptions in a matter-of-fact, nonthreatening manner.

Recognition that a misperception/distortion exists is necessary before client can accept reality and reduce significance of impairment.

Encourage verbalization of fears and anxieties associated with identified stressful life situations. Discuss ways in which client may respond more adaptively in the future.

Verbalization of feelings with a trusted individual may help the client come to terms with unresolved issues. A plan of action formulated with assistance and at a time when anxiety is low may prevent later dysfunctional response by client.

Encourage and give positive feedback for independent self-care behaviors, while gradually withdrawing attention from dependent behaviors.

Lack of attention to maladaptive behaviors discourages their repetition. Positive reinforcement enhances self-esteem and promotes repetition of desirable behaviors.

Collaborative

Administer medications as indicated, e.g.:
    Antidepressants, e.g., clomipramine (Anafranil), or selective serotonin reuptake inhibitors, e.g., fluoxetine (Prozac).

These psychoactive drugs increase the amount of serotonin available for uptake by brain cells, which tends to lessen the individual's bodily preoccupations and lifts their spirits.

NURSING DIAGNOSIS	SELF CARE deficit (specify)
May Be Related to:	Paralysis of body part
	Inability to see, hear, speak
	Pain, discomfort
Possibly Evidenced by:	Inability to bring food from a receptable to the mouth; obtain or get to water sources; wash body or body parts; regulate temperature or flow of water
	Impaired ability to put on or take off necessary items of clothing, obtain or replace articles of clothing, fasten clothing, maintain appearance at a satisfactory level
	Inability to get to toilet or commode (impaired mobility); manipulate clothing for toileting; flush toilet or empty commode; sit on or rise from toilet or commode; carry out proper toilet hygiene

Desired Outcomes/Evaluation Criteria—Client Will:	Display willingness to participate in ADLs.
	Demonstrate techniques/lifestyle changes to meet self-care needs.
	Perform self-care activities independently within level of ability.

ACTIONS/INTERVENTIONS	RATIONALE

Independent

Assess degree of impairment; note level of disability as well as areas of strength.	Establishes client needs and identifies individual potentials.
Encourage client to perform ADLs to own level of ability. Intervene only when client is unable to perform.	Loss of function may be related to unfulfilled dependency needs. Intervening when client is capable of performing independently serves to foster dependency in the client.
Convey a nonjudgmental attitude as nursing assistance with self-care activities is provided. Remember that the physical symptom is real to the client and is not within the client's conscious control.	A judgmental attitude interferes with the nurse's ability to provide therapeutic care for the client, provoking defensiveness that blocks client's willingness to look at own behavior/dynamics.
Provide positive reinforcement for ADLs performed independently.	Enhances self-esteem and encourages repetition of desirable behaviors.
Encourage client to discuss feelings regarding the disability and the need for dependency it creates. Help the client to see the purpose this disability is serving.	Self-disclosure and exploration of feelings with a trusted individual may help client fulfill unmet needs and come to terms with unresolved issues, thus eliminating the need for maladaptive physical responses.
Involve family members in care at level of their ability/willingness.	Feelings of anger toward the client may interfere with ability to provide care in a therapeutic/nonjudgmental manner.

Collaborative

Refer to occupational/physical therapy, community resources/supports.	Involvement with these programs provides role models, enhances client's self-esteem, promoting ability to care for self.

NURSING DIAGNOSIS	SENSORY/PERCEPTUAL alterations (specify)
May Be Related to:	Psychological stress (narrowed perceptual fields caused by anxiety, expression of stress as physical problems/deficits)
	Poor quality of sleep
	Presence of chronic pain
Possibly Evidenced by:	Reported change in voluntary motor or sensory function (e.g., paralysis, anosmia, aphonia, deafness, blindness, loss of touch or pain sensation)
	La belle indifférence (lack of concern over functional loss)

359

Desired Outcomes/Evaluation Criteria—Client Will:	Verbalize understanding of emotional problems as a contributing factor to alteration in physical functioning.
	Identify adaptive ways of coping with stress and community support systems to whom she or he may go for help.
	Demonstrate recovery of lost function.

ACTIONS/INTERVENTIONS	RATIONALE

Independent

Identify gains that the physical symptom is providing for the client (e.g., increased dependency, attention, distraction from other problems).	Helps provide focus on "actual" problem, enhancing appropriateness of interventions and problem resolution.
Assist client with ADLs with which the physical symptom is interfering.	Promotes general well-being, meets comfort and safety needs without undue attention.
Allow client to be as independent as possible without focusing on the disability. Intervene only when client requires assistance.	Encourages client to begin to assume responsibility for self. Giving attention to the use of the maladaptive response reinforces secondary gain, such as dependency.
Encourage client to participate in therapeutic activities to the best of ability. Do not allow client to use disability as an excuse for nonparticipation. Withdraw attention if client continues to focus on physical limitation. Reinforce reality as required while ensuring maintenance of a nonthreatening environment.	Gently confronting reality of client's abilities while minimizing attention to problem helps client begin to accept own responsibility.
Encourage client to verbalize fears and anxieties. Help client recognize that physical symptom appears at times of extreme stress and is a way of coping with that stress.	May be unaware of relationship between physical symptom and emotional stress.
Help client identify positive coping mechanisms that can be used when faced with stressful situations.	Client has been accustomed to using maladaptive coping to retreat from reality and needs to begin to change to more realistic ways of dealing with problems.
Explain/review assertiveness techniques and use role-play to practice use.	Enhances self-esteem and minimizes anxiety in interpersonal relationships.
Identify SO(s), other support systems that can provide assistance to the client.	Satisfactory supports can help client cope with overwhelming stress.

Collaborative

Monitor ongoing assessments, laboratory findings, and other data.	Assures client that possibility of organic pathology is clearly ruled out. Failure to do so may jeopardize client safety.

NURSING DIAGNOSIS	SOCIAL INTERACTION, impaired
May Be Related to:	Inability to engage in satisfying personal relationships
	Preoccupation with self and physical symptoms; altered state of wellness, chronic pain
	Rejection by others due to focus on self/physical symptoms
Possibly Evidenced by:	Preoccupation with own thoughts; repetitive verbalization about self/physical symptoms
	Seeking to be alone; uncommunicative, withdrawn; no eye contact; sad, dull affect
	Absence of supportive significant others(s)—family, friends, social contacts
Desired Outcomes/Evaluation Criteria—Client Will:	Spend time voluntarily with others in group activities.
	Interact with others without apparent discomfort.
	Demonstrate interest in others, while discontinuing use of statements that focus on self/physical symptoms.

ACTIONS/INTERVENTIONS	RATIONALE

Independent

Spend time with client after setting limits on attention-seeking behaviors. Withdraw presence if ruminations about physical symptoms begin.	The nurse's presence conveys a sense of worthwhileness to the client. Lack of reinforcement of maladaptive behaviors may help to decrease their repetition.
Increase amount of time/attention given during times when client is not focusing on physical symptoms.	This separates the person from the behavior and increases feelings of self-worth as unconditional acceptance is experienced by the client without need for the physical symptoms.
Describe client's interpersonal behaviors objectively. Emphasize how the focus on self/physical symptoms discourages relationships with others.	Client may not realize how own behavior is perceived by others/results in alienation.
Assist client in learning assertiveness techniques, especially the ability to recognize the difference between passive, assertive, and aggressive behaviors and the importance of respecting the human rights of others while protecting one's own basic rights.	Use of these techniques enhances self-esteem and facilitates communication and mutual acceptance in interpersonal relationships.
Encourage attendance in group activities after client is interacting appropriately in the 1:1 relationship. Accompany the client the first few times.	As a trusted individual, the nurse provides objective feedback about client's behavior in the group. Subsequent discussion and role-play on a 1:1 basis may help prepare client for future group encounters and may promote success with this endeavor.

Provide positive feedback for any attempts at social interaction in which the client's focus is on others rather than self/physical symptoms.

Positive feedback enhances self-esteem and encourages repetition of desirable behaviors.

NURSING DIAGNOSIS	KNOWLEDGE deficit [LEARNING NEED] regarding condition, prognosis, and treatment needs
May Be Related to:	Strong denial defense system
	Severe level of repressed anxiety
	Preoccupation with self and pain
	Lack of interest in learning
Possibly Evidenced by:	Verbalization of denial statements, such as, "I don't know why the doctor put me on the psychiatric unit, I have a physical problem."
	History of "doctor shopping" for evidence of organic pathology to substantiate physical symptoms
	Lack of follow-through with psychiatric treatment plan
Desired Outcomes/Evaluation Criteria— Client Will:	Verbalize understanding of psychological implications of physical symptoms.
	Report relief from physical symptoms.
	Demonstrate more appropriate coping mechanisms to employ in response to stress.

ACTIONS/INTERVENTIONS	RATIONALE

Independent

Ascertain client's level of knowledge regarding effects of psychological problems on the body. Be aware of degree to which denial defense controls client's behavior.

Knowing what information the individual already has provides a base that is necessary to develop an effective teaching plan for the client. Strong denial system needs to be penetrated before learning can begin.

Assess client's level of anxiety and readiness to learn.

Effective learning does not take place when level of anxiety is moderate to severe. Client's narrowed focus precludes attending to external cues.

Explain purpose and review results of laboratory/ diagnostic testing, as well as aspects of the physical examination.

Client has basic right to knowledge about care. Objective knowledge about physical condition may help to break through the strong denial defense.

Have client keep 2 separate records: (1) a diary of the appearance, duration, and intensity of physical symptoms and (2) a journal of situations that the client finds especially stressful.

Comparison of these records may provide objective data from which to observe the relationship between physical symptoms and stress. Guided therapeutic writing is also a useful tool for monitoring the client's safety and response to interventions.

362

Help client identify needs that are being met through the sick role (e.g., dependency needs, attention seeking, or cover-up for painful conflicts in life situation).

Help client recognize and accept more adaptive means for fulfilling these needs. Practice through role-playing. Demonstrate/encourage use of adaptive methods of stress management (e.g., relaxation techniques, physical exercises, meditation, breathing exercises, autogenics).

Incorporate occupational/recreational therapy activities in treatment plan to help client learn adaptive coping mechanisms.

Encourage participation in Outdoor Education Program, e.g., wall/rock climbing, hiking, caving.

Include family/SO(s) in learning opportunities, assisting them to understand underlying reasons for client's behavior.

Client usually does not realize that the physical symptoms are fulfilling unmet needs. Recognition needs to be achieved before change can occur. Role-play can relieve anxiety by helping client anticipate responses to stressful situations.

These techniques may be employed in an attempt to relieve anxiety and discourage the use of physical symptoms as a maladaptive response. Additionally, exercise therapy need not be aerobic or intensive to stimulate release of endorphins and enhance client's sense of general well-being.

Daily activities can provide opportunities to learn/practice specialized techniques for coping with stress (e.g., decision-making, problem-solving, housekeeping, art/plant therapy, bowling, volleyball, weight lifting).

Involvement in activities that challenge physical and psychological abilities can help the client learn to become more self-aware and confident and increase self-esteem.

Having understanding support from significant other(s) can help client to accept reality of situation and make required changes.

SOMATOFORM DISORDERS: Somatoform Disorders

NURSING DIAGNOSIS

SEXUAL dysfunction, actual/risk for

May Be Related to:

Perceived or actual loss of bodily structure or function

Preoccupation with physical symptoms; total focus on self/chronic pain response

Fear of contracting a serious disease

Possibly Evidenced by (Actual):

Alterations in relationship with SO

Actual/perceived limitation imposed by condition

Change in interest in self/others; sexual indifference

Lack of pleasure/pain [dyspareunia] during intercourse

Inability to achieve or maintain erection

Desire to achieve greater satisfaction in sexual role

Desired Outcomes/Evaluation Criteria—Client Will:

Identify underlying stressors that contribute to the dysfunction.

Discuss concerns/perceptions with partner.

Demonstrate techniques to control stressors.

Verbalize achievement of sexual functioning at a mutually desired level.

363

Independent

Obtain sexual history, including previous pattern of functioning and client's perception of current problem.

Identifies individual need(s) in order to focus therapeutic interventions

Determine pattern of drug use, including type, amount, and frequency of use.

Certain types of drugs can interfere with sexual functioning, e.g., alcohol, tranquilizers, narcotics, antihypertensives, antidepressants.

Identify stressors in client's life. Explore correlation of stressful situations to onset of sexual dysfunction.

Recognition and acceptance of psychological implications (progression beyond the denial defense) need to occur before positive change can be effected.

Be aware of pathophysiology that could negatively affect sexual functioning, e.g., hypertension, diabetes.

Organic pathology as an etiological factor needs to be considered in problem-solving when setting goals and identifying appropriate interventions.

Provide education regarding sexual functioning and alternative methods of fulfillment, as client indicates need and desire for this type of information.

Client may have misinformation about normal bodily functioning that may interfere with sexual fulfillment. Alternative methods may help to meet a need until desired level of functioning is attained.

Include SO in sessions as appropriate.

Input from client's sexual partner will have a significant influence on client's progress. The couple should be treated as a unit. An absence of mutual trust and unwillingness to discuss each other's needs interferes with the goals of remediation.

Collaborative

Refer to appropriate resources, such as clinical specialist, professional sex therapist, or family counselor.

May require individuals with a greater degree of knowledge and expertise in this specialty area to achieve resolution of persistent problem(s).

CHAPTER 11

DISSOCIATIVE DISORDERS

DISSOCIATIVE DISORDERS

DSM-IV
300.12 Dissociative amnesia
300.13 Dissociative fugue
300.14 Dissociative identity disorder
300.15 Dissociative disorder NOS
300.6   Depersonalization disorder

In these disorders a disturbance or alteration exists in the normally integrative functions of identity, memory, or consciousness. The individual blocks off part of his or her life from consciousness during periods of intolerable stress. The stressful emotion becomes a separate entity, as the individual "splits" from it and mentally drifts into a fantasy state.

ETIOLOGICAL THEORIES

Psychodynamics

Selective repression of distressing mental contents from conscious awareness is used as a mechanism for protecting the individual from emotional pain or expressing self in dangerous ways. The stressor(s) may arise from external circumstances or internal sources with onset of symptoms sudden or gradual and of transient or chronic nature. Intrapsychic conflict thus uses denial and "ego splitting" to decrease anxiety.

Physical sensations seen in these disorders may represent forbidden wishes that have been somatized. The use of the defense mechanism of displacement allows the feeling(s) to be directed away from the ego-threatening object toward one less threatening. In psychoanalytic terms, dissociation is a form of denial in which the object denied is part of the self or ego.

Biological

Research on the biological basis of these disorders is increasing as more recognition of the mind-body connection is accepted. It is difficult to determine whether the biological changes (fight-or-flight mechanism) that accompany severe anxiety precede or precipitate the emotional state. Biochemical, physiological, and endocrine systems have an intimate connection with actual physical changes occurring in all body systems via the autonomic nervous system. Some studies have shown EEG abnormalities associated with cerebral mechanisms in the temporal and limbic regions of the brain, which mediate identity formation and a sense of personal boundaries and may affect development of gender and generation boundaries.

Organic causes of pathological dissociative experiences that are known or suspected include temporal lobe epilepsy, sensory deprivation, sleep loss, strokes, encephalitis, and Alzheimer's disease. Drugs may also induce amnesia or depersonalization directly or indirectly in some incidences. However, most dissociative states are not associated with any obvious organic conditions and the diagnosis of dissociative disorder requires that the condition is not due to the direct effects of a substance or a general medical condition.

Family Dynamics

In Systems theory, the family is viewed as a system in which the process (interactions between/among family members) is the prime determinant. Level of differentiation and level of anxiety determine the degree of pathology.

Psychosocial theory states that individuals who develop dissociative disorders have often experienced severe physical, sexual, and/or emotional abuse early in life—stress so severe that the only way to cope with the painful emotions is to detach from them. The child learns to respond to stressful situations in this manner. One parent may be abusive, with the other being a passive participant, not taking care of or protecting the child. Psychiatric diagnoses (especially alcoholism) in close relatives are common, although multiple personality diagnosis is not.

Certain behaviors observed in childhood, though considered normal, may be identified as dissociative, including construction of imaginary playmates, use of different names or ages for themselves, taking on the role of an animal, imagining self as having been adopted or coming from another family, separation from the past, gender confusion, and regressive behavior. Responding to stressful situations with dissociative behaviors then becomes a method of coping for some individuals into adulthood, when there is less control over the dissociative states. The response becomes maladaptive in that the individual escapes from the stressful situation rather than facing it.

CLIENT ASSESSMENT DATA BASE

Activity/Rest

Insomnia

Ego Integrity

Confusion about personal identity, may have assumed a new identity either partial or complete (fugue)
Anxiety responses, report of phobias; fears of going crazy

Neurosensory

Memory lapses/amnesia; disorientation; inability to recall important personal information/specific incidents not due to direct effects of a substance, general medical condition, or ordinary forgetfulness
May report hallucinations, delusions
Mood swings; psychological conflicts; family/peers may describe client's behavior as erratic, unpredictable, or unreliable
Sudden, unexpected travel away from familiar surroundings of work and home, with inability to recall past (fugue)
Persistent/recurrent experiences of feeling detached from own mental processes or body, although reality testing remains intact (depersonalization)
Presence of 2 or more distinct identities or personality states (mean average of 13), with each a fully integrated, complex unit with unique memories, behaviors, and relationships (or may be a personality state that does not have as wide a range of patterns) recurrently taking control of client's behavior, with transition from one personality to another being sudden/associated with psychosocial stress. Alternate personalities vary in their awareness of each other, may be of opposite genders, and are commonly children, although some may be stated to be older than the individual (dissociative identity disorder)
Transient changes in facial expression, voice, and posture; tastes/habits that seem to change quickly or often

Safety

Suicidal feelings/behaviors
Evidence of self-mutilation

Sexuality

History of severe childhood incest, sexual/physical/psychological abuse
Sexually inhibited or promiscuous

Social Interactions

Significant distress or impairment in social, occupation, or other important areas of functioning

Teaching/Learning

More common in women than in men, in persons with some higher education, and in white-collar workers
Age of onset is early childhood, although often not diagnosed until the third decade
Seldom diagnosed upon initial clinical contact (accurate diagnosis may be delayed by a period of months to years)
Substance abuse may be reported (but is not cause of disorder)
Absence of organic brain disorders (e.g., temporal lobe epilepsy)
History of major depression greater than 90% (dissociative identity disorder)

DIAGNOSTIC STUDIES

(Evaluations to rule out an underlying or concurrent disease process are based on individual symptoms.)

Neurological Testing (e.g., EEG and CT/MRI Scans): To rule out organic brain conditions related to trauma, tumor, congenital defects, and temporal lobe epilepsy, symptoms of which often parallel manifestations of dissociative identity disorder.

Psychosocial Assessment, such as Rorschach, Thematic Apperception Test (TAT), Minnesota Multiphasic Personality Inventory (MMPI), Weschler Adult Intelligence Scale (WAIS), Dissociative Experiences Scale (DES), Dissociative Disorders Interview Schedule (DDIS), and Hypnosis or Amobarbital Interviews: As indicated to provide behavioral observation and documentation describing the character, duration, frequency, and precipitation of behavioral changes and client comments or complaints essential to the diagnostic process, as these clients are frequently misdiagnosed initially because of blurring of symptoms that parallel other psychiatric problems—commonly depression, neuroses, personality disorders, and schizophrenia.

Drug Screen: Assess for concomitant substance use.

NURSING PRIORITIES

1. Provide safe environment; protect client/others from injury.
2. Assist client to recognize anxiety.
3. Promote insight into relationship between anxiety and development of dissociative state/other personalities.
4. Support client/family in developing effective coping skills and participating in therapeutic activities.

DISCHARGE GOALS

1. Recognizes potentially dangerous behaviors/personalities and contracts for safety.
2. Client/family are participating in therapeutic regimen.
3. Effective coping skills, understanding of underlying dynamics of condition are demonstrated.

4. Recovers deficits in memory.
5. Major/emerging personality has been chosen and accepted (dissociative identity disorder) or client is managing stress without resorting to dissociation.
6. Plan in place to meet needs after discharge.

NURSING DIAGNOSIS	ANXIETY [severe/panic]/FEAR
May Be Related to:	Maladaptation of ineffective coping continuing from early life
	Unconscious conflict(s); threat to self-concept, threat of death (perceived or actual)
	Unmet needs
	Phobic stimulus
Possibly Evidenced by:	Increased tension; apprehension, fright; restlessness
	Feelings of inadequacy; focus on self or projection of personal perceptions onto the environment
	Verbalized focus of fear, e.g., fear of "going crazy"
	Maladaptive response to stress (dissociating self/fragmentation of the personality)
	Sympathetic stimulation: cardiovascular excitation, superficial vasoconstriction, pupil dilation
Desired Outcomes/Evaluation Criteria—Client Will:	Acknowledge and discuss feelings of anxiety and fear.
	Identify ways to manage anxiety/fear effectively.
	Demonstrate problem-solving skills.
	Use resources effectively.

ACTIONS/INTERVENTIONS	RATIONALE
Independent	
Develop rapport and trust; accept client's verbal expression of feelings/anxieties.	A trusting alliance facilitates early identification of the underlying sources of anxiety and development of an appropriate treatment approach. Learning to turn to trusted others for support helps the client develop healthy methods of dealing with anxiety.
Discuss with the client the availability of assistance in maintaining safety. (Refer to ND: Violence, risk for, directed at self/others.)	Prevents a false assurance of safety, particularly when internal threats to safety may not be readily apparent. Lack of awareness of need/failure to use resources increases the likelihood of isolation and destructive behaviors. **Note:** Expressions of anxiety may represent a very real threat to or from alternate personalities and/or others.

Identify stressor(s) that precipitate severe anxiety. (Refer to ND: Personal Identity disturbance.)

Helps client recognize individual factors precipitating dissociative symptoms (e.g., splitting, fugue, amnesia), which interfere with developments/use of adequate coping skills.

Maintain a neutral approach when confronted by an alternate personality or dissociative state.

Allows essential observation and documentation and promotes a trusting relationship. Also helps the therapist/care provider to avoid consciously or unconsciously promoting fragmentation of the personality. Because dissociative identity disorder has been sensationalized, personnel may be intrigued by manifestations and respond to the client in ways that reinforce the behaviors manifesting the disorder.

Provide support and encouragement during times of depersonalization.

Client experiences fear and anxiety at these times and may fear "going crazy." Acknowledging these feelings will help client deal appropriately with them.

Reduce alterable sources of stress. Provide calm environment; minimize external stimuli. Identify individual causes/precipitators of stress.

Manipulation of the environment to reduce extraneous sources of stress allows the client to recognize and develop skills in managing internal sources of conflict.

Discuss relationship between severe anxiety and depersonalization behaviors.

Awareness of this relationship provides opportunity to define problem, look at options for dealing with stressors in more effective ways.

Explore past experiences and painful situations (e.g., trauma, abuse) that may be repressed.

Traumatic experiences/patterns of behavior may predispose individuals to dissociative disorders.

Provide positive reinforcement and expectations. Role-model desired behaviors.

This client is commonly very suggestible and responsive to the positive expectations and attention of trusted others. Development of healthy coping mechanisms helps in reducing anxiety.

Prepare client for any testing procedures; provide information about the reason for the test and what is to be expected from the results.

An explanation of the processes of each test can allay anxiety. Care needs to be taken that the physical assessment is presented as routine because the client may misperceive the test as indicative of the presence of a physical disorder and may be prone to a psychosomatic or conversion disorder.

Review test results as indicated.

Receiving the results in a timely manner relieves antianxiety. Once organic causes have been ruled out, it is unlikely that extensive examinations and/or testing will have to be repeated, reducing the likelihood that the client might adopt physical symptoms, providing secondary gain.

Observe for/review with client untoward effects/adverse reaction to medication regimen. Monitor level of alertness, vital signs; note urinary retention, dry mouth, blurred vision, parkinson-like symptoms, rigidity, or atypical response (excitability, restlessness, agitation).

Psychoactive medications (sedatives, antianxiety/antipsychotic agents, and antidepressants) frequently produce hypotension and anticholinergic and extrapyramidal symptoms, in addition to the desired effect. Early intervention will alleviate prolonged difficulties and/or serious physical complications and may prevent/lessen anxiety about their presence.

369

Collaborative

Coordinate and develop a combined treatment plan. Facilitate communication among team members.

These clients do better when dealing with one primary provider supported by a cohesive treatment team. Therefore, it is essential that all members of the treatment team work together in planning care to ensure that goals and objectives are in agreement and continuity of care exists. Because these clients are prone to manipulative behaviors and may be resistant to therapy, a coordinated treatment plan prevents dissension between disciplines.

Administer antianxiety medications as indicated, e.g., alprazolam (Xanax), diazepam (Valium).

Antianxiety medications are given with caution for brief periods to allay panic states or disabling anxiety. Caution is essential, as substance abuse is a common complication and also because of the potential for self-destructive behavior.

NURSING DIAGNOSIS	THOUGHT PROCESSES, altered
May Be Related to:	Psychological conflict; severe level of repressed anxiety
	Pattern of trauma/abuse; threat to physical integrity/self-concept
Possibly Evidenced by:	Memory loss/deficit—inability to recall selected events related to a stressful situation, inability to recall events associated with entire life, inability to recall own identity; disorientation
Desired Outcomes/Evaluation Criteria— Client Will:	Verbalize understanding that loss of memory is related to stress.
	Begin discussing stressful situation(s).
	Recover deficits in memory.
	Develop more adaptive coping mechanisms to deal with life stressors.

ACTIONS/INTERVENTIONS	RATIONALE

Independent

Determine degree/extent of memory deficits. Obtain information about client from family/SO, identifying likes, dislikes, important people, activities, music, pets, etc.

Incorporating information about past may aid client in recovering memories.

Expose client to stimuli that represent pleasant experiences from the past, such as smells associated with enjoyable activities and music known to be pleasurable.

Providing pleasurable stimuli can lead client to remembering the past without risk of sudden trauma.

Avoid flooding client with data about past life.

May expose client to painful information from which the amnesia is providing protection. Client may decompensate even further into a psychotic state if recall is too rapid.

Engage in further activities that stimulate life experiences as memory returns.

Encourage client to discuss situations that have been especially stressful and to explore the feelings associated with those times.

Explore more adaptive ways to respond to anxiety.

Supports continued recall in a nonthreatening manner.

Verbalization of feelings in nonthreatening environment may help client come to terms with unresolved issues that may be contributing to the dissociative process.

Dissociative behaviors will no longer be needed when more effective responses are used.

Collaborative

Administer medication as indicated, e.g.: methylphenidate (Ritalin), pemoline (Cylert), bupropion (Wellbutrin).

Anecdotal information suggests that use of agents that increase synaptic levels of dopamine may be beneficial in treating depersonalization disorder when the client is distressed by persistent symptoms.

Prepare for/assist with IV amobarbital (Amytal) therapy.

May help client regain memory in amnesic or fugue state.

NURSING DIAGNOSIS	COPING, INDIVIDUAL, ineffective
May Be Related to:	Personal vulnerability; unmet expectations; inadequate support systems/coping methods
	Multiple stressors/recurrent, overwhelming trauma to the client, usually occurring in the family of origin
Possibly Evidenced by:	Verbalization of inability to cope/problem-solve
	Inappropriate use of defense mechanisms (dissociative states)
	Reports of chronic worry, anxiety, depression, poor self-esteem
	Inability to meet role expectations; divorce and alienation
Desired Outcomes/Evaluation Criteria— Client Will:	Identify ineffective coping behaviors and consequences that are creating problems for the client.
	Meet psychological needs as evidenced by appropriate expression of feelings, identification of options, and use of resources.
	Demonstrate positive coping mechanisms.

ACTIONS/INTERVENTIONS	RATIONALE

Independent

Discuss measures being taken to protect client. Stay with client as needed.

Reassures client of psychological safety/security when dissociative behaviors and/or therapy are frightening to the client. Presence of a trusted person can provide sense of security.

Commit to long-term alliance. Contract with client to refrain from acting on destructive thoughts or ending therapy abruptly. (Refer to ND: Violence, risk for, directed at self/others.)

Encourage discussion and verbalization of stressful situation and exploration of feelings associated with those times. Help client to understand that disequilibrium is to be expected, is understandable, and will resolve as integration occurs.

Demonstrate acceptance during disclosure of painful experiences.

Have client identify methods of coping with stress in the past, the purpose served, and consequences. Determine whether the response was adaptive or maladaptive.

Remain alert to possibility of substance use.

Assist the client to explore alternative coping strategies, evaluating benefits and consequences of each.

Reinforce positive coping techniques.

Provide supportive, insight-oriented therapy; encourage expression of feelings; accept verbal expressions without judgment; encourage recognition of strengths, positive attributes, and progress toward wellness.

Discuss problems of discouragement with slow progress/resolution of problems.

Identify specific conflicts that remain unresolved and problem-solve possible solutions.

Collaborative

Assist client to develop a network of support systems through family, friends, community

These clients often have difficulty developing a therapeutic relationship. Because of high incidence of childhood abuse, client mistrusts authority and has a lifelong habit of "keeping secrets" from self and others.

Ventilation in a nonthreatening environment may help the client to come to terms with issues that may be contributing to the dissociative process. Provides opportunity for client to relive traumatic experiences, purge associated feelings, and accept the memories.

Fear of condemnation and criticism makes such disclosure difficult, even in a trusting relationship, and support provides reassurance that information will be treated tactfully.

As anxiety decreases, client can begin to develop insight into the appropriateness of the response and develop a plan of action for the future. It is important for the client to understand and accept that the dissociative behavior was originally adaptive and allowed the individual to survive an intolerable situation.

A significant percentage of these clients use substances, such as alcohol, as a means of numbing feelings/coping with psychic pain. This can cloud symptomatology and interfere with progress.

Helps the client to learn new ways to problem-solve and make decisions, which will promote development of independence and use of adaptive coping skills.

Promotes repetition of adaptive behaviors. These clients are very responsive to positive attention.

Dissociative symptoms arise from internal conflict. The behaviors protect the client from psychic pain. Subsequently, any stressor can precipitate a like reaction. Insight-oriented therapy in a supportive setting allows the client to confront and resolve past and present painful or fear-inducing events.

Discouraged feelings are inevitable (in face of treatment that may last for years), and client may resort to old, maladaptive coping mechanisms and feel like giving up. (Refer to ND: Violence, risk for, directed at self/others.)

When these underlying conflicts are not resolved, any improvement in coping behaviors may be regarded as temporary.

The tendency to overdependency present in these individuals is antitherapeutic and draining to resources, school/work and church affiliations, as well as health and mental healthcare providers and internal resources.

family, friends, and therapy providers. Development of a large support network and internal resources promotes autonomy.

NURSING DIAGNOSIS	VIOLENCE, risk for, directed at self/others
Risk Factors May Include:	Dissociative state/conflicting personalities
	Depressed mood
	Panic states
	Suicidal behaviors
[Possible Indicators:]	Increased motor activity, pacing, excitement, irritability, agitation
	Self-destructive behaviors, active aggressive suicidal acts/threats; "internal homicide" (in which one personality attempts to kill another personality)
	Substance abuse
Desired Outcomes/Evaluation Criteria— Client Will:	Verbalize understanding of why behavior occurs.
	Demonstrate self-control as evidenced by relaxed posture, nonviolent behavior.
	Express increased self-esteem and meet needs in an assertive manner.
	Use resources and support systems effectively.

ACTIONS/INTERVENTIONS	RATIONALE

Independent

Remain vigilant to behavioral changes that may signal destructive actions. Assess seriousness of suicidal tendency, gestures, threats, or previous attempts. (Use scale of 1–10 and prioritize according to severity of threat, availability of means.)

Client behavior may change abruptly and dramatically. Impulse control may be impaired. (May be no. 1 nursing diagnosis if score is high.)

Structure the environment to reduce stressors, and remove dangerous objects.

Minimizing environmental stimuli to provide calm surroundings may prevent escalation/occurrence of violence.

Help client identify/recognize precipitants to destructive behaviors. Discuss ways to reduce exposure to external stressors such as avoidance when practical.

Permits the client to recognize personally distressing factors, promoting early detection and timely intervention. Allows environmental manipulation to reduce the occurrence of disruptive/injurious behaviors.

Active-listen, and encourage the client to seek restraint and/or support, when self-destructive or violent impulses are present.

A therapeutic alliance promotes client responsibility for behavioral restraint while supplementing internal controls. Ventilation can reduce the need for action.

Arrange protection in presence of multiple personalities for "individual" who is prone to violent behavior. Appoint another personality, usually the primary one, to monitor/control the behavior of the suspect personality.

Usually one personality can be identified as having these behaviors, and use of another personality may keep the violence from occurring.

Assist client to identify alternatives to aggression or self-destructive behaviors (e.g., verbal expression, physical activity, written expression).

Provides a substitute activity in response to overwhelming impulse to enable client to respond to impulses in a nondestructive manner.

Take immediate and decisive action when danger is imminent. Tell client to STOP and/or hold as necessary until client calms down.

The organized approach of a concerned response by caregivers allows for rapid resolution and minimizes potential for injury to the client/staff/others.

Encourage participation in exercise program/physical activities.

Promotes safe and effective way of relieving tension. Enhances sense of general well-being. **Note:** Exercise therapy does not need to be aerobic or intensive to achieve desired effect.

Note presence/degree of depression and reassess periodically, noting suicidal ideation.

Client may become discouraged and depressed, as treatment is a long-term process, possibly in excess of 10 years.

Collaborative

Hospitalize as necessary in inpatient/acute care psychiatric facility.

Usually instituted for differential diagnosis, in response to self-destructive thoughts/behavior, violence or potential violence, and/or psychosomatic complaints or conversion reaction.

Place in isolation and provide physical restraint in a nonpunitive manner. Observe closely/stay with client.

Punishment has no therapeutic value, but external controls are necessary to ensure safety/provide reassurance to client when internal controls fail. Close observation following initial restraint will be necessary to assure the effectiveness of the restraints and that the client is not injured by the restraint (e.g., impaired circulation, aspiration, suffocation, strangulation).

Administer antianxiety/antidepressant medication as indicated.

May be required to reduce anxiety until internal controls are achieved and/or elevate mood to allow client to begin to deal with feelings/situation.

NURSING DIAGNOSIS	PERSONAL IDENTITY disturbance
May Be Related to:	Psychological conflicts (dissociative state[s])
	Threat to physical integrity/self-concept; pattern of childhood trauma/abuse
	Underdeveloped ego
Possibly Evidenced by:	Memory loss (unable to recall selected events/own identity); presence of more than one personality within the individual
	Confusion about sense of self, purpose or direction in life; alteration in preception or experience of the self

Desired Outcomes/Evaluation Criteria—Client Will:	Loss of one's own sense of reality/the external world; poorly differentiated ego boundaries
	Acknowledge threat to personal identity.
	Engage in a therapeutic alliance.
	Integrate threat in a healthy, positive manner (e.g., make commitment to long-term therapy, state anxiety is manageable, make plans for future).
Client With Dissociative Identity Disorder (in addition to above)	Verbalize awareness of all personalities, their thoughts and behaviors (development of co-consciousness).
	Display cooperation among the personalities.
	Demonstrate more stable personalities with resolution of traumatic events, moving toward partial to full integration into one personality.
	Verbalize acceptance of positive feelings toward emerging personality.

ACTIONS/INTERVENTIONS	RATIONALE

Independent

Develop trusting relationship with individual (and "alters" or subpersonalities if present).	Trust is the basis of a therapeutic relationship, but it may be difficult to achieve as client is often demoralized and suspicious, believing life is unjust/hopeless, or even that she or he is evil. In dissociative identity disorder, each of the personalities views itself as a separate entity and must initially be treated as such.
Determine client's perception of the extent of the threat of self-integrity and current response.	Degree of distress perceived by the client will assist in determining therapeutic interventions.
Help client understand/accept reality of the disorder (e.g., other personalities) and meaning of lapses in memory.	May be unaware/lack understanding of condition, resulting in increased anxiety and confusion about self.
Ascertain what client does recall and compare with information obtained from family members/other personalities.	Helps in orienting to realities of past events and assists client toward memory integration.
Share information in small amounts over a period of time. Avoid giving too much information (flooding) at any one time.	Enables client to begin to deal with painful information for which the amnesia has provided protection in the past. Too much material at any one time can be difficult for client to handle, increasing risk of decompensation.
Facilitate identification of stressful situations that precipitate dissociative state/transition from one personality to another. (Refer to ND: Coping, Individual, ineffective.)	Assists client to respond more adaptively and to eliminate the need for separation from self.

375

Encourage client to identify the need the behavior/ each subpersonality serves in the overall identity of the individual.

Knowledge of these unfulfilled needs enables client to face unresolved issues without dissociation and is the first step toward integration of multiple personalities.

Provide psychotherapy with feedback relative to behavioral observations. Encourage journal-keeping (therapeutic writing) and other methods designed to allow gradual insight.

Decreases denial and amnesia, providing an opportunity for client to accept the presence of the disorder and begin to "own" behaviors/ personality components. Acceptance and ownership assist the client in cooperating as a unified identity and with subsequent integration when multiple personalities are present.

Discuss integration of the subpersonalities into a unified identity within the individual and help client understand that all personalities will contribute to the whole.

The idea of total elimination generates fear and defensiveness within alters who function as separate entities.

Collaborative

Plan use of confrontive methods with all team members. Use cautiously.

These methods need to be paced with the individual's ability to benefit therapeutically and planned within the team conference to avoid overstressing the individual and precipitating exacerbation or decompensation.

Use/assist with hypnosis as indicated.

Allows client to become familiar with dissociation and learn how to interrupt/control it. Provides opportunity for client to make traumatic memories/feelings conscious and realize this will not destroy them. May be used to gain access to multiple personalities, helping client to work through and accept realities of positive aspects of each personality and participate in rituals of joining/integration.

Engage in activities that reflect life experiences, using occupational/vocational/recreational/ physical therapy. Begin with pleasurable stimuli (as identified by the client), e.g., events, smells, pets, or music associated with pleasurable activities.

Presents additional stimulation, which may encourage recall of repressed material. Provides opportunity to experience positive feelings that have also been repressed and to work toward beginning to deal with negative feelings/ occurrences.

NURSING DIAGNOSIS	**FAMILY COPING, ineffective: compromised/disabling**
May Be Related to:	Multiple stressors, repeated over period of time
	Temporary family disorganization and role changes; prolonged progression of disorder that exhausts the supportive capacity of significant people
	Significant person with chronically unexpressed feelings of guilt, anger, hostility, and so forth
	High-risk family situation (e.g., recurrent episodes of neglect/abuse, substance abuse)

Possibly Evidenced by:	Significant person describes inadequate understanding or knowledge base that interferes with effective assistive or supportive behaviors
	Expresses despair regarding family reactions/lack of involvement
	Marital conflict (separation/divorce)
	Neglectful care of client in regard to basic human needs; intolerance, abandonment, rejection, desertion
	Distortion of reality regarding the client's health problem, including extreme denial about its existence or severity
Desired Outcomes/Evaluation Criteria— Family Will:	Verbalize more realistic understanding and expectations of the client.
	Identify/verbalize resources within individual members to deal with the situation.
	Provide opportunity for client to deal with situation in own way.
	Remain intact, or separate in healthy way, being supportive of the client and one another.

ACTIONS/INTERVENTIONS	RATIONALE

Independent

Identify contributing factors within the family or environment.	Family and marital dysfunction are extremely likely to occur. These factors contribute to ongoing emotional stress for all family members.
Note family members who are involved with client, e.g., by marriage (husband, children), family of origin (mother/father, siblings, extended family). Complete a genogram.	It is important that all willing family members interacting with client be involved in helping with the therapeutic regimen, to allow for the best possible outcome for client.
Provide client/family education relative to the disorder and treatment plan.	Understanding of problem and that the disorder can be treated reduces anxiety, frustration, and guilt and lets client progress within a supportive environment.
Explore family dynamics. Note denial, enabling/ sabotage behaviors (e.g., denying existence of problems, failure to attend therapy/keeping client from attending).	Other family members may be invested in keeping the "sick" member symptomatic in order to camouflage their own problems.
Provide for client safety within the family setting or arrange for alternative living arrangements if abuse or neglect is an issue. (Refer to CP: Parenting, regarding issues of current abuse/neglect.)	If client remains in family of origin, a diagnosis of dissociative state/dissociative identity disorder should alert personnel to the possibility of abuse/neglect. As the "responsible adult," client may be unable to meet needs of own child(ren)/ family.
Help family respond to client in a manner that reinforces positive behaviors.	Without assistance, the family may provide secondary gain for client's continued illness instead of promoting wellness.

377

Encourage the family to ventilate negative feelings and continue as much as possible with usual daily activities. Discourage family from allowing client to escape responsibilities because of the illness.

Family members are less likely to abandon the affected member if they have an outlet for anger/frustration and are not overburdened in caretaking. Positive expectations from family members promote hope for recovery, enhance self-esteem, and decrease the likelihood of secondary gain.

Collaborative

Refer for additional individual, family, or marriage counseling.

Concurrent psychiatric problems in other family members are common. If client's symptoms are the most florid, that individual has likely been identified as the "sick" family member and others have not sought/received help.

CHAPTER 12

SEXUAL AND GENDER IDENTITY DISORDERS

SEXUAL DYSFUNCTIONS AND PARAPHILIAS

DSM-IV
SEXUAL DESIRE DISORDERS
302.71 Hypoactive sexual desire disorder
302.79 Sexual aversion disorder
SEXUAL AROUSAL DISORDERS
302.72 Female sexual arousal disorder
302.72 Male erectile disorder
ORGASMIC DISORDERS
302.73 Female orgasmic disorder
302.74 Male orgasmic disorder
302.75 Premature ejaculation
SEXUAL PAIN DISORDERS
302.76 Dyspareunia (not due to a general medical condition)
306.51 Vaginismus (not due to a general medical condition)
(Refer to *DSM-IV* manual for sexual dysfunctions due to a general medical condition)
PARAPHILIAS
302.4 Exhibitionism
302.81 Fetishism
302.89 Frotteurism
302.2 Pedophilia
302.83 Sexual masochism
302.84 Sexual sadism
302.82 Voyeurism
302.3 Transvestic fetishism

Sexual disorders include sexual dysfunctions and paraphilias. Sexual dysfunction is defined as persistent impairment/disturbance of a normal or desired pattern in any phase of the sexual response cycle. Paraphilias are more specific disorders in which unusual or bizarre imagery or acts are necessary for realization of sexual excitement. Because many paraphiliac behaviors are illegal in most states, individuals usually come for psychiatric treatment because of pressure from others, partners, or the authorities/judicial system.

ETIOLOGICAL FACTORS

Psychodynamics

Individual causes of sexual desire disorders may include religious beliefs, obsessive-compulsive personality, conflicts with gender identity or sexual preference, sexual phobias, fear of losing control over sexual urges, secret sexual deviations, fear of pregnancy, inadequate grieving following the death of a spouse, depression, and aging-related concerns. Psychological factors may also be involved in arousal disorders.

Psychoanalytical theories state that paraphilias are the product of childhood desires that survive into adulthood in their immature forms because emotional development has been inhibited, distorted, and diverted. These wishes are believed to be universal and are used to achieve arousal and release when ordinary forms of sexual activity are not available. Deviations arise when these immature forms of libido dominate adult sexual life. Fixation is thought to occur in Freud's oral, anal, and phallic phases when corresponding body parts provide sources of instinctual gratification. Conflict arises when an imperfect compromise occurs between these impulses and reality, resulting in fear, which the unconscious perceives as castration.

Behavioral theorists believe any paraphilia/sexual dysfunction can be acquired through conditioning, in which an initial pairing of an object is accidentally associated with/then becomes necessary for sexual release. This need may become generalized to other situations of tension/anxiety.

Biological

Sometimes the cause is clearly biological (e.g., temporal lobe epilepsy that may cause changes in sexual behavior between seizures). It has also been suggested that the problem arises out of interference with brain pathways governing rage and sexual arousal. Sex hormones have been studied. Rat studies have demonstrated that small, properly timed doses of androgens (male hormones) or estrogens (female hormones) in the fetus or newborn can influence sexual behavior. Various organic reasons, medication and other drug use, physical illnesses (most notably diabetes mellitus), surgery (such as prostatectomy), and degenerative neural disorders (e.g., multiple sclerosis) may be involved in sexual desire, arousal, and pain disorders.

It is generally accepted that abnormal hormonal activity and biological (genetic) predisposition interacting with social and family factors influence the development of these fantasies/sexual acts. Although these behaviors may occur in normal sexual activity, when they become the primary source of sexual satisfaction they may result in problems for the individual/others.

Family Dynamics

There appears to be some evidence that paraphilias run in families and may be the result of dysfunctional family interactions and social learning.

Sexual dysfunctions are believed to be influenced by what the individual has learned/not learned as a child within the family system and by values and beliefs that may be based on myths and misconceptions.

CLIENT ASSESSMENT DATA BASE
SEXUAL DYSFUNCTIONS

Neurosensory

Mental Status: Findings may indicate intense distress about situation/condition or coexisting psychiatric disorders
Mood and affect may reveal evidence of increased anxiety and depression

Sexuality

Problems may be lifelong or acquired after a period of normal sexual functioning
May report inhibition or interference with some part of the human response cycle (e.g., low sexual desire, aversion to genital sexual contact, arousal/erectile/orgasmic disturbances, premature ejaculation, genital pain during or after sexual intercourse, and involuntary spasm of the outer third of the vagina interfering with coitus)
May display negative attitude(s) toward sexuality

Social Interactions

Impairment may be noted in marital/conjugal relations but rarely affects job performance

Teaching/Learning

Most commonly occur in early adulthood, although male erectile disorder may surface later in life

PARAPHILIAS

Ego Integrity

May express shame or guilt about behavior
May or may not act on fantasies

Neurosensory

Personality disturbances frequently accompany sexual disorder(s)

Safety

Physical injury may be seen following episodes of sadomasochistic activity

Sexuality

Recurrent, intense sexual urges and fantasies involving the exposure of one's genitals to a stranger that have been acted on, cause severe distress, and may be accompanied by masturbation (exhibitionism)
Use of nonliving object(s) to stimulate recurrent intense sexual urges and sexually arousing fantasies (e.g., female undergarments [fetishism])
Rubbing and touching against a nonconsenting person to invoke recurrent, intense sexual urges and fantasies, with the touching, not the coercive nature of the act, causing sexual excitement (frotteurism)
Sexual activity with a prepubescent child or children (pedophilia)
Participation in the act (real, not simulated) of being humiliated, beaten, bound, or otherwise made to suffer (sexual masochism)
Participation in acts (real, not simulated) in which the psychological or physical suffering (including humiliation) of the victim is sexually exciting to the person (sexual sadism)
Cross-dressing activities (transvestic fetishism)
Observing unsuspecting person(s), usually a stranger, who is naked, in the process of disrobing or engaging in sexual activity (voyeurism)

Social Interactions

May not view self as ill; however, behavior may cause distress for the individual or may bring suffering to others
May be in conflict with partner or society because of behavior
Possible interference with interpersonal/occupational functioning

Teaching/Learning

Occurs mostly in males

Some evidence of occurrence in families of paraphiliacs and of depressed individual; high correlation between pedophiles and family history of pedophilic activity

DIAGNOSTIC STUDIES

As indicated, to rule out physical causes of sexual dysfunction.

Screening for sexually transmitted diseases (STDs) including HIV/AIDS.

NURSING PRIORITIES

1. Assist client to understand the nature of the behavior (disorder/dysfunction).
2. Encourage use of acceptable methods for reduction of anxiety.
3. Help to recognize the legal/interpersonal consequences of paraphilic behaviors.
4. Explore options for change.
5. Encourage involvement of client/family (significant other) in treatment regimen.

DISCHARGE GOALS

1. The nature of the problem and consequences for the individual/family understood.
2. Anxiety reduced/managed in acceptable ways.
3. Options explored and appropriate one(s) chosen.
4. Confidence in own capabilities/sense of self-worth expressed.
5. Participating in treatment program and using community/treatment resources effectively.
6. Plan in place to meet needs after discharge.

NURSING DIAGNOSIS	SEXUAL dysfunction/SEXUALITY PATTERNS, altered
May Be Related to:	Biophysical alteration of sexuality: ineffectual or absent role models; vulnerability; misinformation; physical/sexual abuse
	Lack of significant other
	Loss of sexual desire; disruption of sexual response pattern (e.g., premature ejaculation, dyspareunia)
	Conflicts involving values; conflicts with variant preferences
	Knowledge/skill deficit about alternative responses
Possibly Evidenced by:	Reported difficulties, limitations/changes in sexual behaviors or activities
	Alterations in achieving sexual satisfaction; difficulty achieving desired satisfaction in socially acceptable ways
Desired Outcomes/Evaluation Criteria— Client Will:	Verbalize understanding of sexual anatomy/ function and individual reasons for sexual problems.
	Recognize stressors involved in lifestyle that contribute to dysfunction.

Identify satisfying/acceptable sexual practices and some alternative ways of dealing with sexual expression.

Demonstrate improved communication and relationship skills.

ACTIONS/INTERVENTIONS	RATIONALE

Independent

Obtain sexual history, noting when problem(s) began, degree of anxiety, presence of relationship, conflict between partners, displacement of pattern of arousal to other than the opposite sex, and client desire/need for change.	Identification of individual situation promotes appropriate goal-setting and interventions.
Determine cultural/value conflicts, preexisting problems affecting current situation.	Stress in other areas of life often affects sexual functioning. Client may feel guilt and shame or feel depressed because of sexual difficulties/deviant behavior.
Explore possible drug use.	Substance/prescription drug use may affects sexual functioning/be used to relieve anxiety of sexually deviant behavior.
Avoid making value judgments.	Does not help client deal with the situation or feel better about self.
Determine what client needs/wants to know and provide information accordingly. Review information regarding safety and/or consequences of actions.	Prevents unnecessary repetition of information or presenting information client is not willing to hear. Reviewing necessary information gives client message that it is important and serves as a reminder of own responsibility.
Encourage open discussion of concerns and expression of feelings and assist with problem-solving.	Promotes thinking about causes/results of behavior(s) and resolution of problem.
Provide sex information/education, as necessary.	Lack of knowledge may be significant to underlying problem(s).
Encourage completion of structured homework exercises dependent on behavior and individual needs (e.g., avoidance of coitus/orgasm, use of masturbation, planned progression of intimate activity, diary of feelings/perceptions).	Heightened sensory awareness and improved nonverbal communication with partner in an atmosphere free of demands for sexual performance may resolve sexual dysfunctions. **Note:** Clients without partners may benefit from assertiveness training, self-exploration, permission to fantasize, correction of misconceptions.

Collaborative

Refer for assessment of physical conditions (e.g., presence of diabetes, vascular problems).	Between ⅓ and ½ of clients with sexual dysfunction have a physical condition that interferes with sexual functioning.
Monitor penile tumescence during REM sleep, as indicated.	Impotence can be assessed by noting erectile ability occurring during sleep. Physical conditions are ruled out when erection occurs.

Refer to appropriate resources as necessary (e.g., clinical specialist psychiatric nurse, professional sex therapist, family counselor).

Additional/in-depth counseling, sex therapy may help client come to terms with underlying problems that interfere with recovery. **Note:** Use of sexual surrogates for clients without partners is no longer recommended because of questions of ethics, values, psychological effects, and relevance to normal sexual relations.

NURSING DIAGNOSIS	ANXIETY [moderate to severe]
May Be Related to:	Unconscious conflict about sexual feelings
	Threat to self-concept; threat to role-functioning
	Unmet needs
Possibly Evidenced by:	Increased tension (sexual)
	Feelings of inadequacy
	Fear of unspecified consequences
	Extraneous movements (foot shuffling, hand/arm movements)
	Glancing about; poor eye contact; focus on self
	Impaired functioning; immobility
Desired Outcomes/Evaluation Criteria—Client Will:	Verbalize awareness of feelings of anxiety and report reduction to a manageable level.
	Demonstrate problem-solving skills and use resources effectively.

ACTIONS/INTERVENTIONS	RATIONALE

Independent

Determine degree and precipitants of anxiety.	Sexual activity is usually undertaken to reduce a state of inner tension and pressure. Fear of "failure," of being found out, and/or of disapproval also creates anxiety. Individual may have sought help because of these fears/coming to the attention of the legal system.
Identify client's perception of the threat represented by the situation.	The client may not perceive the behavior as a problem; however, it is the reaction of others and consequences that create anxiety. Circumstances that prevent the client from indulging in paraphilic behavior can lead to intense anxiety.
Assess withdrawn behavior and evaluate for substance use (alcohol, other drugs), sleep disturbances, limited/avoidance of interactions with others.	These behaviors may be used by the client to deal with anxiety/other feelings (e.g., guilt) instead of positive coping mechanisms. Substance use may be a factor in the occurrence of the dysfunction(s).
Note prodromal symptoms of irritability, restlessness, tension, and headache.	In the exhibitionist, these may be the response to abnormal discharges in the temporal lobes.
Encourage appropriate expression of feelings (e.g., crying [sadness], laughing [fear, denial], sweating [fear, anger]).	Suppression of feelings has contributed to difficulties client has in dealing with anxiety and coping appropriately with sexual desires and/or dysfunction.

Provide calm, quiet environment. Display accepting attitude.	Promotes discussion of sensitive sexual issues/concerns. Sexual performance is closely tied to individual sense of self as male or female, making self-disclosure difficult.
Confront the client's illegal behavior without judgment.	Client needs to hear that behavior, not the individual, is not acceptable.
Assist the client to recognize a helpful degree of anxiety and ways to begin to use it.	Moderate degree of anxiety heightens awareness and permits the client to focus on dealing with the problems.

Collaborative

Administer medication as indicated, e.g.: Antiandrogen drugs: medroxyprogesterone (Depo-Provera);	These drugs have been useful for altering sexual behavior, but their use is limited because they suppress desired as well as unwanted sexual responses.
Antidepressants: fluoxetine (Prozac), imipramine (Tofranil), lithium (Eskalith).	Research suggests that some compulsive sexual activity viewed as excessive or out of control (e.g., compulsive masturbation, obsessional fantasies about sex with children, voyeurism) may be an atypical symptom of depression. Sexual desire may be reduced and sexual activity become more normal when antidepressants are used. **Note:** Use Prozac with caution as it may cause sexual dysfunction in some individuals.
Refer to therapy as indicated, e.g.: Psychotherapy;	Psychotherapy may be used to help the client recognize the problem of sadness and isolation caused by the dysfunction and deal with the emotional issues involved. May also be used to help client accept sexual nature when behavior is not damaging/dangerous (e.g., transvestism).
Marital/family therapy;	May resolve problems of communication, which may be major factor in many sexual dysfunction problems.
Behavioral therapy.	Aversion therapy, in which the unwanted sexual act/thought is linked to an unpleasant sensation such as an electric shock or nausea and/or imagining a frightening or disgusting event, is used as negative reinforcement and is designed to extinguish the desire. Desensitization to painful heterosexual coitus is used with limited long-lasting success.

NURSING DIAGNOSIS **May Be Related to:**	**SELF ESTEEM chronic/situational low** Emotional insecurity; lack of self-confidence Biophysical/psychosocial factors (e.g., achievement of sexual satisfaction in deviant ways; failure to perform satisfactorily) Substance use

Possibly Evidenced by:	Verbalization of fear of rejection/reaction by others; negative feelings about body; feelings of helplessness, hopelessness, or powerlessness
	Change in social involvement
	Difficulty accepting positive reinforcement
	Lack of follow-through
	Self-destructive behaviors
Desired Outcomes/Evaluation Criteria— Client Will:	Identify feelings and methods for coping with negative perception of self.
	Verbalize increased sense of self-esteem in relation to current situation (e.g., sees self as a worthwhile person).
	Demonstrate adaptation to events that have occurred by setting realistic goals and actively participating in treatment program.
	Report satisfactory sexual experiences.

ACTIONS/INTERVENTIONS	RATIONALE

Independent

Determine individual behaviors and situation that affect client's self-esteem, as well as client's perception of the threat to self and awareness of own responsibility for dealing with situation.	Failure to perform sexually can affect a person's sense of esteem and self-worth. When the problem is defined as paraphilic, the client may not recognize the sexual behavior as related to current problem(s). Identification of individual circumstances helps in choosing appropriate interventions.
Assess type of sexual dysfunction/problem by asking direct questions (e.g., describe the dysfunction client is experiencing, clarify relationship between partners, presence of power struggle, anger, concern regarding commitment or stability of relationship; preference for nonliving objects, dressing in clothes of the opposite sex, use of physical/mental pain as a source of sexual arousal).	Partners may have very different expectations of the relationship, and sexual disorder may serve to correct power imbalance or maintain emotional distance. Client may not see sexual deviance as a problem but may seek help for feelings of guilt and sadness. Asking directly can promote client recognition of these factors.
Provide information about sexual anatomy/ physiology as needed.	Lack of information and myths/misconceptions are the basis of sexual functioning problems, and accurate knowledge may be crucial to resolution of the problems, motivation for change.
Ascertain if client has ever been arrested.	Pattern of involvement with the law can provide information about extent of the problem.
Determine client motivation for change.	When client accepts the fact that the sexual behavior is responsible for the problems that exist and makes the decision to change, therapy has more chance of being successful. If therapy is court-ordered, possibility for change is less likely but still possible.
Discuss what purpose (positive intention) the behavior serves for the client (e.g., sense of	Identification of the purpose allows opportunity for the client to examine whether the behavior

inadequacy as a male may be met by exhibitionistic behaviors) and what other options might be available to meet needs in more satisfying and socially acceptable ways.

Give positive reinforcement for progress noted.

Permit client to progress at own rate.

Assist client to incorporate changes accurately into self-concept.

Collaborative

Refer to classes (e.g., assertiveness training, positive self-image, communication).

meets the purpose in an adaptive or maladaptive manner.

Encouragement can support development of mature coping behaviors.

Immaturity is believed to be involved in the development of paraphilias, and adaptation to a change in self-concept depends on the significance the individual attaches to the change, how long this behavior has been used, and necessary changes in lifestyle. Learning to see oneself as a capable, competent adult who interacts in an adult sexual manner takes a long time.

Helps client recognize and cope with events/ alterations and sense of loss of control.

Assists with learning skills to promote self-esteem.

NURSING DIAGNOSIS	**FAMILY PROCESSES, altered**
May Be Related to:	Situational crisis (e.g., change in roles/revelation of sexual deviance/dysfunction)
Possibly Evidenced by:	Expressions of confusion about what to do/difficulty coping with situation
	Inappropriate boundary maintenance; family does not demonstrate respect for individuality and autonomy of its members
	Family system does not meet emotional/security needs; does not adapt to change or deal with traumatic experience constructively
	Difficulty accepting/receiving help appropriately
Desired Outcomes/Evaluation Criteria—Family Will:	Express feelings freely and appropriately.
	Demonstrate individual involvement in problem-solving processes directed at appropriate solutions for the situation.
	Encourage and allow involved member ("identified patient") to handle situation in own way, progressing toward independence.

ACTIONS/INTERVENTIONS	RATIONALE

Independent

Determine crisis that has occurred and individual members' perceptions of the situation.	Dysfunction may be perceived as signaling the end of individual's sexual activity. Sexual behavior may have resulted in arrest and be new knowledge to family members.

387

Identify patterns of communication in the family.	Interaction among family members provides information about family dynamics, boundaries, and role expectations and may be indicative of support client may receive.
Assess energy direction, whether efforts at resolution/problem-solving are purposeful or scattered.	Indicative of degree of disorganization family is experiencing.
Note cultural and/or religious factors.	Strong beliefs about sexual expression and deviance/dysfunction influence acceptance or rejection by individuals involved.
Assess support systems available outside the family.	May be needed to help client and family members, if disorganization is severe.
Acknowledge difficulties observed while reinforcing that some degree of conflict is to be expected and can be used to promote growth.	Acceptance of the reality of what is going on helps client and family to feel comfortable/begin to deal with situation.
Emphasize importance of continuous open dialogue between family members.	Promotes understanding of each other's point of view and allows for clarification of misunderstandings/misconceptions.
Identify and encourage use of previously successful coping behaviors.	Family has used these in the past and may have neglected them during the stress of current situation.
Encourage use of stress-management techniques (e.g., appropriate expression of feelings; relaxation exercises, imagery).	Decreases anxiety and promotes opportunity to problem-solve in calm manner.

Collaborative

Refer to additional resources as indicated (e.g., classes, psychologic counseling, family/multifamily group therapy).	Providing information, opportunity to share feelings/concerns with others can be helpful to positive resolution of problems.

(Also refer to CP: Gender Identity, NDs: Family Coping, ineffective: compromised, and Family Coping: potential for growth.)

GENDER IDENTITY DISORDER

DSM-IV
GENDER IDENTITY DISORDERS
302.6   Gender identity disorder in children

302.85 Gender identity disorder in adolescents and adults (specify: sexually attracted to males/females/both/neither)

302.6   Gender identity disorder not otherwise specified (intersex conditions, androgen insensitivity syndrome, or congenital adrenal hyperplasia and gender dysphoria)

313.82 Identity problem (specific to sexual orientation and behavior)

Sexuality is a product of one's genetic identity, gender identity, gender role and sexual orientation. As all of these are independent components, there is a 4×4 interaction that can result in 16 distinct possibilities of sexual identity. In a society in which clear differences between the sexes is the expected norm, any individual challenging this dichotomy is deemed problematic. However, in the mental health arena, sexual orientation is a concern only when the individual experiences persistent and marked distress regarding uncertainty about issues relating to personal identity—in this case, sexual orientation and behavior.

Consensual homosexuality in adults is no longer viewed as a mental disturbance. Homosexual individuals in general have no more psychopathology than heterosexuals, and when they do seek treatment it is for the same reasons as heterosexuals—psychiatric disorders (e.g., bipolar disorder, borderline personality), relationship problems, and stress. Therefore, it is important to avoid mistakenly attributing psychiatric symptoms to the individual's sexual orientation.

In gender identity disorder, the individual does not view himself or herself as homosexual; rather, there is a strong and persistent cross-gender identification and discomfort with one's gender or a sense of inappropriateness in the assigned gender role exists (e.g., a male "trapped" in a female's body). This perception results in clinically significant distress/functional impairments (e.g., social, occupational).

In addition, this plan of care also addresses the diagnosis of Identity Problem for homosexuals who are uncertain about multiple issues relating to their identity, such as sexual orientation and behavior, moral values, friendship patterns, and group loyalties.

ETIOLOGICAL THEORIES

Psychodynamics

The libido is seen as the force that expresses sexual instinct and develops gradually during the oral stage, which focuses on the mouth and lips. The central concern of the anal stage is the anus and the elimination/retention of feces. During the phallic stage, the male is concerned with love of his mother, is jealous of his father, and has castration anxiety (Oedipus complex). The female has penis envy, loves her father, and rejects her mother (Electra complex). This theory focuses on the biological inferiority of women because they do not have penises, with subsequent envy of the male.

Developmental theories suggest that sexuality develops throughout life and especially during the formative years. Confusion about one's individual personality and sexual identity affects the ability to be intimate, interfering with sexual development.

Biological

Although adult endocrine levels are usually normal in individuals who are homosexual, a "hormonal wash" may have occurred at a critical time of embryonic development, sensitizing brain cells in as yet immeasurable ways. Androgen is necessary for masculinization in the fetal male, with the fetus developing as female without the addition of this hormone.

When androgenic influences in the fetal hypothalamus are decreased in the male or increased in the female, homosexuality may occur. Some research sources report that there is a neuroendocrine factor (e.g., that the fetus was exposed to large amounts of androgenic hormones or that the mother may have received synthetic hormones at a crucial fetal developmental period, preventing adequate stimulation for neural differentiation).

Current research allows monitoring of normal fetal exposure to testosterone in utero. When subsequent behavior is linked to this information, we will understand more than has been previously available from studies of abnormal exposure of the fetus to high levels of androgen, overdoses due to drugs, or adrenal malfunction. Research continues into the effect of prenatal brain-sexing on homosexual development. We know that lack of male hormone at a crucial state of male fetal development can lead to a feminine brain in a male body. It is clear that, as with other aspects of behavior, sexual orientation is crucially mediated by hormonal influences on the developing brain in utero. It is believed that abnormal hormones interact with neurotransmitters, the chemicals that direct the construction of the brain, affecting the sex centers, mating centers, and the so-called gender-role centers, which assume their structure at different times of brain development (Moir & Jessel, 1991).

Family Dynamics

Role-modeling of gender-specific behaviors is believed to play a part in the development of these disorders as well as the negative effect of a disturbed relationship with one or both parents. Imprinting and classic conditioning may affect the development of gender identity.

In males with gender identity disorders, a symbiotic relationship appears to exist between mother and child. The father is usually absent, ineffectual, or hostile and is perceived as weak and distant, with the mother seen as strong and protective.

In females with these disorders, the child may not be valued as a girl, or the mother may be absent, depressed, or suffer from other illness, resulting in inadequate mothering. The father may treat the daughter as his little boy, expecting "masculine" behavior.

CLIENT ASSESSMENT DATA BASE

Ego Integrity

Believes feelings/reactions are typical of other sex
May report considerable anxiety and depression, attributable to difficulty of living in role of assigned gender

Hygiene

Exhibits a persistent, marked aversion to wearing gender-appropriate clothing

Neurosensory

Moderate to severe coexisting personality disturbance may be noted
Mental Status: May reveal intense distress (e.g., ego-dystonic homosexuality) about general identity or coexisting psychiatric disorders
Mood and affect may reveal evidence of increased anxiety and depression

Safety

May have been victim of assault
History of suicide attempts

Sexuality

Higher incidence in males than females (may be owing to narrow study base)
Incongruence between assigned gender and the sense of knowing to which gender one belongs

May report a persistent and intense distress about his or her assigned gender and the desire to be/insistence that he or she is of the other gender; belief by males that penis/testes are disgusting/will disappear, or by females that they will not develop breasts/menstruate; or desires medical/surgical intervention to alter sexual characteristics to simulate the other gender

Possible preoccupation with stereotypic activities/toys designed for the opposite gender, and/or repudiation of anatomical structures noted/reported in childhood

Sexual responsiveness/romantic attraction to individual of same gender

Social Interactions

Impairment in social/occupational functioning, often experiencing peer isolation, bullying

May report family alienation

Teaching/Learning

May present at any age; can be identified in childhood but most often in late adolescence or early adulthood, although possibly later

Substance use/abuse

DIAGNOSTIC STUDIES

Psychological testing to rule out concomitant psychiatric conditions.

Screens for sexually transmitted diseases (STDs), including HIV/AIDS.

NURSING PRIORITIES

1. Help client reduce level of anxiety.
2. Promote sense of self-worth.
3. Encourage development of social skills/comfort level with own sexual identity/preference.
4. Provide opportunities for client/family to participate in group therapy/other support systems.

DISCHARGE GOALS

1. Anxiety reduced/managed effectively.
2. Self-esteem/image enhanced.
3. Accepts and is comfortable with identity as established.
4. Client/family are participating in ongoing treatment/support programs.
5. Plan in place to meet needs after discharge.

NURSING DIAGNOSIS	ANXIETY [severe]
May Be Related to:	Ego-dystonic gender identification
	Unconscious conflicts about essential values/beliefs
	Threat to self-concept; unmet needs
Possibly Evidenced by:	Increased tension/helplessness (hopelessness)
	Feelings of inadequacy, apprehension, uncertainty
	Increased wariness; insomnia
	Focus on self; impaired daily functioning

Desired Outcomes/Evaluation Criteria—Client Will:	Verbalize awareness of feelings of anxiety and healthy ways to deal with them.
	Appear relaxed and report anxiety is reduced to a manageable level.
	Demonstrate problem-solving skills and use resources effectively.

ACTIONS/INTERVENTIONS	RATIONALE

Independent

ACTIONS/INTERVENTIONS	RATIONALE
Assess level of anxiety and degree of interference with daily activities/life.	Necessary information to identify the extent of problem for the individual and plan appropriate interventions.
Review drug/substance use history (e.g., prescription/illicit), familial/physiological factors (e.g., mental/physical illness, family disorganization).	Drugs (including alcohol) may have been used to handle anxious feelings in the past. Other factors contribute to anxiety and may affect individual's ability to handle stress of dealing with own identity problems.
Help client identify feelings, conveying empathy and unconditional positive regard. Encourage free expression of feelings in appropriate ways.	Identification of feelings within a safe, therapeutic environment can help the client begin to explore causes of anxiety and begin to move toward acceptance of self as a worthwhile person.
Acknowledge reality of anxiety/fear. (Do not deny or reassure client that everything will be all right.)	Helps client accept own feeling(s) and learn trust in self. Denial of these feelings contributes to increased anxiety. Platitudes lack factual basis, and providing false reassurance can damage trust and may increase client's anxiety.
Provide accurate information to assist client to clarify reality base, reframe sexuality, and delineate boundaries.	Anxiety may be the result of misinterpretation or lack of knowledge about sexuality/gender identity, and client may fantasize unrealistic ideation.
Accept the client as he or she is.	Lack of self-acceptance is the basis of much anxiety, and other's unacceptance increases anxiety.
Identify things client has done previously when feeling nervous/anxious.	Helps client see which previous actions have been beneficial and can be used in this situation, increasing sense of control/capability and allaying anxiety.
Assist with developing program of exercise (e.g., brisk walking, aerobic class).	Strenuous activity releases opiate-like endorphins, which create sense of well-being and decrease anxiety. However, exercise therapy need not be aerobic or intensive to achieve the desired effect.

NURSING DIAGNOSIS	ROLE PERFORMANCE, altered/PERSONAL IDENTITY disturbance
May Be Related to:	Crisis in development, in which person has difficulty knowing/accepting to which gender he or she belongs or to which he or she is attracted

Possible Evidenced by:	Sense of discomfort and inappropriateness about anatomical sex characteristics
	Confusion about sense of self, purpose or direction in life, sexual identification/preference
	Verbalization of desire to be/insistence that person is the opposite gender
	Change in self-perception of role; conflict in roles
Desired Outcomes/Evaluation Criteria—Client Will:	Talk with family/significant other(s) about situation and changes that are occurring/have occurred.
	Develop realistic plans for adapting to new role/role changes as appropriate.
	Verbalize realistic perception and acceptance of self.

ACTIONS/INTERVENTIONS	RATIONALE

Independent

Show acceptance of the client as he or she is presented.	These clients are sensitive to others' beliefs and will pick up on prejudicial feelings. The client needs to be free to express any views/feelings to begin to solve the problems being faced.
Determine type of role dysfunction/distress client is expressing (e.g., ego-dystonic heterosexual/ homosexual feelings, gender dysphoria).	Lack of self-acceptance and conflicting feelings regarding sexual expression requires therapeutic intervention. Lack of public and religious acceptance, few legal protections for same-sex couples along with lack of role clarity/boundaries can create significant stressors for the client. **Note:** When the individual views sexual expression/feelings/behavior as adaptive, a healthy attitude exists, and intervention is unnecessary when behavior is within legal boundaries.
Identify beliefs and values of the individual about hetero/homo/transsexuality. Discuss client's beliefs and ideas in detail, providing information as appropriate.	Client may be ignorant of the facts and base fears on hearsay, prejudice, and religious beliefs. Learning the facts and discussing them with an unbiased person provides an opportunity to make informed decisions. **Note:** Transsexuals who are attracted to members of their own biological gender do not view themselves to be homosexual and may consider the term "gay" or "lesbian" to be an insult.
Explore client's feelings about gender identity (transsexuality) and review options for change (e.g., hormonal therapy, psychotherapy, surgical reassignment).	The client who feels strongly that he or she is in a body of the "wrong" gender needs to have complete information about available choices to help begin to accept self and feel comfortable with the decision. **Note:** Not all transsexuals choose to have surgery.
Ascertain degree of openness client feels about sexual orientation concerns.	Degree to which client previously shared individual situation has an impact on one's level of concern/comfort and degree of conflict present.

393

	The process of sharing or withholding one's situation requires much emotional energy.
Determine presence of support system (e.g., family, social, work).	May feel "different" and isolate self from usual support systems. May be pressured by family/friends to be heterosexual, which creates conflict within self.
Role-play sexual disclosure encounters.	Once the decision to disclose sexuality is made, open discussion and practice of responses is necessary to the success of disclosure.
Assist client to develop strategies to cope with threat to identity.	Provides protection and gives client a sense of control to have thought about/decided on actions that can be taken when feeling threatened.
Assess response of family/SO. (Refer to NDs: Family Coping, ineffective: compromised; Family Coping: potential for growth.)	May be in shock when first learning of client's concerns and then may either reject or rally to support client.
Encourage client to deal with situation in small steps.	Helps client cope with the "larger picture" when in stress overload.
Provide accurate information about threat to and potential consequences for the individual.	Knowledge about gender identity issues helps client assess own situation and make decisions based on fact.
Be aware of one's own biases. Seek assistance/terminate therapeutic role as appropriate.	Personal values/beliefs and conflicts or biases can have a negative impact on the therapeutic relationship and effectiveness of interventions.

Collaborative

Identify available resources/support groups.	Can provide positive role models, opportunity to discuss shared concerns, and facilitate problem-solving. Group therapy/peer support can be especially helpful to adolescent/early adult homosexuals who are struggling with their identity and need support for future life choices.
Refer to professionals who are expert in the field of human sexuality and gender reassignment.	Client needs to be known to the therapist for a period of at least 3–6 months and demonstrate a sense of discomfort with self and a desire to live in the opposite gender role before a major life-changing decision is finalized.
Refer to a therapist who is an expert in the field of gender reassignment for a second opinion when surgery is contemplated.	Because these procedures are not reversible, the client needs to be sure the correct decision has been made and demonstrate success in living in the opposite role for a period of 1–2 years.

NURSING DIAGNOSIS	**SEXUALITY PATTERNS, altered**
May Be Related to:	Ineffective or absent role models
	Conflicts with sexual orientation and/or preferences
	Impaired relationship with a significant other

Possibly Evidenced by:	Verbalizations of discomfort with sexual orientation and/or role
	Lack of information about human sexuality
Desired Outcomes/Evaluation Criteria— Client Will:	Verbalize understanding of sexuality and acceptance of self.
	Demonstrate behaviors directed at lifestyle changes necessary to achieve desired effects.

ACTIONS/INTERVENTIONS

Independent

Have client describe problem in own terms, noting comments of client/SO that may reveal discounting by overt/covert sexual expressions.

Take sexual history, including perception of normal function, use of vocabulary, and concerns about identities/clarifies concerns to be dealt with by the client/nurse.

Note cultural and religious/value factors and conflicts that may exist.

Explore knowledge of alternative sexual responses and expressions.

Inquire about drug use, including OTC/prescription drugs, illicit drugs, and alcohol.

Provide atmosphere in which discussion of sexual problems is encouraged, promoting free expression of feelings.

Encourage discussion of possibilities and alternatives for client situation. (Refer to ND: Role Performance, altered/Personal Identity disturbance.)

Review hormonal therapy as indicated.

Collaborative

Refer to resources as indicated (e.g., homosexual/lesbian support group; LAMBDA, AA, Gay and Lesbian; Common Bond; gender identity clinics, Exodus International).

RATIONALE

It may be difficult for client to talk about situation/express feelings, and client may joke, make oblique remarks, or use sarcasm to convey/cover concerns.

Provides information about level of knowledge about anatomy/physiology of human sexuality and gender identity.

Provides opportunity to give information/discuss resources available to client who may believe thoughts and feelings are sinful, and feel guilty.

May have knowledge gained only in discussions with friends, from myths, and from misconceptions.

Drug use can affect sexual functioning. Additionally, client may use substances to dull pain of indecision/anxiety of identity.

Essential to identification and resolution of problems. Client may have concerns about sexual behavior and diseases, such as AIDS.

Full range of discussion can help client reach a decision about the identity that is comfortable and the course to pursue.

Transsexuals who elect to undergo surgical reassignment, and those who for economic or other reasons choose to live in the transsexual role, usually receive long-term, high-dose estrogen or testosterone therapy. Client needs to understand the implications of hormone therapy before making the decision to pursue this course of therapy.

These organizations are reference groups that provide information/support for homosexuals and families. Information from these groups can help client reach a decision about sexual preference and/or provide support once decision has been made. Exodus International is a Christian-based group that directs efforts to assist the client toward a decision to become heterosexual.

NURSING DIAGNOSIS	FAMILY COPING, ineffective: compromised
May Be Related to:	Inadequate/incorrect information or understanding
	Temporary preoccupation by a significant person who is trying to manage emotional conflicts and personal suffering and is unable to perceive or to act effectively in regard to client's needs
	Temporary family disorganization and role changes
	Client providing little support in turn for the primary person
Possibly Evidenced by:	Client expressing/confirming a concern or complaint about family/SO(s) response to client's gender/sexual concerns
	SO describing preoccupation with own personal reactions to client's situation
	Family attempting supportive behaviors with less than satisfactory results/withdraw support when needed
Desired Outcomes/Evaluation Criteria— Family Will:	Identify resources within itself to deal with situation
	Interact appropriately with client and staff, providing support and assistance as indicated.

ACTIONS/INTERVENTIONS

Independent

Determine individual situation and identify factors that may contribute to difficulty family is having in providing needed assistance/support for the client.

Note behaviors of family members (e.g., withdrawn, rejecting, supportive, willing to learn). (Refer to ND: Family Coping: potential for growth.)

Discuss underlying reasons for behaviors client is expressing/exhibiting.

Encourage each individual to be responsible for own self, not taking on problem(s) of others.

RATIONALE

Individuals may have problems of their own that interfere with ability to extend themselves to the client. Problems of prejudice, myth/misinformation, values may also cause separation between/among family members.

Identifies individual needs and steps to be taken to resolve family disorganization/assist the family in moving toward growth.

Helps family understand and accept the person as having different beliefs/values.

The concept of "who owns the problem" can help clarify issues of who has responsibility for solution of specific problems.

Encourage free expression of feelings and ideas about homosexuality/gender identity issues.	Promotes an atmosphere in which individual can reveal feelings of self-blame, revulsion, confusion and anger, or blaming of other(s). Once these have been expressed, members can move on to resolution.
Provide information as appropriate.	Because much of the problem may center around lack of knowledge, information can help individuals make informed decisions/choices about what is happening.
Discuss options for individuals in regard to client's decision about sexual partner, gender identity/ surgical reassignment (e.g., separation/divorce for spouses, resolution of parent/child issues).	Family members may have difficulty accepting client's alternative sexual expression/sexual reassignment. Individual needs to make decision about willingness to accept other person in altered role. Children of transsexuals have questions such as "Who am I, as the daughter of a father who is now a woman?"
Provide time to talk with family to discuss views/ concerns about situation, feelings toward client's sexual partner.	Opportunity to ventilate feelings, ask questions, and express ideas helps resolve problems.
Assist members to develop effective communication skills (e.g., Active-listening, I-messages, problem-solving process). Provide role model with which the family may identify. Include SO as appropriate.	Helpful in dealing with current situation as well as providing skills that will assist with resolution of future problems. Role-modeling shows individuals that the skills can be helpful to them. Including partner provides opportunity for resolution of conflict, incorporation into family.

Collaborative

Identify/refer to support groups/classes that deal with similar problems, (e.g., Parents/Friends of Lesbians and Gays [PFLAG], gender identity clinics).	Talking with others who have been through similar experiences can provide opportunity for members to learn/accept client.
Refer for marriage counseling as appropriate.	May be needed to help couple decide whether separation/divorce is in the best interests of each person, or whether they want to work out their problems and stay together.

NURSING DIAGNOSIS	FAMILY COPING: potential for growth
May Be Related to:	Individual's basic needs are sufficiently gratified and adaptive tasks effectively addressed to enable goals of self-actualization to surface
Possibly Evidenced by:	Family members attempt to describe growth impact of crisis on their own values, priorities, goals, or relationships
	Family members are moving in direction of health-promoting and enriching lifestyle that supports client's search for self
	Family members choosing experiences that optimize wellness

Desired Outcomes/Evaluation Criteria— Family Will:	Express willingness to look at its own role in the family's growth.
	Verbalize knowledge and understanding of client's gender/sexual orientation.
	Express desire to understand tasks leading to change.

ACTIONS/INTERVENTIONS	RATIONALE
Independent	
Listen to family's expressions of hope, planning, and effect on relationships/life.	Provides clues to opportunities that exist to help family move toward growth and positive relationships. When family members are doing this, client is free to move toward a positive resolution of own life.
Help the family in supporting the client in meeting own needs/making own decision.	Significant other(s) may not have skills/know-how to give support even when desired, and giving information and providing support enables them to learn and grow.
Note expressions of change of values (e.g., "He/she is still my son/daughter even though homosexual/lesbian, or contemplating sex-change surgery.").	Indicators of beginning of acceptance of the situation as it is and willingness to learn and support child.
Provide a role model with which the family may identify.	Modeling of accepting behaviors/communication skills enables family members to learn new ways of interacting with the client.
Discuss importance of open communication and harm secretive behavior produces.	Open communication allows all participants to have access to all information, enhancing resolution of problems/understanding of what is happening.
Encourage open discussions of concerns about lifestyle changes, fear of AIDS and other sexually transmitted diseases.	Individuals may have unexpressed fears, and this provides the opportunity to ask questions and get accurate answers; make informed decisions.
Provide experiences for the family (e.g., involvement with other families facing similar decisions).	Helps them learn ways of assisting/supporting client.
Collaborative	
Refer to community resources (e.g., same-gender, transsexual groups).	Provides ongoing support as client/family make necessary lifestyle changes, go on with their lives.

CHAPTER 13

EATING DISORDERS

ANOREXIA NERVOSA/BULIMIA NERVOSA

DSM-IV
307.1 Anoxexia nervosa
307.51 Bulimia nervosa
307.50 Eating disorders NOS
Binge-eating disorder (proposed, requiring further study)

Anorexia nervosa is an illness of starvation, brought on by severe disturbance of body image and a morbid fear of obesity.

Bulimia nervosa is an eating disorder (binge-purge syndrome) characterized by extreme overeating, followed by self-induced vomiting. It may include abuse of laxatives and diuretics.

Binge-eating is defined as recurrent episodes of overeating associated with subjective and behavioral indicators of impaired control over and significant distress about the eating behavior but without the use of inappropriate compensatory behaviors (e.g., purging, fasting, excessive exercise).

ETIOLOGICAL THEORIES

Psychodynamics

The individual reflects a developmental arrest in the very early childhood years. The tasks of trust, autonomy, and separation-individuation are unfulfilled, and the individual remains in the dependent position. Ego development is retarded. Symptoms are often associated with a perceived loss of control in some aspect of life and may center on fears of sexual maturity/intimacy. Although these disorders affect women primarily, approximately 5% to 10% of those afflicted are men. Additionally, eating disorders are often associated with depression, anxiety, phobias, and cognitive problems.

Biological

These disorders may be caused by neuroendocrine abnormalities within the hypothalamus. Symptoms are linked to various chemical disturbances normally regulated by the hypothalamus. Furthermore, a physiological defect may make it difficult for the individual to interpret sensations of hunger and fullness.

Family Dynamics

Issues of control become the overriding factors in the family of the client with an eating disorder. These families often consist of a passive father, a domineering mother, and an overly dependent child. There is a high value placed on perfectionism in this family, and the child believes she or he must please others and satisfy these standards.

399

CLIENT ASSESSMENT DATA BASE

Activity/Rest

Disturbed sleep patterns (e.g., early morning insomnia; fatigue)

Feeling "hyper" and/or anxious

Increased activity/avid exerciser, participation in high-energy sports

Employment in positions/professions that require control of weight (athletics, such as gymnasts, swimmers, jockeys, wrestlers; modeling, flight attendants)

Circulation

Feeling cold even when room is warm

Low BP; tachycardia, dysrhythmias

Ego Integrity

Powerlessness/helplessness, lack of control over eating (e.g., cannot stop eating/control what or how much is eaten [bulimia]; feeling disgusted with self, depressed, or very guilty after overeating [binge-eating])

Distorted (unrealistic) body image—reports self as fat regardless of weight (denial), and sees thin body as fat; persistent overconcern with body shape and weight—fears gaining weight (females)

Concerned with achieving masculine body build (males), rather than actual weight or weight gain

Stress factors (e.g., family move/divorce, onset of puberty)

High self-expectations

Suppression of anger; emotional states of depression, withdrawal, anger, anxiety, pessimistic outlook

Elimination

Diarrhea/constipation

Decreased frequency of voiding/urine output, urine dark amber (dehydration)

Vague abdominal pain and distress, bloating

Laxative/diuretic use

Food/Fluid

Constant hunger or denial of hunger; normal or exaggerated appetite that rarely vanishes until late in the disorder (anorexia)

Intense fear of gaining weight (female); may have prior history of being overweight (particularly males)

Inordinate pleasure in weight loss, while denying self pleasure in other areas

Refusal to maintain body weight at or above minimal norm for age/height (anorexia)

Recurrent episodes of binge-eating; a feeling of lack of control over behavior during eating binges; minimum average of 2 binge eating episodes a week for at least 3 months (bulimia); ingests large amounts of food when not feeling physically hungry, often consuming as much as 20,000 calories in a 2-hour period; eating much more rapidly than normal in a discrete period of time (e.g., within a 2-hour period), an amount of food that is definitely larger than most people would eat (binge-eating); feels uncomfortably full

Regularly engages in either self-induced vomiting (binge-purge syndrome [bulimia]) independently or as a complication of anorexia or strict dieting or fasting; excessive gum chewing

Weight loss/maintenance of body weight 15% or more below that expected (anorexia) or weight may be normal or slightly above or below (bulimia)

Cachectic appearance; skin may be dry, yellowish/pale, with poor turgor

Preoccupation with food (e.g., calorie-counting, gourmet cooking; hiding food, cutting food into small pieces, rearranging food on plate)

Peripheral edema

Swollen salivary glands; sore, inflamed buccal cavity, erosion of tooth enamel; gums in poor condition; continuous sore throat (bulimia)

Vomiting; bloody vomitus (may indicate esophageal tearing—Mallory-Weiss)

Hygiene

Increased hair growth on body (lanugo); hair loss (axillary/pubic); hair dull/not shiny

Brittle nails

Signs of erosion of tooth enamel; gum abscesses, ulcerations of mucosa

Neurosensory

Appropriate affect, except in regard to body and eating; or depressive affect (depression)

Mental changes: apathy, confusion, memory impairment (brought on by malnutrition/starvation)

Hysterical or obsessive personality style; no other psychiatric illness or evidence of a psychiatric thought disorder present (although a significant number may show evidence of an affective disorder)

Pain/Discomfort

Headaches, sore throat, general vague complaints

Safety

Body temperature below normal

Recurrent infectious processes (indicative of depressed immune system)

Eczema/other skin problems

Abrasions/callouses may be noted on the back of hands (sticking finger down throat to induce vomiting)

Sexuality

Absence of at least 3 consecutive menstrual cycles (decreased levels of estrogen in response to malnutrition)

Promiscuity or denial/loss of sexual interest

History of sexual abuse

Breast atrophy, amenorrhea

Social Interactions

Middle-class or upper-class family background

Passive father/dominant mother, family members enmeshed, togetherness prized, personal boundaries not respected

History of being a quiet, cooperative child

Problems of control issues in relationships, difficult communications with others/authority figures; poor communications within family of origin

Engagement in power struggles

Altered relationships or problems with relationships (not married/divorced), withdrawal from friends/social contacts

Abusive family relationships

Sense of helplessness

May have history of legal difficulties (e.g., shoplifting)

Teaching/Learning

High academic achievement
Family history of higher than normal incidence of depression, other family members with eating disorders (genetic predisposition)
Onset of the illness usually between the ages of 10 and 22
Health beliefs/practices (e.g., certain foods have "too many" calories, use of "health" foods)
No medical illness evident to account for weight loss

DIAGNOSTIC STUDIES

CBC with Differential: Determines presence of anemia, leukopenia, lymphocytosis. Platelets show significantly less than normal activity by the enzyme monoamine oxidase (thought to be a marker for depression).

Electrolytes: Imbalances may include decreased potassium, sodium, chloride, and magnesium.

Endocrine Studies:

Thyroid Function: Thyroxine (T_4) levels usually normal; however, circulating triiodothyronine (T_3) levels may be low.

Pituitary Function: Thyroid-stimulating hormone (TSH) response to thyrotropin-releasing factor (TRF) is abnormal in anorexia nervosa. Propranolol-glucagon stimulation test (studies the response of human growth hormone) reveals depressed level of GH in anorexia nervosa. Gonadotropic hypofunction is noted.

Cortisol: Metabolism may be elevated.

Dexamethasone Suppression Test (DST): Evaluates hypothalamic-pituitary function, dexamethasone resistance indicates cortisol suppression, suggesting malnutrition/depression.

Luteinizing Hormone Secretions Test: Pattern often resembles those of prepubertal girls.

Estrogen: Decreased.

Blood Sugar and Basal Metabolic Rate (BMR): May be low.

Other Chemistries: AST elevated, increased carotene level; decreased protein and cholesterol levels.

MHP 6 Levels: Decreased, suggestive of malnutrition/depression.

Urinalysis and Renal Function: BUN may be elevated; ketones present reflecting starvation; decreased urinary 17-ketosteroids; increased specific gravity (dehydration).

EKG: Abnormal tracing with low voltage, T-wave inversion, dysrhythmias.

NURSING PRIORITIES

1. Reestablish adequate/appropriate nutritional intake.
2. Correct fluid and electrolyte imbalance.
3. Assist client to develop realistic body image/improve self-esteem.
4. Provide support/involve SO, if available, in treatment program to client/SO.
5. Coordinate total treatment program with other disciplines.
6. Provide information about disease, prognosis, and treatment.

DISCHARGE GOALS

1. Adequate nutrition and fluid intake maintained.
2. Maladaptive coping behaviors and stressors that precipitate anxiety recognized.
3. Adaptive coping strategies and techniques for anxiety reduction and self-control implemented.
4. Self-esteem increased.
5. Disease process, prognosis, and treatment regimen understood.
6. Plan in place to meet needs after discharge.

NURSING DIAGNOSIS	NUTRITION: altered, less than body requirements
May Be Related to:	Inadequate food intake; self-induced vomiting
	Chronic/excessive laxative use
Possibly Evidenced by:	Body weight 15% (or more) below expected (anorexia), or may be within normal range (bulimia, binge-eating)
	Pale conjunctiva and mucous membranes; poor skin turgor/muscle tone, edema
	Excessive loss of hair; increased growth of body hair (lanugo)
	Amenorrhea
	Hypothermia
	Bradycardia, cardiac irregularities, hypotension
Electrolyte imbalances	
Desired Outcomes/Evaluation Criteria— Client Will:	Verbalize understanding of nutritional needs.
	Establish a dietary pattern with caloric intake adequate to regain/maintain appropriate weight.
	Demonstrate weight gain toward expected goal range.

ACTIONS/INTERVENTIONS

RATIONALE

Independent

Establish a minimum weight goal and daily nutritional requirements.	Malnutrition is a mood-altering condition leading to depression and agitation and affecting cognitive functioning/decision-making. Improved nutritional status enhances thinking ability, and psychological work can begin.
Involve client with team in setting up/carrying out program of behavior modification. Provide reward for weight gain as individually determined; ignore loss.	Provides structured eating stimulation while allowing client some control in choices. Behavior modification may be effective only in mild cases or for short-term weight gain. **Note:** Combination of cognitive-behavioral approach is preferred for treating bulimia.
Use a consistent approach. Sit with client while eating; present and remove food without persuasion and/or comment. Promote pleasant environment and record intake.	Client detects urgency and reacts to pressure. Any comment that might be seen as coercion provides focus on food. When staff member responds consistently, client can begin to trust her or his responses. The single area in which client has exercised power and control is food/eating, and she or he may experience guilt or rebellion if forced to eat. Structuring meals and decreasing discussions about food will decrease power struggles with client and avoid manipulative games.

403

Provide smaller meals and supplemental snacks, as appropriate.

Make selective menu available and allow client to control choices, as much as possible.

Be alert to choices of low-calorie foods/beverages; hoarding food; disposing of food in various places such as pockets or wastebaskets.

Maintain a regular weighing schedule, such as Monday/Friday before breakfast in same attire, on same scale, and graph results.

Weigh with back to scale (depending on program protocols).

Avoid room checks and other control devices whenever possible.

Provide 1:1 supervision and have the client remain in the dayroom area with no bathroom privileges for a specified period (e.g., 2 hours) following eating, if contracting is unsuccessful.

Monitor exercise program and set limits on physical activities. Chart activity/level of work (pacing, and so on).

Maintain matter-of-fact, nonjudgmental attitude if giving enteral feedings, parenteral nutrition, etc.

Be alert to possibility of client disconnecting tube and emptying parenteral nutrition, if used. Check fluid measurements and tape tubing snugly.

Collaborative

Consult with dietitian/nutritional therapy team.

Refer for dental care.

Provide diet and snacks with substitutions of preferred foods when available.

Administer liquid diet, tube feedings/parenteral nutrition as appropriate.

Gastric dilation may occur if refeeding is too rapid following a period of starvation dieting. **Note:** Client may feel bloated for 3–6 weeks while body readjusts to food intake.

Client who gains self-confidence and feels in control of environment is more likely to eat preferred foods.

Client will try to avoid taking in what is viewed as excessive calories and may go to great lengths to avoid eating.

Provides accurate ongoing record of weight loss/gain. Also diminishes obsessing about changes in weight.

Although some programs prefer client to see the results of weighing, this approach can force the issue of trust in client who usually does not trust others.

External control reinforces client's feelings of powerlessness and are therefore usually not helpful.

Prevents vomiting during/after eating. Client may desire food and use a binge-purge syndrome to maintain weight. **Note:** Purging may occur for the first time in a client as a response to establishment of weight gain program.

Moderate exercise helps maintain muscle tone/weight and combat depression. However, client may exercise excessively to burn calories.

Perception of punishment is counterproductive to promoting self-confidence and faith in own ability to control destiny.

Sabotage behavior is common in attempt to prevent weight gain.

Helpful in determining individual dietary needs and appropriate sources. **Note:** Insufficient calorie and protein intake can lower resistance to infection and cause constipation, hallucinations, and liver damage.

Periodontal disease and loss of tooth enamel leading to caries and loose fillings requires prompt intervention to improve nutritional intake and general well-being.

Having a variety of foods available will enable the client to have a choice of potentially enjoyable foods.

When caloric intake is insufficient to sustain metabolic needs, nutritional support can be used to prevent malnutrition while therapy is continuing. High-calorie liquid feedings may be given as medication, at times separate from meals,

Blenderize and tube feed anything left on the tray after a given period of time if indicated.

Avoid giving laxatives.

Monitor laboratory values, as appropriate (e.g., prealbumin, transferrin, serum protein levels; electrolytes).

Administer medications as indicated, e.g.,
Cyproheptadine (Periactin);

Tricyclic antidepressants, e.g., amitriptyline (Elavil, Endep), imipramine (Tofranil), desipramine (Norpramin); selective serotonin reuptake inhibitors, e.g., fluoxetine (Prozac);

Antianxiety agents, e.g., alprozolam (Xanax);

Antipsychotics, e.g., chlorpromazine (Thorazine);

MAO inhibitors, e.g., tranylcypromine sulfate (Parnate).

Prepare for/assist with electroconvulsive therapy (ECT) if indicated. Discuss reasons for use and help client understand this therapy is not punishment.

Transfer to acute medical setting for nutritional therapy, when condition is life-threatening.

as an alternate means of increasing caloric intake. Enteral feedings are preferred as they preserve GI function and reduce atrophy of the gut. TPN is usually reserved for life-threatening situations.

May be used as part of behavior modification program to provide total intake of needed calories.

Laxative use is counterproductive, as it may be used by client to rid body of food/calories. **Note:** Metamucil/bran may be used to treat constipation.

Identifies therapeutic needs/effectiveness of treatment. Electrolyte imbalances can cause cardiac dysrhythmias, severe muscle spasms, and even sudden death.

A serotonin and histamine antagonist used in high doses to stimulate the appetite, decrease preoccupation with food, and combat depression. Does not appear to have serious side effects, although decreased mental alertness may occur. Lifts depression and stimulates appetite. SSRIs reduce binge-purge cycles and may also be helpful in treating anorexia. **Note:** Use must be closely monitored owing to potential side effects, although side effects from SSRIs are less significant than those associated with tricyclics.
Reduces tension and anxiety/nervousness and may help client to participate in treatment.
Promotes weight gain and cooperation with psychotherapeutic program, however, used only when absolutely necessary because of extrapyramidal side effects.
May be used to treat depression when other drug therapy is ineffective; decreases urge to binge in clients with bulimia.

In rare and difficult cases in which malnutrition is severe/life-threatening, a short-term ECT series may enable the client to begin eating and become accessible to psychotherapy.

The underlying problem cannot be cured without improved nutritional status. Hospitalization provides a controlled environment in which food intake, vomiting/elimination, medications, and activities can be monitored. It also separates the client from SO(s) and provides exposure to others with the same problem, creating an atmosphere for sharing.

NURSING DIAGNOSIS

May Be Related to:

FLUID VOLUME deficit, risk for or actual

Inadequate intake of food and liquids

Consistent self-induced vomiting

Chronic/excessive laxative or diuretic use

Possibly Evidenced by (Actual):	Dry skin and mucous membranes, decreased skin turgor
	Increased pulse rate, body temperature; hypotension
	Output greater than input (diuretic use); concentrated urine/decreased urine output (dehydration)
	Weakness
	Change in mental state
	Hemoconcentration, altered electrolyte balance
Desired Outcomes/Evaluation Criteria—Client Will:	Maintain/demonstrate improved fluid balance as evidenced by adequate urine output, stable vital signs, moist mucous membranes, good skin turgor.
	Verbalize understanding of causative factors and behaviors necessary to correct fluid deficit.

ACTIONS/INTERVENTIONS	RATIONALE
Independent	
Monitor vital signs, capillary refill, status of mucous membranes, skin turgor.	Indicators of adequacy of circulating volume. Orthostatic hypotension may occur, with risk of falls/injury following sudden changes in position.
Monitor amount and types of fluid intake. Measure urine output accurately as indicated.	Client may abstain from all intake, resulting in dehydration, or may substitute fluids for caloric intake, affecting electrolyte balance.
Discuss strategies to stop vomiting and laxative/diuretic use.	Helping client deal with feelings that lead to vomiting and/or laxative/diuretic use may prevent continued fluid loss. **Note:** The client with bulimia has learned that vomiting provides a release of anxiety.
Identify actions necessary to regain/maintain optimal fluid balance (e.g., specific schedule for fluid intake).	Involving client in plan to correct fluid imbalances improves chances for success.
Collaborative	
Review results of electrolyte/renal function test results.	Fluid/electrolyte shifts, decreased renal function can adversely affect client's recovery/prognosis and may require additional intervention.
Administer/monitor IV, TPN; potassium supplements, as indicated.	Used as an emergency measure to correct fluid/electrolyte imbalance. May be required to prevent cardiac dysrhythmias.

NURSING DIAGNOSIS	THOUGHT PROCESSES, altered
May Be Related to:	Severe malnutrition/electrolyte imbalance
	Psychological conflicts (e.g., sense of low self-worth, perceived lack of control)
Possibly Evidenced by:	Impaired ability to make decisions, problem-solve
	Non–reality-based verbalizations
	Ideas of reference
	Altered sleep patterns, e.g., may go to bed late (stay up to binge/purge) and get up early
	Altered attention span/distractibility
	Perceptual disturbances with failure to recognize hunger, fatigue, anxiety and depression
Desired Outcomes/Evaluation Criteria—Client Will:	Verbalize understanding of causative factors and awareness of impairment.
	Demonstrate behaviors to change/prevent malnutrition.
	Display improved ability to make decisions, problem-solve.

ACTIONS/INTERVENTIONS	RATIONALE
Independent	
Be aware of client's distorted thinking ability.	Allows the caregiver to have more realistic expectations of the client and provide appropriate information and support.
Listen to/avoid challenging irrational, illogical thinking. Present reality concisely and briefly.	It is not possible to respond logically when thinking ability is physiologically impaired. The client needs to hear reality, but challenging the client leads to distrust and frustration.
Adhere strictly to nutritional regimen.	Improved nutrition is essential to improved brain functioning. (Refer to ND: Nutrition: altered, less than body requirements.)
Collaborative	
Review electrolyte/renal function tests.	Imbalances negatively affect cerebral functioning and may require correction before therapeutic interventions can begin.

NURSING DIAGNOSIS	BODY IMAGE disturbance/SELF ESTEEM, chronic low
May Be Related to:	Morbid fear of obesity; perceived loss of control in some aspect of life

Possibly Evidenced by:	Unmet dependency needs, personal vulnerability
	Continued negative evaluation of self
	Dysfunctional family system
	Distorted body image (views self as fat even in the presence of normal body weight or severe emanciation)
	Expresses little concern, uses denial as a defense mechanism, and feels powerless to prevent/make changes
	Expresses shame/guilt
	Overly conforming, dependent on others' opinions
Desired Outcomes/Evaluation Criteria— Client Will:	Establish a more realistic body image.
	Acknowledge self as an individual.
	Accept responsibility for own actions.

ACTIONS/INTERVENTIONS	RATIONALE

Independent

Establish a therapeutic nurse/client relationship.	Within a helping relationship, client can begin to trust and try out new thinking and behaviors.
Promote self-concept without moral judgment.	Client sees self as weak-willed, even though part of person may feel a sense of power and control (e.g., dieting/weight loss).
Have client draw picture of self.	Provides opportunity to discuss client's perception of self/body image and realities of individual situation.
State rules clearly regarding weighing schedule, remaining in sight during medication and eating times, and consequences of not following the rules. Without undue comment, be consistent in carrying out rules.	Consistency is important in establishing trust. As part of the behavior-modification program, client knows risks involved in not following established rules (e.g., decrease in privileges). Failure to follow rules is viewed as the client's choice and accepted by the staff in matter-of-fact manner so as not to provide reinforcement for the undesirable behavior.
Respond (confront) with reality when client makes unrealistic statements such as "I'm gaining weight, so there's nothing really wrong with me."	Client may be denying the psychological aspects of own situation and is often expressing a sense of inadequacy and depression.
Be aware of own reaction to client's behavior. Avoid arguing.	Feelings of disgust, hostility, and infuriation are not uncommon when caring for these clients. Prognosis often remains poor even with weight gain because other problems may remain. Many clients continue to see themselves as fat, and there is also a high incidence of affective disorders, social phobias, obsessive-compulsive symptoms, drug abuse, and psychosexual dysfunction. Nurse needs to deal with own response/feelings so they do not interfere with care of the client.

Assist client to assume control in areas other than dieting/weight loss (e.g., management of own daily activities, work/leisure choices).

Feelings of personal ineffectiveness, low self-concept, and perfectionism are often part of the problem. Client feels helpless to change and requires assistance to problem-solve methods of control in life situations. Helps direct energy away from eating/body image to other life-enhancing and personally satisfying activities.

Help client formulate goals for self (not related to eating) and create a manageable plan to reach those goals, a single goal at a time, progressing from simple to more complex.

Client needs to recognize ability to control other areas in life and may need to learn problem-solving skills in order to achieve this control. Setting realistic goals fosters success.

Discuss the meaning of illness and effect of these behaviors.

Giving up an illness that has helped form the individual's personal identity, the unconscious benefit of the "sick role," and the overvalued beliefs about an ideal body and the benefits of thinness must be addressed before the client can confront the full role the illness has played in the client's life.

Assist client to confront sexual fears. Provide sex education as necessary.

Major physical/psychological changes in adolescence can contribute to development of eating disorders. Feelings of powerlessness and loss of control of feelings (particularly sexual) and sensations lead to an unconscious desire to desexualize themselves. Clients often believe that these fears can be overcome by taking control of bodily appearance/development/function. **Note:** Some clients with anorexia believe staying small and emaciated will help keep them childlike (and therefore sexually unappealing), whereas clients with binge-eating disorders wish to remain obese, believing excess body fat will lessen sexual attraction.

Determine history of sexual abuse and institute appropriate therapy.

Client may use eating as a means of gaining control in life when sexual abuse has been experienced.

Note client's withdrawal from and/or discomfort in social settings.

May indicate feelings of isolation and fear of rejection/judgment by others. Avoidance of social situations and contact with others can compound feelings of worthlessness.

Encourage client to take charge of own life in a more healthful way by making own decisions and accepting self as is at this moment (including inadequacies and strengths).

Client often does not know what she or he may want for self. Parents (usually mother) often make decisions for client. Client may also believe she or he has to be the best in everything and holds self responsible for being perfect.

Let client know that it is acceptable to be different from family, particularly mother.

Developing a sense of identity as separate from family and maintaining sense of control in other ways, besides dieting and weight loss, is a desirable goal of therapy/program.

Involve in personal development program, preferably in a group setting. Provide information about proper application of makeup and grooming.

Learning about methods of enhancing personal appearance may be helpful to long-range sense of self-concept/image. Feedback from others can promote feelings of self-worth.

409

Suggest disposing of "thin" clothes as weight gain occurs. Recommend consultation with an image consultant.	Provides incentive to at least maintain and not lose weight. Removes visual reminder of thinner self. Positive image enhances sense of self-esteem.
Use interpersonal psychotherapy approach rather than interpretive therapy.	Interaction between persons is more helpful for the client to discover feelings/impulses/needs from within own self. Client has not learned this internal control as a child and may not be able to interpret or attach meaning to behavior. **Note:** Cognitive therapy is usually more effective for clients diagnosed as bulimic or binge-eaters but may not be useful for anorectic clients during the period of acute hospitalization.
Encourage client to express anger and acknowledge when it is verbalized.	Important to know that anger is part of self and as such is acceptable. Expressing anger may need to be taught to client, because anger is often considered unacceptable in the family, and therefore client does not express it.
Assist client to learn strategies other than eating for dealing with feelings. Have client keep a diary of feelings, particularly when thinking about food.	Feelings are the underlying issue, and clients often use food instead of dealing with feelings appropriately. Therapeutic writing helps client recognize feelings and how to express them clearly and directly.
Assess feelings of helplessness/hopelessness.	Lack of control is a common/underlying problem for this client and may be accompanied by more serious emotional disorders. **Note:** 54% of clients with anorexia have a history of major affective disorder, and 33% have a history of minor affective disorder.
Be alert to suicidal ideation/behavior.	Intensity of anxiety/panic about weight gain, depression, hopeless feelings may lead to suicidal attempts, particularly if client is impulsive.

Collaborative

Involve in group therapy.	Provides an opportunity to talk about feelings and try out new behaviors.
Refer to occupational/recreational therapy.	Can develop interests and skills to fill time that has been occupied by obsession with eating. Involvement in recreational activities encourages social interactions with others and promotes fun and relaxation.
Encourage participation in directed activities (e.g., bicycle tours, wilderness adventures, such as Outward Bound Program).	Although exercise is often used negatively by these clients (i.e., for weight loss/control), directed activities provide an opportunity to learn self-reliance, enhance self-esteem, and realize that food is the fuel required by the body to do its work.
Refer to therapist trained in dealing with sexuality.	May need professional assistance to accept self as a sexual adult.

NURSING DIAGNOSIS	FAMILY PROCESSES, altered
May Be Related to:	Issues of control in family
	Situational/maturational crises
	History of inadequate coping methods
Possibly Evidenced by:	Dissonance among family members; family needs not being met
	Family developmental tasks not being met
	Ill-defined family rules, functions, and roles
	Focus on "identified patient" (IP); family member(s) acting as enablers for IP
Desired Outcomes/Evaluation Criteria— Family Will:	Demonstrate individual involvement in problem-solving processes directed at encouraging client toward independence.
	Express feelings freely and appropriately.
	Demonstrate more autonomous coping behaviors with individual family boundaries more clearly defined.
	Recognize and resolve conflict appropriately with the individuals involved.

ACTIONS/INTERVENTIONS	RATIONALE
Independent	
Identify patterns of interaction. Encourage each family member to speak for self. Do not allow 2 members to discuss a third without that member's participation.	Helpful information for planning interventions. The enmeshed, overinvolved family members often speak for each other and need to learn to be responsible for their own words and actions.
Discourage members from asking for approval from each other. Be alert to verbal or nonverbal checking with others for approval. Acknowledge competent actions of client.	Each individual needs to develop own internal sense of self-worth. Individual often is living up to others' (family's) expectations rather than making own choices. Acknowledgment provides recognition of self in positive ways.
Listen with regard when the client speaks.	Sets an example and provides a sense of competence and self-worth in that the client has been heard and attended to.
Encourage individuals not to answer to everything.	Reinforces individualization and return to privacy.
Communicate message of separation, that it is acceptable for family members to be different from each other.	Individuation needs reinforcement. Such a message confronts rigidity and opens options for different behaviors.
Encourage and allow expression of feelings (e.g., crying, anger) by individuals.	Often these families have not allowed free expression of feelings and will need help and permission to learn and accept this.

411

ACTIONS/INTERVENTIONS	RATIONALE

Prevent intrusion in dyads by other members of family.

Inappropriate interventions in family subsystems prevent individuals from working out problems successfully.

Reinforce importance of parents as a couple who have rights of their own.

The focus on the child with an eating disorder is very intense and often is the only area through which the couple interact. The couple needs to explore their own relationship and restore the balance within it to prevent its disintegration.

Prevent client from intervening in conflicts between parents. Help parents identify and solve their marital differences.

Triangulation occurs in which a parent-child coalition exists. Sometimes the child is openly pressed to align with 1 parent against the other. The symptom or behavior (eating disorder) is the regulator in the family system, and the parents deny their own conflicts.

Be aware of and confront sabotage behavior on the part of family members.

Feelings of blame, shame, and helplessness may lead to unconscious behavior designed to maintain the status quo.

Collaborative

Refer to community resources, such as family group therapy, parents' groups, as indicated; and Parent Effectiveness classes.

May help reduce overprotectiveness, support/facilitate the process of dealing with unresolved conflicts and change.

NURSING DIAGNOSIS	SKIN INTEGRITY, impaired, risk for or actual
May Be Related to:	Altered nutritional state; edema
	Dehydration/cachectic changes (skeletal prominence)
Possibly Evidenced by:	Dry/scaly skin with poor skin turgor; tissue fragility
	Brittle/dry hair
	Dry rash, reports of itching, dermal abrasions (from scratching)
Desired Outcomes/Evaluation Criteria— Client Will:	Verbalize understanding of causative factors and relief of discomfort.
	Identify and demonstrate behaviors to maintain soft, supple, intact skin.

ACTIONS/INTERVENTIONS	RATIONALE

Independent

Observe for reddened, blanched, excoriated areas.

Indicators of increased risk of breakdown requiring more intense treatment.

Encourage bathing every other day instead of daily.

Frequent baths contribute to skin dryness.

Use skin cream twice a day and always after bathing.

Lubricates skin and decreases itching.

Massage skin gently, especially over bony prominences.

Improves skin circulation, enhances skin tone.

Discuss importance of frequent change of position, need for remaining active.

Emphasize importance of adequate nutrition/fluid intake. (Refer to ND: Nutrition: altered, less than body requirements.)

Enhances circulation and perfusion to skin by preventing prolonged pressure on tissues.

Improved nutrition and hydration will improve skin condition.

NURSING DIAGNOSIS	KNOWLEDGE deficit (LEARNING NEED) regarding condition, prognosis, self care and treatment needs
May Be Related to:	Lack of exposure to/unfamiliarity with information resources; misinterpretation Lack of interest in learning Learned maladaptive coping skills
Possibly Evidenced by:	Verbalization of misconception Preoccupation with extreme fear of obesity and distortion of own body image Refusal to eat, binging/purging Abuse of laxatives/diuretics; excessive exercising Expression of desire to learn more adaptive ways of coping with stress or of relationship of current situation and behaviors Inappropriate behaviors (e.g., apathy)
Desired Outcomes/Evaluation Criteria— Client Will:	Verbalize awareness of and plan for lifestyle changes to maintain desired weight. Identify relationship of signs/symptoms (e.g., weight loss, tooth decay) to behaviors of not eating/binge-purging. Assume responsibility for own learning. Seek out sources/resources to assist with making identified changes. Formulate plan to meet individual goals for wellness.

ACTIONS/INTERVENTIONS

RATIONALE

Independent

Determine level of knowledge and readiness to learn.

Note blocks to learning (e.g., physical/intellectual/ emotional).

Review dietary needs, answering questions as indicated. Encourage inclusion of high-fiber foods and adequate fluid intake.

Learning is easier when it begins where the learner is.

Malnutrition, family problems, drug abuse, affective disorders, obsessive-compulsive symptoms can interfere with learning, requiring resolution before effective learning can occur.

Client/family may need assistance with planning for new way of eating. As constipation may occur when laxative use is curtailed, dietary

413

	considerations may prevent need for more aggressive therapy.
Discuss consequences of behavior.	Sudden death may occur owing to electrolyte imbalances; suppression of the immune system and liver damage may result from protein deficiency; or gastric rupture may follow binge-eating/vomiting.
Encourage the use of relaxation and other stress-management techniques (e.g., visualization, guided imagery, biofeedback).	New ways of coping with feelings of anxiety and fear will help client manage these feelings more effectively, assisting in giving up maladaptive behaviors of not eating/binging-purging.
Assist with establishing a sensible exercise program. Caution regarding overexercise.	Exercise can help develop a positive body image and combats depression (release of endorphins in the brain enhances sense of well-being). Client may use excessive exercise as a way of controlling weight.
Provide written information for client/SO(s).	Helpful as reminder of and reinforcement for learning.
Discuss need for information about sex and sexuality.	Because avoidance of own sexuality is an issue for this client, realistic information can be helpful in beginning to deal with self as a sexual being.
Refer to National Association of Anorexia Nervosa and Associated Disorders, Overeaters Anonymous, and other local resources.	May be a helpful source of support and information for client and SO(s).

SAMPLE CLINICAL PATHWAY:
Eating Disorders Program ELOS: 28 days Behavioral Unit

ND and categories of care	Time dimension	Outcomes/actions	Time dimension	Outcomes/actions	Time dimension	Outcomes/actions
Altered Nutrition: less than body requirements R/T inadequate intake, self-induced vomiting, laxative use	Ongoing	Gain 3lb/wk as indicated	Day 2–28	Consume at least 75% of food provided at each meal	Day 15–28	Demonstrate ability to select foods to meet at least 80% of nutritional needs
Risk for fluid volume deficit	Ongoing	Be free of signs/symptoms of dehydration; Display balanced I & O	Day 2–28; Day 3	Ingest at least 1500 ml fluid/day; Vital signs WNL	Day 22–28; Day 28	Refrain from self-induced vomiting; Be free of signs/symptoms of malnutrition with all laboratory results WNL
Referral	Day 1 & PRN	Dietitian				
Diagnostic studies	Day 1	Electrolytes, CBC, BUN/Cr, Thyroid function, UA, ECG as indicated	Day 14	Repeat selected studies as appropriate		
Additional assessments	Day 1–2	Vital signs/I & O q shift	Day 3–7	V.S. q AM	Day 8–28	As indicated
	Day 1	Weight on admission	Day 7, 14	Wt. 7:30 AM same clothes		
	Day 1–28	Types and amount of food/fluid intake; Behavior/purging following meals; Level of activity				
Medications Allergies: _____	Day 1–28	Periactin; Tricyclic anti-depressant; Vitamin supplement				
Action/therapies	Day 1 & PRN	Orient to unit and schedule; Engage in behavior modification program	Day 7–14	Review principles of nutrition; foods for maintenance of wellness	Day 21–28	Discuss how to incorporate nutritional plan into lifestyle and home setting

continued

Eating Disorders Program ELOS: 28 days Behavioral Unit—*continued*

ND and categories of care	Time dimension	Outcomes/ actions	Time dimension	Outcomes/ actions	Time dimension	Outcomes/ actions
Action /Therapies continued		Determine minimum weight goal and initial nutritional needs	Day 7–28	Involve mother/SO as appropriate in nutritional counseling and planning for future		
	Day 1–3	Assist client with formulation of behavioral contract and monitoring of cooperation				
	Day 1–7	Administer tube feeding/blenderized food as indicated				
	Day 1–21	Bathroom locked for 1 hr following meals				
	Day 1–28	Provide social setting for meals				
Ineffective denial R/T presence of overwhelming anxiety-producing feelings, learned response pattern, personal/family value system	Ongoing	Participate in behavior modification program and adhere to unit policies	Day 8–28	Attend and contribute to group sessions	Day 18–28	Verbalize acceptance of reality that eating behaviors are maladaptive
	Day 2–28	Cooperate with therapy to restore nutritional well-being	Day 14	Develop trusting relationship with at least one staff member on each shift		Demonstrate ability to cope more adaptively
						Identify ways to gain control in life situation
						Refrain from use of manipulation of others to achieve control
					Day 28	Plan in place to meet needs postdischarge

	Day		Day		Day	
Referrals	Day 5 (or when physical condition stable)	Psychologist Social worker Psychodramatist	Day 8–28	Group psychotherapy sessions	Day 25	Community resource contact person(s)
Additional assessments	Ongoing	Degree and stage of denial Perception of situation	Day 5–7	Readiness to participate in group sessions	Day 8–28	Degree/quality of involvement in group sessions
	Day 1–17	Ability to trust Use of manipulation to achieve control	Day 7–28	Congruence between verbalizations and behaviors (insight)		
Actions/therapies	Day 1 & PRN	Review privileges and responsibilities of behavior modification and consequences of behaviors	Day 3/ongoing	Discuss eating disorder and consequences of eating behavior	Day 21	Discuss role of support groups/community resources
		Encourage expression of feelings	Day 5–28	Promote involvement in unit activities	Day 21–28	Involve family (as appropriate) in long-range planning for meeting individual needs
	Day 1/ ongoing	Avoid agreeing with inaccurate statements/ perceptions Provide positive feedback for desired insight/behaviors Set limits on maladaptive behavior	Day 8–28	Support interactions with family members Encourage interactions in group sessions		
	Day 2–28	Attend therapy sessions on a daily basis				
Body Image disturbance/ Chronic Low Self Esteem R/T perceived loss of control unmet dependency needs, personal vulnerability, negative evaluation of self	Day 7	Acknowledge that attention will not be given to discussion of body image and food	Day 21	Acknowledge misperception of body image as fat Verbalize positive self-attributes	Day 28	Demonstrate realistic body image and self-awareness Verbalize acceptance of self, including "imperfections" Acknowledge self as sexual adult

continued

417

Eating Disorders Program ELOS: 28 days Behavioral Unit—continued

ND and categories of care	Time dimension	Outcomes/actions	Time dimension	Outcomes/actions	Time dimension	Outcomes/actions
Referrals	Day 1 (or when physical condition stable)	Therapists: Occupational, Recreational, Music, Art	Day 14	Image consultant	Day 28	Therapist (to address pertinent issues such as sexuality post-discharge)
Additional assessments	Day 1–7	Suicide ideation/behaviors	Day 8	Individual strengths/weaknesses		
	Day 3	Sexual history including abuse	Day 8–28	Congruency of feelings/perceptions with actions		
	Day 3–28	Perceptions of body image				
		Family patterns of interaction				
Actions/therapies	Day 1	Develop therapeutic relationship	Day 7	Compare actual measurements of client's body with client's perceptions	Day 14	Instruct in personal appearance and grooming
	Day 1–28	Support responsibility for self in family setting	Day 7–9	Assist with planning to meet individual goals	Day 14–28	Identify alternative coping strategies for dealing with feelings
		Provide positive feedback for participation and independent decision-making	Day 7–28	Clarify misconceptions of body image	Day 14–28	Have client keep diary of feelings, especially when thinking of food
		Confront sabotage behavior by family members	Day 8–10	Review general wellness needs		Role-play new behaviors for dealing with feelings and conflicts
	Day 3–5	Encourage control in areas other than diet	Day 8–28	Discuss human behavior and interactions with family/others—transactional analysis (TA)	Day 21–28	Provide sex education reflecting individual sexuality and needs
	Day 4–6	Support development of goals not related to eating		Involve in physical activity/exercise program		

Adapted from Townsend, MC: Psychiatric Mental Health Nursing, ed 2. FA Davis, Philadelphia, 1996.

OBESITY

DSM-IV
316.00 *Psychological factors affecting medical condition—maladaptive health behaviors*

Obesity is defined as an excess accumulation of body fat at least 20% over average weight for age, sex, and height. Although considered to be a type of eating disorder, obesity is a general medical condition coded on Axis III, with psychological factors that adversely affect the course and treatment of the medical condition, creating additional health risks for the individual.

ETIOLOGICAL THEORIES

Psychodynamics

Food is substituted by the parent for affection and love. The child harbors repressed feelings of hostility toward the parent, which may be expressed inward on the self. Because of a poor self-concept, the person has difficulty with other relationships. Eating is associated with a feeling of satisfaction and becomes the primary defense.

Biological

These disorders may arise from neuroendocrine abnormalities within the hypothalamus, which cause various chemical disturbances. Familial tendencies have been identified, but obesity is not clearly identified as being hereditary. People who are overweight have more fat cells than thin people and are known to be less active. Although overeating has long been believed to be the cause of obesity, research has not borne this out. Another popular theory has identified carbohydrates as the fattening substance. Currently, a high intake of fat in the diet is being identified as the reason for weight gain/inability to lose weight. The set-point theory proposes that people are programmed to maintain a certain level of weight to protect fat stores. Studies reveal that leptin regulates body weight by telling the body how much fat is being stored. Obese individuals often have higher leptin levels, suggesting a failure of the body to respond to leptin. This may represent a deficiency of receptor sites or inadequate amounts of glucagon-like peptide-1 (GPL-1), which may impair the leptin signaling pathway.

In recent research, genetics, metabolic changes placing some people at risk, and the way the body stores fat all play a part in the problems of obesity. Rather than a single, simple cause, obesity appears to be the result of a complex system reflecting all these factors.

Family Dynamics

Parents act as role models for the child. Maladaptive coping patterns (overeating) are learned within the family system and are supported through positive (or even negative) reinforcement. Family systems may sabotage efforts at changing any part of the system to maintain the status quo.

CLIENT ASSESSMENT DATA BASE

Activity/Rest

Fatigue, constant drowsiness
Inability/lack of desire to be active or engage in regular exercise
Increased heart rate/respirations with activity; dyspnea with exertion

Circulation

Hypertension, edema

419

Ego Integrity

Weight may/may not be perceived as a problem
Perception of body image as undesirable
Cultural/lifestyle factors affecting food choices; value for thinness/weight
Eating relieves unpleasant feelings (e.g., loneliness, frustration, boredom)
Reports of SO's resistance/demands regarding weight loss (may sabotage client's efforts)

Food/Fluid

Normal/excessive ingestion of food
History of recurrent weight loss and gain
Experimentation with numerous types of diets (yo-yo dieting) with varied/short-lived
    results
Weight disproportionate to height; endomorphic body type (soft/round)
Failure to adjust food intake to diminishing requirements (e.g., change in lifestyle from
    active to sedentary, aging)

Pain/Discomfort

Pain/discomfort on weight-bearing joints or spine

Respiration

Dyspnea with exertion
Cyanosis, respiratory distress (sleep apnea, pickwickian syndrome)

Sexuality

Menstrual disturbances, amenorrhea

Social Interactions

Family/significant other(s) may be supportive or resistant to weight loss (sabotage client's
    efforts)

Teaching/Learning

Problem may be lifelong or related to life event
Family history of obesity
Concomitant health problems may include hypertension, diabetes, gallbladder and
    cardiovascular disease, hypothyroidism

DIAGNOSTIC STUDIES

Metabolic/Endocrine Studies: May reveal abnormalities (e.g., hypothyroidism,
    hypopituitarism, hypogonadism, Cushing's syndrome [increased cortisol or glucose
    levels], hyperglycemia, hyperlipidemia, hyperuricemia, hyperbilirubinemia). The
    cause of these disorders may arise out of neuroendocrine abnormalities within the
    hypothalamus, which result in various chemical disturbances.
Anthropometric measurements: Measures fat-to-muscle ratio.

NURSING PRIORITIES

1. Help client identify a workable method of weight control incorporating needed
   nutrients/healthful foods.
2. Promote improved self-concept, including body image, self-esteem.
3. Encourage health practices to provide for weight control throughout life.

DISCHARGE GOALS

1. Healthy pattern for eating and weight control identified.
2. Weight loss toward desired goal established.
3. Positive perception of self verbalized.
4. Plan in place to meet needs for future weight-control.

NURSING DIAGNOSIS	NUTRITION: altered, more than body requirements
May Be Related to:	Food intake that exceeds body needs
	Psychosocial factors
	Socioeconomic status
Possible Evidenced by:	Weight of 20% or more over optimum body weight; excess body fat by anthropometric measurements
	Reported/observed dysfunctional eating patterns; intake more than body requirements
Desired Outcomes/Evaluation Criteria—Client Will:	Identify inappropriate behaviors and consequences associated with overeating or weight gain.
	Demonstrate change in eating patterns and involvement in individual exercise program.
	Display weight loss with optimal maintenance of health.

ACTIONS/INTERVENTIONS	RATIONALE
Independent	
Review individual factors for obesity (e.g., organic or nonorganic).	Identifies/influences choice of interventions.
Implement/review daily food diary (e.g., caloric intake, types of food, eating habits).	Provides the opportunity for the individual to focus on/internalize a realistic picture of the amount of food ingested and corresponding eating habits/feelings. Identifies patterns requiring changes and/or a base on which to tailor the dietary program.
Discuss emotions/events associated with eating.	Helps to identify when client is eating to satisfy an emotional need rather than physiological hunger.
Formulate an eating plan with the client.	Although there is no basis for recommending one diet over another, a good reducing diet should contain foods from all food groups with a focus on low-fat intake. It is helpful to keep the plan as similar to client's usual eating pattern as possible. A plan developed with and agreed to by the client is more apt to be successful. **Note:** It is important to maintain adequate protein intake to prevent loss of lean muscle mass.

Develop nutritional plan using knowledge of individual's height, body build, age, gender, individual patterns of eating, and energy and nutrient requirements.

Standard tables are subject to error when applied to individual situations, and circadian rhythms/lifestyle patterns need to be considered.

Emphasize the importance of avoiding fad diets.

Elimination of needed components can lead to metabolic imbalances (e.g., excessive reduction of carbohydrates can lead to fatigue, headache, instability and weakness, and metabolic acidosis [ketosis] interfering with effectiveness of weight loss program).

Discuss need to give self permission to include desired/craved food items in dietary plan.

Denying self by excluding desired/favorite foods results in a sense of deprivation and feelings of guilt/failure when individual succumbs to temptation. These feelings can sabotage weight loss. Knowing that it is important to include small portions of these foods can prevent negative feelings and promote cooperation with weight loss program.

Identify realistic increment goals for weekly weight loss.

Reasonable weight loss (1–2 pounds/wk) results in more lasting effects. Excessive/rapid loss may result in fatigue and irritability and ultimately lead to failure in meeting weight loss goals. Motivation is more easily sustained by meeting "stair-step" goals.

Weigh periodically as individually indicated, and obtain appropriate body measurements.

Provides information about effectiveness of therapeutic regimen and visual evidence of success of client's efforts. During hospitalization for controlled fasting, daily weight measurement may be required. Weekly weight measurement is more appropriate after discharge.

Determine current activity levels and plan progressive exercise program (e.g., walking) tailored to individual goals and choice.

Exercise furthers weight loss by burning calories and reducing appetite, increasing energy, toning muscles, and enhancing sense of well-being and accomplishment. Client's commitment enables the setting of more realistic goals and adherence to the plan.

Develop an appetite reeducation plan with the client.

In these clients, signals of hunger and fullness often are not recognized, have become distorted, or are ignored.

Emphasize the importance of avoiding tension at mealtimes and not eating too quickly.

Reducing tension provides a more relaxed eating atmosphere and encourages more leisurely eating patterns. This is important because a period of time is required for the appestat mechanism to recognize that the stomach is full.

Encourage client to eat only at a table or designated eating place and to avoid standing while eating.

Techniques that modify behavior may be helpful in avoiding diet failure.

Discuss restriction of salt intake and diuretic drugs if used.

Water retention may be a problem because of increased sodium intake, as well as the result of fat metabolism.

Reassess caloric requirements every 2–4 weeks to determine need for adjustment. Be aware of

Changes in weight and exercise will necessitate changes in diet. As weight is lost, changes in

plateaus when weight remains stable for periods of time.

metabolism occur. Plateaus can create distrust and accusations of "cheating" on caloric intake, which are not helpful. Client may need additional support at this time.

Collaborative

Consult with dietitian to determine caloric/nutrient requirements for individual weight loss.

Individual intake can be calculated by several different formulas, but weight reduction is based on the basal caloric requirement for 24 hours, depending on client's sex, age, current/desired weight, and length of time estimated to achieve desired weight.

Provide medications as indicated:
Appetite-suppressant drugs, e.g., diethylpropion (Tenuate), mazindol (Sanorex);

May be used with caution/supervision at the beginning of a weight loss program to support client during stress of behavioral/lifestyle changes. They are only effective for a few weeks and may cause problems of tolerance/dependence in some people.

Hormonal therapy, e.g., thyroid (Euthroid);

May be necessary when hypothyroidism is present. When no deficiency is present, replacement therapy is not helpful and may actually be harmful. **Note:** Other hormonal treatments, such as human chorionic gonadotropin (hCG), although widely publicized, have no documented evidence of value.

Vitamin, mineral supplementation.

Obese individuals have large fuel reserves, but are often deficient in vitamins and minerals.

Hospitalize for fasting regimen and/or stabilization of medical problems.

Aggressive therapy/support may be necessary to initiate weight loss, although fasting is not usually a treatment of choice. Client can be monitored more effectively in a controlled setting to minimize complications such as postural hypotension, anemia, cardiac irregularities, and decreased uric acid excretion with hyperuricemia.

Refer for evaluation of surgical options (e.g., gastric partitioning, bypass), as indicated.

May be necessary to assist the client lose weight when obesity is life-threatening.

NURSING DIAGNOSIS	BODY IMAGE disturbance/SELF ESTEEM, chronic low
May Be Related to:	Biophysical/psychosocial factors, such as client's view of self (slimness is valued in this society, and negative messages may be received when thinness is stressed)
	Family/subculture encouragement of overeating
	Control, sex, and love issues
Possibly Evidenced by:	Verbalization of negative feelings about body (mental image often does not match physical reality); expressions of shame/guilt

	Rejection of positive feedback and exaggeration of negative feedback about self
	Feelings of hopelessness/powerlessness; fear of rejection/reaction by others
	Lack of follow-through with diet plan; verbalization of powerlessness to change eating habits; hesitancy to try new things
	Preoccupation with change (attempts to lose weight)
Desired Outcomes/Evaluation Criteria— Client Will:	Verbalize a more realistic self-image.
	Demonstrate beginning acceptance of self as is, rather than an idealized image.
	Acknowledge self as an individual who has responsibility for own self.
	Seek information and actively pursue appropriate weight loss.

ACTIONS/INTERVENTIONS	RATIONALE
Independent	
Determine client's view of being fat and what it does for the individual.	Mental image includes our ideal and is usually not up to date. Fatness and compulsive eating behaviors may have deep-rooted psychological implications (e.g., compensating for lack of love and nurturing, or a defense against intimacy).
Provide privacy during care activities.	Individual usually is sensitive/self-conscious about body.
Have client recall coping patterns related to food in family of origin and explore how these may affect current situation.	Parents act as role models for the child. Maladaptive coping patterns (overeating) are learned within the family system and are supported through positive reinforcement. Food may be substituted by the parent for affection and love, and eating is associated with a feeling of satisfaction, becoming the primary defense.
Determine relationship history and possibility of sexual abuse.	May contribute to current issues of self-esteem/patterns of coping.
Identify client's motivation for weight loss and set goals.	May harbor repressed feelings of hostility, which may be expressed inward on the self. Because of a poor self-concept, client often has difficulty with relationships. **Note:** When losing weight for someone else, client is less likely to be successful/maintain weight loss.
Be alert to myths the client/SO may have about weight and weight loss.	Beliefs about what an ideal body looks like or unconscious motivations can sabotage efforts at weight loss. Some of these include the feminine thought of "If I become thin, men will pursue me or desire/rape me"; the masculine counterpart of "I don't trust myself to stay in control of my feelings"; as well as issues of strength, power, or the "good cook" image.

Have client keep a journal noting feelings that lead to compulsive eating.	Awareness of emotions that lead to overeating can be the first step in behavior change (e.g., people often eat because of depression, anger, and guilt).
Develop strategies for doing something besides eating for dealing with feelings (e.g., talking with a friend).	Replacing eating with other activities helps to retain old patterns and establish new ways to deal with feelings.
Graph weight on a weekly basis.	Provides ongoing visual evidence of weight changes (reality orientation).
Promote open communication, avoiding criticism/judgment about client's behavior.	Supports client's own responsibility for weight loss; enhances sense of control, and promotes willingness to discuss difficulties/setbacks and problem-solve. **Note:** Distrust and accusations of "cheating" on caloric intake are not helpful.
Outline/clearly state responsibilities of client and nurse.	It is helpful for each individual to understand area of own responsibility in the program to avoid misunderstandings.
Be alert to binge-eating, and develop strategies for dealing with these episodes (e.g., substituting other actions for eating).	The client who binges experiences guilt about it that is counterproductive because negative feelings may sabotage further weight loss.
Encourage client to use imagery to visualize self at desired weight and to practice handling new behaviors.	Mental rehearsal is very useful to help client plan for and deal with anticipated change in self-image or deal with occasions that may arise (family gatherings, special dinners) in which confrontations with food will occur.
Provide information about the use of makeup, hairstyles, and ways of dressing to maximize figure assets.	Enhances positive feelings of self-esteem, promotes improved body image.
Encourage buying clothes instead of food treats as a reward for weight loss.	Properly fitting clothes enhance the body image as small losses are made and the individual feels more positive. Waiting until the desired weight loss is reached can become discouraging.
Suggest client dispose of "fat clothes."	Removes the "safety valve" of having clothes available "in case" the weight is regained. Retaining fat clothes can convey the message that the weight loss will not occur/be maintained.
Help staff be aware of and deal with own feelings when caring for client.	Judgmental attitudes, feelings of disgust, anger, and weariness can interfere with care/be transmitted to client, reinforcing negative self-concept/image.
Help client identify positive self-attributes. Focus on strengths/past accomplishments (unrelated to physical appearance).	It is important that self-esteem not be tied solely to size of the body. Client needs to recognize that obesity need not interfere with positive feelings regarding self-concept and self-worth.

Collaborative

Refer to community support and/or therapy group.	Support groups can provide companionship, increase motivation, decrease loneliness and social ostracism, and give practical solutions to common problems. Group therapy can be helpful in dealing with underlying psychological concerns.

425

NURSING DIAGNOSIS	SOCIAL INTERACTION, impaired
May Be Related to:	Verbalized or observed discomfort in social situations
	Self-concept disturbance
Possibly Evidenced by:	Reluctance to participate in social gatherings
	Verbalization of a sense of discomfort with others
Desired Outcomes/Evaluation Criteria—Client Will:	Verbalize awareness of feelings that lead to poor social interactions.
	Be involved in achieving positive changes in social behaviors and interpersonal relationships.

ACTIONS/INTERVENTIONS	RATIONALE

Independent

ACTIONS/INTERVENTIONS	RATIONALE
Review family patterns of relating and social behaviors. Assess weight issues among family of origin, especially mother/father.	Social interaction is primarily learned within the family of origin. When inadequate patterns are identified, actions for change can be instituted.
Encourage client to express feelings and perception of problems.	Helps client identify and clarify reasons for difficulties in interacting with others (e.g., client may feel unloved/unlovable or insecure about sexuality).
Assess client's use of coping skills and defense mechanisms.	May have coping skills that will be useful in the process of weight loss. Defense mechanisms used to protect the individual may contribute to feelings of aloneness/isolation, or resistance to change.
Have client list behaviors that cause discomfort.	Identifies specific concerns and suggests actions that can be taken to effect change.
Involve in role-playing new ways to deal with identified behaviors/situations.	Practicing these new behaviors lets client become comfortable with them in a safe environment.
Discuss negative self-concepts and self-talk (e.g., "No one wants to be with a fat person," "Who would be interested in talking to me?").	May be impeding positive social interactions.
Encourage use of positive self-talk such as telling oneself "I am OK" or "I can enjoy social activities and do not need to be controlled by what others think or say."	Positive strategies enhance feelings of comfort and support efforts for change.

Collaborative

ACTIONS/INTERVENTIONS	RATIONALE
Refer for ongoing family or individual therapy as indicated.	Client benefits from involvement of family/SO to provide support and encouragement.

NURSING DIAGNOSIS	KNOWLEDGE deficit [LEARNING NEED] regarding condition, prognosis, self care and treatment needs
May Be Related to:	Lack of/misinterpretation of information
	Lack of interest in learning, lack of recall
	Inaccurate/incomplete information presented

Possibly Evidenced by:	Questions/request for information about obesity and nutritional requirements
	Verbalization of problem with weight reduction
	Inadequate follow-through with previous diet and exercise instruction
Desired Outcomes/Evaluation Criteria—Client Will:	Assume responsibility for own learning.
	Begin to look for information about nutrition and ways to control weight.
	Verbalize understanding of need for lifestyle changes to maintain/control weight.
	Establish individual goal and plan for attaining goal.

ACTIONS/INTERVENTIONS	RATIONALE

Independent

Determine level of nutritional knowledge and what client believes is most urgent need.	Necessary to know what additional information to provide. When client's views are listened to, trust is enhanced.
Identify individual holistic long-term goals for health (e.g., lowering blood pressure, controlling serum lipid and glucose levels).	A high-relapse rate at 5-year follow-up suggests obesity cannot be reliably reversed/cured. Shifting the focus from initial weight loss/percentage of body fat to overall wellness may enhance rehabilitation.
Provide information about ways to maintain satisfactory food intake in settings away from home.	"Smart" eating when dining out or when traveling helps client maintain weight and desired level while still enjoying social outlets.
Identify other sources of information (e.g., books, tapes, community classes, groups).	Using different avenues of accessing information will further client's learning. Involvement with others who are also losing weight can provide support.
Emphasize necessity to continue follow-up care/counseling, especially when "plateaus" occur.	As weight is lost, metabolism changes, interfering with further loss by creating a "plateau" as the body activates a survival mechanism, attempting to prevent "starvation." This requires new strategies and aggressive support to help client continue weight loss.
Identify alternatives to chosen activity program to accommodate weather, travel, and so on. Discuss use of mechanical devices/equipment for reducing weight.	Promotes continuation of program. **Note:** Fat loss occurs on a generalized overall basis, and there is no evidence that spot-reducing or mechanical devices aid in weight loss in specific areas. However, specific types of exercise or equipment may be useful in toning specific body parts.
Discuss necessity of good skin care, especially during summer months.	Prevents skin breakdown/yeast infections in moist skinfolds.
Identify alternative ways to "reward" self/family for accomplishments or to provide solace.	Reduces likelihood of relying on food to deal with feelings.
Encourage involvement in social activities that are not centered on food (e.g., bike ride/nature hike, attending musical event, group sporting activities, window shopping).	Provides opportunity for pleasure and relaxation without "temptation." Activities/exercise may also use calories to help maintain desired weight.

427

CHAPTER 14

ADJUSTMENT DISORDERS

ADJUSTMENT DISORDERS

DSM-IV
ADJUSTMENT DISORDERS (SPECIFY IF ACUTE/CHRONIC)
309.24 With anxiety
309.0 With depressed mood
309.3 With disturbance of conduct
309.4 With mixed disturbance of emotions and conduct
309.28 With mixed anxiety and depressed mood

The essential feature of adjustment disorders is a maladaptive reaction to an identifiable psychosocial stressor that occurs within 3 months of the onset of the stressor. (The reaction to the death of a loved one is not included here, as it is generally diagnosed as bereavement.) The stressor also does not meet the criteria for any specific Axis I disorder or represent an exacerbation of a preexisting Axis I or Axis II disorder.

The response is considered maladaptive because social or occupational functioning is impaired or because the behaviors are exaggerated beyond the usual expected response to such a stressor. Duration of the symptoms for more than 6 months indicates a chronic state. By definition, an adjustment disorder must resolve within 6 months of the termination of the stressor or its consequences. If the stressor/consequences persist (e.g., a chronic disabling medical condition, emotional difficulties following a divorce, financial reversals resulting from termination of employment, or a developmental event such as leaving one's parental home, retirement), the adjustment disorder may also persist.

ETIOLOGICAL THEORIES

Psychodynamics

Factors implicated in the predisposition to this disorder include unmet dependency needs, fixation in an earlier level of development, and underdeveloped ego.

The client with predisposition to adjustment disorder is seen as having an inability to complete the grieving process in response to a painful life change. The presumed cause of this inability to adapt is believed to be psychic overload—a level of intrapsychic strain exceeding the individual's ability to cope. Normal functioning is disrupted, and psychological or somatic symptoms occur.

Biological

The presence of chronic disorders is thought to limit an individual's general adaptive capacity. The normal process of adaptation to stressful life experiences is impaired, causing increased vulnerability to adjustment disorders. A high family incidence suggests a possible hereditary influence.

The autonomic nervous system discharge that occurs in response to a frightening impulse and/or emotion is mediated by the limbic system, resulting in the peripheral effects of the autonomic nervous system seen in the presence of anxiety.

Some medical conditions have been associated with anxiety and panic disorders, such as abnormalities in the hypothalamic-pituitary-adrenal and hypothalamic-pituitary-thyroid axes; acute myocardial infarction; pheochromocytomas; substance intoxication and withdrawal; hypoglycemia; caffeine intoxication; mitral valve prolapse; and complex partial seizures.

Family Dynamics

The individual's ability to respond to stress is influenced by the role of the primary caregiver (her or his ability to adapt to the infant's needs) and the child-rearing environment (allowing the child gradually to gain independence and control over own life). Difficulty allowing the child to become independent leads to the child having adjustment problems in later life.

Individuals with adjustment difficulties have experienced negative learning through inadequate role-modeling in dysfunctional family systems. These dysfunctional patterns impede the development of self-esteem and adequate coping skills, which also contribute to maladaptive adjustment responses.

CLIENT ASSESSMENT DATA BASE

(Symptoms of affective, depressive, and anxiety disorders are manifested dependent on the individual's specific response to a stressful situation.)

Activity/Rest

Fatigue
Insomnia

Ego Integrity

Reports occurrence of personal stressor/loss (e.g., job, financial, relationship) within past 3 months
May appear depressed and tearful and/or nervous and jittery
Feelings of hopelessness

Neurosensory

Mental Status: Depressed mood, tearful, anxious, nervous, jittery
Attention and memory span may be impaired (depends on presence of depression, level of anxiety, and/or substance use)
Communication and thought patterns may reveal negative ruminations of depressed mood or flight of ideas/loose associations of severely anxious condition

Pain/Discomfort

Various physical symptoms such as headache, backache, other aches and pains (maladaptive response to a stressful situation)

Safety

Anger expressed inappropriately
Involvement in high-risk behaviors (e.g., fighting, reckless driving)
Suicidal ideations may be present

429

Social Interactions

Difficulties with performance in work/social setting, when no difficulties had been experienced prior to the occurrence of the stressor
Socially withdrawn/refuses to interact with others (e.g., isolates self in own room)
Reports of vandalism, reckless driving, fighting, defaulting on legal responsibilities, violation of the rights of others or age-appropriate norms and rules
May display manipulative behavior (e.g., testing limits, playing individuals/family members against each other)

Teaching/Learning

Academic difficulties, failure to attend class/complete course work
Substance use/abuse possibly present

DIAGNOSTIC STUDIES

Diagnostic studies and psychological testing as indicated to rule out conditions that may mimic or coexist (e.g., endocrine imbalance, cardiac involvement, epilepsy, or a differential diagnosis with affective, anxiety, conduct, or antisocial personality disorders).
Drug Screen: Determine substance use.

NURSING PRIORITIES

1. Provide safe environment/protect client from self-harm.
2. Assist client to identify precipitating stressor.
3. Promote development of effective problem-solving techniques.
4. Provide information and support for necessary lifestyle changes.
5. Promote involvement of client/family in therapy process/planning for the future.

DISCHARGE GOALS

1. Relief from feelings of depression and/or anxiety noted, with suicidal ideation reduced.
2. Anger expressed in an appropriate manner.
3. Maladaptive behaviors recognized and rechanneled into socially accepted actions.
4. Client involved in social situations/interacting with others.
5. Ability and willingness to manage life situations displayed.
6. Plan in place to meet needs after discharge.

NURSING DIAGNOSIS	ANXIETY [moderate to severe]
May Be Related to:	Situational/maturational crisis
	Threat to self-concept; threat (or perceived threat) to physical integrity
	Unmet needs; fear of failure
	Dysfunctional family system; unsatisfactory parent/child relationship resulting in feelings of insecurity
	Fixation in earlier level of development
Possibly Evidenced by:	Overexcitement/restlessness; increased tension; insomnia

	Feelings of inadequacy; fear of unspecified consequences
	Poor eye contact, focus on self; difficulty concentrating
	Continuous attention-seeking behaviors; selective inattention
	Sympathetic stimulation; numerous physical complaints
Desired Outcomes/Evaluation Criteria—Client Will:	Verbalize awareness of feelings of/indicators of increasing anxiety.
	Demonstrate/use appropriate techniques to interrupt escalation of anxiety.
	Appear relaxed and report anxiety is reduced to a manageable level.

ACTIONS/INTERVENTIONS

RATIONALE

Independent

Establish a therapeutic nurse/client relationship. Be honest, consistent in responses, and available. Show genuine positive regard.

Honesty, availability, and unconditional acceptance promote trust, which is necessary for the development of a therapeutic relationship.

Provide activities geared toward reduction of tension and decreasing anxiety (e.g., walking or jogging, musical exercises, housekeeping chores, group games/activities).

Tension and anxiety can be released safely, and physical activity may provide emotional benefit to the client through release in the brain of morphine-like substances (endorphins) that promote sense of well-being.

Encourage client to identify true feelings and to acknowledge ownership of those feelings.

Anxious clients often deny a relationship between emotional problems and their anxiety. Use of the defense mechanisms of projection and displacement are exaggerated.

Maintain a calm atmosphere and approach to client.

Can help to limit transmission of anxiety to/from client.

Assist client to recognize specific events that precede onset of elevation in anxiety. Provide information about signs and symptoms of increasing anxiety and ways to intervene before behaviors become disabling.

Recognition of precipitating stressors and a plan of action to follow should they recur provides client with feelings of security and control over similar situations in the future. This in itself may help to control anxiety response.

Offer support during times of elevated anxiety. Provide physical and psychological safety. (Refer to ND: Violence, risk for, directed at self/others.)

Presence of a trusted individual may provide needed security/client safety.

Collaborative

Administer medications as necessary, e.g., benzo-diazepines: alprazolam (Xanax).

Antianxiety medications induce a calming effect and work to maintain anxiety at a manageable level while providing the opportunity for client to develop other ways to manage stress.

431

NURSING DIAGNOSIS	VIOLENCE, risk for, directed at self/others
Risk Factors May Include:	Depressed mood, hopelessness, powerlessness; inability to tolerate frustration; rage reactions
	Low self-esteem; unmet needs
	Negative role modeling; lack of support systems
	Substance use/abuse; history of previous suicide attempts
[Possible Indicators:]	Increased motor activity (pacing, excitement, irritability, agitation)
	Muscle tension (e.g., clenched fists, tense facial expressions, rigid posture, tautness)
	Hostile, threatening verbalizations; provocative behavior (argumentative, dissatisfied, overreactive, hypersensitive)
	Suicide ideation
Desired Outcomes/Evaluation Criteria— Client Will:	Verbalize understanding of behavior and precipitating factors.
	Participate in care and meet own needs in an assertive manner.
	Rechannel anger/hostile feelings into socially acceptable behaviors.
	Demonstrate self-control as evidenced by relaxed posture, absence of violent behavior, etc.
	Use resources/support systems in an effective manner.

ACTIONS/INTERVENTIONS	RATIONALE
Independent	
Observe client's behavior frequently during routine activities and interactions; avoid appearing watchful and suspicious.	Close observation is required so that intervention can occur if required to ensure the safety of others. Instilling suspicion may provoke aggressive behaviors.
Ask client direct questions regarding intent, plan, and availability of the means for self-harm. Evaluate and prioritize on a scale of 1–10 according to severity of threat, availability of means.	Direct questions, if presented in a caring, concerned manner, provide the necessary information to assist the nurse in formulating an appropriate plan of care for the suicidal client.
Provide a safe environment: reduce stimuli (e.g., low lighting, few people, simple decor, low noise level).	A stimulating environment may increase agitation and provoke aggressive behavior.
Remove potentially dangerous objects, such as straps, belts, ties, sharp objects, glass items, and drugs, as indicated.	External control of environment aids in preventing impulsive actions at a time when client lacks own internal controls.

Secure contract from client that she or he will not harm self and will seek out staff member if suicidal ideations emerge.

A contract encourages the client to share in the responsibility of own safety. A degree of control is experienced, and the attitude of acceptance of the client as a worthwhile individual is conveyed.

Promote verbalizations of honest feelings. Through exploration and discussion, help client identify symbols of hope in own life.

May be difficult for client to express negative feelings. Verbalization of these feelings in a nonthreatening environment may help client come to terms with unresolved issues and identify reasons for wanting to change life/continue living.

Help client identify true source of anger/hostility and underlying feelings.

Because of weak ego development, client may be using the defense mechanism of displacement. Helping the client to recognize this in a nonthreatening environment may help reveal unresolved issues so that they may be confronted, regardless of the discomfort involved.

Convey an attitude of acceptance toward the client. Impart a message that it is not the client but the behavior that is unacceptable.

Promotes feelings of self-worth. These feelings are further enhanced as person and behavior are viewed separately, communicating unconditional positive regard.

Explore with client alternative ways of handling frustration/pent-up anger that channel hostile energy into socially acceptable behavior (e.g., brisk walks, jogging, physical exercises, volleyball, punching bag, exercise bike).

Physically demanding activities help to relieve pent-up tension. **Note:** Exercise need not be aerobic or intensive to achieve therapeutic effect.

Maintain a calm attitude toward the client if behavior escalates. Have sufficient staff available to convey a show of strength to the client if it becomes necessary.

Anxiety is contagious and can be transferred from person to person. A calm attitude provides client with a feeling of safety and security. A display of strength provides reassurance for the client that the staff is in control of the situation and will provide physical security for the client, staff, and others.

Be alert to increased potential for suicidal action as mood elevates.

Client may mobilize self for suicidal attempt as decrease in depression results in increased energy and motivation.

Collaborative

Administer medication as indicated, e.g.:
   Tricyclic drugs: amitriptyline (Elavil), desipramine (Norpramin), doxepin (Sinequan), imipramine (Tofranil); selective serotonin reuptake inhibitors (SSRIs): fluoxetine (Prozac), sertraline (Zoloft), paroxetine (Paxil); monoamine-oxidase inhibitors: isocarboxazid (Marplan), phenelzine (Nardil);

Antidepressant medication may elevate the mood, as it increases level of energy and decreases feelings of fatigue.

   Benzodiazepines: diazepam (Valium), chlordiazepoxide (Librium), alprazolam (Xanax).

Antianxiety medication may provide needed relief from anxious feelings, inducing a calming effect and inhibiting aggressive behavior.

433

NURSING DIAGNOSIS

May Be Related to:

Possibly Evidenced by:

Desired Outcomes/Evaluation Criteria—Client Will:

COPING, INDIVIDUAL, ineffective

Situational/maturational crises

Dysfunctional family system; negative role modeling; inadequate support systems

Unmet dependency needs; low self-esteem; retarded ego development

Inability to cope/problem-solve

Chronic worry, depressed/anxious mood

Alteration in societal participation; manipulation of others

Inability to meet role expectations; increased dependency; refusal to follow rules of the unit

Numerous physical complaints

Destructive behavior, substance abuse

Assess the current situation accurately.

Identify ineffective coping behaviors and consequences.

Meet psychological needs as evidenced by appropriate expression of feelings, identification of options, and use of resources.

Refrain from manipulating others for own gratification.

ACTIONS/INTERVENTIONS	RATIONALE

Independent

Explain rules of the unit/therapeutic relationship and consequences of lack of cooperation. Set limits on manipulative behavior. Be consistent in enforcing the consequences when rules are broken and limits tested.

Negative reinforcement may work to decrease undesirable behaviors. Consistency among all staff members is vital if intervention is to be successful.

Ignore negative behaviors when possible and provide feedback when positive behaviors are noted, encouraging client to acknowledge own success.

Negative behaviors diminish when they provide no reward of attention. When client gives self positive feedback, inner rewards are enhanced.

Encourage client to discuss angry feelings. Help client identify the true object of the hostility. Provide physical outlets for healthy release of the hostile feelings (e.g., punching bags, pounding boards). Involve in outdoor recreation program, if available.

Verbalization of feelings with a trusted individual may help client work through unresolved issues. Physical exercise provides a safe and effective means of releasing pent-up tension, as well as of developing self-confidence and trust in others.

Take care not to reinforce dependent behaviors.

Independent accomplishment and positive reinforcement enhance self-esteem and encourage repetition of desirable behaviors.

Allow client to perform as independently as possible and provide feedback. Help client recognize aspects

Recognition of personal control, however, minimal diminishes the feeling of powerlessness

of life over which a measure of control is maintained/possible. (Refer to ND: Powerlessness.)

Give minimal attention to the physical condition if client is coping through numerous somatic complaints and organic pathology has been ruled out. Increase attention when client is not focusing on physical complaints.

Discuss the negative aspects of substance abuse as a response to stress. Help client recognize difficult life situations that may be contributing to use of substances.

Assist with problem-solving process. Suggest alternatives, and help client to select more adaptive strategies for coping with stress.

Encourage client to learn relaxation techniques, use of imagery.

Collaborative

Refer client to substance rehabilitation program if problem is identified.

and decreases the need to manipulate others.

Organic pathology must always be considered. Failure to do so may place the client in physical jeopardy. Lack of attention to maladaptive behaviors may decrease their repetition. Positive reinforcement encourages desirable behaviors.

Denial of problems related to substance use is common. Client needs to recognize relationship between substance use and personal problems before rehabilitation can begin.

Because of level of anxiety and delayed development, client may require assistance in determining which methods of coping are most individually appropriate. Increased anxiety interferes with client's problem-solving ability.

These skills can be helpful in developing new coping methods to deal with/reduce stress.

A greater likelihood of success can be expected if client seeks professional assistance with this problem.

NURSING DIAGNOSIS	ADJUSTMENT, impaired [when stressor is a change in health status]
May Be Related to:	Change in health status requiring modification in lifestyle (e.g., development of chronic disease/disability, changes associated with aging process)
	Assault to self-esteem
	Inadequate support systems
Possibly Evidenced by:	Verbalization of nonacceptance of health status change
	Difficulty in problem-solving, decision-making, or goal-setting; lack of future-oriented thinking
	Lack of movement toward independence
Desired Outcomes/Evaluation Criteria—Client Will:	Recognize reality of situation and individual needs/options.
	Assume personal responsibility for care, problem-solve needs.
	Initiate necessary lifestyle changes.
	Plan for future needs/changes.

435

ACTIONS/INTERVENTIONS	RATIONALE

Independent

Encourage client to talk about lifestyle before the change in health status.	It is important to identify the client's strengths so that they may be used to facilitate adaptation to change or loss that has occurred.
Discuss coping mechanisms that were used at stressful times in the past. Help client to discuss the change/loss and particularly to express anger associated with it.	Some individuals may not realize that anger is a normal stage in the grieving process. If it is not released appropriately, it may be turned inward on the self, leading to pathological depression.
Have client express fears associated with the change/loss or the resulting alteration in lifestyle that has occurred.	Change often creates a feeling of disequilibrium, and the individual may respond with fears that are irrational or unfounded. Client may benefit from feedback that corrects misperceptions about how life will be with the change in health status.
Assist with activities of daily living as required, but encourage independence to the limit that client's ability will allow. Give positive feedback for activities accomplished independently.	Independent accomplishments and positive feedback enhance self-esteem and encourage repetition of desired behaviors. Successes also provide hope that adaptive functioning is possible and decrease feelings of powerlessness.
Help client with decision-making regarding incorporation of change or loss into lifestyle. Identify an individual's ability to solve problems and make appropriate decisions.	The high degree of anxiety that usually accompanies a major lifestyle change often interferes with problems created by the change or loss.
Discuss alternative solutions, weighing potential benefits and consequences of each alternative. Support client's decisions.	Client may need help with this process to progress toward successful adaptation.
Role-play stressful situations that might occur in relation to the health status change.	Decreases anxiety and provides a feeling of security for the client by preparing a plan of action with which to respond appropriately when a stressful situation occurs.
Provide information regarding the physiology of the change in health status and necessity for optimal wellness. Encourage client and family to ask questions. Provide printed material explaining the change.	Helps client and family understand what has happened, clarifies information, and provides opportunity to review information at individual's leisure.

Collaborative

Refer to resources within the community (e.g., self-help/support groups, public health nurse, counselor, or social worker).	Provides assistance in adapting to the change in health status.

NURSING DIAGNOSIS	GRIEVING, dysfunctional
May Be Related to:	*Real or perceived loss of any concept of value to the individual; bereavement overload (cumulative grief from multiple unresolved losses, excluding the death of a loved one)*

Possibly Evidenced by:	Absence of anticipatory grieving; thwarted grieving response to loss
	Feelings of guilt generated by ambivalent relationship with the lost concept/person
	Idealization of the lost concept; difficulty in expressing loss; denial of loss
	Excessive anger, expressed inappropriately; labile affect
	Developmental regression
	Alterations in concentration and/or pursuit of tasks
Desired Outcomes/Evaluation Criteria—Client Will:	Express emotions appropriately.
	Demonstrate progress in dealing with stages of grief at own pace.
	Carry out activities of daily living independently.
	Express feeling of hope for the future.

ACTIONS/INTERVENTIONS	RATIONALE
Independent	
Determine stage of grief in which client is fixed. Identify behaviors associated with this stage.	Accurate baseline assessment data are necessary to choose appropriate interventions/provide effective care and evaluate progress. (Most depressed people are fixed in the anger stage, with the anger directed inward on the self.)
Convey an accepting attitude; encourage client to express self openly.	An accepting attitude enhances trust and communicates to the client that you believe the client is a worthwhile person, regardless of what may be expressed.
Encourage client to express anger. Avoid defensive response if initial expression of anger is displaced on nurse/therapist. Assist client to explore angry feelings and direct them toward the intended object/person or other loss.	Verbalization of feelings in a nonthreatening environment may help client come to terms with unresolved issues related to the loss.
Encourage participation in large motor activities.	Physical activity provides a safe and effective method for discharging pent-up tension/anger.
Provide information about the stages of grief and the behaviors associated with each stage. Help client understand that feelings, such as anger directed toward the loss, are appropriate during the grief process.	Knowledge of the acceptability of the feelings associated with normal grieving may help relieve some of the guilt that these responses generate.
Encourage client to review relationship with loss. With support and sensitivity, point out reality of the situation in areas where misrepresentations are expressed.	Client needs to give up idealized perception and accept both positive and negative aspects about the loss before resolution of grief can occur.

437

Help client determine methods for more adaptive coping with the experienced loss. Provide positive feedback for strategies identified and decisions made.

Feelings of depression may interfere with client's problem-solving ability, resulting in need for assistance. Positive feedback enhances self-esteem and encourages repetition of desirable behaviors.

Collaborative

Determine client's perception of spiritual needs as support in the grieving process. Involve chaplain or appropriate spiritual leader as indicated.

Some individuals derive great strength from spiritual support. This strength may be used by the client in the task of grief resolution.

NURSING DIAGNOSIS	HOPELESSNESS
May Be Related to:	Lifestyle of helplessness (repeated failures, dependency)
	Incomplete grief work of losses in life
	Lost belief in transcendent values/God
Possibly Evidenced by:	Verbal cues/despondent content (e.g., "I can't," sighing)
	Apathy/passivity, decreased response to stimuli
	Lack of initiative, nonparticipation in care or decision-making when opportunities are provided
Desired Outcomes/Evaluation Criteria—Client Will:	Recognize and verbalize feelings.
	Demonstrate independent problem-solving techniques to take control over life.
	Verbalize acceptance of life situations over which one does not have control.

ACTIONS/INTERVENTIONS	RATIONALE

Independent

Identify use of maladaptive behaviors/defense mechanisms (e.g., withdrawal, substance use, regression).	Personal attempts to overcome feelings of hopelessness may have resulted in ineffective/harmful behaviors. Recognizing the behaviors provides opportunity for change.
Encourage client to explore and verbalize feelings and perceptions.	Identification of feelings underlying behaviors helps client to begin process of taking control of own life.
Identify individual signs of hopelessness, (e.g., decreased physical activity, social withdrawal).	Helps to individualize interventions, focus attention on areas of need.
Express hope to client in positive, low-key manner.	Even though client feels hopeless, it can be helpful to hear positive expressions from others.
Help client identify areas of life situation that are under own control.	Client's emotional condition may interfere with ability to problem-solve. Assistance may be required to perceive the benefits and consequences of available alternatives accurately.

438

Encourage client to assume responsibility for own self-care (e.g., setting realistic goals, scheduling activities, making independent decisions).

Providing the client with choices increases feelings of control. **Note:** Unrealistic goals set the client up for failure and reinforce feelings of hopelessness.

Help client identify areas of life situation that are not within ability to control. Discuss feelings associated with this lack of control.

Client needs to identify and resolve feelings associated with inability to control certain life situations before level of acceptance can be achieved.

NURSING DIAGNOSIS	SELF ESTEEM disturbance [specify]
May Be Related to:	Maturational transitions
	Unmet dependency needs; retarded ego development
	Repeated negative feedback, diminished self-worth
	Dysfunctional family system
Possibly Evidenced by:	Self-negating verbalization, inability to deal with events; difficulty accepting positive feedback
	Lack of eye contact; nonassertive/passive behaviors; indecision, difficulty making decisions
	Hesitancy to undertake new tasks; fear of failure
	Social isolation; nonparticipation in therapy
	Manipulation of one staff member against another
	Self-destructive ideas /behavior
Desired Outcomes/Evalution Criteria—Client Will:	Identify feelings and underlying dynamics for negative perception of self.
	Demonstrate behaviors/lifestyle changes to promote positive self-esteem.
	Accept recognition for personal accomplishments/abilities.
	Verbalize increased sense of self-worth.

ACTIONS/INTERVENTIONS

RATIONALE

Independent

Discuss goals, making sure they are realistic. Plan activities in which success is likely.

Achievement/success enhance self-concept.

Convey unconditional positive regard for the client. Promote understanding of acceptance for client as a worthwhile human being.

Unconditional acceptance of an individual serves to counteract feelings of worthlessness by reinforcing that individual is worthy of another person's respect.

Spend time with client both on a 1:1 basis and in group activities.

Conveys that the nurse sees the client as someone worth spending time with.

439

Assist client to identify positive aspects of self and develop plans for changing the characteristics viewed as negative.

Individuals with low self-esteem often have difficulty recognizing positive attributes. They may also lack problem-solving skills and require assistance to formulate a plan for implementing the desired changes.

Encourage and support client in confronting the fear of failure by attending therapy activities and undertaking new tasks. Offer recognition of successful endeavors and positive reinforcement for attempts made.

Recognition and positive reinforcement enhance self-esteem and encourage repetition of desirable behaviors.

Help client avoid ruminating about past failures. Withdraw attention if client persists.

Lack of attention to these undesirable behaviors may discourage their repetition. Client needs to focus on positive attributes if self-esteem is to be enhanced.

Minimize negative feedback to client. Enforce limit setting in matter-of-fact manner, imposing previously established consequences for unacceptable behavior.

Negative feedback can be extremely threatening to a person with low self-esteem, possibly aggravating the problem. Consequences need to convey unacceptability of the behavior but not the person.

Encourage independence in the performance of personal responsibilities, as well as in decision-making related to own self-care. Offer recognition and praise for accomplishments.

The ability to perform self-care activities independently enhances self-concept. Positive reinforcement encourages repetition of desirable behaviors.

Support client in critical examination of feelings, attitudes, and behaviors. Help client understand that it is acceptable for attitudes and behaviors to differ from those of others, as long as they do not become intrusive.

The need for judging the behavior of others diminishes as client increases self-esteem through greater self-awareness and the achievement of self-acceptance.

NURSING DIAGNOSIS	**SOCIAL INTERACTION, impaired**
May Be Related to:	Unmet dependency needs; retarded ego development
	Negative role-modeling
	Low self-concept
Possibly Evidenced by:	Verbalized/observed discomfort in social situations; use of unsuccessful/dysfunctional social interaction behaviors
	Verbalized or observed inability to receive or communicate a satisfying sense of belonging, caring, interest
	Exhibits behaviors unacceptable for age, as defined by dominant cultural group
Desired Outcomes/Evaluation Criteria—Client Will:	Verbalize awareness of factors resulting in difficulty in forming satisfactory relationships with others.
	Identify feelings that lead to poor social interactions.

Interact with staff and peers with little/no indication of discomfort.

Participate in group activities appropriately and willingly.

Identify/develop effective social support system.

ACTIONS/INTERVENTIONS	RATIONALE

Independent

Establish 1:1 relationship with client, which serves as role model for testing new behaviors.

Client needs to learn to interact appropriately with nurse, so that behaviors may then be generalized to others.

Encourage client to engage in activities out of room/home.

Decreases opportunity for client to isolate self.

Offer to attend initial group interactions with client. Provide feedback for appropriate interactions.

Presence of a trusted individual may provide a feeling of security and decrease the anxiety generated by difficult social situation. Positive reinforcement enhances self esteem and encourages repetition of desirable behaviors.

Act as role model for client through appropriate interactions with client and others.

Because of weak ego development, client is inclined to imitate the actions of those individuals admired or trusted.

Establish schedule of group activities for client.

It is through these group interactions, with positive and negative feedback from peers, that client learns socially acceptable behavior.

NURSING DIAGNOSIS	FAMILY PROCESSES, altered
May Be Related to:	Situational/maturational crisis
Possibly Evidenced by:	Needs of family members not being met; confusion within family system regarding how needs should be met
	Impaired family communication; dissonance among family members
	Impairment of family decision-making process; family developmental tasks not being fulfilled
	Reduced/restricted social involvement
Desired Outcomes/Evaluation Criteria—Family Will:	Express feelings freely and appropriately.
	Develop effective patterns of communication, encouraging honest input from all members.
	Identify source(s) of dysfunction and effectively problem-solve to achieve desired resolution.
	Demonstrate pattern of functioning improved from premorbid state, having gained knowledge and achieved growth from crisis situation.

441

ACTIONS/INTERVENTIONS	RATIONALE

Independent

Assess family developmental stage, communication patterns, and extent of dysfunction.

Identifies specific needs and provides direction for care.

Meet with the total family group as often as possible.

The family as a system operates as a single unit. Each member affects, and is affected by, all other members. Therapy is most effective when directed toward the functioning of the family system.

Construct a client/family genogram.

Genograms help identify emotional closeness among family members over several generations. Family process is clarified, and configuration and dynamics are clearly illustrated.

Assist family to identify true source of conflict. Help them recognize that "identified patient's" adjustment disorder may be a way to avoid confronting the real problem.

Conflict creates high levels of anxiety within the family system. Common defense mechanisms such as denial, displacement, projection, and rationalization are used by the family to decrease anxiety and avoid conflict.

Encourage family members to set goals and identify alternatives. Support efforts directed toward positive change. Assist with necessary modifications of original plan.

Life crises interfere with family decision-making and problem-solving abilities. Assistance with this process may be required to promote adaptation and growth.

Promote separation and individuation and clear, functional boundaries between/among members.

Emotional connectedness among family members (enmeshment) discourages individual growth and ability to function autonomously.

Help client-family identify actions/problem-solve for potential life crises.

Anticipatory guidance/knowing what to expect and having a plan of action for management of situations may help to avert a crisis in the future.

Collaborative

Involve family in group therapy.

Interacting with others in family/multifamily groups can help identify dysfunctional patterns and assist in learning new skills and solutions for family problems.

Refer family to other resources, such as support groups, classes (e.g., parenting/assertiveness training).

Sharing with others who have had similar experiences can provide support and assist family members to learn new ways to deal with situation.

CHAPTER 15

PERSONALITY DISORDERS

ANTISOCIAL PERSONALITY DISORDER

DSM-IV
301.7 Antisocial personality disorder

"Sociopath" and "psychopath" are terms often used to describe the individual with antisocial personality. As deceit and manipulation are central features of the disorder, it is extremely difficult to treat. Imprisonment has been society's major method for controlling the most dangerous behaviors.

ETIOLOGICAL THEORIES
Psychodynamics

Psychodynamically, this individual remains fixed in an earlier level of development. Because of parental rejection or indifference, needs for satisfaction and security remain unmet, and the ego is underdeveloped. Because of a lack of ego strength, behavior is id directed and results in the need for immediate gratification. An immature supergo allows this individual to pursue gratification, regardless of means and without experiencing feelings of guilt.

Biological

Genetic involvement has been implicated in studies that showed that individuals with antisocial personality, and their parents, showed excessive EEG abnormalities when these examinations were conducted on both groups. Some research suggests that a variant of the D_4 dopamine receptor gene (D_4DR) appears more frequently in individuals who report high levels of "novelty seeking." People scoring high on this characteristic are often judged to be excitable, quick-tempered, and seek out thrilling sensations/situations—features associated with antisocial personality disorder. However, no clear effect on personality has been demonstrated at this time. (Despite genetic or environmental factors, sociopaths choose their lifestyle; therefore, it is up to them to choose to change it.)

Family Dynamics

Family functioning has been implicated as an important factor in determining whether or not an individual develops this disorder. The following circumstances may predispose to the disorder: absence of parental discipline (teaching/guidance), extreme poverty, removal from the home, growing up without parental figures of both sexes, erratic and inconsistent limit-setting, being "rescued" each time the person is in trouble (never having to suffer the consequences of own behavior), and maternal deprivation.

CLIENT ASSESSMENT DATA BASE

Circulation

Heart Rate: Slight increase may be demonstrated when anticipating stress (correlates with electrodermal responses indicating minimal anxiety)

Ego Integrity

Lacks motivation for change, often not seeking therapy voluntarily (unless client can no longer tolerate the mess he or she has made of own life or is facing long-term imprisonment)
Absence of feelings of guilt/shame
Use of aliases

Neurosensory

Mental Status: Personality appears charming, engaging, and is usually intelligent; demeanor is often a pretense intended to deceive or facilitate exploitation of others; manipulation is style of operating (e.g., needs and demands immediate gratification); low tolerance level results in feelings of frustration when desires are not immediately gratified
    Mood: Adaptive to individual's intended goal, mood may range from charming and pleasant to intensely angry
    Affect: Emotional reactions may be erratic and extreme, with lack of concern for other people's feelings
    Thought Processes: Client is preoccupied with own interests and has grandiose expressions of own importance, poor insight/judgment, and impulsivity or failure to plan ahead
Signs of personal distress possibly evident (e.g., tension and poor tolerance for boredom)
Lacks emotional attachment to others—even parents
Displays preference for stimulation rather than isolation

Safety

Experiences low level of autonomic arousal and responds to dangerous or painful stimuli with minimal anxiety
Reckless disregard for safety of self/others
May be homeless—living on the streets or from others' charity

Sexuality

Early, aggressive, sexual acting-out behaviors

Social Interactions

Occurs most frequently in lower socioeconomic populations
Family may be dysfunctional with little positive interaction; may be history of violence in the home
Displays chronic antisocial behavior incompatible with the value system of general society (e.g., lying, stealing, fighting, frequent conflicts with the law, conning others for personal profit or pleasure)
Repeatedly violates the rights of others without remorse (i.e., is indifferent to or rationalizes behavior [is thought to be without a conscience])
Rejects authority, has contempt for morality, does not learn from the past, and does not care about the future
Significant impairment in social, marital, and occupational/military functioning (generally has poor employment history, fails to honor financial obligations)

Teaching/Learning

More prevalent in males (with onset in childhood) than females (with onset at puberty)
History/evidence of conduct disorder with onset before age 15 with antisocial behaviors occurring since age 15 and usually diminishing after age 30, when the individual seems to "mellow out"/get tired of situation
Alcohol/substance abuse

DIAGNOSTIC STUDIES

EEG: Abnormally higher amounts of slow-wave activity, reflecting a possible deficit in inhibitory mechanisms, which may lessen impact of punishment.
Aversive Stimuli: Tends to be slower in learning to avoid shock, associated with a lower than normal level of physiological arousal; heightened ability to tune out aversive stimuli.
Psychopathy Checklist: Recently developed rating scale identifies 2 sets of characteristics (impulsiveness and instability; callousness, egocentricity, and limitation of capacity for anxiety) that are useful in predicting client outcome and likelihood of future violent crime activity.
Drug Screen: Determines substance use

NURSING PRIORITIES

1. Limit aggressive behavior; promote socially acceptable responses.
2. Develop a trusting relationship.
3. Assist client to learn healthy ways to deal with anxiety.
4. Increase sense of self-worth.
5. Promote development of alternate, constructive methods of interacting with others.

DISCHARGE GOALS

1. Self-control maintained.
2. Assertive behaviors used to gain desired responses.
3. A trusting relationship initiated.
4. Anxiety recognized and diminished/managed.
5. Client/family involved in ongoing therapy/support groups.
6. Plan in place to meet needs after discharge.

NURSING DIAGNOSIS	VIOLENCE, risk for, directed at others
Risk Factors May Include:	Contempt for authority/rights of others (antisocial character)
	Inability to tolerate frustration; need for immediate gratification; easy agitation
	Vulnerable self-esteem; inability to verbalize feelings
	Use of maladjusted coping mechanisms including substance use
	Negative role modeling; suspiciousness of others
[Possible Indicators:]	Body language (muscle tension, facial expression, rigid posture); increased motor activity, irritability, agitation

	Hostile, threatening verbalizations (boasting of prior abuse of others); possession of destructive means
	Becoming assaultive when angry; choice of aggression to meet needs; overt and aggressive acts
	Substance abuse
Desired Outcomes/Evaluation Criteria— Client Will:	Verbalize understanding of why behavior occurs, its consequences, and how it affects outcome(s).
	Develop and use assertive/nonaggressive, socially acceptable behaviors to gratify needs and interact with others.
	Demonstrate self-control as evidenced by relaxed posture and manner.

ACTIONS/INTERVENTIONS	RATIONALE

Independent

Convey accepting attitude toward client. Work on development of trust. Be honest, keep all promises, and convey message that the behavior, not the client, is unacceptable.	Feelings of rejection are undoubtedly familiar to client. An attitude of acceptance promotes feelings of self-worth. Trust is the basis of a therapeutic relationship. **Note:** Major obstacles in working with this client lie in an inherent inability to form a trusting, open relationship with a therapist.
Maintain low level of stimuli in client's environment (low lighting, few people, simple decor, low noise level).	A stimulating environment may increase agitation and promote aggressive behavior.
Provide structured environment, set firm limits (e.g., consistent schedule, ward rules, expectations of the client for cooperating. Involve client in process and follow through with consequences).	Individuals with antisocial personality disorder often function better in a controlled setting. Structure discourages escalation of aggressive behaviors and facilitates therapeutic intervention by reducing the anxiety caused by ambiguity.
Encourage verbalization of feelings and provide outlet for expression.	Increases client's self-awareness of feelings and stressors.
Help client identify the true object of his or her hostility (e.g., "You seem to be upset with . . .").	Because of weak ego development, client may be misusing the defense mechanism of displacement. Helping client recognize this in a nonthreatening manner may reveal unresolved issues so that they may be confronted.
Note distortions of the truth, manipulation. Confront client with these behaviors in a calm but firm manner, pointing out discrepancies in statements and behaviors.	Confronting unacceptable behaviors helps to increase client's awareness of own feelings and the effect these feelings and behaviors have on others.
Monitor escalating behaviors (e.g., increased psychomotor activity, threats, attempts to intimidate). Isolate if observed to be losing control.	Client can become dangerous very quickly with or without provocation. Early detection provides opportunity to alter behavior before violence occurs.

446

Be aware of prior history of violent behavior, seriousness of homicidal tendency, gestures, threats. (Use scale 1–10 and prioritize according to severity of threat, availability of means.)

Therapist needs to be aware of client's style of acting and behaviors to provide a safe environment and protect client and others.

Remove all dangerous objects from client's environment, as appropriate.

Decreases availability of "means" that can compromise safety of client/others.

Remain calm and nonaggressive in communicating with client. Avoid responding to client's verbal hostility with anger.

Anger is released through others. Not responding to client's anger breaks cycle, providing opportunity for change.

Assist client to identify when feelings of loss of control began and to identify events that led to this situation.

Recognition of these events provides an opportunity for resolution/adaptation of more effective behaviors. **Note:** These individuals have often been victims of child abuse and need to deal with these feelings.

Explore with client how aggressive, destructive behaviors have affected interpersonal relationships (e.g., with children, spouse, parents, peers).

Needs to realize own role and responsibility in personal interactions.

Discuss ways to detect potentially provocative/volatile situations before becoming involved. Help client learn to anticipate situations that usually result in anger, and develop a plan to handle anger before losing control.

These clients tend to tune out aversive stimuli and need to increase awareness of environment to avoid becoming involved in volatile situations. Restructuring helps to eliminate old behavioral patterns that result in acting out. A plan of action provides client with a feeling of control.

Review with client the benefits of using assertive behaviors and the consequences of aggression. Ask client to identify situations when aggression was used and discuss/role-play alternate methods for handling those situations.

Consequences serve as the best motivation for changing behavior. Client needs a rehearsed plan of action to aid in handling situations differently.

Encourage client to engage in healthy outlets for anger (e.g., telling other person in an assertive manner, use of large motor skill activities/relaxation techniques).

Developing new ways of reacting is essential to breaking the maladaptive pattern of responding.

NURSING DIAGNOSIS	**COPING, INDIVIDUAL, ineffective**
May Be Related to:	Very low tolerance for external stress
	Lack of experience of internal anxiety such as guilt or shame
	Personal vulnerability; unmet expectations; conflict; difficulty delaying gratification
	Inadequate support systems
	Multiple life changes
Possibly Evidenced by:	Inability to cope, problem-solve; choice of aggression and manipulation to handle problems and conflicts
	Inappropriate use of defense mechanisms (e.g., denial, projection)

Desired Outcomes/Evaluation Criteria—Client Will:	Chronic worry, anxiety, depression; poor self-esteem
	High rate of accidents; destructive behavior toward self (substance use/abuse) or others
	Identify maladaptive coping behaviors and consequences.
	Verbalize awareness of own positive coping abilities.
	Demonstrate increased tolerance for external stress and meet needs with assertive behaviors.
	Verbalize feelings congruent with behavior.

ACTIONS/INTERVENTIONS	RATIONALE
Independent	
Provide outlet for expression of feelings/concerns. Assist client to recognize anxiety by describing feeling states.	Individual needs to get in touch with own feelings, accept ownership of them, and be responsible for them before he or she can begin to change behavior. Identifying sources of fears and anxieties increases understanding and self-awareness of feelings, which facilitates appropriate actions.
Assist to identify/recognize early warning signs of increased anxiety.	Becoming aware of feelings provides opportunity for client to apply new skills that aid in controlling/reducing anxiety and impulsive actions.
Explore anxiety-producing situations. Help to formulate possible reasons for feelings.	Clarifying basis of anxious feelings may help eliminate unnecessary worry. Establishing a possible cause-effect relationship provides opportunity for insight.
Discuss present patterns of coping with feelings and effectiveness of these mechanisms.	Client needs to become aware that present patterns are self-destructive as well as harmful to others.
Investigate pattern of attempting to control environment through anger and intimidation and use of denial and projection.	Increases client's awareness of inappropriate mode of interaction and the consequences.
Provide information about constructive, effective coping strategies (e.g., discussing feelings with staff, running or jogging, relaxation techniques).	Client has likely not learned effective coping skills and needs information to begin to replace maladaptive skills/modify stressors.
Confront client with manipulative and intimidating behaviors when they occur.	Helps reinforce the need to stop this pattern.
Explore the implications/consequences of continuing antisocial activities.	Needs to be constantly aware of the direction life is taking and the effect these behaviors have on society and self.
Discuss the importance of being responsible for own actions and not blaming others for own behaviors.	Individuals with antisocial personality disorder tend to externalize blame onto others and do not accept responsibility for own actions.

Give positive feedback when client demonstrates use of constructive alternatives.

Evaluate with client effectiveness of new behaviors and discuss modifications.

Discuss fears or anxieties of others' responses to client's new behaviors, and client's feelings concerning these responses. Role-play anticipated experiences.

Encourage participation in unit activities, groups, outdoor education program (e.g., hiking, wall/rock climbing, caving).

Acknowledge difficulties of therapy and slow progress. Discuss likelihood of discouragement and ways to deal with these feelings.

Enhances self-esteem and reinforces acceptable behaviors.

If client's new methods of coping are not working, assistance will be needed to reassess and develop new strategies.

Gives client a sense of what might be expected from others and how to respond, helping to alleviate fears. Using role-play provides the opportunity for experiencing new ways of responding.

Interaction with others provides opportunities for client to begin to experience success, feel good about self, get needs met in positive ways. Exercise therapy also expends energy and increases release of endorphins, enhancing sense of general well-being.

Difficulty in developing therapeutic relationship, degree of impairment, and need for total life restructuring require prolonged intervention.

NURSING DIAGNOSIS

May Be Related to:

Possibly Evidenced by:

Desired Outcomes/Evaluation Criteria—Client Will:

SELF ESTEEM, chronic low

Lack of positive feedback; repeated negative feedback

Unmet dependency needs; retarded ego development

Dysfunctional family system

Acting-out behaviors, such as excessive use of alcohol and other drugs, sexual promiscuity

Feelings of inadequacy/diminished self-worth; inability (difficulty) accepting positive reinforcement

Nonparticipation in therapy

Acknowledge self as an individual who has responsibility for own actions.

Verbalize a sense of worthwhileness.

Make healthy choices regarding management of/be involved in meeting own care needs.

Demonstrate prosocial functioning.

Recognize and incorporate change into self-concept in accurate manner without negating self-esteem.

ACTIONS/INTERVENTIONS	RATIONALE

Independent

Encourage verbalization of feelings of inadequacy, worthlessness, fear of rejection, and need for acceptance from others.	Client may relate acting-out behaviors to a poor self-concept, and acceptance of reality of own behaviors in relation to others' reactions can assist decision to change.
Assist client to identify positive aspects about self related to social skills, work abilities, education, talents, and appearance.	Helps to build on positive aspects of personality and use them to improve self-concept.
Provide clear, consistent, verbal/nonverbal communication. Be truthful and honest.	Client's perception is keen and can instantly detect insincerity.
Explore the relationship between feelings of inadequacy and aggressive behaviors, use of drugs, sexual promiscuity.	Provides opportunity for client to understand relationship between low self-esteem and ineffective measures taken to "feel" better.
Discuss how companions are chosen. Ask if these people reinforce client's own antisocial activities/ values.	Helps client see how much peers can influence thinking and thereby reinforce antisocial behavior.
Ask client to describe interpersonal relationships, their quality and depth. If relationships are superficial, discuss how this came about.	Individuals with antisocial personality disorder have great difficulty forming close relationships. Exploring early relationships with parents or siblings may provide insight into the problem.
Review ways to improve the quality of interaction with others.	Learning to recognize/respect feelings of others in relation to own helps client develop more satisfactory relationships.
Help client identify positive aspects of the self and develop ways to change the characteristics that are socially unacceptable.	Individuals with low self-esteem often have difficulty recognizing their positive attributes. They may also lack problem-solving ability and require assistance to formulate a plan for implementing the desired changes.
Minimize negative feedback to client. Enforce limit-setting in a matter-of-fact manner, imposing previously established consequences for violations.	Negative feedback can be extremely threatening to a person with low self-esteem, possibly aggravating the problem. Consequences should convey unacceptability of the behavior but not of the person.
Encourage independence in the performance of personal responsibilities and in decision-making related to own self-care. Offer recognition and praise for accomplishments.	Positive reinforcement enhances self-esteem and encourages repetition of desirable behaviors.
Provide instruction about assertiveness techniques, especially the ability to recognize the differences between passive, assertive, and aggressive behaviors and the importance of respecting others' human rights while protecting one's own basic human rights.	These techniques increase self-esteem while enhancing the ability to form satisfactory interpersonal relationships.
Identify individual goals for therapy and activities to enhance feelings of success and self-esteem. Suggest keeping a journal of these activities.	Focusing on practical realities helps the client to move ahead step by step. Journaling can assist client to connect actions with changes that occur, to promote continuing positive change.

NURSING DIAGNOSIS	FAMILY COPING, ineffective: compromised/disabling
May Be Related to:	Family disorganization and role changes
	Client providing little support in turn for the primary person
	Prolonged disability progression that exhausts the supportive capacity of significant people
	Highly ambivalent family relationships; history of abuse/neglect in the home
Possibly Evidenced by:	Expressions of concern or complaint about significant other's response to client's problem
	Significant person reporting preoccupation with personal reactions regarding condition
	Significant person displaying protective behavior disproportionate (too little or too much) to client's abilities or need for autonomy
Desired Outcomes/Evaluation Criteria— Family Will:	Identify/verbalize resources within individual members to deal with the situation.
	Interact appropriately with the client/each other, providing support and assistance as indicated.
	Provide opportunity for client to deal with situation in own way.
	Express feelings openly and honestly.

ACTIONS/INTERVENTIONS	RATIONALE
Independent	
Identify behaviors/interactions of family members. Note factors affecting abilities of family members to provide needed support.	Provides information about patterns within family and whether they are helpful to resolution of current problems. Personality disorder/mental illness of other family members inhibits coping abilities.
Listen to comments and expressions of concern of client/SOs, noting nonverbal behaviors and/or responses.	Provides clues to underlying feelings, unconscious motivations/defenses.
Discuss basis for client's behavior(s).	Helps family begin to understand and accept/deal with unacceptable actions.
Assist family and client to understand who "owns" the problem and who is responsible for resolution.	When each individual begins to assume responsibility for own actions, each one can begin to problem-solve without expectation that someone else will take care of him or her.
Encourage free expression of feelings, including frustration, anger, hostility, and hopelessness.	Expression of feelings can be the beginning of recognition and resolution of short-/long-term problems.

451

| Set limits on acting-out and impulsive behaviors, and determine safety of home situation. | Family members need to understand that acting out angry feelings is not acceptable. Identification of factors/behaviors in the home situation can lead to alternative actions to prevent harm to client/family members. |
| Help family members identify coping skills being used and how these skills are/are not helping them to deal with the situation. | Identification of what is helpful and what is not will allow for learning new ways to cope with behaviors/situation. |

Collaborative

| Refer to additional resources as needed (e.g., family therapy, financial counseling, spiritual advisor, social services). | May need further assistance to help with resolution of current/long-term problems. May need to remove client/family members to ensure safety. |

NURSING DIAGNOSIS	SOCIAL INTERACTION, impaired
May Be Related to:	Factors contributing to the absence of satisfying personal relationships (e.g., inadequate personal resources [shallow feelings], immature interests, underdeveloped conscience, unaccepted social values)
Possibly Evidenced by:	Difficulty meeting expectations of others; lack of belief that rules pertain to them
	Sense of emptiness/inadequacy covered up by expressions of self-conceit, arrogance, and contempt
	Use of unsuccessful social interaction behaviors; behavior unaccepted by dominant cultural group
Desired Outcomes/Evaluation Criteria— Client Will:	Identify causes and actions to correct isolation.
	Express increased sense of self-worth.
	Participate willingly in activities/programs without use of manipulation.
	Demonstrate behavior congruent with verbal expressions.

ACTIONS/INTERVENTIONS	RATIONALE

Independent

| Note expressions of hopelessness/worthlessness (e.g., "I'm a loser," "It's fate."). | These may be the only genuine emotions this individual feels and may be expressed in subtle ways when failures can no longer be denied. Although these feelings may be dismissed quickly, this may be the time when the client is most accessible to change. |
| Listen to expressions of feelings and "insight," pointing out discrepancies between what is said versus behaviors. | Client may be very good at saying what others want to hear. However, behavior is the ultimate determinant of real change. It is almost impossible |

Confront expressions of powerlessness, inability to control situation or make a difference in relationship/commitments.

Consistent confrontation with reality of how client's behavior affects interactions with and trust of others may force client to begin to look at own responsibility for problems in these areas. This person's refusal to accept criticism and/or projection of failure as the fault of others make it difficult to change behavior.

for this person to understand the feelings of others.

Encourage client to make requests/ask for what is wanted in a clear, straightforward manner and express feelings clearly to others.

As needs are met by direct action, client may begin to see the value of this approach.

Explore client's need for immediate gratification.

Client needs to understand own feelings in order to work on resolution.

Ask client to describe feelings when someone says "no." Review with client feelings regarding authority and violating rights of others.

Client often experiences pleasure through antisocial behaviors and needs to gain insight regarding personal motives.

Discuss with client thoughts and fantasies present before committing crimes. Ascertain how much planning went into the crimes. Did the client "experience the crime mentally" before commission?

Antisocial behavior may lead to involvement in criminal activity. Fantasizing about crime plays a large role in eventual commission. In order to restructure cognitive processes, client needs to break this pattern.

Have client discuss thoughts/feelings about family, peers, authority figures, opposite sex, violence, and victims. Give feedback on the "correctness" of thinking process.

Reinforces positive values or attitudes and exposes problem areas in thinking process. This is important for cognitive restructuring.

Help client recognize behaviors that do not get intended response and discuss possible modifications.

These individuals have difficulty interpreting others' feelings and need guidance in this area.

Collaborative

Involve in group activities (e.g., occupational/vocational therapy, psychotherapy, outdoor education program, codependency meetings).

Provides opportunity for interaction with others to learn new behaviors, gain support for change, reduce dependence on manipulation of others.

453

BORDERLINE PERSONALITY DISORDER

DSM-IV

301.83 Borderline personality disorder

"Borderline" has been used to identify clients who seem to fall on the border between the standard categories of neuroses or psychoses. The term has been refined to indicate a client with a pervasive pattern of instability of interpersonal relationships, self-image, affect, and control over impulses beginning in early adulthood, and includes such factors as feelings of abandonment, impulsivity, reactivity of mood, chronic feelings of emptiness, and problems with anger.

ETIOLOGICAL THEORIES

Psychodynamics

Unconscious processes that are believed to shape personality are set in motion by drives or instincts that are then influenced by conflicts among them as well as instinctual wishes and demands of reality. Defensive maneuvers are unconsciously developed to protect against anxiety arising from this conflict. This personality is seen as a painstaking but poorly constructed defense.

It is also seen as resulting from a fixation of libido at stages of psychosexual development associated with certain body parts. Although it is difficult to agree on how personality is formed, severe personality disorders are believed to begin early in childhood and milder forms are thought to be influenced by factors during later development.

Biological

Personality is believed to have a hereditary basis known as "temperament" and biological dispositions that affect mood and level of activity (e.g., cranky, placid, self-contained, outgoing, impulsive, cautious). There is little agreement about how this affects the development of personality disorders.

Family Dynamics

The child's social environment, particularly that within the family, is assumed to be the main force that shapes personality. The theory of object relations provides a basis for personality development and an explanation of the dynamics that manifest the borderline characteristics. The individual with borderline personality may be fixed in the rapprochement phase of development (18–25 months of age). In this phase, the child is experiencing increasing autonomy, while still requiring "emotional refueling" from the mothering figure. Because the mother feels threatened by the child's efforts at independence, she strives to keep the child dependent. Nurturing and emotional support become bargaining tools. They are withheld when the child exhibits independent behaviors and are used as rewards for clinging, dependent behaviors. This engenders a deep fear of abandonment in the child that persists into adulthood as the child continues to view objects (people) as parts—either good or bad. This is called "splitting," which is the primary dynamic of borderline personality.

Current studies suggest that borderline personality disorders are strongly associated with a history of physical or sexual abuse by family members, and incest may be a major reason for the disproportionate ratio (2:1) of female clients.

CLIENT ASSESSMENT DATA BASE

Ego Integrity

Markedly disturbed/distorted sense of self
Experiences ambivalence toward being independent; does not like to be alone (frantic
    attempts to avoid real or imagined abandonment)

Reports feelings of emptiness and boredom; depression, sadness
May conform to current companions, sharing beliefs and values based on imitation

Food/Fluid

Binge eating may be reported (impulsivity)

Neurosensory

Mental Status:
  Behavior: May be erratic, impulsive, intense, clinging; may indulge in
    unpredictable/impulsive behaviors (e.g., irresponsible spending, reckless driving,
    gambling, substance abuse)
  Mood: Marked reactivity of mood (e.g., intense episodes of anxiety, irritability,
    dysphoria)
  Emotions: Intense emotions with rapid, unpredictable, strong mood swings; quick to
    anger (may be intense, inappropriate), lacks ability to control; may exhibit hostile
    attitude
  Affect: May appear genuine but not necessarily be appropriate to the situation
  Thought Processes: Displays overall poor reality base with difficulty making decisions;
    engages in concrete "all-or-nothing"/black-or-white thinking; lacks insight and does
    not learn from past experience; unable to form long-term goals or values
Magical thinking, difficulty in identifying the self; severely impaired self-concept
Lying and fabrication habitual, almost delusional
Self-centered, often to the point of narcissism, inordinantly hypersensitive, and inflexible;
    relationships may be transient, shallow, and/or demanding, with little flexibility and
    unstable interpersonal behavior; may use and exploit others; lacks empathy for others
Major defense mechanism used is projection (seeing in others those attitudes one fails to see
    in self)
May border on neuroses and psychoses, exhibiting transient psychotic symptoms when
    experiencing extreme stress; transient episodes of paranoid ideation or severe
    dissociative symptoms
May be associated with other personality disorders that have histrionic, narcissistic,
    schizotypal, or antisocial features

Safety

May reveal evidence of self-mutilative acts, usually nonlethal actions (e.g., cutting, burning)
History of recurrent suicidal behavior, gestures, threats

Sexuality

May present a profound disturbance in gender identity
Sexual promiscuity
Possible history of incest/sexual abuse

Social Interactions

Significant impairment in social, marital, and occupational functioning
Interpersonal relationships unstable and intense, alternating between extremes of
    overidealization and devaluation
Frequently attempts to provoke guilt in others, making endless demands
History of recurrent physical fights

Teaching/Learning

More prevalent in females
Substance abuse (especially alcohol) may be reported
Higher incidence found in families with history of both chronic schizophrenia and major
    affective disorders

455

DIAGNOSTIC STUDIES

P-300: A change in brain electrical activity that occurs in most people about 300 milliseconds after they perceive a tone, light, or other signal indicating that they have to perform a task; may be abnormal, smaller than average, and slightly delayed.

CSF5-HIAA (5-hydroxyindoleacetic acid): Decreased in some clients.

Prolacting Response: Diminished response to serotonin-releaser fenfuramine.

Drug Screen: Identifies substance use.

NURSING PRIORITIES

1. Limit aggressive behavior; promote socially acceptable responses.
2. Encourage assertive behaviors to attain sense of control.
3. Assist client to learn healthy ways of controlling anxiety/developing positive self-concept.
4. Promote development of effective coping skills.
5. Help client learn alternate, constructive methods of interacting with others.

DISCHARGE GOALS

1. Impulsive behavior(s) recognized and controlled.
2. Establishes goals and asserts control over own life.
3. Problem-solving techniques used constructively to resolve conflicts.
4. Interacts with others in socially appropriate manner.
5. Client/family involved in behavioral therapy/support programs.
6. Plan in place to meet needs after discharge.

NURSING DIAGNOSIS	VIOLENCE, risk for, directed at self or others/SELF-MUTILATION, risk for
Risk Factors May Include:	Use of projection as a major defense mechanism
	Pervasive problem with negative transference
	Feelings of guilt/need to "punish" self, distorted sense of self
	Inability to cope with increased psychological/physiological tension in a healthy manner
[Possible Indicators:]	Vulnerable self-esteem
	Easily agitated, angry when frustrated (may become assaultive)
	Provocative behavior: argumentative, dissatisfied, overreactive, hypersensitive; use of unprovoked anger, hostility toward others
	Choice of maladjusted ways of getting needs met (e.g., splitting, projection, provocation, depression)
	Self-mutilative acts; substance abuse
Desired Outcomes/Evaluation Criteria— Client Will:	Verbalize understanding of why behavior occurs.
	Recognize precipitating factors.

Demonstrate self-control, using appropriate, assertive coping skills.

Clarify feelings of negative transference and eliminate the use of projection.

ACTIONS/INTERVENTIONS	RATIONALE

Independent

Establish therapeutic nurse/client relationship. Maintain a firm, consistent approach.	Building rapport and trust is imperative, although difficult, for this client.
Determine negative transference feelings and clarify the actual source of anger, hostility.	Heightens self-awareness of these feelings to assist with resolution.
Help identify how much anger is "elicited" by significant other(s) and how much results from own unresolved feelings.	Becoming aware of the use of projection helps break this maladjusted pattern. **Note:** Feelings of anger and hostility, not depression, are more often the basis for destructive behaviors/suicidal acts.
Intervene immediately in a nondefensive manner when acting-out occurs. Set firm, consistent limits.	Intervention is critical to prevent dangerous situation for client or others. Therapeutic milieu helps client manage self and develop self-control. Environmental safety provides external control until internal control is regained.
Make an agreement or "no harm" contract to discuss angry or hurt feelings when they begin, instead of "internalizing" and displacing anger/hurt onto others and acting on the feelings.	Agreeing not to engage in violent behaviors involving self, others, or property promotes safety and enhances feelings of self-worth by having client assume control of own behavior. Helps client learn to work through feelings as they occur, to prevent intensification and promote resolution.
Encourage client to evaluate situations in which angry feelings develop. Discuss whether the amount of anger is appropriate to the actual event.	Needs to listen to recognize/assess inappropriate, unwarranted anger directed at others.
Explore what client expects from others, and self, in interpersonal relationships.	Helps client learn to define roles and recognize own responsibility in the situation.
Define expectations and rules of the situation clearly, and state what the client can/cannot do.	Structure reduces ambiguity and anxiety, providing sense of security and minimizing escalation of violent behavior.
Determine prior suicidal gestures/attempts. Evaluate seriousness of suicidal expressions/ideation. Use scale of 1–10 and prioritize according to seriousness of threat, availability of means, timing of previous attempts, current age.	It is important to take suicidal threats seriously, listening carefully to underlying messages and providing a safe environment to prevent client from following through on plan, especially when scale is in upper range. **Note:** Risk of suicide completion is highest during first few years after initial presentation, declining as client ages.
Provide close supervision, as indicated.	Allows for early recognition of escalating behavior and timely intervention.
Note substance use/withdrawal. (Refer to Ch. 6, for specific plan of care, as appropriate.)	Substance use, especially alcohol, increases likelihood of suicide 6-fold.

457

Provide care for client's wounds, if self-mutilation occurs, in a matter-of-fact manner. Do not offer sympathy or provide additional attention.

Additional attention and sympathy can provide positive reinforcement for the maladaptive behavior and may encourage its repetition. A matter-of-fact attitude can convey empathy/concern.

Collaborative

Have client participate in group therapy sessions with feedback given by peers.

Group setting aids in promoting diffusion of anger; provides insight as to how negative, aggressive behaviors affect others, making feedback easier to digest.

Support substance withdrawal. Refer to support group (e.g., Alcohol/Narcotics Anonymous).

Provides assistance to enable client to maintain abstinence.

Administer medication as indicated, e.g., carbamazepine (Tegretol), tranylcypromine (Parnate).

May reduce frequency of impulsive/self-destructive acts while other therapeutic interventions are initiated.

NURSING DIAGNOSIS	ANXIETY [severe to panic]
May Be Related to:	Unconscious conflicts (experience of extreme stress)
	Perceived threat to self-concept; unmet needs
Possibly Evidenced by:	Easy frustration and feelings of hurt
	Abuse of alcohol/other drugs
	Transient psychotic symptoms (disorganized thinking; misinterpretation of environment, interference with ability to think clearly and logically)
	Performing self-mutilating acts
Desired Outcomes/Evaluation Criteria— Client Will:	Verbalize awareness of feelings of anxiety and healthy ways to deal with them.
	Recognize warning signs of increasing anxiety and validate perceptions before drawing conclusions.
	Develop and implement effective methods for decreasing anxiety.
	Report anxiety reduced to manageable level.
	Use resources effectively.

ACTIONS/INTERVENTIONS	RATIONALE

Independent

Maintain open communication and provide consistency of care.

Provides for accurate information and reduces anxiety.

Assess escalating anxiety and observe client contact with reality (e.g., presence/development of resultant inability to think clearly).

Underlying feelings of worthlessness, inadequacy, powerlessness can lead to increasing anxiety with psychotic symptoms, delusions/hallucinations,

Note rapid changes in behavior (e.g., from cooperative to angry, demanding, argumentative).

Monitor for substance use; note physical symptoms of abuse (e.g., slurred speech, mood swings, dilated/constricted pupils, abnormal vital signs, needle marks).

Provide information in brief, clear, calm manner.

Maintain calm, quiet, nonstimulating environment.

Correct misinterpretations of environment as expressed by the client.

Encourage client to identify events that precipitate stress/anxious feelings (e.g., real or anticipated anxiety about relationships with others).

Explore how client has dealt with these feelings, including times when substances were taken to relive tension, anxiety.

Have client keep an "anger journal" describing when anger occurs, how it is handled, and outcome of situation.

Assist in learning to identify early warning signs that anxiety is escalating and request intervention before it becomes overwhelming.

Ask client to describe events/feelings preceding cutting or hurting self. Explore ways to relieve anxiety without self-damaging acts. (Refer to ND: Violence, risk for, directed at self or others/Self-Mutilation, risk for.)

Identify constructive ways of releasing tension (e.g., jogging, talking with nurse/therapist, use of relaxation/imagery techniques), involvement in outdoor education programs (e.g., hiking, wall/rock climbing, caving).

Discuss fears involving interactions with parents, spouse, children, or significant other(s).

Encourage client to develop a relationship with more than 1 person.

disorganized thinking, confusion, altered communication patterns. (Refer to CP: Delusional Disorder.)

Need for immediate gratification can lead to frustration and changes in behavior, which may indicate loss of touch with reality.

May cloud symptomatology, potentiate erratic behavior, and interfere with progress, requiring therapeutic intervention.

Specific instructions and expectations about what is happening help client maintain contact with reality.

Auditory and visual stimulation may increase labile affect and potential for acting-out.

Confronting misperceptions honestly, with a caring and accepting attitude, provides a therapeutic orientation to reality and preserves client's feelings of dignity and self-worth.

Helps to establish a cause-effect relationship, enhancing awareness and promoting change.

Provides an understanding of the relationship between anxiety and drug use.

When reviewed periodically with primary nurse/therapist, therapeutic writing can provide insight into development of feelings, effectiveness of response and create opportunity to develop new coping strategies.

Promotes development of internal control.

Provides knowledge for adapting new effective coping skills and breaking the pattern of self-destructive acts.

Client needs to learn constructive methods of coping to replace the maladjusted behaviors that have been used. Note: Exercise does not need to be aerobic or intensive to achieve therapeutic effect.

Knowledge of specific fear may provide insight into problem areas.

Helps client to achieve object constancy. (Client may feel abandoned when therapist leaves and have a feeling that the person ceases to exist.)

Dependency can be avoided, and client can begin to develop independent activities in this atmosphere.

459

Collaborative

Administer medications as indicated:
    Antipsychotics, e.g., haloperidol (Haldol),
        thiothixine (Navane), thioridazine (Mellaril);

    Antidepressants.

May help reduce anxiety, hostility, ideas of
    reference, illusions, increasing receptiveness to
    other therapeutic approaches.
A number of agents have been used with varying
    success to help alleviate symptoms of severe
    depression.

NURSING DIAGNOSIS	SELF ESTEEM, chronic low/PERSONAL IDENTITY disturbance
May Be Related to:	Lack of positive feedback; unmet dependency needs
	Retarded ego development/fixation at an earlier level of development
Possibly Evidenced by:	Difficulty identifying self or defining self-boundaries; feelings of depersonalization, derealization
	Extreme mood changes; lack of tolerance of rejection or being alone
	Unhappiness with self, striking out at others
	Performance of ritualistic, self-damaging acts, such as "cutting veins and watching the blood flow to cleanse the soul"; belief in need to punish self
Desired Outcomes/Evaluation Criteria— Client Will:	Verbalize a sense of worthwhileness.
	Demonstrate increased self-worth/respect with reduction in frequency of punishing/mutilative behaviors.
	Use "I" self-image to promote good interpersonal relationships.

ACTIONS/INTERVENTIONS	RATIONALE

Independent

Encourage client to describe and verbalize feelings about self.

Aids in assessing in which areas negative feelings are most intense.

Provide safe, supportive environment to discuss issues of abuse/incest and ownership of behaviors. (Refer to CP: Problems Related to Abuse or Neglect.)

Studies suggest a high percentage of these clients may be victims of physical/sexual abuse, which is a significant factor in the development of the disorder. Failure to address these issues potentiates continued problems with relationships and self-destructive acts.

Explore client's need to punish self. When did this begin, and what events precipitated these acts?

May help to establish a cause-effect relationship for feelings of low self-esteem.

Discuss what stressors usually bring on anger/depression. Explore ways to deal with feelings before they become overwhelming.

Note attitude of superiority, arrogant behaviors, exaggerated sense of self, resentment, and anger.

Note personality traits such as extreme shyness, chaotic impulsiveness, chronic irascibility, antisocial tendencies, refusal of treatment for substance abuse.

Encourage client to verbalize feelings of insecurity and need for constant reassurance from others.

Discuss feelings of worthlessness and how these feelings relate to need for acceptance by others.

Identify situations in which client pushed others away. Help client to look at reality of behavior in context of this situation.

Identify positive, realistic behaviors the client possesses.

Give feedback regarding nonverbal behaviors.

Encourage increased sense of responsibility for own behaviors.

Define sexual identity and what areas create confusion, fears.

Assess knowledge of human sexuality and supply needed information.

Information can be used to learn and implement effective methods to prevent onset of depression, destructive acts.

Indicative of attempt to compensate for feelings of worthlessness, inadequacy, and powerlessness.

Research suggests these traits are associated with poor outcomes. Recognition of this provides opportunity to deal with these issues, possibly influencing therapeutic efforts in a positive manner to improve individual response.

Provides insight into sources of insecurities which affect image of self as worthwhile individual.

Gives client the message that life cannot be spent trying to meet others' expectations.

Pattern of relationships has often been one of approach-avoidance conflicts characterized by intense feelings, crises, and stormy episodes. Fearing engulfment, client pushes others away, then, fearing abandonment, tries to draw them back in. Awareness of this pattern of behavior and underlying dynamics provides opportunity for change.

Helps client begin to look at possibility of making desired changes to meet needs in a more satisfying way.

Increases awareness of the possibility of double messages that client may be giving.

Use of projection has enabled client to blame others for own problems/consequences of behavior.

Helps client assess possible learning needs or which direction to take in alleviating anxiety.

Provides information appropriate to learning needs.

NURSING DIAGNOSIS	POWERLESSNESS
May Be Related to:	Lifestyle of helplessness; need for control (history of abuse/incest as a child)
Possibly Evidenced by:	Becoming enraged and hurt
	Manipulative behavior; self-centered and hypersensitive attitude
	Provoking guilt in others; making endless demands; using and exploiting others
	Ambivalence toward being independent; alternating clinging and distancing behaviors

Desired Outcomes/Evaluation Criteria— Client Will:	Express sense of control over present situation and future outcome.
	Develop a sense of being in charge of own life.
	Interact with others without abusing or violating their rights.
	Make choices related to and be involved in care.

ACTIONS/INTERVENTIONS	RATIONALE

Independent

Develop alliance with the client and assist to overcome fear of closeness and intimacy.	This individual is generally frightened by close relationships; an alliance demonstrates that it is possible to trust. **Note:** Evidence indicates incest/physical abuse in childhood are strongly associated with a poor outcome and high rates of suicide/violent crime.
Identify behaviors used to gain control of others (e.g., manipulation, attempts to influence, intimidate).	Increases awareness of modes of interaction that are used to get own way and feel in control of the situation.
Explore areas of life in which client is feeling inadequate or having no control.	Provides insight into feelings that are necessary for learning adaptive behaviors.
Encourage verbalization of how feelings of anger, hurt, and loss of control relate to desire to strike out at others.	Enhances understanding of how the use of projection has become a pervasive pattern.
Confront inconsistencies in statements; discuss what needs these statements serve.	Reinforces that lying and manipulation are maladaptive and lead to feelings of low self-esteem.
Recognize client manipulations and respond differently.	Redirection stops the manipulation, allowing for straight, congruent communication.
Provide opportunities to learn how to get needs met in an acceptable, truthful way.	Promotes inner strength and adaptive functioning.
Ask client to discuss feelings about someone in life who seems self-centered. Compare behaviors.	By comparing behaviors, client may understand how others perceive self-centeredness and the feelings about these behaviors.
Help client learn to listen to others and consider their feelings by putting self in their place.	Promotes feelings of empathy for others.
Encourage client to participate in developing treatment plan.	Aids in promoting a sense of control over life and helps client assume greater responsibility for own life.
Role-play desired behaviors (e.g., appropriate anger, admitting mistakes, shared humor).	Avoiding angry confrontations, maintaining sense of humor help client learn new ways of control.

NURSING DIAGNOSIS	COPING, INDIVIDUAL, ineffective
May Be Related to:	Use of maladjusted defense mechanisms (e.g., projection, denial, externalizing)

Possibly Evidenced by:	Chronic feelings of emptiness, boredom
	Repetitive use of ineffective coping strategies
	Inability to cope, problem-solve, or ask for assistance
	Not learning from previous experiences
	Inappropriate use of defense mechanisms (e.g., projection, manipulation)
	Relief of anxiety through destructive acts (sexual promiscuity, impulsive spending, gambling, substance abuse)
Desired Outcomes/Evaluation Criteria—Client Will:	Identify ineffective coping behaviors and consequences.
	Verbalize awareness of own coping abilities.
	Meet psychologic needs as evidenced by appropriate expression of feelings, identification of options, and effective use of resources.
	Verbalize feelings congruent with behavior.

ACTIONS/INTERVENTIONS

Independent

Ask client to describe present coping patterns and their consequences.

Have client identify problems and perceptions of their cause.

Promote development of effective ways to deal with stress, anger, frustration.

Develop with client/have client sign a behavioral contract to include minimum standards of acceptable behaviors, management of anger.

Discuss ways of dismissing feelings of boredom and assist client to understand that these feelings can be controlled.

Be aware of attempts to split staff. Avoid manipulative games and be consistent in dealing with the client.

Confront manipulative and other maladaptive behaviors.

RATIONALE

Recognizing which defenses are maladjusted, ineffective, and destructive provides opportunity to effect change.

Exposes problem areas in thinking process and possible cognitive distortions.

Client will need help in learning new behaviors, e.g., appropriate expression of anger, "I-messages."

Fosters collaborative relationship between client and nurse that can be generalized to others as progress is made. Encourages client to assume control of own behavior and, as specified outcomes are achieved, enhances sense of self-worth and encourages repetition of successful behaviors.

Client needs to get in touch with own feelings and own/be responsible for them before they can be resolved.

Staff-splitting can be a major problem. Client may behave in one way (quiet/cooperative) with some staff and in another way (angry/demanding) with others.

Consistent confrontation removes the reward and reinforces need for the client to adopt new behavior and to stop directing anger at others. Consistency in approach provides a stable environment and reinforces sense of trust.

463

Give feedback on how effectively client is handling situations and discuss suggestions for improvement.	May need assistance and guidance in modifying behaviors that are not working.
Give positive feedback when client demonstrates use of appropriate, constructive behaviors.	Reinforces use of positive techniques, enhances self-esteem.
Evaluate antisocial behaviors and resulting problems. (Refer to CP: Antisocial Personality.)	Destructive behaviors may lead to legal involvements and other problems in which client needs to learn new behaviors.
Encourage client to discuss issues related to family. Involve family in therapeutic process when possible.	High incidence of incest/physical abuse is associated with the diagnosis of borderline personality disorder. Additionally, clients whose families accept and support them demonstrate more positive outcomes.

Collaborative

Involve entire team in planning and evaluating care.	When team is committed to a single approach and information is shared by all, issues of splitting and countertransference can be minimized.

NURSING DIAGNOSIS	SOCIAL ISOLATION
May Be Related to:	Immature interests; unaccepted social behavior
	Inadequate personal resources
	Inability to engage in satisfying personal relationships
Possibly Evidenced by:	Alternating clinging and distancing behaviors
	Difficulty meeting expectations of others
	Experiencing feelings of difference from others
	Expressed interests inappropriate to developmental age
	Exhibiting behavior unaccepted by dominant cultural group (including sexual promiscuity)
Desired Outcomes/Evaluation Criteria— Client Will:	Identify causes and actions to correct isolation.
	Verbalize willingness to be involved with others.
	Participate in activities at level of desire.
	Express increased sense of self-worth.

ACTIONS/INTERVENTIONS	RATIONALE

Independent

Determine presence of factors contributing to sense/ choice of isolation.	Identification of individual factors allows for developing appropriate plan of care/ interventions.
Differentiate isolation from solitude and aloneness.	The latter are acceptable or by choice, and this differentiation helps client identify which is applicable to self so steps to deal with problem can be taken.

Let client know the nurse will not abandon her or him.

Ask client to identify significant other(s) with whom she or he can talk. If there is no one, ascertain how this came about.

Examine guilt feelings involving significant other(s). Discuss how these feelings occurred.

Discuss/define fears about being alone. Develop a schedule to "practice" being alone a few minutes each day, gradually increasing the time.

Identify how fears, anxieties have affected quality and depth of interpersonal relationships.

Develop a plan of action with client (e.g., look at available resources, support risk-taking behaviors).

Discuss ways to identify and confront inappropriate behaviors. Talk about how others may respond to these behaviors, and suggest ways client can deal with them. Use role-play to practice new skills.

Encourage client to identify positive, realistic behaviors currently being used.

Collaborative

Encourage involvement in classes/group therapy (e.g., assertiveness, vocational, sex education), psychotherapy.

Client is often fearful that the therapist will become angry or discouraged and give up.

Aids in seeing a pattern of interaction that is ineffectual.

May have unrealistic guilt feelings that need resolution before work on the relationship can begin.

Provides knowledge for developing adaptive coping skills and desensitizes person to feelings of anxiety.

Reinforces a sense that projection does indeed cripple relationships.

Structure of a plan with support of a trusted person helps client try out new behaviors.

When plan is agreed on, client is involved and willing to look at behaviors that create problems in relationships. Provides a beginning to develop more appropriate ways to interact with others.

As client recognizes that there are already some positive behaviors to build on, self-confidence is enhanced, and client may be willing to take more risks.

Provides opportunity to learn social skills, enhance sense of self-esteem, and promote appropriate social involvement.

PASSIVE-AGGRESSIVE PERSONALITY DISORDER

DSM-IV
301.9 Personality disorder NOS
Passive-Aggressive personality disorder (negativistic personality disorder)—provided for further study.

This disorder is characterized by a pervasive pattern of passive resistance, expressed indirectly rather than directly, to demands for adequate social/occupational performance, with the individual viewing the future as negatively as they view the present.

ETIOLOGICAL THEORIES

Psychodynamics

These clients are unaware that ongoing difficulties are the result of their own behaviors. They experience conscious hostility toward authority figures but do not connect their own passive-resistant behaviors with hostility or resentment. They do not trust others, are not assertive, are intentionally inefficient, and try to "get back" at others through aggravation. Anger and hostility are released through others, who become angry and may suffer because of the client's inefficiencies. This disorder can lead to more serious psychological dysfunctions such as major depression, dysthymic disorder, and alcohol and other drug abuse/dependence.

These behaviors, although not disturbing to the client, are disturbing to those in the environment who interact with the client. Therapy is not usually sought, but the client is generally referred for help by family members.

Biological

Personality disturbance is attributed to constitutional abnormalities. There may be a biological base to behavioral and emotional deviations, and researchers hope to demonstrate a correlation between chromosomal and neuronal abnormalities and a person's behavior.

Family Dynamics

Theories of development implicate environmental factors occurring in the very early years of the child's life. Feelings of rejection or inadequate nurturing by the primary caregiver result in anger that is then turned inward on the self. Depression is common.

CLIENT ASSESSMENT DATA BASE

Ego Integrity

Feels cheated, unappreciated, misunderstood
Chronically complains to others
Blames others for failures

Neurosensory

Covert aggressive behaviors chosen over self-assertive behaviors
Passive resistance to demands (to increase or maintain certain level of performance) through behaviors such as dawdling, stubbornness, procrastination, and "forgetfulness"
Mental Status:
　Behavior: May not appear uncomfortable in social situations but is cold and indifferent, reflecting stiff perfectionism; superficial bravado

Mood and Affect: Displays a seriousness with difficulty expressing warm feelings, may sulk and pout, passively acquiesce/conform; harbors unspoken resentment

Emotion: Displays/reports anxiety, depression; expresses sense of low self-worth, lack of self-confidence; may be dependent and passive

Thought Processes: Views world in a negativistic manner but fails to connect behavior to others' reactions; feels resentful, and believes others are being unfair; sees the world as a hostile and unfair environment

Overtly ambivalent

Social Interactions

Habitually "forgets" commitments, arrives late for appointments

Authority figures (e.g., parents, teachers, superiors at work) may be focus of discontent-criticizing/voicing hostility with minimal provocation

Demands for adequate performance are met with resistance expressed indirectly (e.g., procrastination, forgetfulness, intentional inefficiency)

Pervasive social/occupational ineffectiveness

Strained interpersonal relationships; difficulty adjusting to close relationships

Envious/resentful of peers who are successful

DIAGNOSTIC STUDIES

Drug Screen: Identifies substance use.

NURSING PRIORITIES

1. Assist client to learn methods to control anxiety and express anger appropriately.
2. Promote effective, satisfying coping strategies.
3. Promote development of positive self-concept.
4. Encourage client/family to become involved in therapy/support programs.

DISCHARGE GOALS

1. Feelings of anger, hostility resolving.
2. Assertive techniques being learned and used.
3. Self-esteem increased.
4. Client/family involved in therapy programs.
5. Plan in place to meet needs after discharge.

NURSING DIAGNOSIS	ANXIETY [moderate to severe]
May Be Related to:	Unconscious conflict; unmet needs; threat to self-concept
	Difficulty in asserting self directly; feelings of resentment toward authority figures
Possibly Evidenced by:	Difficulty resolving feelings/trusting others
	Passive resistance to demands made by others
	Extraneous movements: foot-shuffling, hand/arm movements
	Irritability, argumentativeness

Desired Outcomes/Evaluation Criteria—Client Will:	Define and use effective methods for decreasing anxiety.
	Demonstrate effective problem-solving skills.
	Report anxiety is reduced to a manageable level.
	Use resources effectively.

ACTIONS/INTERVENTIONS	RATIONALE

Independent

ACTIONS/INTERVENTIONS	RATIONALE
Encourage direct expression of feelings. Help client to recognize when open, honest feelings are not being expressed.	Client has established a pattern of expressing feelings indirectly through covert aggression. Needs to learn to express feelings directly as they occur.
Explore situations that lead to feelings of anger, hostility. Discuss possible causes.	Client needs to gain insight into areas that cause resentment and anger in order to plan resolution.
Examine feelings toward authority figures. Discuss how these feelings come about.	Authority figures are a common target for client's aggression. May have started in early childhood, leaving multiple unresolved conflicts.
Assist client to be in tune with own feelings and increasing internal anxiety. Encourage journaling.	Client is often unaware that responses are consequences of anxiety. Therapeutic writing can help client become aware and identify feelings.
Discuss fears concerning intimate relationships. Does client feel betrayed by significant other(s)?	Inability to trust is a significant problem for this client. Examining situations in past provides opportunity for insight.
Review how the inability to express feelings has resulted in covert acting-out behaviors.	Important for establishing the correlation between hostility and covert maneuvers.
Aid client in establishing a possible cause-and-effect relationship of "forgetfulness," dawdling, procrastination, etc. to internal resentment toward the person making demands.	Important for heightened awareness of own feelings and behaviors manifested.
Encourage client to recognize need to act-out with covert aggression to "get back" at others. Together develop effective methods to alter response.	Client is not always aware of own feelings/needs, and assistance in redirecting aggression can help client to change behaviors.
Support verbalization of feelings in an assertive manner instead of using flight response.	Client needs to learn to face issues directly, using assertive techniques.
Discuss client's fears regarding new assertive behaviors. Help define ways to alleviate these fears. Role-play anticipated situations.	Self-assertion is a new experience for this client. Discussing fears about self-assertion and participating in role-play help to diminish these fears.
Explore with client how often anger is displaced onto others because client believes the real target of the anger cannot be approached.	Reinforces need for client to deal directly with target of feelings.
Explain "pressure cooker" effect of "stuffing" feelings.	This individual usually has established a lifelong pattern of internalizing feelings, and this eventually leads to exploding inappropriately. Education is necessary to understand relationships between/among thoughts, feelings, and behavior.

468

Define methods of expression that effectively control anxiety (e.g., relaxation, use of "I-messages").

This is a new approach for the client, who therefore needs guidance in learning effective anxiety control.

Give positive feedback for new behaviors. Discuss any needed modifications.

Provides reassurance and encourages repetition of newly learned skills. Client may have difficulty trusting own judgment.

Involve family/SO(s) in treatment plan and practice (role-play) sessions.

Longstanding patterns of interaction need to be changed to enable client and SO(s) to develop new style of communication/behavior.

NURSING DIAGNOSIS	COPING, INDIVIDUAL, ineffective
May Be Related to:	Inability to cope, problem-solve; inadequate coping method (does not use self-assertive behaviors)
	Personal vulnerability
	Unrealistic perceptions; unmet expectations
	Lack of recognition of relationship between passive-aggressive behaviors and internal anxiety
Possibly Evidenced by:	Use of maladaptive, temporary relief behaviors that do not last or really satisfy; lack of assertive behaviors
	Real issues remaining unaddressed and unresolved
	Maneuvers such as dawdling, procrastination, stubbornness, forgetfulness, habitual tardiness
	Difficulty meeting basic needs
	Alteration in societal participation
Desired Outcomes/Evaluation Criteria— Client Will:	Identify ineffective coping behaviors and consequences.
	Develop and implement repertoire of coping strategies that are based on problem-solving techniques and that provide effective relief of conflicts.

ACTIONS/INTERVENTIONS

RATIONALE

Independent

Discuss present patterns of coping and evaluate their effectiveness.

Client needs to recognize pattern and see that current coping methods do not bring positive results.

Help client identify how passive-resistant behaviors are maladaptive relief behaviors.

Needs to associate behaviors with an attempt to gain relief from anxiety and hostility.

Confront client with what needs the behaviors are really serving when forgetfulness and procrastination are used.

Confrontation heightens awareness of problem, of providing stimulus for change to get needs met in more constructive ways.

469

Review what unmet needs are and why present coping patterns do not afford lasting relief.

Discourage client from justifying current automatic relief behaviors. Point out the inadequacies of these behaviors.

Encourage client to identify examples of situations when the client felt imposed upon or angered but did not speak up. Discuss alternate ways to handle those situations.

Suggest client ask family members/SO(s) to verbalize when they feel imposed on or angered by client's behavior.

Ask client to discuss how it feels when others are habitually forgetful and do not keep commitments.

Discuss importance of following through with what is promised. Give feedback on how passive-resistant behaviors affect others.

Provide information about problem-solving techniques to provide base for effective, satisfying coping behaviors.

Give positive feedback when client demonstrates use of adaptive skills and makes suggestions for improvement.

Brings to light that client's needs are really not being satisfied.

Client will have difficulty changing old behaviors and has already spent a lifetime justifying them to self.

Promotes understanding that avoidance of dealing directly with anger often leads to a negative outcome. Realization is crucial to learning new coping skills.

Helps develop new awareness and opportunity to change old ineffective ways of responding.

Developing empathy may help break this pattern.

Client needs to realize how destructive the behaviors can be and how difficult it is to maintain intimate relationships with family/SO(s).

Helps client learn to think through problems and arrive at well-thought-out solutions that are successful.

Aids in reinforcing positive behaviors.

NURSING DIAGNOSIS	SELF ESTEEM, chronic low
May Be Related to:	Retarded ego development
	Unmet dependency needs; early rejection by significant other(s)
	Lack of positive feedback
Possibly Evidenced by:	Lack of self-confidence; feelings of inadequacy, fear of asserting self
	Dependency on others
	Directing frustrations toward others by using covert aggressive tactics
	Not accepting own responsibility for what happens as a result of maladaptive behaviors
	Not verbalizing negative feelings and working through them.
Desired Outcomes/Evaluation Criteria—Client Will:	Verbalize a sense of worthwhileness.
	Use assertive, effective behaviors to interact with others.
	Actively participate in program(s) to develop positive self-esteem.

ACTIONS/INTERVENTIONS	RATIONALE

Independent

Encourage client to describe self and perceived inadequacies and how these relate to others. Note whether client compares self to others and, if so, in what terms.

Negative self-image often comes from comparing oneself unfavorably to others.

Assess client's self-concept. Determine if client is realistic about strengths and limitations.

May not have accurate perceptions of own strengths and shortcomings.

Encourage client to make adjustments in thinking if expectations of self and others are unrealistic.

Cannot improve self-esteem if expectations are not realistic or achievable.

Discuss how evaluations by others might have negatively affected the client.

Individuals are often hypersensitive to others' comments and allow them to stick as a "label."

Explore past relationships. Determine if client feels let down or hurt by significant other(s).

Client may be hanging on to old pain that needs to be worked through or let go.

Help client learn how to express feelings assertively (e.g., "I feel hurt, angry, rejected, discounted, etc.").

Expressing feelings assertively is self-enhancing. This mode of interaction promotes more comfortable relationships.

Explain that willingness to take some risks by allowing others to get close is necessary, even though it may mean getting hurt.

Taking risks and experiencing success can do much to enhance self-esteem. Likewise, knowledge that one can survive failure can enhance confidence in ability to handle difficult situations as they arise.

Discuss specific objectives for self-improvement and enhancing relationships.

Client needs to take action on newly gained knowledge in order to achieve success.

Encourage client to learn more about others to gain a clearer perspective of their motives and feelings.

Client uses defense mechanism of projection of own feelings on others. Anger and hostility can be diffused by gaining more information about others and their situations.

Ask client to describe what is defined as success in others and perceptions of what made them successful, and compare with own life successes.

May already have qualities for success but has overshadowed them with negative feelings.

Explore how the desired attributes can be adopted and put into practice.

Helps client apply goals to daily life situations.

Encourage client to accept self with strengths and liabilities and learn to like self.

Self-acceptance is necessary to build self-esteem and improve relationships with others.

NURSING DIAGNOSIS	POWERLESSNESS
May Be Related to:	Interpersonal interaction
	Lifestyle of helplessness; dependency feelings
	Difficulty connecting own passive-resistant behaviors with hostility or resentment
Possibly Evidenced by:	Experiencing conscious hostility toward authority figures

<table>
<tr>
<td></td>
<td>Releasing anger and hostility through others, who may become angry or suffer because of client's inefficiencies</td>
</tr>
<tr>
<td></td>
<td>Getting back at others through aggravation</td>
</tr>
<tr>
<td>Desired Outcomes/Evaluation Criteria—
Client Will:</td>
<td>Express sense of control over present/future outcomes.</td>
</tr>
<tr>
<td></td>
<td>Verbalize resolution of hostile feelings.</td>
</tr>
<tr>
<td></td>
<td>Use assertive (instead of aggressive) behaviors to deal with feelings, anxiety-producing situations, and interactions with others.</td>
</tr>
</table>

ACTIONS/INTERVENTIONS	RATIONALE

Independent

Examine hostile feelings toward authority figures. Determine when this hostility began and what painful experiences have occurred because of those in authority.	A major dynamic for this personality disorder is resentment of authority and the resulting sense of powerlessness. It helps the nurse to know what experiences client has had that led to this situation, especially relationship with primary caregiver during early years, when client may have felt particularly helpless.
Explore areas of life in which client feels inadequate or has a sense of no control.	Provides insight into feelings, which is necessary for learning adaptive behaviors.
Identify covert aggressive behaviors used to gain control of others.	Increases awareness of mode of interaction used and attempts to maintain sense of own control.
Encourage verbalization of how feelings of anger, hurt, and loss of control relate to desire to strike out at others.	Enhances understanding of how use of covert aggression has become a pervasive pattern.
Provide opportunity to learn how to get needs met in an acceptable, assertive manner.	Promotes inner strength and adaptive functioning, enhancing sense of control.
Assist client to learn to listen to others and consider their feelings by putting self in their place.	Promotes empathy for others and sense of own self-worth.
Have client assist in developing treatment plan.	Aids in promoting a sense of control and involvement in own care/future. This sense of participation enhances cooperation.

CHAPTER 16

OTHER CONDITIONS THAT MAY BE A FOCUS OF CLINICAL ATTENTION

PSYCHOLOGICAL FACTORS AFFECTING MEDICAL CONDITION

DSM-IV
316 (Psychological factors) affecting medical condition
Choose name based on nature of/most prominent factor:
   Mental disorder affecting medical condition
   Psychological symptoms affecting medical condition
   Personality traits or coping style affecting medical condition
   Maladaptive health behaviors affecting medical condition
   Stress-related physiological response affecting medical condition
   Unspecified psychological factors affecting medical condition
(Refer to *DSM-IV* listing for specific definitions.)

These disorders represent a group of ailments in which emotional stress is a contributing factor to physical problems (coded on Axis III) involving an organ system under involuntary control. Any organ system may be affected, depending on the individual's susceptibility. The result is the development or exacerbation of, interference with therapy for, and/or delayed recovery from a medical condition.

Lists of related medical conditions are subject to change as research progresses because to date a clear psychological-biological connection has been implied but not yet scientifically proved.

ETIOLOGICAL THEORIES

Although the etiology of psychosomatic disorders is unknown, an individual's emotional state and life circumstances are believed to significantly affect the onset, form, and course of psychosomatic illness. The interaction of psychological, social, and biological factors becomes evident as physical symptoms appear and diminish in direct relationship to the amount of stress the person is experiencing. Psychophysiological disorders do occur without known psychological components, but these disorders usually require some genetic predisposition to respond to stress pathologically.

473

Psychodynamics

Thought to center around issues of unresolved dependency conflicts, undischarged aggressive feelings, repressed anger, hostility, resentment, and anxiety, these conflicts are expressed somatically. Physiological responses correspond to unconscious emotional conflict instead of directly through verbalization, indicating inadequate or maladaptive defense mechanisms.

Interpersonal theory proposes that individuals with specific personality traits are predisposed to develop or precipitate certain disease processes (e.g., those who are dependent may develop asthma); depression has been linked to cancer and aggressiveness to chest pain or dysrhythmias.

Biological

A new field of psychoneuroimmunology is developing around research of the biological factors that underlie these illnesses. The immune response can be affected by behavior modification. Skills are being taught to help people modify responses that are thought to lead to illness.

In extensive stress studies, it was found that specific physiological responses under direct control of the pituitary/adrenal axis occurred in response to stress. When these stress responses are prolonged, psychosomatic disorders can develop. The specific organ system involved and type of psychosomatic disorder the individual develops may be genetically determined.

The Selye stress theory proposes three levels of response: the alarm reaction, the stage of resistance, and the stage of exhaustion. This is called the general adaptation syndrome, and these responses to stress have an effect on physical functioning. The belief of the individual regarding the degree of stress is related to the effect of the stressor on the physiological condition.

Family Dynamics

Children who grow up observing the attention, increased dependency, or other secondary gain an individual receives because of illness see these behaviors as a desirable response and subsequently imitate them. The dysfunctional family system may use these psychophysiological problems to cover up interpersonal conflicts. Anxiety is thus shifted from the conflict to the ailing member. As anxiety decreases, conflict is avoided, and positive reinforcement is given for the symptoms of the sick person.

CLIENT ASSESSMENT DATA BASE

(These clients present a pattern of anxiety and problems of coping with stress that occurs in their lives. Data obtained depend on organ system involved.)

Atherosclerotic Heart Disease

Activity/Rest

May exhibit an abrupt, fast-talking presentation, with constant movement (e.g., jiggling knees or tapping fingers)
Reports work overload, lack of vacations
Often "too busy" to notice quiet, beautiful surroundings

Circulation

Elevated blood pressure, tachycardia, palpitations, angina

Ego Integrity

Measures success by material goods/personal accomplishments; intense need to compete and win, even if competing with a child

Multiple life stressors
Poor anger management

Neurosensory

Mental Status: Psychological factors linking stress and personality traits include ongoing emotional turmoil/anger, and overexertion

May feel a need to do everything in a hurry and become impatient if asked to wait (e.g., may not tolerate waiting in lines)

Driving, idealistic, dominant, compulsive individual, with passive-aggressive tendencies, strict superego, feelings of insecurity, and difficulty managing anger

Social Interactions

May be overdutiful to job; with social contacts/events related to employment
Hostile, angry, and aggressive toward others

Teaching/Learning

Higher incidence in males
Risk factors most frequently reported: cigarette smoking, hypertension, elevated serum cholesterol and triglyceride levels, left ventricular hypertrophy, diabetes, and age

Gastrointestinal Bleeding/Irritable Bowel Conditions

Activity/Rest

Fatigue

Ego Integrity

May express an intense need for perfection and feelings of not having enough control over stressors and environment

Precipitating stressors center on real or feared threats to significant interpersonal relationships or deaths

Elimination

Diarrhea (with/without blood)

Food/Fluid

History of multiple stomach complaints (e.g., gastritis/ulcers, hyperacidity; heartburn, reflux; food intolerances)

Weight loss, pallor, anemia

Neurosensory

Mental Status: Longstanding feelings of anxiety, repressed anger, difficulty expressing anger/hostility directly, resentment, and a sense of helplessness, with difficulty in coping; highly developed superego, conscientious/dutiful; insecurity/nervousness; compulsivity, especially regarding punctuality and neatness; timidity, obstinacy, hyperintellectualism, lack of humor

May perceive even the slightest criticism as rejection and feel a loss of self-esteem, and respond by using avoidance or by becoming suspicious

Pain/Discomfort

Reports of pain ranging from mild to severe

Social Interactions

Difficulty in interpersonal relationships/dependency on others

Ambivalence/hypersensitivity toward significant others who have been a source of hurt or perceived rejection

Feeling hurt or humiliated and unable to/not inclined to meet the demands of those on whom they feel dependent

Teaching/Learning

Other affected family members possible, revealed in family history

Can occur at any age

Essential Hypertension

Activity/Rest

Fatigue, sleep disturbances

Circulation

Chronic high blood pressure with no known organic origin

Dizziness, nervousness, palpitations

Ego Integrity

May report emotional trauma, presence of stressful situations in daily life; controlled emotionality

Increased incidence in urban areas rather than in rural or tropical areas (may reflect a more relaxed lifestyle)

Food/Fluid

Obesity, sensitivity to salt

Neurosensory

Mental Status: Conflicted over expression of hostile and aggressive feelings, struggle with dependency vs. achievement needs; tends to hold anger in and to feel guilty if anger is expressed, inhibits aggressive wishes, may show greater reactivity to stressful stimuli, even in normal situations

Pain/Discomfort

Headaches

Social Interactions

Feelings of isolation

Teaching/Learning

More prevalent in black population; onset usually in early adult life (mean age in early 30s)

Bronchial Asthma

Neurosensory

Mental Status: Dependent, meek, sensitive, nervous, compulsive, and perfectionistic; anxiety, anger, depression, tension, frustration, and anticipation of a pleasurable event can contribute exacerbation of symptoms

Feelings of insecurity and oppression, insufficient superego, compulsiveness, overdutiful attitudes, tendency to be passive-aggressive

May be shy, irritable, impatient, stubborn, and tyrannical at times

Respiratory

Wheezing, shortness of breath
Restlessness, cyanosis
Hyperventilation, sighing, hiccups
Smoking in the home

Social Interactions

Strong correlation between asthma attacks and tension in the home/estranged relationships with parents

Teaching/Learning

Can occur at any age (1/3 are children; 2/3 of these are boys)
Respiratory infections/induced emotionally possibly triggering or exacerbating attacks

Migraine Headache

Activity/Rest

Fatigue

Food/Fluid

Nausea, vomiting

Neurosensory

Sensitivity to light/noise; visual disturbances; sensory/motor disturbances (e.g., tingling of face, hands; staggering gait)
Mental Status: Compulsive/perfectionistic, conscientious, intelligent, neat, inflexible, rigid, resentful; experiences guilt feelings

Pain/Discomfort

Head pain, unilateral or bilateral; aching, throbbing
Associated Symptoms: nausea/vomiting photosensitivity

Other Symptoms/Conditions That May be Noted:

Genitourinary: Menstrual and urinary disturbances; dyspareunia, impotence
Musculoskeletal: Joint stiffness/pain, backache, muscle cramps, tension headaches
Skin: Pruritus, cutaneous inflammation (neurodermatitis), excessive sweating (hyperhidrosis)
Others: Autoimmune diseases, manifested as rheumatoid arthritis, systemic lupus of erythematosus, myasthenia gravis, and pernicious anemia, etc.

DIAGNOSTIC STUDIES

Dependent on specific presenting condition/symptoms.

NURSING PRIORITIES

1. Encourage verbalization of feelings and stressors.
2. Assist client to develop coping skills and assertiveness techniques to reduce/manage anxiety.

477

3. Promote development of positive self-esteem.
4. Help client accomplish a sense of autonomy and independence.

DISCHARGE GOALS

1. Assertive techniques used as a more productive, effective means of expression.
2. Stress management methods used to reduce anxiety.
3. Positive self-esteem that satisfies client's needs without compromising self/others is displayed.
4. Client/family involved in group therapy/community support programs.
5. Plan in place to meet needs after discharge.
   Note: This plan of care deals with the psychiatric component of these conditions. Ongoing evaluation of physical condition is required to ensure timely intervention and client well-being. The user is referred to a medical/surgical resource (such as Doenges, Moorhouse, Geissler: *Nursing Care Plans: Guidelines for Planning and Documenting Patient Care,* F.A. Davis, Philadelphia, 1997) for physiological considerations.

NURSING DIAGNOSIS	ANXIETY [moderate to severe]
May Be Related to:	Internalized feelings of inadequacy, resentment, frustration, anger; negative self-talk
	Inability to obtain relief from stress; unmet needs
	Perceived threat to self-concept
Possibly Evidenced by:	Stimulation of the "fight-or-flight" reaction; sympathetic stimulation, increase in blood pressure/somatic complaints
	Focus on self
	Denial of relationship between physical symptoms and emotional problems
Desired Outcomes/Evaluation Criteria— Client Will:	Verbalize understanding of relationship between feelings of anxiety and physical symptoms.
	Develop effective methods for decreasing anxiety.
	Report anxiety reduced to manageable level.
	Experience marked decrease in somatic symptoms.

ACTIONS/INTERVENTIONS	RATIONALE
Independent	
Use gentle, supportive therapeutic approach to develop a positive rapport.	Skill of the therapist is crucial. Care needs to be taken to avoid alienating the client.
Be cautious in using confrontational techniques or making demands for achievement.	Client has low tolerance for stress. It is most critical not to exacerbate onset of symptoms.
Explore situations that lead to feelings of anger, resentment. Identify possible causes and explore stressors or events that trigger illness.	Helps client define problem areas and begin to establish goals to work through them.

Discuss ways to stop escalation of anxiety.	Client reacts to stress psychologically and needs to learn to control/deal effectively with emotional responses.
Assist client to learn to be in tune with feelings and recognize situations that cause increase in anxiety.	Client may be out of touch with body and not aware of feelings; therefore, he or she does not experience "signal anxiety," which helps client recognize beginning development of anxiety so steps can be taken for control.
Encourage direct expression of feelings. Help client to recognize times when the feelings are internalized.	The client who internalizes feelings is not always aware of doing that and may have trouble even identifying feelings.
Identify the amount of anxiety experienced if not perceiving self as "perfect" in job performance and interpersonal relationships.	May put pressure on self to be "perfect," while at the same time not recognizing/accepting feelings and resultant anxiety, which is then expressed in physical illness.
Examine possible cause-effect relationship between internalizing feelings and somatic symptoms.	Client needs to see the relationship between physical discomfort and turning feelings inward, so steps can be taken to intervene/deal more appropriately with the stress.
Help client relate pattern of resurgence of symptoms and stressful life situations. Have client keep a diary of appearance, duration, and intensity of physical symptoms. Maintain a separate record of stressful situations and compare with diary entries.	Reinforces the fact that client does transfer stress to body (e.g., GI upset, tension headache, chest pain, respiratory distress) and needs to learn how to stop this unhealthy reaction. Guided therapeutic writing not only serves as a release for anxiety and stress but may also provide objective data from which to observe the relationship between physical symptoms and stress.
Help client recognize difference between assertive and aggressive behaviors. Instruct in assertiveness techniques. Discuss importance of respecting rights of others while protecting one's own basic rights.	Assertiveness training is of utmost importance for the client who does not know how to directly express self, in order to defuse inner tension and relieve resulting physiological effects of anxiety. Also promotes self-esteem and may improve ability to form satisfactory interpersonal relationships.
Demonstrate/encourage use of relaxation, visualization, imagery techniques (e.g., progressive relaxation, meditation).	Studies show that these techniques decrease anxiety and work to moderate the stimulation of the sympathetic nervous system.
Explore possible recreational activities (e.g., brisk walks/jogging, volleyball, bowling, swimming).	Physical activity (exercise therapy) is very effective for relieving and rechanneling stress productively, and it provides opportunity to develop new skills to dissipate anxiety.

Collaborative

Evaluate appropriateness of/refer for hypnotherapy.	This form of relaxation therapy (which requires a qualified therapist) allows the client to access the subconscious mind to experience deep relaxation and work through emotional conflicts.

NURSING DIAGNOSIS	COPING, INDIVIDUAL, ineffective
May Be Related to:	Personal vulnerability
	Inadequate repertoire of coping mechanisms
	Compelling, intense desire to compete and win, excessive need to achieve success
	Feeling pressured to hurry, preoccupation with the urgency of passing time; work overload, too many deadlines; no vacations
	Unrealistic perceptions; unmet expectations
Possibly Evidenced by:	Inability to cope/problem-solve or to ask for help
	Internalizing stress/buildup of frustration; failure to obtain relief from and/or not resolving negative feelings; inadequate discharge of aggressive feelings/desires
	Use of maladaptive coping methods; use of passive-aggressive maneuvers
	Somatic symptoms, rise in blood pressure
Desired Outcomes/Evaluation Criteria— Client Will:	Develop and implement repertoire of coping strategies based on problem-solving techniques.
	Use assertive techniques in place of passive-aggressive, maladaptive behaviors.
	Demonstrate a more moderate lifestyle.
	Verbalize understanding of health risks.

ACTIONS/INTERVENTIONS	RATIONALE
Independent	
Assist client to identify present coping patterns and the consequences/effectiveness of behaviors.	A realistic picture of how effective current mechanisms are provides insight and enables client to acknowledge ineffectiveness of these methods and begin to look at healthy alternatives.
Help client identify/understand unmet needs and how present coping patterns relate to relief of anxiety.	Developing a keen sense of self-awareness and how these factors are interrelated provides opportunity for change.
Demonstrate/practice problem-solving techniques. Encourage client to think through problems, identify goals for own care.	Learning to arrive at thought-out solutions provides base for effective, satisfying coping behaviors. Personal involvement in own care provides a feeling of control, increases chances for positive outcome, and enhances self-esteem.
Ask client to give examples of situations when resentment and anger were felt but were not expressed. Discuss/role-play alternate ways to handle those situations.	Behavior rehearsal helps client to learn how to handle troublesome situations much more effectively.

480

Examine how needs are expressed, passively or aggressively.	Client may not be aware of use of passive or aggressive approach. Awareness offers choice to change behavior.
Have client identify and discuss personal dynamics. Determine if personal dynamics are used to prevent guilt or win approval.	Many interactions may be based on trying to relieve guilt or to please others while ignoring own wishes.
Confront with behaviors that are used to prevent rejection or disapproval by others.	Increases self-awareness of maladaptive pattern(s).
Encourage client to assume control over own reactions to stressful events, even though the circumstances cannot always be controlled.	The client can learn to control how much a stressful event affects feelings, behavior, and becoming upset by changing the way these events are viewed.
Identify competitive behaviors and explore reasons for feeling a compulsion to achieve/win.	Realization that the compulsive drive for achievement can be strong enough to endanger health may provide stimulus for change.
Evaluate the effect these compulsive feelings have had on physical and emotional health.	Heightens awareness of the possible toll on health, longevity.
Explore how these behaviors have affected interpersonal relationships.	Client may be intolerant of others and aggressive in relationships, resulting in problems interacting with others.
Help client identify what needs are really being met by competitive behaviors.	Recognition of own self-esteem needs provides opportunity to meet these needs in a more direct/successful manner.
Discuss consequences of "driving" oneself and how to moderate lifestyle to reduce stress.	Reinforces the negative effects of continuing an intense lifestyle.
Discuss importance of leisure time and how to develop and use it. Explain how pacing oneself can be a more productive and efficient use of time.	Client has not been accustomed to taking time out to relax, and learning how to relax and enjoy recreation can relieve anxiety and promote effective coping.

NURSING DIAGNOSIS	POWERLESSNESS
May Be Related to:	Unresolved dependency conflicts; sacrificing own wishes for others
	Feelings of insecurity, resentment; repression of anger and aggressive feelings
Possibly Evidenced by:	Lack of a sense of control in stressful situations
	Difficulty expressing self directly and assertively
	Passive/docile or aggressive behavior
	Internalization of stress/increased anxiety expressed through somatic symptoms, elevated blood pressure
Desired Outcomes/Evaluation Criteria— Client Will:	Recognize and work through feelings of insecurity, resentment.

Use assertive behaviors to deal with feelings, anxiety-producing situations, and interactions with others.

Verbalize awareness of self-control and how stress is handled in situations over which client does not have control.

Report less frequent episodes of illness with fewer physical complaints.

ACTIONS/INTERVENTIONS	RATIONALE
Independent	
Have client describe events that lead to feeling inadequate or having no control.	Helpful in identifying sources of frustration and defining problem areas so action can be taken.
Examine together how client feels when not "perfectly" competent or adequate in performance.	Client may be self-deprecating and believe he or she has failed unless self is perceived as "perfect."
Assess client's attitude toward making mistakes (e.g., ability to admit and accept, or feelings of inadequacy and worthlessness).	When client indulges in self-punishment, he or she needs to learn a rational way of thinking about mistakes. Failure is seldom a catastrophe and often leads to learning important lessons when the client is open to the opportunity.
Discuss how worry and anxiety prevent dealing with problems efficiently and cause more feelings of incompetency.	Worry and anxiety can prevent objective evaluation of a situation and lead to poor judgment.
Encourage client to do the feared activity. Provide support for these efforts.	Avoiding dreaded events increases unnecessary fears and causes further loss of self-confidence. Confronting the situation provides opportunity for client to test reality, consequences, and ability to cope with whatever happens, thus increasing self-confidence.
Discuss behaviors that are self-defeating and explore new, productive behaviors (e.g., looking at problem as a challenge instead of a threat, developing a sense of commitment to something, and gaining a sense of control over own life).	Past solutions to problems may not be relevant at this time, and previous failed experiences are not sufficient reason to discount their reevaluation.
Ask client to describe significant others' behaviors that are perceived as intimidating and how fear of these behaviors can be overcome.	Identifying successful actions to use can improve self-esteem. As self-confidence is gained, the client will be less easily intimidated.
Explain how a lack of self-confidence in one's own judgment and abilities can result in feeling powerless in stressful situations.	Loss of self-confidence serves only to "immobilize"/prevent using effective mechanisms in dealing with problems.
Use role-playing techniques to demonstrate how to assert feelings and help client learn direct self-expression when faced with frustration or aggression.	Behavior rehearsal is an effective way to practice self-expression/learn to deal with troublesome situations, get the desired need met, and enhance sense of control.
Have client describe people seen as dynamic or powerful individuals and how they achieved personal power. Explore how client can achieve these desired attributes.	Helps client to clearly define goals and values and look at how these relate to own self.

482

Examine sources of resentment. Identify what has been done to resolve these feelings and whether an effort has been made to get information to justify resentment.

More information can diffuse an angry or resentful response. Situations are not always as they appear, and an individual's perceptions may be distorted. Checking out reality can help the client decide on appropriate followup/response.

Encourage client to be open and direct in verbal expression. Confront when guarding of feelings is noted.

Learning new ways of expression is difficult. Reinforcing open/direct expression promotes continuation of activity.

Assess client's pattern of response to aggression or frustration, and together evaluate the effectiveness of these responses.

Client first needs to recognize own pattern of maladaptive defense mechanisms to learn new adaptive responses.

Examine situations that produce anger or guilt in client and discuss what triggers these feelings.

Unresolved guilt and anger lead to feelings of frustration or powerlessness.

Discuss causes of difficulty in making own needs known to others and fears surrounding these issues.

The client does not assert own needs and either passively accepts things as they are or ineffectively tries to assert control, increasing feelings of powerlessness. Discussion and awareness provide opportunity for change.

Explore guilt feelings when expressing anger and ways to work through this problem.

Client needs to learn that it is acceptable to feel and express anger appropriately.

Examine causes of hostility and how these feelings can be adequately discharged (e.g., pounding pillows, yelling appropriately; expressing feelings assertively, not aggressively, to the other person).

Client may be harboring undischarged hostility that needs resolution or release instead of allowing these feelings to affect body negatively (e.g., increased blood pressure, tension headache).

Ask client to verbalize how and why feelings of helplessness and dependency began. Discuss ways to put these feelings into perspective.

Being aware of emotional dependency and how these dynamics originate provides opportunity to change behavior/outcomes.

Explore with client fears of loss/rejection and evaluate together how realistic these concerns are.

May tend to exaggerate slight criticism into unrealistic fears.

Help client think through concerns about loss/ rejection and identify ways to deal with them.

Client needs to learn to accept the positive and negative aspects of relationships without becoming dysfunctional.

Have client identify what will happen if client functions independently. Help client learn how to use own capabilities.

Functioning autonomously and capitalizing on own strengths promote client's sense of control over own life/outcomes.

NURSING DIAGNOSIS	**SELF ESTEEM disturbance [specify]**
May Be Related to:	Lack of positive feedback, repeated negative feedback resulting in diminished self-worth
	Dysfunctional family system; unmet dependency needs
	Retarded ego development
	Unrealistic expectations of self and/or others
	Belief that individual should be "perfect"
Possibly Evidenced by:	Not expressing needs directly, lacking self-confidence, being dependent, not verbalizing/not working through negative feelings
	Feelings of worthlessness

483

Desired Outcomes/Evaluation Criteria—Client Will:	Verbalize view of self as a worthwhile, important person who functions well both interpersonally and occupationally.
	Demonstrate self-confidence by setting realistic goals and actively participating in life situations.
	Experience a decrease in somatic symptoms.

ACTIONS/INTERVENTIONS

Independent

Assess client's strengths and limitations and compare with client's own assessment of self.

Discuss client's goals. Are they what the client really wants or are they what the client thinks they "should" or "ought" to be?

Explain why it is necessary to take risks in order to build self-esteem.

Encourage client to explore feelings about criticism from others. Discuss ways to cope with these feelings and how to accept disapproval from others without experiencing a sense of failure.

Identify what needs are being met by preoccupation with neatness and orderliness. Relate these needs to self-esteem needs.

Discuss possible feelings of ambivalence toward significant other(s) who have been a source of disappointment, rejection, or loss.

Explore expectations family and/or significant others hold for client.

Assist client to identify realistic needs for change in relation to self, family/significant other(s).

Reinforce client's ability to assume responsibility and rely on own abilities.

RATIONALE

An accurate picture of the client's sense of self-worth is important in developing the plan of care.

Typically tends to ignore own wishes and do what client thinks others expect.

Self-confidence is built on taking risks and learning from success and/or failure.

May have unrealistic feelings when criticized and needs to learn how to apply constructive criticism for personal growth rather than becoming devastated. Helps to develop confidence in own abilities and judgment despite what others think.

Client more than likely experiences a sense of failure if unable to keep environment perfect.

Often experiences ambivalent feelings toward significant others, owing to inability to deal with negative feelings directly and having a fear of rejection if negative feelings are expressed.

Client may be trying to meet unrealistic expectations, further increasing sense of failure and anxiety.

Without guidance, may misinterpret/block needs, setting self up for failure.

Needs emotional support and encouragement to become self-reliant.

NURSING DIAGNOSIS	ROLE PERFORMANCE, altered
May Be Related to:	Chronic illness
	Situational crisis, conflicts
	Developmental crisis regarding values/beliefs
Possibly Evidenced by:	Changes in usual patterns of responsibility; inability (perceived/actual) to resume role

484

Desired Outcomes/Evaluation Criteria—Client Will:	Change in own/other's perception of role Assumption of dependent role Verbalize realistic perception of role expectations/obligations. Assume role-related responsibility.
Client and Family Will:	Initiate plan for conflict resolution.

ACTIONS/INTERVENTIONS	RATIONALE

Independent

Determine client's usual role within the family system. Identify roles of other family members.	Accurate data base is required to formulate appropriate plan of care for client.
Assess specific disabilities related to role expectations. Note relationship of disability to actual physical condition.	It is necessary to determine the validity of the client's/family's role expectations in light of client's physical ability to make realistic plans to modify role and encourage adaptation.
Encourage client to discuss conflicts evident within the family system. Identify how client and other family members have responded to this conflict.	Identifies specific stressors, as well as adaptive and maladaptive responses within the system, so that individualized assistance can be provided in an effort to initiate change.
Assist client to identify feelings associated with family conflict, the subsequent exacerbation of physical symptoms, and the accompanying disabilities.	Client may be unaware of the relationship between physical symptoms and emotional problems. An awareness of the correlation is the first step toward effecting change.
Help client identify changes he or she would like to occur within the family system.	Involving client helps to focus thinking on positive ways to adapt to problems in the family.
Encourage family participation in effort to resolve the conflict for which the client's sick role provides relief.	Input from the individual(s) who will be directly involved in the change will increase the likelihood of a positive outcome. (Refer to ND: Family Coping, ineffective: compromised/disabling.)
Involve all family members in the plan for change as well as knowledge of benefits, consequences, selection, and methods for implementation of alternatives.	Family may require assistance with this problem-solving process. When all members are involved, chances for success are enhanced.
Ensure that client has accurate perception of role expectations within family system. Use role-play to practice areas associated with role that client perceives as painful.	Repetition through practice may help to desensitize client to the anticipated distress.
Discuss more adaptive coping strategies that may be used to prevent interference with performance of role during times of stress.	As client is able to understand the relationship between exacerbation of physical symptoms and existing conflict, more effective skills can be used.

NURSING DIAGNOSIS	FAMILY COPING, ineffective: compromised/disabling)
May Be Related to:	Inadequate or incorrect information or understanding by a primary person

Possibly Evidenced by:	Prolonged disease progression that exhausts supportive capacity of significant other(s)
	Significant person with chronically unexpressed feelings of guilt, anxiety, hostility, despair
	Client providing little support for primary person
	Client expresses despair regarding family reactions/lack of involvement
	Intolerance/abandonment; psychosomatic tendency
	Taking on illness signs of client
	Distortion of reality regarding the client's health problem
	Significant other(s) display protective behavior disproportionate (too little or too much) to client's abilities or need for autonomy
Desired Outcomes/Evaluation Criteria—Family Will:	Identify/verbalize resources within themselves to deal with situation.
	Interact appropriately with the client and each other, providing support and assistance as indicated.
	Verbalize knowledge and understanding of illness.
	Participate actively in treatment program.

ACTIONS/INTERVENTIONS	RATIONALE
Independent	
Explore past relationships and feelings about successes and failures.	May help identify a pattern of interacting that may be counterproductive and lead to failure.
Discuss precipitating stresses regarding real or feared threats to significant personal relationships.	Unrealistic fears may be dictating relationships.
Determine extent of "enabling" behaviors evidenced by family members; explore with family/client.	"Enabling" is doing for the client what he or she needs to do for own self. People want to be helpful and do not want to feel powerless to help their family member to be well. When the family members' roles are to "help" the client stay ill, they need to learn new ways of interacting to attain/maintain health for each individual.
Help client develop communication skills that enable needs to be met by using assertive expressions (e.g., "I-messages").	Using assertive, direct communication can make significant differences in communicating needs and having these needs met in more effective ways.
Explore possible negative feelings or fears caused by feeling compelled to meet demands of others.	May frustrate own wishes to please others owing to fear of rejection or loss of the relationship.
Discuss ways of handling troublesome situations by using newly learned coping skills.	Having a plan for handling situations before they arise helps increase successful interactions.

486

Give positive feedback for efforts toward using constructive new behaviors.

Client/family members may lack self-confidence and require emotional support and assurance of capability.

Collaborative

Refer to support groups, family therapy, if indicated.

May need additional assistance to promote healthy ways of interacting and assist client/family members to deal effectively with illness/improve quality of life.

PROBLEMS RELATED TO ABUSE OR NEGLECT

DSM-IV
IF FOCUS OF ATTENTION IS ON THE VICTIM [SURVIVOR]:
995.52 Neglect of child
995.53 Sexual abuse of child
995.54 Physical abuse of child
995.81 Physical abuse of adult
995.83 Sexual abuse of adult
IF FOCUS OF ATTENTION IS ON THE PERPETRATOR [OFFENDER] OR ON THE RELATIONAL UNIT IN WHICH BEHAVIOR OCCURS:
V61.21 Neglect; physical or sexual abuse of child (specify)
V61.12 (Physical or sexual abuse of adult by partner)
V62.83 (Physical or sexual abuse of adult by person other than partner)

Abuse affects all populations and is not restricted to specific socioeconomic or ethnic/cultural groups. Although "violence" means the use of force or physical compulsion to abuse or damage, the term "abuse" is much broader and includes physical or mental maltreatment and neglect that result in emotional, physical, or sexual injury. In the case of children, the disabled, or elderly, abuse can result from direct actions or omissions by those responsible for the individual's care. Additionally, one's perception of abuse is affected by cultural and religious practices, values, and biological predispositions. The problem can be generational, with victimizers often being victims of abuse themselves as children.

Violence is not a new problem; in fact, it is probably as old as humankind. However, in the United States, medicine has focused on these issues only since 1946. Therefore, the parameters of abuse are being identified and redefined on what seems to be an almost daily basis. For example, until recently women and children were considered the personal property of men and they did not own property or have rights of their own. Women viewed themselves as sexual objects and were expected to subjugate themselves/defer to the will of men. Harsh treatment of children was justified by the belief that corporal and/or excessive punishment was necessary to maintain discipline and instill values. Changes in societal beliefs and the enactment of new laws have done little to curb abuse. Today, battering is the single most common cause of injury to women, and there has been an increase in the incidence of child abuse and neglect-related fatalities reported to child protection service agencies in the United States. Whether these statistics represent an increase in incidents or are the result of changing attitudes and/or better reporting is much debated. The Centers for Disease Control and Prevention has declared violence to be a public health problem.

This plan of care addresses the problems of abuse and neglect in both adults and children and includes both the person who offends and the survivor of the offense.

ETIOLOGICAL THEORIES

Psychodynamics

Psychoanalytical theory suggests that unmet needs for satisfaction and security result in an underdeveloped ego and a poor self-concept in the individuals involved in violent episodes. Aggression and violence supply the offender with a sense of power and prestige that boosts the self-image and provides a significance or purpose to the individual's life that is lacking. Some theorists have supported the hypothesis that aggression and violence are the overt expressions of powerlessness and low self-esteem. The same dynamics promote acceptance in the person who is the victim of violence.

Biological

Various components of the neurological system have been implicated in both the facilitation and inhibition of aggressive impulses. The limbic system in particular appears to be involved. In addition, higher brain centers play an important role by constantly interacting with the aggression centers. Various neurotransmitters, such as epinephrine, norepinephrine, dopamine, acetylcholine, and serotonin, may also play a role in facilitation and inhibition of aggressive impulses. This theory is consistent with the "fight-or-flight" arousal in response to stress.

Some studies suggest the possibility of a direct genetic link; however, the evidence for this has not been firmly established. Organic brain syndromes associated with various cerebral disorders have been linked to violent behavior. Particularly, areas of the limbic system and temporal lobes, brain trauma, and diseases such as encephalitis and disorders such as epilepsy have been implicated in aggressive behavior.

Family Dynamics

Child abuse is often the consequence of the interactions of parental vulnerabilities (e.g., mental illness, substance abuse); child vulnerabilities (e.g., low birth weight, difficult temperament); a particular developmental stage, such as toddler, adolescence; and social stressors (e.g., lack of social supports, young parental age, single parenthood, poverty, minority ethnicity, lack of acculturation, exposure to family violence).

Learning theory states that children learn to behave by imitating their role models, usually parents, although as they mature they are influenced by teachers, friends, and others. Individuals who were abused as children or whose parents disciplined them with physical punishment are more likely to behave in a violent manner as adults. Television and movies are believed to have an influence on developing both adaptive and maladaptive behavior. Some theorists believe that individuals who have a biological influence toward aggressive behavior are more likely to be affected by external models than those without this predisposition.

The influence of culture and social structure cannot be discounted. Difficulty in negotiating interpersonal conflict has led to a general acceptance of violence as a means of solving problems. When individuals/groups of people discover they cannot meet their needs through conventional methods, they are more likely to resort to delinquent behaviors. This may contribute to a subculture of violence within society.

CLIENT ASSESSMENT DATA BASE

Activity/Rest

Sleep problems (e.g., sleeplessness or oversleeping, nightmares, sleepwalking, sleeping in strange place [avoiding offender])
Fatigue

Ego Integrity

Negative self-appraisal, acceptance of self-blame/making excuses for the actions of others
Low self-esteem (offender/survivor)
Feelings of guilt, anger, fear and shame, helplessness, and/or powerlessness
Minimization or denial of significance of behaviors (most prominent defense mechanism)
Avoidance or fear of certain people, places, objects; submissive, fearful manner (particularly in presence of offender)
Report of stress factors (e.g., family unemployment; financial, lifestyle changes; marital discord)
Hostility toward/mistrust of others
Threatened when partner shows signs of independence or shares self/time with others (offender)

Elimination

Enuresis, encopresis
Recurrent urinary infections
Changes in tone of sphincter

Food/Fluid

Frequent vomiting; changes in appetite: anorexia, overeating (survivor)
Changes in weight; failure to gain weight appropriately/signs of malnutrition, repeated
    pica (neglect)

Hygiene

Wearing clothing that covers body in a manner inappropriate for weather conditions
    (abuse), or that is inadequate to provide protection (neglect)
Excessive/anxiety about bathing (abuse); dirty/unkempt appearance (neglect)

Neurosensory

Behavioral extremes (very aggressive/demanding conduct); extreme rage or passivity and
    withdrawal; age-inappropriate behavior
Mental Status:
    Memory: Blackouts, periods of amnesia; reports of flashbacks
    Disorganized thinking; difficulty concentrating/making decisions
    Inappropriate affect; may be hypervigilant, anxious, depressed
Mood swing—"dual personality," extremely loving, kind, contrite after battering episode
    (offender)
Pathological jealousy; poor impulse control; limited coping skills; lacks empathy (offender)
Rocking, thumb sucking, or other habitual behavior; restlessness (survivor)
Psychiatric manifestations (e.g., dissociative phenomena including multiple personalities
    (sexual abuse); borderline personality disorder [adult incest survivors])
Presence of neurological deficits/CNS damage without external injuries evident (may
    indicate "shaken baby" syndrome)

Pain/Discomfort

Dependent on specific injuries/form of abuse
Multiple somatic complaints (e.g., stomach pain, chronic pelvic pain, spastic colon,
    headache)

Safety

Bruises, bite marks, skin welts, burns (e.g., scalding, cigarette), bald spots, lacerations,
    unusual bleeding, rashes/itching in the genital area; anal fissures, skin tags,
    hemorrhoids, scar tissue, changes in tone of sphincter
Recurrent injuries; history of multiple accidents, fractures/internal injuries
Description of incident incongruent with injury, delay in seeking treatment
Lack of age-appropriate supervision, inattention to avoidable hazards in the home (neglect)
Intense episodes of rage directed at self or others
Self-injurious/suicidal behavior; involvement in high-risk activities
History of suicidal behavior of family members

Sexuality

Changes in sexual awareness or activity, including compulsive masturbation, precocious
    sex play, tendency to repeat or reenact incest/abuse experience; excessive curiosity
    about sex; sexually abusing another child; promiscuity; overly anxious/ inhibited about
    sexual anatomy or behavior
May display feminine sex-role stereotypes; confusion about sexuality (male survivors); may
    have unconscious homosexual tendencies (male offenders of incest)
Reports of decreased sexual desire (as adult), erectile dysfunction, premature ejaculation,
    and/or anorgasmia; dyspareunia, vaginismus; flashbacks during intercourse; inability
    to engage in sex without anxiety

Episodes of marital rape or forced intercourse

Impaired sexual relationship between parents (incest)

Parent/female careprovider aware or strongly suspects incestual behavior, may be grateful not to be focus of partner's sexual demands

Obstetrical history of preterm labor, abruptio placentae, spontaneous abortions, low birth weight, fetal injury/death (1 in 6 pregnant women are battered during pregnancy); lack of prenatal care until 3rd trimester (abused women twice as likely to delay care)

Vaginal bleeding; linear laceration of hymen, vaginal mucosa

Presence of STDs, vaginitis, genital warts, or pregnancy (especially child)

Social Interactions

Multiple family/relationship stressors reported

Household members may include step-relatives or a paramour

History of frequent moves/relocation

Few/no support systems

Lacks knowledge of appropriate child-rearing practices (child abusers)

Inability to form satisfactory peer relationships; withdrawal in social settings; inappropriate attachment to imaginary companion

Very possessive, perceives partner as a possession; repeatedly insults/humiliates partner, strives to isolate partner from others/keeps partner totally dependent, challenges partners honesty, uses intimidation to achieve power/control over partner (offender)

Lack of assertive communication skills; difficulty negotiating interpersonal conflicts

Cheating, lying; low achievement or drop in school performance

Running away from home/relationship

Parent may interfere with child's normal peer relationships to prevent exposure (incest)

Memories of childhood may contain blank periods, excessive fantasizing/daydreaming; report of violence/neglect in family of origin

Family Interaction Pattern: Less verbally responsive, increased use of direct commands and critical statements, decreased verbal praise or acknowledgment, belittling, denigrating, scapegoating, ignoring; significant imbalance of power/use of hitting as control measure, patterns of enmeshment, closed family system; one parent domineering, impulsive; other partner passive, submissive

Teaching/Learning

May be any age, race, religion/culture, or educational level; from all socioeconomic groups (usual child profile is under age 3 or perceived as different due to temperamental traits, congenital abnormalities, chronic illness)

Learning disabilities include attention-deficit disorders, conduct disorders

Delay in achieving developmental tasks, declines on cognitive testing; brain damage, habitual truancy/absence from school for nonlegitimate reasons (neglect)

Substance abuse by individuals involved in abuse/neglect, or other family member(s) (most often cocaine, crack, amphetamines, alcohol)

Use of multiple healthcare providers/resources (limits awareness of repeated nature of problem); lack of age-appropriate health screening/immunization, dental care, absence of necessary prostheses, such as eyeglasses, hearing aid (neglect)

DIAGNOSTIC STUDIES

Physical and Psychological Testing

Dependent on individual situation/needs

Screening Tests (e.g., Child Behavior Checklist): Elevated scores on the internalization scale reveal behaviors described as fearful, inhibited, depressed, overcontrolled or undercontrolled, aggressive, antisocial.

NURSING PRIORITIES

1. Provide physical/emotional safety.
2. Develop a trusting therapeutic relationship.
3. Enhance sense of self-esteem.
4. Improve problem-solving ability.
5. Involve family/partner in therapeutic program.

DISCHARGE GOALS

1. Physical/emotional safety maintained.
2. Trusting relationship with one person established.
3. Self-growth and positive approaches to problems evident.
4. Client/SOs participating in ongoing therapy.
5. Plan in place to meet needs after discharge.

NURSING DIAGNOSIS	TRAUMA, risk for
Risk Factors May Include:	Dependent position in relationship(s)
	History of previous abuse/neglect
	Lack or nonuse of support systems/resources
Possibly Evidenced by:	[Not applicable; presence of signs and symptoms establishes an *actual* diagnosis.]
Desired Outcomes/Evaluation Criteria— Client Will:	Be free of injury/signs of neglect.
Client/Family Will:	Recognize need for/seek assistance to prevent abuse.
	Identify and access resources to assist in promoting a safe environment.

ACTIONS/INTERVENTIONS	RATIONALE

Independent

Note age/developmental level of survivor, mentation, agility, physical abilities/limitations.	Children under 3, those perceived as having different temperament, or those with congenital problems/chronic illness are at increased risk of being abused/neglected. Additionally, the elderly who are dependent on others because of age/ infirmities or individuals with significant disabilities are also at risk. Those who are incapable of meeting their own needs/directing their personal affairs may require alternate placement/court-ordered advocate.
Review physical complaints/injuries including those that suggest possibility of sexual abuse (e.g., bladder infection, bruises in the genital area, reports of aggression or inappropriate sexual behavior). Note affect and demeanor.	The visible evidence of physical abuse/neglect makes it more easily recognized. Although these clients display signs of emotional involvement, inappropriate affect, and behaviors such as withdrawal, acting out, or suicidal gestures in the absence of physical evidence of abuse/neglect,

Identify individual concerns of client.

Interview offender(s)/family in a nonjudgmental manner, displaying tact and professional concern for individual(s).

Maintain objectivity and avoid blame or accusations during interview process.

Use open-ended questions with gentle, caring manner. Speak at individual's level (e.g., child vs. adult, or developmentally disabled individual). Provide privacy as indicated by age, circumstances of the situation.

Use techniques of play therapy to obtain information from children. Videotape session(s) as appropriate.

Note sequence of events as related by parent(s)/caregivers or partner, paying particular attention to inconsistencies and contradictory reports.

---

suggests presence of emotional abuse. Child sexual abuse is particularly difficult to diagnose. Although the signs noted here are not definitive, they suggest need for further investigation.

Concerns will vary dependent on individual circumstances and affect choice of interventions, possible options.

Can provide insight into risks to client and potential for repetition of behavior. The need for power over or control of survivor, excessive jealousy/overpossessiveness, frequency of verbal arguments that can escalate to violence, substance abuse, severity of past injuries inflicted, history of forced or threatened sexual acts, and/or threats to kill client (especially when offender indicates a belief he or she cannot live without partner) greatly increases the level of concern for survivor's safety and choice of interventions.

Individuals will be defensive and may react with hostility and anger, or may withdraw, making it difficult to obtain accurate information. Initially, offender may not be known, and even if family is not involved in situation, members may feel guilt that they did not protect the survivor. Avoiding blame promotes open communication and therapeutic interactions and may enhance the investigation process.

Survivor and parent/family members will respond more positively to caring approach and be more available for help to correct underlying problems when dealt with in this way. **Note:** Care must be taken to avoid leading the child survivor, or suggesting answers to questions. As these individuals are vulnerable, they are suggestible and may provide answers to "please" the therapist, resulting in questionable information.

The child may be afraid to tell/be unable to adequately verbalize what has happened. Play therapy is a nonthreatening method of observation/Active-listening that allows for free expression of the child's feelings and perceptions without undue influence from adults. Videotaping allows various parties (legal and counseling) to view the same data, reducing risk of misinterpretation and negating need for child to submit to repeated questioning, which may color data over time. In addition, this can provide safeguards for both therapist and survivor.

May reveal reality of what happened. Offender(s)/family members are upset and afraid about what has happened/the potential consequences and may try to cover up circumstances of injury.

493

Evaluate family and home environment. Note particularly areas of stress related to abusive occurrence.	Provides clues to need for change to prevent further problems. Families who move their residence frequently and are socially isolated, and stepfamilies are at greater risk. Children who have been separated from parents because of prematurity or neonatal illness also may be more at risk, owing in part to problems with bonding and situational stressors (e.g., financial concerns, demands of caregiving role).
Identify individual risk factors for recidivism of abuse/neglect.	Offender's resistance to ongoing therapy, substance abuse, immaturity, and narcissistic personality traits increase risk that violent behavior will recur.
Help adult survivor develop a safety plan incorporating available personal and community resources.	Typically, these individuals have few/are separated from support systems and require assistance to identify options and initiate a plan. Additionally, availability of resources such as women's shelters, counseling services, or ombudsman for the elderly/disabled varies according to locality.
Discuss importance of involved adults participating in therapeutic program. Identify consequences of abusive behaviors.	Without outside intervention, the behavior is likely to continue. Loss of family (divorce, separation, restraining order, alternate placement), loss of property/income, possible loss of job, as well as potential for incarceration can occur. Studies indicate skilled specialized counseling has a success rate of 50%–75% in eliminating violent behavior.

Collaborative

Follow correct procedures and be familiar with reporting protocols of institution/community.	Legal obligations vary from state to state, but most states have mandatory reporting of suspected child abuse and some have added mandatory reporting for adults as well. Sensitive handling of this procedure can provide protection for the client and direct families to the help they need to promote improved functioning.
Arrange for home-based interventions (e.g., visiting nurse, First Visitor, Bright Beginnings) as indicated.	Home visitation/support provides opportunity for teaching/modeling of effective child rearing behaviors, ongoing monitoring of home situation, and early identification of/intervention for developing problems to help maintain the family unit.
Refer to individual/family therapy.	As in the case of violent behavior, involved individuals need to distinguish between validity of emotions and the inappropriateness of behavior. Violence is the choice of the offender, is under his or her control, and is his or her sole responsibility although the dynamics of relationship(s) may be a factor.
Refer individuals to substance abuse program, as appropriate.	Substance abuse has a negative impact on the therapeutic process and increases likelihood that behavior will recur/continue.

494

NURSING DIAGNOSIS	SELF ESTEEM, chronic low
May Be Related to:	Personal vulnerability, feelings of abandonment, circular process of self-negation
	Life choices perpetuating failure/abuse
Possibly Evidenced by:	Self-negating verbalization, expressions of shame/guilt
	Evaluating self as unable to deal with events
	Rationalizing away/rejecting positive feedback and exaggerating negative feedback about self
	Hesitancy to try new things/situations; nonassertive/passive, indecisive, or overly conforming behaviors
Desired Outcomes/Evaluation Criteria— Client Will:	Verbalize understanding of negative evaluation of self and reasons for this problem.
	Participate in treatment program to promote change in self-evaluation.
	Demonstrate behaviors/lifestyle changes to promote positive self-esteem.
	Verbalize increased sense of self-esteem in relation to current situation.

ACTIONS/INTERVENTIONS	RATIONALE
Independent	
Develop therapeutic relationship. Be attentive, validate client's communication, provide encouragement for efforts, maintain open communication, use skills of Active-listening and "I-messages."	Promotes self-esteem by validating the individual as a worthwhile person who has important things to say and has value in the situation. This relationship may be slow to develop because client's feelings of betrayal will influence ability to trust others as well as herself or himself. **Note:** Males who have been sexually abused may have difficulty with self-disclosure to male therapists, and young children may fear being seduced by male therapist or be concerned that female therapist will not act in a protective manner.
Note body language and hypervigilant attitude.	After period of testing reliability of caregiver/therapist, client may begin to relax vigilance, indicating initiation of trust relationship and openness to progress in therapy.
Assess content of negative self-talk.	"Damaged goods" syndrome and self-blame for what has occurred are common. Additionally, this may be reinforced by negative responses by individuals/peers, hostility from family members, and inner feelings of shame/guilt. Depending on severity, this will likely be the initial focus of therapy once survivor safety is assured.

495

Discuss survivor's perceptions of self related to what is happening. Confront misconceptions.

Client frequently believes she or he is "lacking" or in some way causing the behavior in the other person. Gently confronting these misperceptions can help client accept the reality that she or he is *not* responsible for the other's behavior.

Emphasize need for client to avoid comparing self to others.

Pattern has been established to make unfavorable comparisons, and stopping this thought process is a step toward increasing client's self-esteem.

Be aware that people are not programmed to be rational—rather, it is a learned behavior/skill.

In order to develop positive self-esteem, individual needs to seek information/facts, choose to learn, choose to think rather than merely accepting/reacting to what is happening, to respect self and value honesty.

Confront client's tendency to minimize situation. Discuss impact of abuse/neglect on individual.

Gentle confrontation can help the client begin to accept the reality of what has happened. Giving up the "fantasy" of "things as you wish they were" provides a stronger base for client to build on, enhancing likelihood of successful outcome.

Proceed with caution when helping client recall/ investigate areas of life that have been forgotten.

While the concept of repression has long been accepted in psychology, the phenomenon of "false memories" has raised questions regarding the validity of what is remembered. The suggestion of questioning and the client's own misperceptions and fantasies can lead to inaccurate conclusions and accusations that may be damaging to the client and family.

Identify what behavior does for client (positive intention, i.e., maintains dependent position, creates sense of power). Ask what options are available to the client/SO.

Promotes awareness of why things are the way they are and provides a starting point for making changes.

Set limits on aggressive or problem behaviors, such as acting out, suicide preoccupation, or rumination. (Refer to ND: Violence, risk for, directed at self/ others.)

These behaviors diminish self-esteem, and continuation of them interferes with recovery. Rumination locks client into a circular path rather than allowing individual to move forward and "get on" with life.

Discuss inaccuracies in self-perception with client/ SO(s). Help client to recognize view of self as "the victim."

Client may not see positive aspects of self that others see, and bringing it to awareness may help change perception. Dwelling on/sense of being "the victim" can interfere with sense of worth and impede recovery.

Have client list current/past successes and strengths. Provide feedback using positive "I-messages" rather than praise.

Helps develop internal sense of self-worth, new coping behaviors. The use of praise is external control and may be rejected by the individual.

Discuss past choices, helping client identify future options. Avoid blaming client; assuring client that his or her decision was the best that could be made at the time.

Negative view of self and perceived lack of options can interfere with client taking control of own life and developing new behaviors to prevent future abusive situations. **Note:** Appropriately attributing responsibility for the abuse to other(s)/accepting responsibility for own actions as appropriate, is an important part of healing, allowing client to stop self-criticism and begin self-nurturing and protection.

Help client identify goals that are personally achievable and supportive of self.	Provides direction for client to work toward. **Note:** Clients not only need to feel differently about themselves but also need to treat themselves differently.
Allow client to progress at own rate.	Adaptation to a change in self-concept depends on its significance to individual, disruption of lifestyle, and length of illness/debilitation. **Note:** Emotional abuse (e.g., rejecting, terrorizing, ignoring, isolating, or corrupting) may have continued for a prolonged period of time before being diagnosed and therefore may be more pervasive and more difficult to overcome than physical abuse.
Involve in activities/exercise program.	Provides opportunities to practice new skills and promotes socialization; helps relieve anger/stress and enhance sense of general well-being.
Encourage development of social/vocational skills.	Participation in classes/activities/hobbies that client enjoys or would like to experience promotes successful accomplishments, enhancing self-worth. Also provides options for increased independence and future options.
Give positive reinforcement for progress noted.	Helps client accept self as a worthwhile person. Positive words of encouragement support development of coping behaviors.
Evaluate educational placement.	Special program may be needed to help client overcome educational deficiencies and catch up to appropriate grade level/obtain GED, etc.
Identify family dynamics past and present.	Family interactions contribute to development of self-esteem in family members and provide clues to problems contributing to abuse.
Provide age-/situation-appropriate bibliotherapy.	Reading information supplements and supports other therapeutic intervention.

Collaborative

Provide therapy in a team setting and seek peer consultation as appropriate.	Opportunity for open discussion increases therapist's awareness of personal feelings regarding abuse behavior/victimization of client, overidentifying with client, merging with the criminal justice system's (society's) need for retribution or need to "rescue" client, which could lead to countertransference problems and interfere with the progress of therapy. **Note:** This concern may be of greater significance when survivor is a child who has been sexually abused and the therapist has discomfort regarding own sexuality and unconscious childhood fantasies.
Involve in classes such as assertiveness training, positive self-image, communication skills.	Assists with learning skills to promote self-esteem.
Provide information about available community programs and opportunities for involvement.	Influencing one's community through volunteer or paid service (e.g., abuse prevention programs or as a survivor advocate) allows individual to be

proactive and view self as a contributing member of society, aiding in client's own recovery process.

Refer to clinical nurse specialist, psychologist/ psychiatrist, group therapy is indicated.

Type, severity, frequency, duration, and age of individual at time of abuse affect recovery. Client may require long-term and/or specialized therapy, such as hypnosis. Additionally, group therapy provides an opportunity for sharing own healing with other survivors/offenders and learn new skills to enhance sense of self-worth.

NURSING DIAGNOSIS	POWERLESSNESS
May Be Related to:	Legitimate dependency on other(s) (child, elderly, disabled individual), personal vulnerability
	Interpersonal interaction (e.g., misuse of power, force, abusive relationships)
	Lifestyle of helplessness (e.g., repeated failures, dependency)
Possibly Evidenced by:	Verbal expressions of having no control
	Reluctance to express true feelings, fearing alienation from caregiver(s)
	Apathy (withdrawal, resignation, crying), passivity; anger
Desired Outcomes/Evaluation Criteria— Client Will:	Express sense of control over future.
	Identify areas over which individual has control.
	Engage in problem-solving activities.

ACTIONS/INTERVENTIONS	RATIONALE
Independent	
Identify circumstances of individual situation contributing to client's sense of powerlessness.	Promotes understanding of factors involved and enables client to begin to develop sense of control over self and future.
Determine client locus of control.	Client who believes problems are caused by others (external) will need to begin to accept own responsibility for being in charge of self. Making a decision to take control of own life is crucial to making changes needed to support growth.
Help client identify factors that are under own control.	Provides a starting point for client to begin to assume control over own life.
Identify use of manipulative behavior and reactions of client, SO(s), and healthcare providers.	Manipulation is used for management of powerlessness because of distrust of others, fear of loss of power/control, fear of intimacy, and search for approval. This can interfere with personal and therapeutic relationships.

498

Discuss needs openly with client. Set agreed-on routines for meeting identified needs.

Identify when flashbacks are problem for survivor and how they may be minimized.

Collaborative

Refer to assertiveness program.

Promotes meeting needs directly and decreases the need for client to use manipulation.

May occur with fatigue or stress and generally intensify feelings of loss of control. Avoidance of individual "triggers" may reduce occurrence.

As client learns these skills and becomes more active/assertive in relationships, she or he is more likely to set limits on the behaviors of others, express feelings more openly/directly, and take control of own life in a healthy manner.

NURSING DIAGNOSIS	COPING, INDIVIDUAL, ineffective
May Be Related to:	Situational/maturational crises
	Overwhelming threat to self, personal vulnerability
	Inadequate support systems
Possibly Evidenced by:	Verbalization of inability to cope/ask for help
	Chronic worry, anxiety, depression, poor self-esteem
	Inability to problem-solve, lack of assertive behaviors
	Inappropriate use of defense mechanisms (e.g., denial, withdrawal)
	High illness rate, destructive behavior toward self/others
Desired Outcomes/Evaluation Criteria— Client Will:	Assess the current situation accurately (related to age, individual condition).
	Identify ineffective coping behaviors and consequences.
	Verbalize feelings congruent with behavior.

ACTIONS/INTERVENTIONS

RATIONALE

Independent

Help client separate issues of vulnerability from blame.

Active-listen and identify client perceptions/ understanding of current situation. Evaluate decision-making ability.

Client blames self/others for situation without looking at own responsibility for victim stance. Although this does not excuse abuse, client needs to change victim behaviors to gain control of self.

Client often enters the healthcare system in response to a crisis. This is an opportunity to help the client look at reality of abuse and begin to make changes.

499

Identify previous methods of dealing with life problems. Note use of denial.

Provides clues to coping skills that can be used for personal growth. Denial is the most prominent defense mechanism used by client/family members to protect against shame/guilt and to preserve intactness of the family, and it must be dealt with before progress can be made.

Encourage verbalization of fears and anxieties and expression of feelings of denial, depression, and anger. Let client know that these are normal reactions.

Expressing feelings helps client to become aware of the feelings, recognize and deal with what is happening.

Encourage and support client in evaluating lifestyle. Assess stressors and make plan for necessary change.

Identifying areas of life that promote abusive reactions/interactions helps client make changes in coping methods to prevent recurrences.

Collaborative

Refer to appropriate resources as indicated by individual situation (e.g., support groups, AA, psychotherapy, spiritual resources).

May need additional therapy/group involvement to learn new coping skills.

NURSING DIAGNOSIS	VIOLENCE, risk for, directed at self or others
Risk Factors May Include:	Negative role modeling, developmental crises
	History of abuse
	Rage reactions; suicidal behavior
	Organic brain syndrome; temporal lobe epilepsy
[Possible Indicators:]	Anger, rage; fear of others
	Increasing anxiety level, motor activity
	Hostile threatening verbalizations; body language indicating effort to control behavior
	Overt and aggressive acts
	Expressed intent/desire to harm self/others; self-destructive behaviors, substance abuse
Desired Outcomes/Evaluation Criteria— Client Will:	Acknowledge realities of the situation.
	Verbalize understanding of why behavior occurs.
	Identify precipitating factors/responses.
	Demonstrate new skills/methods for dealing with own responses.

ACTIONS/INTERVENTIONS

RATIONALE

Independent

Determine underlying dynamics of individual situation (e.g., pattern of abuse, contributing factors to violent behavior, relationship of involved persons [parent/child, spouse or lover], family pattern of communication.)

Necessary to determine needs/safety concerns.

Note signs of suicidal/homicidal intent (e.g., statements of intent/threats, development of a plan, giving away belongings, possession of means).

Allows for initiation of safety measures to protect client/others. **Note:** Association between suicidal behavior and physical abuse may be related to modeling of aggressive behavior within family/exposure to suicidal behavior of family member(s) as well as biological risk in family for disorders associated with suicide (e.g., substance abuse and affective or impulsive conduct disorders).

Determine client's perception of self, impact of abuse on life, and future expectations.

May see self as useless, damaged goods without hope for positive change/productive future, which may result in feelings of hopelessness and the perception of lacking options. Depth of rage and extent of feelings of powerlessness may predict potential for violent behavior.

Explore death fantasies when expressed (e.g., "They'll be sorry.").

Discussion of fantasies helps client look at reality of ideas and begin to deal with them.

Note coping behaviors being used currently by the client (e.g., denial, helplessness, rage reaction).

Provides information about mechanisms client uses to maintain the status quo, which may also increase risk for violent behavior.

Acknowledge reality of suicide/homicide as an option. Discuss consequences of actions if individual were to follow through on intent. Ask how it will help client resolve problems.

Acknowledging feelings helps the client begin to look at what might happen if actions were acted on, own ability to control self and make choices regarding recovery.

Encourage appropriate expression of feelings. Acknowledge reality and normalcy of these feelings. Set limits on acting-out behaviors.

Promotes awareness of feelings and ability to deal with them in acceptable ways.

Accept client's anger without reacting on an emotional basis.

Client's anger is directed at situation and those involved, not at healthcare provider, so remaining separate from the client allows therapist to be helpful to the resolution of the anger.

Contract with client for safety.

Provides parameters to help client deal with destructive thoughts/actions and helps to keep client safe.

Assist client to learn new coping skills (e.g., assertive rather than nonassertive/aggressive behavior, effective parenting techniques).

Promotes sense of self-worth and ability to control own actions/situation.

Collaborative

Administer antidepressants as indicated.

Helps client deal with feelings of sadness and hopelessness and move forward in therapy. Age of client and nature of abusive situation affect depth of client's depression.

Refer to inpatient program as appropriate.

May require more intensive therapy to deal with covert forms of self-destructive behavior (e.g., substance abuse, heavy risk-taking/runaway behavior).

Refer to community resources (e.g., social services, AA, others), as appropriate.

Helps attain/maintain recovery program.

NURSING DIAGNOSIS	FAMILY PROCESSES, altered [dysfunctional]/PARENTING, altered
May Be Related to:	Situational crises (e.g., economic, illness, change in roles), developmental transitions [loss/gain of family member(s), blending of families]
	Poor role model, lack of support systems; unrealistic expectation for self, infant, partner
	Physical/psychosocial abuse of nurturing figure
Possibly Evidenced by:	Family system does not meet its members' physical, emotional, spiritual, or security needs
	Inability of family members to relate to each other for mutual growth and maturation
	Rigidity in functions, rules, roles; verbalization of inability to control child, resentment toward child, unresolved disappointment in gender or physical characteristics of child
	Inattention to child needs, inappropriate caretaking behaviors, history of child abuse or abandonment, incidence of physical/psychological trauma
Desired Outcomes/Evaluation Criteria— Family/Parent Will:	Express feelings freely and appropriately.
	Demonstrate individual involvement in problem-solving process.
	Engage in appropriate parenting behaviors.

ACTIONS/INTERVENTIONS	RATIONALE
Independent	
Determine composition of family, developmental stage, presence/involvement of extended family, use of special supports.	Helps identify problem areas/strengths to formulate plans to change abusive situation. Lack of/ineffective use of support systems increases risk of recidivism.
Review type, severity, duration of problem, and contribution of, as well as impact on, individual family members.	Affects choice of interventions. Abuse is an act of commission, whereas neglect is considered an act of omission. These behaviors indicate the presence of problems with relationships and/or parenting skills and individual problems such as inability to deal with stressors, substance abuse, mental illness, cognitive limitations, or criminality. Even if the behavior is the result of a single individual, all family members may be involved in the denial/coverup or even passive condoning of the behavior. Additionally, all family members will be affected by the disclosure of the behavior.
Assess boundaries of family members such as whether members share family identity, have little sense of individuality, seem emotionally distant/ not connected with one another.	These factors are critical to understanding individual family dynamics and developing strategies for change. Family that pressures survivor to heal quickly/forgive offender, blames

Discuss parenting techniques and parents' expectations. Review developmental levels of children.	individual for causing pain by disclosing situation, fails to acknowledge significance of abuse, or minimizes/negates need for counseling is nonsupportive and will likely impede recovery process.
	Ineffective parenting and unrealistic expectations contribute to abuse. Understanding normal responses, progression of developmental milestones may help parents cope with changes. (Refer to ND: Growth and Development, altered.)
Note cultural and religious factors.	Beliefs about family roles, parenting style, and religious beliefs may contribute to participation in/acceptance of practices that are seen as abusive.
Discuss negative mode of individual interactions. Emphasize importance of continuous, open dialogue between family members using therapeutic communication skills.	Promotes successful interactions to break cycle of abuse. Keeping family secrets is destructive and can impede the change process.
Determine current "family rules." Identify areas of needed change.	Rules may be imposed by adults rather than through a democratic process involving all family members, leading to conflict and angry confrontations. Setting positive family rules with all family members participating can promote a functional family.
Identify and encourage use of previously successful coping behaviors.	Everyone has positive ways of dealing with life stressors, and when these are identified and supported they can help to change abusive situation.
Discuss therapeutic concept of forgiveness for covert acts as well as acts of omission.	Forgiving others and oneself takes time, but can free individuals from the past, allowing them to move forward with life. Although forgiving does not condone the actions, it may help heal relationships.
Acknowledge realities of situation and inability to change others.	Family may not change, or relationship may be permanently destroyed. Individual needs to go forward with own life and healing process.

Collaborative

Encourage family participation in multidisciplinary team conference/group therapy as appropriate.	Participation in family and group therapy for 13–18 months increases likelihood of success as interactional issues (e.g., marital conflict, scapegoating of the abused child) can be addressed/dealt with. Involvement with others can help family members to experience new ways of interacting and gain insight into their behavior, providing opportunity for change.
Refer to classes (e.g., Parent Effectiveness), specific disease/disability support groups (including substance abuse resources)/spiritual advisor as indicated.	Can assist family to effect positive change/ enhance conflict resolution. Parents may require positive role modeling to learn nonpunitive child-rearing techniques. Presence of substance abuse problems requires all family members to seek support/assistance in dealing with situation to promote a healthy outcome.

503

Refer family to community programs/resources (e.g., support/psychotherapy groups, social services as needed).

When the individual is willing to accept responsibility for past behavior, self-help organizations help families overcome stigma of situation and achieve greater self-esteem while providing professionally supervised treatment. **Note:** High dropout rates have been reported when abusive parents are referred to traditional community mental health clinics. Parents often view authority figures with suspicion and mistrust and require more personal approaches (e.g., 24-hour availability of counselors, evening and after-hours appointments).

NURSING DIAGNOSIS	GROWTH AND DEVELOPMENT, altered
May Be Related to:	Inadequate caretaking (physical/emotional neglect or abuse)
	Indifference, inconsistent responsiveness, multiple caretakers
	Environmental and stimulation deficiencies
Possibly Evidenced by:	Delay or difficulty in performing skills (including self-care or self-control activities) appropriate for age
	Altered physical growth
	Loss of previously acquired skills, precocious or accelerated skill attainment
	Flat affect, listlessness, decreased responses
Desired Outcomes/Evaluations Criteria— Child Will:	Perform motor, social, and/or expressive skills typical of age group, within scope of individual capabilities.
	Perform self-care and self-control activities appropriate for age/development level.
Parents/Caregivers Will:	Verbalize understanding of developmental delay/deviation and plan(s) for intervention.

ACTIONS/INTERVENTIONS	RATIONALE

Independent

Determine existing condition(s) that contribute to developmental deviation. Note severity/pervasiveness of situation.	May be long-term physical/emotional abuse, situational disruption, or inadequate assistance during period of crisis or transition. Identifying individual situation of abuse/neglect guides choice of interventions.
Ascertain nature of parenting/caretaking activities and parents' expectations of the child (e.g., inadequate, inconsistent, unrealistic/insufficient expectations; lack of stimulation, inappropriate responsiveness and limit-setting).	Provides information about needs of family/child. Parents' unrealistic expectations of the abilities/independence needs of the child may lead to demands for behavior that the child is unable to accomplish or may interfere with the

Identify developmental age/stage of child, expected skills/activities using authoritative texts (e.g., Gesell) or assessment tools (e.g., Draw-a-Person, Denver Developmental Screening Test).

Provide information regarding normal growth and developmental process and appropriate expectations for individual child.

Note significant stressful events that have occurred recently in the family.

Avoid blame when discussing contributing factors.

Support attempts to maintain or return to optimal level of self-control or self-care activities.

Involve parents/caregivers in role-play, group activities.

Provide list/copies of pertinent reference materials.

Collaborative

Consult appropriate professional resources (e.g., occupational/rehabilitation/speech therapists, special education teacher, job counselor).

Encourage attendance at appropriate educational programs (e.g., Parent Effectiveness classes, infant stimulation sessions, nurturing programs).

developmental process. **Note:** Conflict may especially arise during the preschool and teen years, when separation issues are paramount.

Baseline information notes areas of deviation, skills affected, whether pervasive or one area of difficulty. Helps determine options/appropriate interventions.

Helps parents/caregivers to develop realistic expectations about child's abilities and potential.

Losses and separation such as the death of a parent, divorce, or unemployment may tax the supportive abilities of the parents/caregivers.

Parents usually feel inadequate and blame themselves for being "a poor parent." **Note:** Adding blame will not be helpful for changing behavior.

Providing assistance enables parents to progress in learning new skills and helping child develop to fullest potential.

Provides opportunities to practice new behaviors, enhance self-confidence and sense of self-worth.

Bibliotherapy provides information to encourage questions and additional learning.

A team approach is necessary to coordinate an individual plan of care to optimize child's growth and development.

Participation in these activities will provide parent with new skills to promote effective coping and enable avoidance of abusive/neglectful behaviors.

NURSING DIAGNOSIS	SEXUAL dysfunction/SEXUALITY PATTERNS, altered
May Be Related to:	Ineffectual or absent role models; impaired relationship with a significant other
	Vulnerability
	Physical/psychosocial abuse (e.g., harmful relationships)
	Misinformation or lack of knowledge
Possibly Evidenced by:	Verbalization of a problem; reported difficulties, limitations, or changes in sexual behaviors or activities
	Inability to achieve desired satisfaction
	Conflicts involving values
	Seeking of confirmation of desirability

Desired Outcomes/Evaluation Criteria—Client Will:	Verbalize understanding of sexual anatomy/function.
	Identify individual reasons/stressors contributing to situation.
	Discuss satisfying/acceptable sexual practices.
	Demonstrate improved communication and relationship skills.

ACTIONS/INTERVENTIONS	RATIONALE

Independent

Discuss client's perceptions of sexuality as learned in family/relationships. Ask client about past abuse/sexual abuse during history taking.	Gives permission to the client to talk about sex and in a safe environment. Many abused individuals feel guilty about sharing family secrets, fear reaction of others, and are concerned that they will not be believed.
Determine usual pattern of functioning and level of desire as well as vocabulary used by the client.	Provides information about how client views sexual activity and areas of lack of knowledge/misinformation.
Identify sexual problems present for the client, e.g., using sex as a weapon to control/dominate partner; avoiding/afraid of sex; or engaging in promiscuous behavior, seeing sex as an obligation; fear, anger, or disgust with touching (particularly sexual touching); feeling emotionally distant during sexual activity; painful intercourse; or orgasmic difficulty.	Sexual abuse is demonstrated in many different ways depending on the extent, duration, and presence of threat/fear of violence. Survivors and offenders require long-term therapy to change attitudes about sex, sense of self as a person/sexual being, and general feelings related to the abuse.
Identify cultural, religious, and/or value factors and conflicts present.	Beliefs/values of client will affect view of what has happened and feelings about situation, influencing therapeutic treatment program.
Note substance use/abuse.	May affect sexual function/satisfaction, requiring therapeutic intervention.
Avoid making value judgments and be aware of own feelings and response to client expressions, revelations, and/or concerns.	Judgments and negative responses do not help client to cope with situation and may result in client withdrawing and not talking further.
Provide information about anatomy/physiology and individual situation according to client needs.	Lack of accurate knowledge may contribute to problems client is experiencing.
Note coping style exhibited.	Client may use repetition and reenactment of the molestation/abuse incident(s) or may avoid sexual stimuli.
Encourage use of higher-level defenses (e.g., repression, sublimation, and intellectualization) by limit-setting, education, interpretation, and desensitization.	Successful intervention focuses on having the survivors become gradually aware of the painful memories and verbalize them instead of acting them out or avoiding them. **Note:** Goal of therapy is to free individual of emotional anesthesia and the sense of living a "lie," allowing client to begin to feel trust and tolerate intimacy.

Set limits on seductive behavior when displayed. Help client distinguish the difference between acceptable and unacceptable behaviors.

The difference between acceptable physically affectionate behavior and behavior with sexual intent, as well as respect for own and others bodily privacy, needs to be learned. The sexually abused child may have difficulty differentiating affectionate from sexual relationships and may be aroused by routine physical or psychological closeness.

Help client learn to say "No" to sex.

It is difficult for survivors to learn to say "Yes" to sex until they can learn to say "No" at any time.

Encourage careful selection of future sexual partner and delaying sexual activity until a friendship is established. Suggest investigation of new partner's past involvement with the criminal system in regard to abusive behavior.

Helps incest/abuse survivors develop a positive sexual experience. Individuals heal best in relationships high in emotional intimacy and support and low in expectations of sexual interaction. Past behavior/involvement with the justice system can provide clues to future problems that may be anticipated.

Encourage client to share thoughts/concerns with partner.

Appropriate self-disclosure in current/future relationships will help couple develop positive relationship.

Identify sights, sounds, smells, and types of touch that are associated with the event/trigger flashbacks for the survivor. Discuss ways to minimize flashbacks/deal with triggers.

Triggers can cause the feelings and fears to recur. Reexperiencing the event in a flashback is a traumatic occurrence and affects current relationship/intimacy.
Avoiding or learning to deal with triggers helps individual to remain in the safety of the present. For example, a specific sexual position may trigger anxious feelings/flashbacks. Sexual partner "allowing" survivor to take control, choose alternate position can lessen these feelings, promoting trust and enhancing emotional growth.

Tell the client that recovery is possible.

May believe that problems will last forever, and it can be reassuring to hear that therapy can help the client gain a positive, healthy perspective on sex and engage in positive relationships.

Collaborative

Refer to clinical nurse specialist, professional sex therapist, family counseling as appropriate.

Problems may be deep-seated and require specialized/prolonged therapy.

507

PREMENSTRUAL DYSPHORIC DISORDER
(Premenstrual Syndrome)

DSM-IV
Premenstrual dysphoric disorder (provided for further study)

Recommended for further systematic clinical study and research, Premenstrual Dysphoric Disorder (popularly called PMS) is characterized by multiple symptom clusters occurring during the menstrual cycle, becoming progressively disabling. Some research suggests these symptoms may be a delayed effect of hormonal changes earlier in the menstrual cycle, or the result of an independent cyclical mood disorder that is synchronized with the menstrual cycle. Although the physical symptoms produce discomfort, the mood change or premenstrual negative affect symptoms are often more distressing, interfering with familial, social, and work-related activities. The condition usually improves after the onset of menses; however, for some women, symptoms persist through and after menses. The symptoms cannot result solely from cyclic or environmental stress but may be enhanced by these stressors. This diagnosis is not used when the person is experiencing a late luteal phase exacerbation of another disorder, such as major depression, panic disorder, or dysthymia.

ETIOLOGICAL THEORIES
Psychodynamics

Although etiology is not understood, symptoms are believed to be related to the interaction of psychological, social, and biological factors. Underlying personality and psychiatric conditions contribute to how any particular individual deals with these physical problems. An individual's past and present negative attitudes toward menstruation are likely to influence the symptomatology of Premenstrual Dysphoric Disorder. Emotion is the result of complex interactions between hormonal changes and cognitive variables. Hormonal changes during the menstrual cycle are likely to increase the female's susceptibility to negative psychological experiences rather than to cause such experiences.

Biological

Although not completely understood, it may be related to the alterations (fluctuations) in estrogen and progesterone and the fluid-retaining action of estrogen during the menstrual cycle. Estrogen excess/deficiency, progesterone deficiency, vitamin deficiency, hypoglycemia, and fluid retention have all been proposed to contribute to Premenstrual Dysphoric Disorder. In addition, levels of androgen, adrenal hormones, and prolactin have been hypothesized to be important in the etiology of this syndrome. Finally, an increase in prostaglandins secreted by the uterine musculature has been implicated in accounting for the pain associated with this disorder.

Family Dynamics

The behaviors associated with this disorder may be learned through modeling during the socialization process. Children may observe and identify with this behavior in significant adults and incorporate it into their own responses as they grow up. Positive reinforcement in the form of primary or secondary gains for these behaviors may perpetuate the learned patterns of disability.

CLIENT ASSESSMENT DATA BASE
Activity/Rest

Decreased interest in usual activities; lack of regular exercise

Sleep disorders (hypersomnia, insomnia)
Fatigue, lethargy; restlessness

Circulation

Heart pounding/palpitations
Increased sweating/diaphoresis

Ego Integrity

Changes in body image (e.g., feeling fat, ugly)
Anxiety, feelings of being unable to cope, sense of loss of control/powerlessness
Mood swings; irritability, frustration, crying spells

Elimination

Urinary frequency or retention, oliguria; recurrent cystitis
Constipation; diarrhea

Food/Fluid

Increased appetite/food craving (e.g., sugar)
Nausea, vomiting
Poor nutritional habits; overeating
Difficulty maintaining a stable weight/transient weight gain
Abdominal bloating
Swelling of extremities, generalized edema

Neurosensory

Headaches (classic migraine)
Dizziness or fainting, vertigo, syncope
Paresthesias of extremities; trembling
Visual disturbances; ringing in ears
Aggravation of seizure activity
Mental Status
  Decreased concentration, forgetfulness, confusion
  Sense of depersonalization
  Nervous tension, impatience, anger, hostility, aggressiveness
  Personality changes (mood swings) not unlike Jekyll and Hyde (e.g., feeling happy or
    serene during the follicular phase of the menstrual cycle and tense, irritable, and
    depressed beginning any time in the luteal phase but primarily during the last week),
    occurring during most menstrual cycles and ceasing at the onset of the menstrual
    period
  Irrational thought processes involving guilt or suicide

Pain/Discomfort

Abdominal cramping
Breast tenderness, joint and muscle stiffness/pain, backache

Respiration

Nasal congestion
Hoarseness
Aggravation of asthmatic episodes

509

Safety

Skin changes: acne, neurodermatitis; easy bruising
Conjunctivitis
Suicidal ideation/attempts

Sexuality

Intolerance or multiple side effects to birth control pills (however, a small percentage of
    women report improvement in condition)
Breast swelling
Changes in sexual drive
History of pregnancy-induced hypertension

Social Interactions

Interference with the quality of life (home, social, and work)
Difficulty with relationships
Nagging behavior/interactions

Teaching/Learning

Age of onset may be any time after menarche but may not be noticeable until the 20s (may
    not seek treatment until 30s or 40s, when the symptoms worsen)
May have close female relative(s) with similar problems
Alcohol/other drug intolerance or addictions

DIAGNOSTIC STUDIES

As indicated by individual situation, dependent on age, medication, therapy, family history, and symptomatology and may include testing to rule out general medical conditions that may present with dysphoria and fatigue exacerbated during the premenstrual period (e.g., seizure disorders, thyroid/other endocrine disorders, cancer, systemic lupus erythematosus, anemias, endometriosis, and various infectious processes).

Measurement of Circulating Reproductive Hormones and/or Daily Self-Rating: Determines the timing of luteal and follicular phases in women who have had a subtotal hysterectomy.

Serum Progesterone and Estradiol 17 (Midluteal Phase): Assesses inadequate luteal phase.

Serum Prolactin and TSH: Rules out pituitary/thyroid abnormalities in client with galactorrhea.

Adrenal Suppression Test: Locates source of androgen excess and serves as a guide for therapy for clients with hirsutism.

Abraham Menstrual System Questionnaire (MSQ), the Dalton Diagnostic Checklist (or Similar Premenstrual Symptoms Worksheet), and Calendar of Premenstrual Symptoms (Minimum 2 Months): Self-reporting tools to determine cycles of symptoms and degree of impairment.

Psychological Assessment: Minnesota Multiphasic Personality Inventory (MMPI) administered twice—once during the follicular phase of the menstrual cycle and again during the luteal phase (preferably the client's most critical day) of the menstrual cycle to identify psychological components and degree of impairment.

NURSING PRIORITIES

1. Provide emotional support and relief of symptoms.
2. Present information about condition/healthcare needs and resources.
3. Encourage adoption of a lifestyle promoting health and diminishing premenstrual symptoms.

DISCHARGE GOALS

1. Assertive behavior/stress-management techniques used to manage problems.
2. PMS condition understood and sources for assistance are identified.
3. Lifestyle changes to promote health/diminish symptoms implemented.
4. Family/SO participating in treatment process.
5. Plan in place to meet needs after discharge.

NURSING DIAGNOSIS	ANXIETY [moderate to panic]
May Be Related to:	Cyclic changes in female hormones affecting other systems
Possibly Evidenced by:	Increased tension; apprehension, jitteriness
	Impaired functioning, feelings of inability to cope/loss of control; depersonalization
	Somatic complaints
Desired Outcomes/Evaluation Criteria—Client Will:	Verbalize awareness of feelings of anxiety.
	Identify healthy ways to deal with feelings.
	Appear relaxed and report anxiety is reduced to a manageable level.
	Use resources/support systems effectively.

ACTIONS/INTERVENTIONS	RATIONALE
Independent	
Assess level of anxiety and degree of interference with daily activities/interpersonal relationships.	Degree to which this disorder is affecting life will indicate need for/type of intervention.
Review history and have client maintain a premenstrual symptom calendar, noting occurrence of nervous tension, mood swings, irritability, and anxiety.	Identifies established patterns of symptoms, allowing for proactive intervention to break cycle of increasing irritability, muscle tension, and escalating feelings of anxiety.
Review with client the premenstrual worksheet, confidential personal data sheets, and Life Events Stress Scale.	Joint evaluation of all the data, noting the interaction between life stress and premenstrual symptoms, is essential to making a correct diagnosis and developing an appropriate treatment program.
Encourage client to acknowledge and express feelings, accepting client's perception of the situation.	Listening to the client promotes feelings of worthwhileness and normalcy, thereby reducing anxiety.
Have client keep a diary of feelings and precipitating factors.	Guided therapeutic writing helps client become more in tune with own body/responses, enhancing ability to intervene/control situation.
Demonstrate/encourage use of stress-reduction techniques, relaxation and visualization skills.	Enhances ability to relax and flow with the discomfort/pain, provides sense of control, and helps to reduce anxiety.

511

Recommend involvement in regular aerobic exercise program such as fast walking, jogging, dancing as individually appropriate.

Provides outlet for tension and promotes release of endorphins, which improve mood and increases sense of general well-being. **Note:** Exercise therapy need not be intensive to achieve desired effect

Help client use anxiety to promote understanding and deal with situation.

A moderate degree of anxiety can be helpful to heighten awareness, and when client learns to use this, problem-solving can be enhanced.

Identify helpful resources/people (e.g., physicians, nurse practitioners/clinicians, psychiatrist/ psychologist, lay support groups).

Professionals who specialize in this disorder can assist client to accept self-feelings as reality-based and begin to identify necessary lifestyle changes.

Collaborative

Administer medications, as indicated:
    Antianxiety, e.g., alprazolam (Xanax), diazepam (Valium);

May be used for short-term control of anxiety.
Dose may be increased as necessary to prevent panic attacks during the luteal phase.

B complex vitamins, especially B_6;

Helpful in reducing feelings of irritability, fatigue, anxiety, and depression.

Calcium carbonate (Os-Cal, Titrilac).

Recent investigational study suggests that most women experience significant reeducation in pain and emotional symptoms while using this product.

Refer client who does not respond to treatment regimen within 3 months for further evaluation of premature menopause, hypoglycemia, diabetes, hypothyroidism, polycystic ovaries, and ovarian failure, as indicated.

Although $1/3$ of clients seeking treatment respond to an initial multifaceted, nonhormonal treatment regimen within 3 months, it is important to rule out hormonal abnormalities, as the client will respond best to treatment for specific need.

NURSING DIAGNOSIS	PAIN, chronic
May Be Related to:	Changes in estrogen/progesterone levels; increased secretion of prostaglandins
	Vitamin deficiency; hypoglycemia
	Fluid retention
Possibly Evidenced by:	Reports of headache, breast tenderness; lower abdominal pain, backache
	Nervousness and irritability; changes in sleep patterns
	Physical and social withdrawal
Desired Outcomes/Evaluations Criteria— Client Will:	Initiate individually appropriate lifestyle changes.
	Verbalize relief from pain/discomforts associated with condition.
	Actively engage in routine ADLs and social activities.

ACTIONS/INTERVENTIONS	RATIONALE

Independent

Note and record type, duration, and intensity of pain.

Determination of the characteristics of pain is necessary to formulate an accurate plan.

Recommend comfort measures (e.g., back rub, warm bath, heating pad) with a matter-of-fact approach that does not provide added attention to the pain behavior.

May serve to provide some temporary relief of pain. Secondary gains from solicitous response may provide nontherapeutic reinforcement to the behavior.

Encourage adequate rest and sleep. Recommend avoiding stressful activity during the premenstrual period.

Fatigue exaggerates associated symptoms. Stress elicits heightened symptoms of anxiety during this period, affecting perception of pain.

Discuss/demonstrate with activities and techniques that distract from focus on self and pain, such as visual or auditory distractions, guided imagery, breathing exercises, massage, application of heat or cold, and other relaxation techniques.

Use of techniques described may help to reduce muscle tension, refocus attention, and provide a sense of control, thus preventing the discomfort from becoming disabling.

Provide positive reinforcement for times when client is not focusing on self and personal discomfort and is functioning independently.

May encourage repetition of desired independent behaviors while eliminating the secondary gain of dependency for the client.

Support use of biofeedback techniques.

May be useful in relieving tension and reducing severity of headaches.

Collaborative

Provide medication as indicated:

When other measures are insufficient to bring about relief, symptomatic drug therapy may be necessary/useful.

Premsyn PMS;

Nonprescription drug containing acetaminophen (for pain relief), pyrilamine (antihistamine for relief of tension, cramps, and irritability), and pamabrom (a mild potassium-sparing diuretic for water related symptoms), which has been effective in treating mild to moderate PMS.

Diuretics, e.g., hydrochlorothiazide (Esidrix, HydroDIURIL), furosemide (Lasix);

Provides relief from discomfort of bloating and edema when fluid retention is extreme and does not respond to other measures (e.g., diet and sodium restriction).

Nonsteroidal antiinflammatory agents, e.g., ibuprofen (Motrin);

May be effective for relief of pain due to increased prostaglandin secretion.

Propranolol (Inderal), naproxen (Naprosyn);

May be used for prophylactic treatment of migraine.

Muscle relaxants, diazepam (Valium);

Useful in relieving severe muscular tension.

Bromocriptin (Parlodel);

Although studies do not show clear benefit, some women report control of pain of mastodynia and other premenstrual symptoms that may be caused by elevated prolactin, although side effects (especially nausea) may preclude use in some clients.

Vitamin E supplement;

May reduce breast tenderness.

Sumatriptan (Imitrex).

Highly effective in the treatment of acute migraine attack.

OTHER CONDITIONS: Premenstrual Dysphoric Disorder

513

NURSING DIAGNOSIS

COPING, INDIVIDUAL, ineffective

May Be Related to:

Personal vulnerability; threat to self-concept

Multiple stressors (premenstrual symptoms) repeated over period of time

Poor nutrition

Work overload, lack of leisure activities

Possibly Evidenced by:

Verbalization of difficulty coping/problem-solving or inability to ask for help

Emotional/muscular tension; chronic fatigue, insomnia; lack of appetite or overeating

High illness rate

Inability to meet role expectations; alteration in societal participation

Desired Outcomes/Evaluation Criteria—Client Will:

Identify ineffective coping behaviors and consequences.

Meet psychological needs as evidenced by appropriate expression of feelings, identification of options, and use of resources.

Participate in ongoing treatment program.

ACTIONS/INTERVENTIONS

RATIONALE

Independent

ACTIONS/INTERVENTIONS	RATIONALE
Assess current functional level/coping ability, noting substance use, smoking habits, eating patterns.	Identifies needs and appropriate interventions for individual situation.
Note understanding of current situation and previous methods of dealing with life problems.	Provides information about how the client views what is happening and provides opportunity for her to look at previous methods of coping that may be helpful now.
Determine effect(s) of problem on client's relationships/family. Include partner/SOs in process, as appropriate.	Destructive impact of symptoms can seriously undermine family systems, resulting in alienation, divorce. Including family promotes open communication and provides opportunity for increased understanding and problem-solving.
Identify extent of feelings and situations when loss of control occurs. Discuss/problem-solve behaviors to protect self/others (e.g., call support person, remove self from situation).	Recognition of potential for harm to self/others and development of plan enables client to take effective actions to meet safety needs.
Discuss importance of learning new coping strategies and developing more supportive relationships.	Realization that past behaviors have contributed to current situation/lack of support may provide impetus for change.
Encourage client to reduce or shift workload and social activities during the premenstrual period as part of a total stress-management program.	Coping realistically with life stresses, and reducing responsibility may relieve stress and therefore help relieve symptoms.

514

Have client identify most troublesome symptoms, which may persist after initial therapy trials.

If other measures are inadequate/unsuccessful, pharmacologic treatment may be needed to enhance coping abilities.

Collaborative

Review psychological assessments such as MMPI and clinical interview. (First MMPI should be taken during the follicular phase, second during the most critical day of the luteal phase.)

MMPI results can show very different patterns of emotional and personality functioning between those two phases. Evaluation of these tests can determine the difference in emotional overlay and psychological functioning. Consideration of these results is essential to an accurate picture of an individual's dynamics, coping skills, and stresses, which play such a significant role in this problem.

Provide counseling with review of previous month's diary, evaluating symptoms and effects of therapy, as well as client relationship(s).

This opportunity for assessing ongoing problems and making needed changes helps both client and nurse to know whether program is successful.

Administer medications as indicated, e.g.
    Hormonal manipulation: oral contraceptive, progesterone vaginal suppositories or injections;

May be useful for some clients to relieve premenstrual symptoms when nonpharmacological measures have not been effective.

    Tricyclic antidepressants: amitriptyline (Elavil);

Used for depression that does not respond as other symptoms are resolved.

    Prostaglandin inhibitors: NSAIDs (e.g., Motrin), steroids;
    Lithium carbonate (Eskalith);

Relieves dysmenorrhea.

May be used in the presence of affective lability when other treatments have not been successful.

    Gonadotropin-releasing hormone agonist (GnRHa): nafarelin (Synarel).

GnRHa has recently been shown to help some women with severe symptoms. Therapy is expensive and extreme. Estrogen and progesterone therapy must be implemented to allow safe use of GnRHa regimen.

Encourage participation in support group, psychotherapy, marital counseling on a regular basis.

May help client/family members learn effective coping strategies and support indicated lifestyle changes.

NURSING DIAGNOSIS	KNOWLEDGE deficit [LEARNING NEED] regarding condition, prognosis, self care and treatment needs
May Be Related to:	Lack of exposure to, misinterpretation of/unfamiliarity with resources
	Inaccurate/incomplete information presented
Possibly Evidenced by:	Verbalization of the problem; request for information; statement of misconception
	Inappropriate or exaggerated behaviors (e.g., hysterical, hostile, agitated)
	Exacerbation of symptoms

ACTIONS/INTERVENTIONS	RATIONALE
Independent	
Determine client's/SO's knowledge of PMS and misconceptions about condition.	Identifies individual needs and provides opportunity to clarify misunderstandings.
Provide written and verbal information about condition.	Provides different methods for accessing/reinforcing information and enhances opportunity for learning/understanding.
Encourage client to limit/stop smoking.	Smoking decreases the absorption of vitamins and may sustain PMS symptoms.
Suggest participation in regular exercise program.	Exercise therapy increases the release of certain neurotransmitters in the brain (endorphins) that are important in regulation mood.
Encourage client to do breast self-exam regularly. Demonstrate procedure and provide instructional brochure.	Although this is important for *all* women to perform, clients with PMS may have a higher incidence of breast cancer.
Review medication regimen, importance of followup visits to healthcare provider.	Understanding enhances cooperation and promotes ongoing evaluation/adjustment of treatment program.
Suggest client continue diary activity, recording symptoms and interventions used, and response.	Useful in determining effectiveness of therapy/need for change.
Have client keep a nutritional survey/record entire food and liquid intake for 3 months.	Assists in determining whether the client's diet is a contributing/aggravating factor. (Commercial computer analysis may be available for interpretation of the survey.)
Discuss recommended diet plan, e.g.,	Beginning an early self-help program may relieve clinical symptoms and encourage the client emotionally.
Limit red meat to 3 ounces/day, reduce intake of fats, especially saturated fats;	Decreases arachidonic acid, which helps balance PGE_1 ("good") with PGE_2 ("bad") prostaglandin, improving many premenstrual symptoms.
Limit dairy products to 2 servings a day;	Excessive dairy products block the absorption of magnesium.
Increase intake of complex carbohydrates (vegetables, legumes, cereals, and whole grains) and foods containing linoleic acid (e.g., safflower oil);	Stimulates insulin release in a less abrupt and more sustained manner. Although the value of linoleic acid has not been proven, some women have found it to be helpful for the relief of PMS symptoms.

Decrease intake of refined and simple sugars;	Reduces possibility of rapid release of insulin, which could lower blood sugar and initiate craving for sweets, thus creating a vicious cycle. Additionally, excess sugar is thought to cause nervous tension, palpitations, headache, dizziness, drowsiness, and excretion of magnesium in the urine, thus preventing the body from breaking down sugar for energy.
Decrease salt intake to below 3 g/day, but not less than 0.5 g/day;	Insulin prevents the kidneys from excreting salt; however, too little salt stimulates norepinephrine and causes sleep disturbances. Salt restriction also prevents edema.
Limit intake of methylxanthines (coffee and chocolate) and alcohol (1 or 2 drinks a week).	These substances can increase breast tenderness, pain, and may negate the therapeutic effect of vitamins. Alcohol can cause reactive hypoglycemia and fluid retention, and may be the biggest reason for treatment failure.
Review need for complete vitamin therapy program, such as Optivite.	Women with this disorder tend to eat more junk food and to be too busy to eat a well-balanced diet; therefore, the client may be deficient in vitamins and minerals, which act as cofactors in a number of chemical reactions in the body and are involved in making, using, and excreting hormones.
Refer to available support groups/research centers.	Provides additional resources to understand and deal with condition.

Bibliography

General

Books

Berkow, R (ed): The Merck Manual, ed 16. Merck Research Laboratories, Rahway, NJ, 1992.

Capers, DF: Culture and Nursing Practice: An Applied View. Holistic Nursing Practice, 6(3). Aspen, Frederick, MD, April 1992.

Cox, HC, et al: Clinical Applications of Nursing Diagnosis, ed 3. FA Davis, Philadelphia, 1997.

Deglin, J, and Vallerand, AH: Davis's Drug Guide for Nurses, ed 5. FA Davis, Philadelphia, 1997.

Doenges, ME, and Moorhouse, MF: Nurse's Pocket Guide: Nursing Diagnoses with Interventions, ed 5. FA Davis, Philadelphia, 1996.

Doenges, M, Moorhouse, MF, and Geissler, A: Nursing Care Plans, Guidelines for Planning and Documenting Patient Care, ed 4. FA Davis, Philadelphia, 1997.

DSM-IV. American Psychiatric Association, Washington, DC, 1994.

Gorman, LM, Sultan, DF, and Raines, ML: Davis's Manual of Psychosocial Nursing for General Patient Care. FA Davis, Philadelphia, 1996.

Hays, J, and Larson, K: Interacting with Patients. Macmillan, New York, 1963.

Hyman, SE, and Tesar, GE: Manual of Psychiatric Emergencies, ed 3. Little, Brown, Boston, 1994.

Moir, A, and Jessel, D: Brain Sex. Dell, New York, 1991.

Nursing Diagnoses: Definitions and Classification. NANDA, Philadelphia.

Shader, RI (ed): Manual of Psychiatric Therapeutics, ed 2. Little, Brown, Boston, 1994.

Thomas, CL (ed): Taber's Cyclopedic Medical Dictionary, ed 18. FA Davis, Philadelphia, 1997.

Townsend, MC: Drug Guide for Psychiatric Nursing, ed 2. FA Davis, Philadelphia, 1994.

Townsend, MC: Nursing Diagnosis in Psychiatric Nursing: A Pocket Guide for Care Plan Construction, ed 4. FA Davis, Philadelphia, 1997.

Townsend, MC: Psychiatric Mental Health Nursing: Concepts of Care, ed 2. FA Davis, Philadelphia, 1996.

Articles

Anderson, LN, and Clarke, JT: De-escalating verbal aggression in primary care settings. The Nurse Practitioner 21(10):10, October 1996.

Canatsey, K, Bermudez, L, and Roper, JM: The homicidal patient: When a plan of care violates standards of care. J Psychosoc Nurs 32(11):13, November 1994.

Cashin, A: Seclusion: The quest to determine effectiveness. J Psychosoc Nurs 34(11):17, November 1996.

Calfee, BE: Documenting suicide risk. Nursing 96 26(7):17, July 1996.

Maier, GJ: Managing threatening behavior: The role of talk down and talk up. J Psychosoc Nurs 34(6):25, June 1996.

Maxfield, M, and Pennington, E: Behavior management training for long-term care staff: A note of caution. J Psychosoc Nurs 34(12):37, December 1996.

McGihon, NN: Writing as a therapeutic modality. J Psychosoc Nurs 34(6):25, June 1996.

Medina, J: Genetic study of human behavior. Its progress and limitations. Harvard Mental Health Letter 12(10):4, April 1996.

Shames, KH: Harness the power of guided imagery. RN 59(8):49, August 1996.

Shinkarovsky, L: Hyponotherapy, not just hocus-pocus. RN 59(6):55, June 1996.

No author: Suicide—Part II. Harvard Mental Health Letter 13(6):1, December 1996.

Chapter 1

Books

American Managed Behavioral Healthcare Association Quality Improvement and Clinical Services Committee, Performance Measures for Managed Behavioral Healthcare Program. AMBHA, Washington, DC, PERMS 1.0, 1–27, August 1995.

Restak, R: The Brain Has a Mind of Its Own. Harmony Books, New York, 1991.

Articles

Anthony, WA: Managed care outcomes—"In recovery, with places to be and symptom free." Psychiatr 19(2):73, February 1995.

Bailey, KP: Preparing for prescriptive practice. J Psychosoc Nurs 34(1):16, January 1996.

Carter, R: Don't forget the mentally ill. *The Denver Post*, p 1E, Sunday, August 22, 1993.

Cowan, PJ: Women's mental health issues, reflections on past attitudes and present practices. J Psychosoc Nurs 34(4):20, April 1996.

Comas-Diaz, L and Greene, B: Women of color: Integrating ethnic and gender identities in psychotherapy. J Psychosoc Nurs 34(8):52, August 1996.

Dawson, PJ: The impact of biological psychiatry on psychiatric nursing. J Psychosoc Nurs 34(8):28, August 1996.

DeMasi, ME, et al: Specifying dimensions of recovery. Paper presented at 6th Annual National Conference on State Mental Health Agency Services Research and Program Evaluation, Arlington, VA, February 1996.

Gordon, S, and Fagin, CM: Preserving the moral high ground. Am J Nurs 96(3):31, March 1996.

Harding, CM, and Zahniser, JH: Empirical corrections of seven myths about schizophrenia with implications for treatment. Acta Psychiatr Scand 1994: 90(Suppl 384): 140–146. Copyright Munksgaard, Printed in Denmark.

Hardy, B: If men are really from Mars and women are really really from Venus, then how are you changing your psychosocial care? J Psychosoc Nurs 34(8):50, August 1996.

Henderson, VA: Some observations on the health care 'industry.' Am J Nurs 96(3):16M, March 1996.

Iglehart, JK, and Iglehart, K: Health policy report—Managed care and mental health. N Engl J Med 334(2):131, January 1996.

Klinkenberg, WD, and Calsyn, RJ: Aftercare and rehospitalization of people with severe mental illness. J Psychosoc Nurs 34(8):51, August 1996.

Lee, S: Clinical pathways for case management. Continuing Care 14(6):12, July/August 1995.

McCrone, SH: The impact of the evolution of biological psychiatry on psychiatric nursing. J Psychosoc Nurs 34(1):38, January 1996.

Plante, TC: Getting physical, does exercise help in the treatment of psychiatric disorders? J Psychosoc Nurs 34(3):38, March 1996.

Robinette, AL: PCLNs: Who are they? How can they help you? Am J Nurs 96(7):48, July 1996.

Schaffer, I, et al: Dialogue. Behavioral Healthcare Tomorrow, p 40, September/October 1995.

Southwick, K: The most costly mental illness. Managed Healthcare, p 13, June 1995.

Weissman, SM: Damaged care for mental ills. Legal Times, p 36, March 4, 1996.

Zander, K: Case management in acute care: Making the connections. The Case Manager 2 (20):40, 1991.

Zander, K: Managed care within acute care settings: Design and implementation via nursing case management. Health Case Supervisor 6(2):27, 1988.

No author: Mental health services in a managed care era. Nurs Trends and Issues 1(6):4, December 1997.

Chapter 2

American Nurses Association: Nursing: A Social Policy Statement. Pub Code NP-63 3SM, 12/80, Kansas City, MO, 1980.

American Nurses Association: Standards of Nursing Practice. Pub Code NO-41, 10M 1:77, Kansas City, MO, 1991.

Statement on Psychiatric-Mental Health Clinical Nursing Practice and Standards of Psychiatric-Mental Health Clinical Nursing Practice. American Nurses Publishing, Washington, DC, 1994.

Books

Doenges, ME, and Moorhouse, MF: Application of Nursing Process and Nursing Diagnosis: An Interaction Text, ed 2. FA Davis, Philadelphia, 1995.

Shore, LS: Nursing Diagnosis: What It Is and How To Do It, A Programmed Text. Medical College of Virginia Hospitals, Richmond, VA, 1988.

Articles

Brooks, KL (ed): Critical thinking in clinical practice. Holistic Nursing Practice 7(3), April 1993.

Chapter 3

Books

Bates, B: A Guide to Physical Examination, ed 5. JB Lippincott, Philadelphia, 1991.

Lampe, SS: Focus Charting, ed 4. Creative Nursing Management, Minneapolis, 1986.

Articles

Wheeland, RM: Focus charting: In a psychiatric facility. J Psychosoc Nurs 31(12):15, December 1993.

Chapter 4

Books

Gordon, T: Teaching Children Self-Discipline, At Home and At School. Random House, New York, 1989.

Articles

Berthier, ML, Bayes, A, and Tolosa, EA: Magnetic resonance imaging in patients with concurrent Tourette's disorder and Asperger's syndrome. J Am Acad Child Adolesc Psychiatry 32(3):633, May 1993.

Blair, DT, and Ramones, VA: The undertreament of anxiety: Overcoming the confusion and stigma. J Psychosoc Nurs 34(6):9, June 1996.

Buchalter, G: To break the silence. Parade Magazine, p 13, August 4, 1996.

Campbell, M, et al: Lithium in hospitalized aggressive children with conduct disorder: A double-blind and placebo-controlled study. J Am Acad Child Adolesc Psychiatry 34(4):445, April 1995.

Capps, L, et al: Parental perception of emotional expressiveness in children with autism. J Consult Clin Psychol 61(3):475, January 1993.

DeLong, R, and Nohria, C: Psychiatric family history and neurological disease in autistic spectrum disorders. Dev Med Child Neurol 36(5):441, May 1994.

Earle, KA, and Forquer, SL: Use of seclusion with children and adolescents in public psychiatric hospitals. Am J Orthopsychiatry 65(2):238, April 1995.

King, W: New treatments aid autistic kids. The Denver Post, p 21A, May 30, 1996.

Locke, J, and Straus, GD: Psychiatric hospitalization of adolescents for conduct disorder. Hosp & Community Psychiatry 45(9):925, Sept 1994.

Offord, DR, and Bennett, KJ: Conduct disorder: Long-term outcomes and intervention effectiveness. J Am Acad Child Adolesc Psychiatry 33(8):1069, October 1994.

Restall, G, and Magill-Evans, J: Play and preschool children with autism. Am J Occupa Ther, 48 (2):113, February 1994.

Piven, J, et al: An MRI study of brain size in autism. Am J Psychiatry, 152(8):1145, August 1995.

Rogers, SJ, Ozonoff, S, and Maslin-Cole, C: Developmental aspects of attachment in young children with pervasive developmental disorders. J Am Acad Child Adolesc Psychiatry 32(6):1274, November 1993.

Ryan, R: Treatment-resistant chronic mental illness: Is it Asperger's syndrome? Hospital & Community Psychiatry 43(8):807, August 1992.

Straus, G, Chassin, M, and Lock, J: Can experts agree when to hospitalize adolescents? 145th Annual Psychiatric Association, J Am Acad Child Adolesc Psychiatry 34(2):418, April 1995.

Volkmar, FR, and Rutter, M: Childhood disintegrative disorder: Results of the DSM IV Autism field trial. J Am Acad Child Adolesc Psychiatry 34(8):1092, August 1995.

Webster-Stratton, C: Advancing videotape parenting training: A comparison study at University School of Nursing, Parenting Clinic, Seattle. US J Consult & Clin Psychol 62(3):583, June 1994.

Wolraich, ML, Wilson, DB, and White, JW: The effect of sugar on behavior or cognition in children. JAMA, 274(20):1617, November 22–29, 1995.

No author: Attention deficit disorder—part I. Harvard Mental Health Letter 11(10):1, April 1995.

No author: Attention deficit disorder—part II. Harvard Mental Health Letter 11(11):1, May 1995.

No author: Bedwetting traced to genetic flaw. Science News 148(7):11, August 12, 1995.

No author: Panic attacks and panic disorder—part I. Harvard Mental Health Letter, 12(10):1, April 1996.

No author: Pain attacks and panic disorder—part II. Harvard Mental Health Letter 12(11):1, May 1996.

No author: Some ADHD kids ride bipolar express. Science News 150(7):111, August 17, 1996.

Chapter 5

Books

Early Identification of Alzheimer's Disease and Related Dementias: Clinical Practice Guideline. US Department of Health and Human Services, Public Health Service Agency for Health Care Policy and Research, Rockville, MD, 1996.

Articles

Aplin, CT: Group therapy for family caregivers of patients with Alzheimer's. Awareness 24(1):27, Fall 1996.

Bonnel, WB: Not gone and not forgotten: A spouse's experience of late-stage Alzheimer's disease. J Psychosoc Nurs 34(8):23, August 1996.

Burney-Puckett, M: Sundown syndrome: Etiology and management. J Psychosoc Nurs 34(5):40, May 1996.

Corliss, J: Alzheimer's in the news. HealthNews 2(15):1, October 29, 1996.

Engel, K and Frame, MW: Ethical and legal guidelines when counseling HIV/AIDS clients: Guidelines for counselors. Awareness 24(1):22, Fall 1996.

Fackelmann, K: Forecasting Alzeheimer's disease: Brain scans and writing samples may predict dementia. Science News 149(20):312, May 18, 1996.

Hall, GR: Acute confusion in the elderly. Nursing 26(7):32, July 1996.

Matteson, MA, Linton, AD, and Barnes, SJ: Cognitive developmental approach to dementia. Image: J of Nurs Scholarship 28(3):233, Fall 1996.

Montgomery, D: The benefits of wandering. Nursing96 26(6):24, June 1996.

Peterson, RC, et al: More on APOE-4. Harvard Mental Health Letter 12(5):7, November 1995.

Ruppert, RA: Caring for the lay caregiver. Am J Nurs 96(3):40, March 1996.

Weiner, MF: What new treatments for Alzheimer's disease are being explored? The Harvard Mental Health Letter 13(1):8, July 1996.

No author: Vitamin E and Alzheimer's disease. HeathNews 3(7):1, May 27, 1997.

Chapter 6

Articles

Gorman, M: The five phases of behavioral change. Am J Nurs 96(7):16, July 1996.

No author: A longer-lasting opioid antagonist. Am J Nurs 96(9):54, September 1996.

No author: Treatment of alcoholism—part I. Harvard Mental Health Letter 13(2):1, August 1996.

No author: Treatment of alcoholism—part II. Harvard Mental Health Letter 13(3):1, September 1996.

No author. Treatment of drug abuse and addiction—part I. Harvard Mental Health Letter 12(2):1, August 1995.

Chapter 7

Books

Moir, A, and Jessel D: Brain Sex. Dell, New York, 1991, Epilogue.

Articles

Benes, FM: Altered neural circuits in schizophrenia. Harvard Mental Health Letter 13(5):5, November 1996.

Bower, B: New culprits cited for schizophrenia. Science News 149(5):68, February 3, 1996.

Fisher, DB: Overcoming schizophrenia. J Psychosoc Nurs 34(9):33, September 1996.

Green, AI, and Patel, JK: The new pharmacology of schizophrenia. Harvard Mental Health Letter 13(6):5, December 1996.

Littrell, K: Olanzapine: A new atypical antipsychotic. J Psychosoc Nurs 34(8):41, August 1996.

McCay, E, Ryan, K, and Amey, S: Mitigating engulfment: Recovering from a first episode of psychosis. J Psychosoc Nurs 34(11):40, November 1996.

Meggison, J, et al: Rh and schizophrenia. Harvard Mental Health Letter 12(11):6, May 1996.

Susser, E, et al: Schizophrenia and the hunger winter. Harvard Mental Health Letter 12(11):7, May 1996.

Zook, R: Take action before anger builds. RN 59(4):46, April 1996.

No author: Genetic hint to schizophrenia. Science News 147(19):297, May 13, 1995.

No author: Schizoaffective disorder. Harvard Mental Health Letter 13(4):1, October 1996.

Chapter 8

Books

Depression in Primary Care, vol 1: Detection and Diagnosis. US Department of Health and Human Service, Public Health Service Agency for Health Care Policy and Research, Rockville, MD, April 1993.

Depression in Primary Care, vol 2: Treatment of Major Depression. US Department of Health and Human Services, Public Health Service Agency for Health Care Policy and Research, April 1993.

Articles

Badger, TA: Living with depression, family members' experiences and treatment needs. J Psychosoc Nurs, 34(1): 21, January 1996.

Bower, B: Depression: Rates in women, men. Science News 147(22):346, June 3, 1995.

Bower, B: Virus may trigger some mood disorders. Science News 147(9):132, March 4, 1995.

Lesseig, DZ: Primary care diagnosis and pharmacologic treatment of depression in adults. Nurse Pract 21(10): 72, October 1996.

Petty, F: What is the role of GABA in mood disorders. Harvard Mental Health Letter, 13(5):8, November 1996.

Pollack, LE: Information seeking among people with manic-depression illness. Image: J Nurs Scholarship 28(3):259, Fall 1996.

Pollack, LE: Inpatients with bipolar disorder: Their quest to understand. J Psychosoc Nurs 34(6):19, June 1996.

No author: Depression's effects run deep. HealthNews 2(16):5, November 19, 1996.

No author: Depressive and manic-depressive illness fact sheet. J Psychosoc Nurs 34(8):7, August 1996.

No author: Manic depression—DNA links. Science News 149(14):221, April 6, 1996.

No author: The relationship between serotonin and depression. Am J Psychiatry 153(2):174, February 1996.

No author: Suicide—part I. Harvard Mental Health Letter 13(5):1, November 1996.

Chapter 9

Books

Dollar, J, and Miller, N: Personality and Psychotherapy. McGraw-Hill, New York, 1950.

Articles

Brown, P, and Yanatis, J: Personal space intrusion and PTSD. J Psychosoc Nurs 34(7):23, July 1996.

Blair, DT, and Ramones, VA: The undertreatment of anxiety: Overcoming the confusion and stigma. J Psychosoc Nurs 34(6):9, June 1996.

Blair, DT, and Ramones, VA: Understanding vicarious traumatization. J Psychsoc Nurs 34(11):24, November 1996.

Bower, B: Trauma syndrome traverses generations. Science News 149(20):310, May 18, 1996.

Herbert, JD, and Mueser, KT: What is EMDR? Harvard Mental Health Letter 12(2):1, August 1995.

Spear, HL: Anxiety, when to worry, what to do. RN 59(7):40, July 1996.

Spencer, VE: Combined therapies in OCD. J Psychosoc Nurs 34(7):37, July 1996.

Zook, R: Take action before anger builds. RN 59(4):46, April 1996.

No author: Panic attacks and panic disorder—part I. Harvard Mental Health Letter, 12(10):1, April 1996.

No author: Pain attacks and panic disorder—part II. Harvard Mental Health Letter, 12(11):1, May 1996.

No author: Obsessive-compulsive disorder. Harvard Mental Health Letter 12(5):1, November 1995.

No author: Prediction and early detection of post-traumatic stress disorder in injured trauma survivors. Am J Psychiatry 153(2):219, February 1996.

No author: Post-traumatic stress disorder—part I. Harvard Mental Health Letter 12(1):1, June 1996.

No author: Post-traumatic stress disorder—part I. Harvard Mental Health Letter 13(12):1, July 1996.

Chapter 10

Articles

Bower, B: Deceptive appearances, imagined physical defects take an ugly personal toll. Science News 148(3):40, July 15, 1995.

Smith, GR, Rost, K, and Kashner, M: First aid for somatizers. Harvard Mental Health Letter, 12(2):6, August 1995.

Chapter 11

Articles

Curtin, SL: Recognizing multiple personality disorder. J Psychosoc Nurs 31(2):29, February 1993.

Stafford, LL: Dissociation and multiple personality disorders: A challenge for psychosocial nurses. J Psychosoc Nurs 31(1):15, January 1993.

Chapter 12

Books

Hyde, J: Understanding Human Sexuality, ed 4. McGraw-Hill, New York, 1990.

Moir, A, and Jessel, D: Brain Sex. Dell, New York, 1991, Chapter 8.

Articles

Beemer, B: Gender dysphoria update. J Psychosoc Nurs 34(4):12, April 1996.

Friedman, RC, and Downey, JI: Psychodynamically oriented therapy for gays and lesbians. Harvard Mental Health Letter 12(5):4, November 1995.

Rubinstein, G: Homosexuality and psychotherapists: A lingering prejudice? Harvard Mental Health Letter 12(11):6, May 1996.

No author: Paraphilias: The dark side of sexual desire. Sex Over Forty 15(9):1, February 1997.

Chapter 13

Articles

Amara, A, and Cerrato, PL: Eating disorders still a threat. RN 59(6):30, June 1996.

McGown, A, and Whitbread, J: Out of control! The most effective way to help the binge-eating patient. J Psychosoc Nurs 34(1):30, January 1996.

Travis, J: Obesity researchers feast on two scoops. Science News 149(1):6, January 6, 1996.

Zerbe, KJ: Eating disordered men require diverse treatment. The Menninger Letter 3(9):4, September 1995.

No author: Childhood sexual abuse and eating disorders. Harvard Mental Health Letter 11(10):7, April 1995.

Chapter 15

Articles

Bower, B: Gene tied to excitable personality. Science News 149(1):4, January 6, 1996.

Bower, B: New data challenge personality gene. Science News 150(18):279, November 2, 1996.

No author: Borderline personality. Harvard Mental Health Letter 10(11):1, May 1994.

Chapter 16

Articles

Chuong, CJ, and Gibbons, WE: Premenstrual syndrome: Update on therapy. Med Aspects of Human Sexuality 24(5):58, May 1990.

Dahlen, P: Working with adult survivors of childhood sexual trauma: An empowerment model. Awareness 24(1):18, Fall 1996.

Draucker, CB, and Petrovic, K: Healing of adult male survivors of childhood sexual abuse. Image J Nurs Sch 28(4):325, Winter 1996.

Foster, T: Munchausen's syndrome: We've met it head on. RN 59(8):17, August 1996.

Limandri, BJ, and Tilden, VP. Nurses' reasoning in the assessment of family violence. Image: J Nurs Sch 28(3):247, Fall 1996.

Lynch, SH: Elder abuse: What to look for, how to intervene. Am J Nurs 97(1):27, January 1997.

McFarlane, J, Parker, B, and Soeken, K: Abuse during pregnancy: Associations with maternal health and infant birth weight. Nurs Res 45(1):37, January/February 1996.

Palmer, L: The impact of child sexual abuse on the children of survivors. J Psychosoc Nurs 34(10):42, October 1996.

Schmidt, PJ, et al: PMS after menstruation. Harvard Mental Health Letter 8(7):5, January 1992.

Taylor, DL: Evaluating therapeutic change in symptom severity at the level of the individual woman experiencing severe PMS. Image: J Nurs Sch 26(1)25, Spring 1994.

Wilkinson, AK: Spousal abuse/homicide a current issue in health risk management. J Psychosoc Nurs 34(10):12, October 1996.

Winslow, EH: Looking out for the abused pregnant woman. Am J Nurs 96(7):54, July 1996.

No author: Post-traumatic stress disorder—part I. Harvard Mental Health Letter 13(1)1, July 1996.

No author: The mind, the body, and the immune system: Part I. Harvard Mental Health Letter 8(7):1, January 1992.

No author: The mind, the body, and the immune system: Part II. Harvard Mental Health Letter 8(8):1, February 1992.

No author: What is late luteal phase dysphoric disorder and why is there a controversy surrounding it? Harvard Mental Health Letter 6(8):8, February 1990.

Appendix 1: Therapeutic and Nontherapeutic Techniques in the Nurse/Client Relationship

Communication in the nurse/client relationship is a skill that promotes understanding and problem-solving for the client. Relating is the desired communication pattern in the establishment of a nurse/client relationship. It is an experience, or series of experiences, characterized by meaningful dialogue between two human beings, in which each individual is aware of, and experiences, openness with, closeness to, and understanding of the other. Every comment made to the client can be evaluated as having therapeutic or nontherapeutic value in that it either contributes to the client's emotional growth or reinforces the illness. Being aware of the potential impact of comments, limiting the frequency of nontherapeutic words, and conscious use of therapeutic communication techniques can provide this meaningful type of dialogue.

THERAPEUTIC TECHNIQUES

1. Silence—absence of verbal communication
2. Accepting—giving indication of reception: "Yes." "Uh hmm." "I follow what you said."
3. Giving recognition—acknowledging, indicating awareness: "Good morning, Mr. D."
4. Offering self—making oneself available: "I'll stay here with you."
5. Giving broad openings—allowing the client to take the initiative in introducing the topic: "Is there something you'd like to talk about?"
6. Offering general leads—giving encouragement to continue: "Go on . . ." "And then . . .?"
7. Placing the event in time or in sequence—clarifying the relationship of events in time: "What seemed to lead up to . . ."
8. Making observations—verbalizing what is perceived: "You appear tense."
9. Encouraging description of perceptions—asking the client to verbalize what he or she perceives: "What is happening?"
10. Encouraging comparison—asking that similarities and differences be noted: "Was it something like . . .?" "Have you had similar experiences?"
11. Restating—repeating the main idea expressed: Client: "I can't sleep, I stay awake all night." Nurse: "You have difficulty sleeping."
12. Reflecting—directing back to the client questions, feelings, and ideas: Client: "Do you think I should tell the doctor . . .?" Nurse: "Do *you* think you should?"
13. Focusing—concentrating on a single point: "This point seems worth looking at more closely."
14. Exploring—delving further into a subject or idea: "Tell me more about that."
15. Giving information—making available the facts the client needs: "My name is . . ." "Visiting hours are . . ."
16. Seeking clarification—seeking to make clear that which is not meaningful or that which is vague. "I'm not sure that I follow."
17. Presenting reality—offering for consideration that which is real: "I see no one else in the room."
18. Voicing doubt—expressing uncertainty as to the reality of the client's perceptions: "Isn't that unusual?"
19. Seeking consensual validation—searching for

mutual understanding, for accord in the meaning of words: "Tell me whether my understanding of it agrees with yours."

20. Verbalizing the implied—voicing what the client has hinted at or suggested: Client: "I can't talk to you or to anyone. It's a waste of time." Nurse: "Is it your belief that no one understands?"

21. Encouraging evaluation—asking the client to appraise the quality of his experiences. "What are your feelings in regard to . . .?"

22. Attempting to translate feelings into words—seeking to verbalize the feelings that are being expressed only indirectly: Client: "I'm dead." Nurse: "Are you suggesting that you feel lifeless?" or "Is it that life seems without meaning?"

23. Suggesting collaboration—offering to share, to strive, to work together with the client for his or her benefit: "Perhaps you and I can discuss and discover what produces your anxiety."

24. Summarizing—organizing and summing up that which has gone before: "Have I got this straight?" "You've said that . . ."

25. Encouraging formulation of a plan of action—asking the client to consider kinds of behavior likely to be appropriate in future situations: "What could you do to let your anger out harmlessly?"

NONTHERAPEUTIC TECHNIQUES

1. Reassuring—indicating that there is no cause for anxiety: "I wouldn't worry about . . ."

2. Giving approval—sanctioning the client's ideas or behavior: "That's good."

3. Rejecting—refusing to consider or showing contempt for the client's ideas or behavior: "Let's not discuss . . ."

4. Disapproving—denouncing the client's behavior or idea: "That's bad."

5. Agreeing—indicating accord with the client: "That's right."

6. Disagreeing—opposing the client's ideas: "That's wrong."

7. Advising—telling the client what to do. "I think you should . . ."

8. Probing—persistent questioning of the client: "Now tell me about . . ."

9. Challenging—demanding proof from the client: "But how can you be President of the United States?"

10. Testing—appraising the client's degree of insight: "Do you still have the idea that . . .?"

11. Defending—attempting to protect someone or something from verbal attack: "This hospital has a fine reputation."

12. Requesting an explanation—asking the client to provide the reasons for thoughts, feelings, behavior, and events: "Why do you think that?"

13. Indicating the existence of an external source—attributing the source of thoughts, feelings, and behavior to others or to outside influences: "What makes you say that?"

14. Belittling feelings expressed—misjudging the degree of the client's discomfort: Client: "I have nothing to live for . . . I wish I was dead." Nurse: "Everybody gets down in the dumps."

15. Making stereotyped comments—offering meaningless cliches, trite expressions: "It's for your own good." "Keep your chin up."

16. Giving literal response—responding to a figurative comment as though it were a statement of fact: Client: "I'm an Easter egg." Nurse: "What shade?"

17. Using denial—refusing to admit that a problem exists. Client: "I'm nothing." Nurse: "Of course you're something. Everybody is somebody."

18. Interpreting—seeking to make conscious that which is unconscious; tell the client the meaning of his experience. "What you really mean is . . ."

19. Introducing an unrelated topic—changing the subject: Client: "I'd like to die." Nurse: "Did you have visitors this weekend?"

Adapted from Hays, JS, and Larson, K: Interacting with Patients. Macmillan, New York, 1963, pp 7–37.

Appendix 2: Suicide Assessment Tool

Intensity of risk can be rated on a scale of 1 to 10 (low 1 to 3, moderate 4 to 7, or high 8 to 10) depending on the subjective/objective data collected.

BEHAVIOR AND APPEARANCE

- Direct verbal statements ("I wish I were dead.")
- Indirect verbal statements ("You won't see me when you come back to work" or asking about specific suicide methods)
- Giving away possessions
- Agitation
- Sudden changes in eating, sleeping, or usual activities
- Neglecting appearance or hygiene
- Drawing up a will
- Refusing medications

MOOD AND/OR EMOTIONS

- Depression or despair
- Sudden lifting of depression, sudden elevation in mood
- Apathy
- Hopelessness
- Helplessness
- Anxiety
- Bitter anger

THOUGHTS, BELIEFS, AND PERCEPTIONS

- Disorganization, chaotic, irrational thinking

- Tunnel vision—inability to see options other than death
- Poor judgment
- Persecutory delusions and hallucinations, especially commands
- Excessive guilt or self-blame
- Low self-esteem

RELATIONSHIPS AND INTERACTIONS

- Social isolation; withdrawal; feeling alone and abandoned
- Recent loss of significant person through death or separation
- Recent tumultuous termination or interruptions of psychiatric treatment

PHYSICAL RESPONSES

- Chronic debilitating illness
- Unrelieved pain
- Terminal illness
- Recent, catastrophic loss of physical abilities

PERTINENT HISTORY

- History of suicide attempts
- Self-destructive behavior, such as drug abuse, reckless acts, or self-mutilation
- Family history of suicide attempts or depression
- Psychiatric illness
- Recent significant loss

ASSESSING SUICIDE LETHALITY

1. Do you think about hurting or killing yourself? If yes, please explain.
2. Do you have a plan? How have you considered doing it? If yes, please explain.
3. Do you think you may or will do something to act on your thoughts? If yes: Where and when? Do you think you have control over your own behavior?
4. Do you have the means available (e.g., rope [could be a rolled-up sheet], gun, saved-up pills)?
5. Have you ever tried to harm yourself in the past? If yes: How? Did you expect to survive?
6. Are you willing to contract or notify therapist/counselor whenever you think you may act on these thoughts?

Our side of the contract is to be available and actively help you during these times. If client denies having a suicide plan, ask about other plans for the future and support systems.

1. What do you see yourself doing in a week, in a month, and in 1 year from now?
2. Do you feel optimistic or pessimistic about the future?
3. Do you have family members or friends with whom you can freely discuss your problems?

Adapted from Gorman, LM, Sultan, DF, and Raines, ML: Davis's Manual of Psychosocial Nursing for General Patient Care. FA Davis, Philadelphia, 1996.

Appendix 3: Classification of NANDA Nursing Diagnoses by Gordon's Functional Health Patterns*

HEALTH PERCEPTION—HEALTH MANAGEMENT PATTERN
Altered health maintenance
Effective management of individual therapeutic regimen
Ineffective management of individual therapeutic regimen
Ineffective management of therapeutic regimen: community
Ineffective management of family therapeutic regimen
Health management deficit (specify)
Noncompliance (specify)
High risk for noncompliance (specify)
Health-seeking behaviors (specify)
Risk for infection
Risk for injury (trauma)
Risk for poisoning
Risk for suffocation
Altered protection

NUTRITIONAL-METABOLIC PATTERN
Adaptive capacity, intracranial: decreased
Altered nutrition: potential for more than body requirements or high risk for obesity
Altered nutrition: more than body requirements or exogenous obesity
Altered nutrition: less than body requirements or nutritional deficit (specify)
Ineffective breastfeeding
Effective breastfeeding
Interrupted breastfeeding
Ineffective infant feeding pattern
Risk for aspiration

Impaired swallowing or uncompensated swallowing impairment
Altered oral mucous membrane
Risk for fluid volume deficit
Fluid volume deficit
Fluid volume excess
Risk for impaired skin integrity or high risk for skin breakdown
Impaired skin integrity
Impaired tissue integrity
Risk for altered body temperature
Ineffective thermoregulation
Hyperthermia
Hypothermia

ELIMINATION PATTERN
Constipation or intermittent constipation pattern
Colonic constipation
Perceived constipation
Diarrhea
Bowel incontinence
Altered urinary elimination pattern
Functional incontinence
Reflex incontinence
Stress incontinence
Urge incontinence
Total incontinence
Urinary retention

ACTIVITY-EXERCISE PATTERN
Risk for activity intolerance
Activity intolerance (specify level)
Fatigue
Impaired physical mobility (specify level)

Risk for disuse syndrome
Total self-care deficit (specify level)
Self-bathing-hygiene deficit (specify level)
Self-dressing-grooming deficit (specify level)
Self-feeding deficit (specify level)
Self-toileting deficit (specify level)
Altered growth and development: self-care skills
    (specify)
Diversional activity deficit
Impaired home maintenance management (mild,
    moderate, severe, potential, chronic)
Infant behavior, disorganized
Risk for disorganized infant behavior
Potential for enhanced organized infant
    behavior
Dysfunctional ventilatory weaning response
    (DVWR)
Inability to sustain spontaneous ventilation
Ineffective airway clearance
Ineffective breathing pattern
Impaired gas exchange
Decreased cardiac output
Altered tissue perfusion (specify)
Dysreflexia
Risk for peripheral neurovascular dysfunction
Altered growth and development

SLEEP-REST PATTERN
Sleep-pattern disturbance

COGNITIVE-PERCEPTUAL PATTERN
Pain
Chronic pain
Acute confusion
Chronic confusion
Sensory-perceptual alterations: input deficit or
    sensory deprivation
Sensory-perceptual alterations: input excess or
    sensory overload
Unilateral neglect
Impaired environmental interpretation
    syndrome
Impaired thought processes
Knowledge deficit (specify)
Decisional conflict (specify)

SELF-PERCEPTION-SELF-CONCEPT PATTERN
Fear (specify focus)
Anxiety
Mild anxiety
Moderate anxiety
Severe anxiety (panic)
Fatigue
Hopelessness
Powerlessness (severe, low, moderate)
Self-esteem disturbance

Chronic low self-esteem
Situational low self-esteem
Body image disturbance
Risk for self-mutilation
Personal identity confusion

ROLE-RELATIONSHIP PATTERN
Anticipatory grieving
Dysfunctional grieving
Disturbance in role performance
Social isolation or social rejection
Social isolation
Impaired social interaction
Altered growth and development: social skills
    (specify)
Relocation stress syndrome
Altered family processes
Altered family process: alcoholism
Altered parenting
Risk for altered parent-infant-child
    attachment
Risk for altered parenting
Parental role conflict
Caregiver role strain
Risk for caregiver role strain
Impaired verbal communication
Altered growth and development:
    communication skills (specify)
Risk for loneliness
High risk for violence

SEXUALITY-REPRODUCTIVE PATTERN
Sexual dysfunction (specify type)
Altered sexuality patterns
Rape trauma syndrome
Rape trauma syndrome: compound reaction
Rape trauma syndrome: silent reaction

COPING-STRESS TOLERANCE PATTERN
Coping, ineffective (individual)
Defensive coping
Ineffective denial or denial
Impaired adjustment
Post-trauma response
Family coping: potential for growth
Ineffective family coping: compromised
Ineffective family coping: disabling
Ineffective community coping
Potential for enhanced community coping
Risk for self-mutilation
Risk for violence directed at others
Risk for violence self-directed

VALUE-BELIEF PATTERN
Spiritual distress (distress of the human spirit)
Potential for enhanced spiritual well-being

528

*Based on Gordon, M: Manual of Nursing Diagnosis 1997–1998.
Mosby-Yearbook Inc., St. Louis, 1997, p xviii, with permission.

Index of Nursing Diagnoses